TYPE 1 DIABETES

A Guide for Children, Adolescents, Young Adults — and Their Caregivers

EVERYTHING YOU NEED TO KNOW TO BECOME AN EXPERT ON YOUR OWN DIABETES

RAGNAR HANAS, MD, PHD

Forewords by Stuart Brink, MD,
and Jeff Hitchcock

MARLOWE & COMPANY

NEW YORK

TYPE 1 DIABETES:
A Guide for Children, Adolescents, Young Adults — and Their Caregivers

Copyright © 2005 by Ragnar Hanas, MD, PhD, Uddevalla, Sweden.

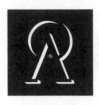

AVALON
publishing group incorporated

Marlowe & Company
An Imprint of Avalon Publishing Group Incorporated
245 West 17th Street o 11th Floor
New York, NY 10011-5300

This is the third English-language edition of this book, which has been previously published, in two earlier editions, in Sweden and the United Kingdom, and distributed in the United States, under the title *Type 1 Diabetes in Children, Adolescents and Young Adults*. The first English-language edition was published by the author in 1998; the second was published by Class Health in 2004. The first printing of this third edition: June 2005.

Illustrations and figures are reproduced with the permission of respective copyright owner (see page 354).

NOTICE

For dosages and applications mentioned in this book, the reader can be assured that the author has taken great lengths to ensure that the indications reflect the standard of knowledge at the time this work was completed. However, insulin needs and diabetes treatment must be individually tailored for each and every person with diabetes. Treatment methods and dosages may change. Advice and recommendations in this book cannot be expected to be generally applicable in all situations and always need to be supplemented with individual assessment by a diabetes team. The author and the publishers do not accept any legal responsibility or liability for any errors or omissions, or the use of the material contained herein and the decisions based on such use. Neither the author nor the publishers will be liable for direct, indirect, special, incidental or consequential damages arising out of the use, or inability to use, the contents of this book.

Library of Congress Cataloging-in-Publication Data is available.

ISBN 1-56924-396-4

9 8 7 6 5 4 3 2 1

Designed by David Penfold and Ragnar Hanas

Printed in the United States of America

Contents

**To my children
Mikael, Malin and Marie**

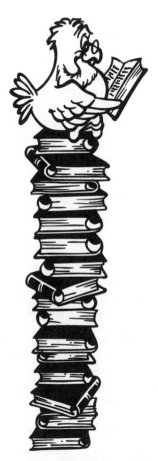

You may well feel that there is an overwhelming amount of knowledge you must take in, but nobody expects you to memorize the entire contents of this book. If you use it as a reference, and read a little at a time, you will gradually get to grips with the information it contains.

Acknowledgments

I am greatly indebted to the children and teenagers with diabetes and their parents who have contributed with experiences, tips, knowledge and drawings, to the diabetes nurses Pia Hanas, Elsie Johansson, Kristin Lundqvist, Ann-Sofie Karttunen and Catarina Andreasson for their many valuable contributions in discussions and clinical work, to my colleagues, collaborators and friends in Sweden and within ISPAD (International Society of Pediatric and Adolescent Diabetes) for joining me in increased efforts of intensive diabetes treatment and to Mats Bergryd for believing in the idea of writing a comprehensive diabetes manual for young people with diabetes and their parents. Without you there would have been no book.

My deep appreciation goes to Dr. Kenneth Strauss for his enthusiastic and continued support of the book, to Dr. Peter Swift, Dr. Charles Fox, Nancy Jones (mother of a child with diabetes), and Janette Apsley, RN, for reviewing and critically reading the second English edition. Many thanks to the dietitians Ellen Aslander, Carmel Smart, and Sheridan Waldron for their comments on the diet chapter. My sincere thanks to my editor Richenda Milton-Thompson, my publisher Dick Warner, and Judith Wise at Class Publishing for their endless patience in transforming my first English edition into a professional publication and to Matthew Lore at Marlowe & Company and Dr. Stuart Brink, Dr. Robyn Houlden and Gary Scheiner, MS, CDE, for constructive criticism that helped me in the Americanization of this third edition.

I am grateful to Louis Nitka for letting me use his drawings on pages 16 and 266 in the book. Illustrations and figures are all reproduced with the permission of the respective copyright owner. A full list is given on page 354.

For dosages and applications mentioned in this book, the reader can be assured that the author has gone to great lengths to ensure that the indications reflect the standard of knowledge at the time this work was completed. However, insulin needs and diabetes treatment must be individually tailored for each and every person with diabetes. Advice and recommendations in this book cannot be expected to be generally applicable in all situations and always need to be supplemented by individual assessment on the part of a diabetes team. The author cannot accept any legal responsibility or liability for any errors or omissions, or the use of the material contained herein and the decisions based on such use. Neither will the author be liable for direct, indirect, special, incidental or consequential damages arising out of the use, or inability to use, the contents of this book.

The use of general descriptive names, trade names, trademarks, etc. in this publication, even if not specifically identified, does not imply that these names are not protected by the relevant laws and regulations. NovoRapid, NovoLog, Levemir, Actrapid, Insulatard, Monotard, Mixtard, Ultratard, Penset, Novolin and Velosulin BR Human insulins are trademarks of Novo Nordisk A/S. Humulin, Humutard, Humaject and Humalog insulins are trademarks of Eli-Lilly & Co. Lantus, Insuman Infusat, Insuman Rapid, Insuman Basal and Insuman Comb insulins are trademarks of Sanofi-Aventis. The indwelling catheter Insuflon is a trademark of Unomedical, Denmark.

Preface

The number of children and adolescents with type 1 diabetes in the world is steadily increasing. There would appear to be something in the environment causing this, as genetic changes are not this rapid in humans. By contrast, the number of young adults developing type 1 diabetes seems to be constant, or even decreasing in some places. This would suggest that a particular group of individuals tend to get type 1 diabetes, but some environmental factor or factors are now causing it to appear earlier in the lifespan. Generally speaking, countries with a higher standard of living also have a high percentage of children with type 1 diabetes. In the US approximately 0.25% and in Canada close to 0.4% of all children can expect to develop diabetes before the age of 15 years. In Finland, the country where it is now most common, this figure is 0.6%.

A great deal of effort is put into research to find the causes of diabetes and to find a cure for this condition. In the meantime, however, we need to make life with diabetes as manageable as possible for our children, and young people. Since I wrote the first edition of this book in 1998, a great deal has happened in the area of insulin treatment. New analogs, both rapid-acting and long-acting, have been developed. These are opening up new possibilities for designing and "tailoring" individual insulin regimens, the better to fit the life of each individual.

Extensive advice on how to use these analogs is now included in the book, and in this third Americanized edition, rapid-acting insulin is the first choice of insulin treatment, as it is in Sweden. Insulin pumps are quickly becoming more widely used by young people, so the chapter on this topic has been updated extensively. The chapter on research and new developments covers the latest news, including the promising results of islet cell transplantation. Sections on diabetes organizations have been added, and you will find new topics such as driving safely with diabetes as well as basic advice on carbohydrate counting. Altogether, the amount of material contained in this book has increased by 27% since the first edition.

I am always so impressed by the huge motivation that whole families put into the learning process. On being told their child has diabetes, they often go to an astonishing amount of effort to make life as good as possible for their child, learning to live with this new condition. Within a couple of weeks, they are able to manage everyday situations in relation to diabetes quite well on their own. In about a years's time, after having experienced the events of an ordinary family life including birthday parties, vacations and sports events but also infections, gastroenteritis and other things that can complicate life, they will have taken over the reins and become their own diabetes experts. It is from families like these that I have learned how to deal with diabetes in such a way that Professor Johnny Ludvigsson's saying becomes true: "It is not fun getting diabetes, but you must be able to have fun even while having diabetes".

I hope that this new, updated edition will make living with diabetes considerably easier for children, teenagers and young adults. Let me know your views and impressions of the contents of this book so that, together, we can improve the treatment of diabetes.

Ragnar Hanas, MD, PhD, Consultant Pediatrician
Department of Pediatrics, Uddevalla Hospital
S-451 80 Uddevalla, Sweden
E-mail: ragnar.hanas@vgregion.se

Foreword by Dr. Stuart Brink

The second edition of Dr Hanas' book remains our favorite diabetes teaching manual at the New England Diabetes and Endocrinology Center (NEDEC). It is comprehensive, witty and informative while at the same time paying particular attention to the psychosocial issues of a chronic condition. Type 1 diabetes is increasing around the world. It affects young children, school age children, teenagers and young adults. It is essential that physicians, nurses, dietitians and other support personnel are well informed for type 1 diabetes to be recognized and treated correctly. It requires health care professionals to work together as a team to support not only those who have this disease but also their family members.

Most importantly, type 1 diabetes is unique because it requires not only excellent health care providers but informed patients, parents and friends. This is a disease where knowledge is a critical component of care. Not just knowledge, but up-to-date knowledge which brings research findings directly to providers and patients and facilitates the use of such knowledge for self-care. This manual provides such information for those who must live with type 1 diabetes. Such self-management skills are not so easy to elucidate, and even more difficult to put into practice.

The simple "rules" of diabetes suggest that too little insulin, too much food, too little activity or major illness or emotional upheaval cause high blood glucose, while too much insulin, too little food and/or too much activity cause hypoglycemia. After all is said and done, the application of these few bits of information explains all of what we need to know about diabetes. However, the details and the intricacies as well as the variations of the themes of these "rules" are what diabetes self-management is all about. The application of such knowledge allows the possibility of excellent glucose control while the inability to afford such care or the misapplication of such knowledge is associated with both acute and chronic complications of type 1 diabetes mellitus.

The psychosocial aspects of self-care and the interplay with family issues are important concepts woven into the text. When appropriate self-care is not taking place, psychosocial problems are often a key to understanding why problems persist. Acknowledging such a dilemma and applying research about empowerment and education coupled with the knowledge of the importance of improving diabetes care is a critical component of getting better results. What Dr Hanas does so well is to start with these basic premises and build the pieces of the self-care treatment puzzle step-by-step so that everyone involved with such care can understand what needs to be done, why it needs to be done and how it may be achieved. He does not offer dogmatic suggestions but rather options to consider under different real life circumstances. In fact, this second edition, like the first, accomplishes its goal of a diabetes teaching manual with attention to detail and application of clinical as well as research findings. School teachers, guidance counselors, therapists and all members of the diabetes medical community should have this book in their armamentarium as should those living with diabetes.

Stuart Brink

Stuart Brink, MD, Associate Clinical Professor of Pediatrics, Tufts University School of Medicine
New England Diabetes & Endocrinology Center
NEDEC, 40 Second Avenue Suite #170
Waltham MA, 02451-1136 USA

Foreword by Jeff Hitchcock

My daughter was diagnosed with type 1 diabetes in September 1989 by Allen Glasgow, a pediatric endocrinologist. My wife and I were fortunate, because Dr. Glasgow gave us the confidence to care for our daughter and to know that, through proper care, "You can make a huge difference in her life," as he put it.

From the beginning, it was clear to me that successfully managing type 1 diabetes was as much about information as it was about insulin. Parents who care for a child with diabetes must become experts on the condition and its treatment. We must learn how insulin works. We must learn about carbohydrates, proteins, and fats, and how each impacts our child's blood glucose levels after a meal. We must learn about exercise and glycogen and the delayed low blood glucose levels that can occur hours afterwards. We must figure out how to deal with our child's diabetes at school and other times when we may not be there to help. We must keep up with advances in care strategies and tools to help them. And we must learn all of this while continuing to nurture and care for the child's other, non-diabetes needs. After all, children with diabetes are still children.

This task — becoming an expert in type 1 diabetes — is daunting, to say the least. Most of us who have a child with diabetes are not medical professionals. Yet we are all asked to become, in effect, our child's diabetes doctor — to help them grow up healthy in spite of their diabetes.

In the first weeks after diagnosis, we are bombarded with information from our child's diabetes team. Slowly, we learn the basics, the life support skills of blood glucose monitoring and insulin injections. We learn about meal planning, perhaps even carbohydrate counting. We no longer feel anguish when we check blood glucose levels or give an insulin injection. Then, one day, we make our first insulin dose adjustment without the help of the diabetes team, marking a transition to independence that signals the beginning of our journey to becoming the expert in our child's diabetes.

From that independence day forward, we grow to know more about our child's diabetes than anyone else. We learn about how they react to various insulins and doses, how specific foods raise their blood glucose levels, and which exercises impact them the most. And to help us, we seek out more information, more resources, and other parents. It is often said, "When the student is ready, the teacher will appear." For anyone caring for someone with type 1 diabetes, that teacher is Dr. Ragnar Hanas. Dr. Hanas will be there, speaking to you through his book, *Type 1 Diabetes: A Guide for Children, Adolescents, Young Adults — and Their Caregivers.*

Both comprehensive and very easy to read, Dr. Hanas offers one of the few "must have" diabetes care books. Parents who have a child with diabetes, as well as teens and adults with type 1 diabetes, will find this book to be an indispensable resource. You'll refer to it often as your child grows and as you seek to learn more about your child's or your own diabetes care. And as you do, you'll find yourself appreciating the care and commitment that Dr. Hanas brings to helping you learn how to become an expert in your own diabetes.

Jeffrey S. Hitchcock

Jeff Hitchcock founded Children with Diabetes (www.childrenwithdiabetes.com) in 1995 to help other families and to help his daughter Marissa meet other kids with diabetes. Jeff continues to serve as president of CWD and spends all his time working to help families who have kids with diabetes.

Introduction

"If you want something done right, do it your-self." This is a wise old saying, but of course you need to know how to do it as well. If you have diabetes, you will need a thorough under-standing of the disease and how to manage it. As anyone living with diabetes knows, it is an illness that is with you 24 hours of every day.

Traditionally, doctors have decided on the doses of insulin, and the times it could be given. Patients took the insulin as prescribed, neither less, nor more. But for 20 years now, we have been doing the opposite at our clinic. We begin by teaching the fundamentals of diabetes man-agement to our young patients. Then, gradually,

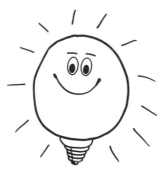

The diabetes clinic will often function as an information center where the diabetes team can pass on good ideas from one family to another.

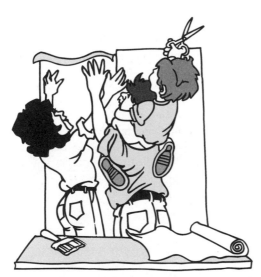

The underlying theme of this book is: "If you want some-thing done right, do it yourself". You are the only one who can be relied upon to be there 24 hours a day, and after a while you will be the greatest authority on your own dia-betes. Learning to care for your diabetes from scratch, like learning anything else, is a matter of trial and error. And during the process, you are bound to make some mistakes. However, you can learn from each one of these, indeed you will learn more from your own mis-takes than from the mistakes other people have made.

we delegate more and more of the daily respon-sibility for diabetes care to the young people themselves, and where appropriate also to par-ents and other family members.

Usually, it takes about a year for someone to experience most of the day-to-day situations that can be affected by diabetes. These may include vacations, birthdays, parties, heavy exercise and periods of sickness. As you become more confident, you will begin to draw upon your own experiences and discover things about your condition that your diabetes team will find it helpful to know about. This sort of free exchange of information not only helps us to help you. It also enables the clinic to function as an information centre, passing on suggestions and knowledge from one family to another.

Knowledge changes over time. What was advis-able 5 to 10 years may not necessarily apply today. At one time I would hear from families whom I had just informed about some new development, "Well, we have been doing it that way for years, but we didn't dare tell anyone". Nowadays we share knowledge and learning with each other instead.

This book deals with type 1 diabetes in children, teenagers and young adults. It does not address the treatment of type 2 diabetes, except in the briefest of ways. It describes methods of treating diabetes that are common in North America as well as much of Europe and elsewhere in the world. However, the methods used may vary from one center to another. The goal is to find a way of treating your diabetes effectively. There may be more than one way of reaching this goal.

Don't try to read the book from cover to cover, or memorize it. Use it as a reference book instead. A number of Latin medical terms are included, but their meaning should be obvious from the context, so you will not need to learn them unless you particularly want to. If you find some parts of the book difficult to understand, especially on the first reading, please don't let this discourage you. When you come back and read the text a second time, and when you have more experience of living with diabetes, it will all begin to fit together. More detailed information, aimed at those who want to learn a little bit more, can be found in the boxes in the text.

The small numbers raised above the lines of text (superscript) indicate the references which back up a particular piece of information. A full list of references, for those who are interested, is given at the end of the book.

Remember that you can learn things in many different ways. We usually arrange lessons around one aspect of diabetes at a time where we sit down with the whole family. However, you may also learn a great deal from a spontaneous conversation with a nurse, for example. The nurse's intonation, body language and expression may give you as much information as the spoken words. So, while you will be given official information during your more formal lessons, you will also hear unofficial views and additional information from other health professionals, fellow patients and others. Be aware of their body language, what they say and how they say it, and perhaps more importantly what they do not say. This type of information is also available from every day contact with doctors. Body language can make more impact than words, and many people find that if it comes to a choice between remembering official information or informal information, they usually find it easier to remember informal information.[504]

If a member of your family has already been in contact with diabetes (perhaps through a relative or colleague) they may well have a clearly defined view of what diabetes is like. It is important to remember that this experience is not at all the same as having diabetes yourself or in your immediate family. Also, the treatment regime is likely to be quite different for someone who has just been diagnosed com-

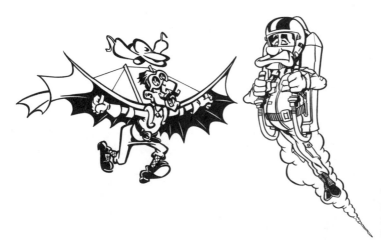

"It is time to replace the old mistakes with more modern ones."

Grönköping's Weekly

"The ability to think differently today than yesterday is what separates the wise from the stubborn."

John Steinbeck

We must be humble. What we look upon today as established knowledge, may appear as something quite different tomorrow.

pared to that for a person who has had diabetes for a number of years.

Many people are preoccupied by concerns about the future and the possible difficulties that may lie ahead. Your diabetes team will give you straightforward information about complications that might occur, and how to postpone them as long as possible or even avoid them. Our policy is to tell all there is to tell, not leaving any information out. Sometimes there is no straight answer to a question but we will tell you as much as we know.

During the first few weeks, you will need to get to know yourself all over again, and your parents will need to redefine their relationship with you too. You now know you have diabetes. To begin with, having to take this knowledge on board may make you scared about all sorts of aspects of your life. You may feel anxious and insecure, since you don't yet know how to tackle the different situations that daily life throws at you. But you will soon get to know

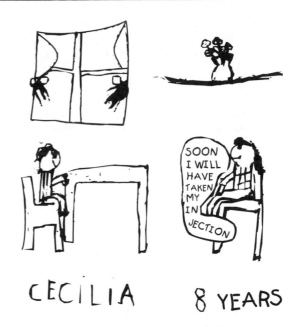

CECILIA   8 YEARS

yourself or your child in this new situation and you will gradually feel more confident about getting on with your life.

Getting to grips with diabetes

Managing diabetes involves lifelong treatment with insulin, but also permanent changes to your daily routine. Diabetes care includes both medical treatment and education. We want young people with diabetes, and their parents, to feel that they can assume responsibility for their own treatment and take charge of their own life. You can control your diabetes rather than let your diabetes control you. Once your diabetes has become manageable, so will other aspects of your life.

When you first find out you have diabetes

In Sweden and many other countries,[58] newly diagnosed diabetes is usually treated in hospital, where patients stay 1-2 weeks on the ward. In a few centers in the UK [733] and many centers in the US [134] it is more usual to start your insulin treatment on an outpatient basis unless you are ill with ketoacidosis (see page 29). Now that health care costs are continually increasing, outpatient treatment at this stage is becoming more common.[137] This approach requires the diabetes team to be "on call" on a 24 hour basis for back up while you are getting used to coping with insulin treatment.[137] The long-term glucose control, which is measured by the level of a substance known as A1C, appears to be just as good in patients who are treated as outpatients initially as in hospitals.[733] Whichever approach

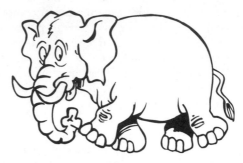

"When a problem is too large and seems unsolvable, don't forget that you can eat an elephant, assuming it is cut it into small enough pieces".

Slavic saying

The first week is often chaotic, and it may be hard to understand how all the different facts fit together. Try to concentrate on one piece of information at a time. By the end of the second week, everything will be becoming much clearer, and you will begin to understand how it all fits together.

you encounter, it is essential that you feel able to approach members of the diabetes team on a daily basis during the first week or two. It is their job to ensure you have the basic understanding and self-confidence necessary to give yourself the required doses of insulin.

The insulin requirement changes daily, and early on, the insulin dose will need to be revised continuously. During the first few days, patients need high doses of insulin, which will then be reduced by degrees. Many people feel much better immediately, and find they become ravenously hungry. This is natural if you consider that most young people who have been recently diagnosed with diabetes will have been insulin deficient for several weeks before the diabetes was discovered, and are likely to have lost some weight. They can usually have as much food as they want at this stage, regulating the doses of insulin instead. The appetite usually settles down after a few weeks.

Keep a list of your questions to avoid problems recalling them when visiting us at the diabetes clinic.

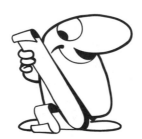

During the first few days, many young people (and their parents too) may experience a feeling of disorientation. If you are in this situation, you may have difficulty taking in the fact that you actually have diabetes. You will need time to examine your feelings and adjust gradually to this strange new situation that now faces you and the rest of your family. At this stage, you will probably find your doctors and nurses spend most of their time with you simply listening and answering questions. Then they will move on by degrees to teaching you more about diabetes. Most things will be new and you will often find them difficult to understand initially but, bit by bit, the different pieces of information will fall into place. By the end of the second week, you will be beginning to understand how insulin and blood glucose affect each other. You will discover that your blood glucose level fluctuates frequently, and that a perfect blood glucose level is a rare thing, even for those people whose diabetes is very closely supervised.

Parents can find they lose touch with each other if one is spending much more time than the other with the child. It is essential that both

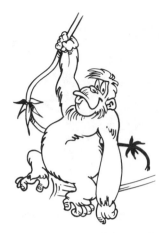

You will be feeling much better after a week or two with insulin. Now is the time to tell your friends at home and at school or work that you have diabetes. Then they will know and need not ask when you do something they don't understand, such as taking a blood glucose test. Even if you are worried about telling them, it often feels better once it is done.

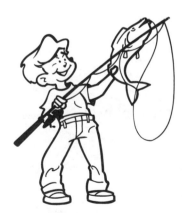

"Give a man a fish and he will not go hungry that day. Teach him how to fish and he will not be hungry for the rest of his life."

Chinese saying

It is important that you get used to handling your own (or your child's) diabetes early on. If you understand "why and how", you will be better prepared to meet different situations in life in harmony with your diabetes.

parents participate as much as possible in the daily care of the child with newly diagnosed diabetes. Taking time off work may help provide sufficient time to focus on diabetes care needs if this is possible.

Most people find that managing diabetes at home is easier than they had anticipated. To feel confident caring for yourself (or, in the case of parents, for your young child) at home, you should know what to do if the blood glucose level falls too low (see "Treating hypoglycemia" on page 60).

You will have time during the early weeks to meet a dietitian several times, as well as a specialist diabetes educator who can help you with many practical issues. Diabetes is an illness that can cause a lot of inconvenience, even in the most "normal" and well-adjusted families.

It can prove very valuable if you are able to see a child psychologist to discuss any difficulties that might arise. This way, if you do run into problems later on, you will already have an established contact should you wish to seek help.

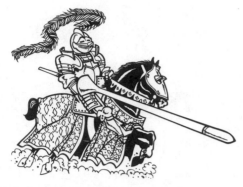

Knowledge and self confidence are your best armor when you are confronted with other people's opinions about diabetes. They will help you to recognize and deal with the prejudice and out of date views that, unfortunately, you are likely to meet. It is important for patients and health professionals to help each other spread better knowledge and understanding about diabetes.

Very young children

In the case of a baby or very young child having diabetes, the teaching will be directed at the parents, for obvious reasons. It is important, however, that children are given every opportunity to learn about diabetes themselves, and are given an increasing amount of responsibility for managing their illness as they grow. One way of helping to achieve this is by including young children in a diabetes camp. Children who have reached or who are approaching the age of puberty should be encouraged to take an active part in managing their diabetes from the start. Parents' self-help groups can also be very helpful, so do ask if there are any in your area.

Our goal is for all children with diabetes, however young they were when diagnosed, to be able to take the greater proportion of responsibility for their diabetes before they enter puberty. If this applies to you, you can then begin to recognize diabetes as your own illness (not something your mom or dad uses to get you to do what they tell you). Then you can direct your energies towards other areas of life.

Routine check-ups

After the initial phase, you are likely to see your diabetes health care team for a check-up every second to third month. At these check-ups, your diabetes team can tell how your glucose control has been over the previous 2-3 months by measuring a substance in your blood called A1C (see page 104). It is important that you realize from the start that it is not possible to achieve perfect blood glucose levels every day. Everyone with diabetes has high blood glucose levels every now and then and, with the methods of treatment available today, this should not cause you too many problems. What is important is that your average blood glucose level is acceptable. More information about this will be found later in this book.

Older teenagers often prefer to come by themselves to their check-ups, or perhaps with a friend or partner for company. If you are in a steady relationship, it is very important that your partner comes with you when you visit your diabetes healthcare team. You may see the dietitian during team visits, but you can also contact him or her directly for further informa-

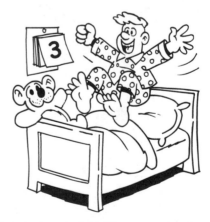

Hurrah, today is my birthday! This is a day for celebrating. For once you can be a bit more relaxed about routines and rules. Young people should be allowed to remember their birthdays and other special occasions as joyful and happy days, without undue restrictions.

tion. Once a year, you will usually have a more thorough check-up, including a full physical examination. Several additional tests (mainly blood tests) may be included in your annual check-up (see page 300).

You need to be aware that the way your body changes during adolescence will affect your diabetes. During puberty your body will need a lot more insulin (see page 192). It is important to know when to increase the doses.

Living the life you choose

Diabetes is a chronic illness that will affect you every day for the rest of your life. Try to become friends with your diabetes (or at least not to see it as an enemy) since you can't escape it and there is no currently known cure. It will probably be easier to manage diabetes well if you have a life with some sort of regular routine. If you are accustomed to a lifestyle that is neither regular nor predictable, you may find it more difficult (though by no means impossible) to combine this with diabetes.

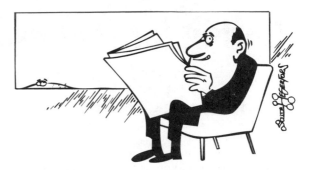

"It is much easier to have a strong opinion if you don't know all the facts involved".

You and your family will find that many people you come in contact with think they know a great deal about diabetes. Often their knowledge about diabetes treatment is far from up to date. Be a bit skeptical when you hear generalized statements about diabetes, especially early on before you have your own knowledge and experience to rely upon.

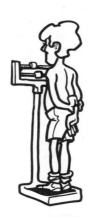

We check your weight and height at every visit to make sure that you continue to grow as well as you did before having diabetes. If you don't get enough insulin you will lose weight and may even experience growth retardation. If, on the other hand, you get too much insulin (and food) you will gain too much weight.

It is essential, however, that from the very beginning you plan how to carry on with your life in a manner that suits you. Don't let your diabetes dictate the type of life you should live. A lot of people find themselves thinking: "I can't do such and such any more, now that I have diabetes. But I used to enjoy it so much before my diagnosis". However, most activities are not only "allowed", but you can do them perfectly well. Nothing is absolutely forbidden, but you would be wise to think things through more carefully than you used to, in all sorts of situations. It is important to experiment and learn by trial and error. If you choose the life you want to live, it is our job as diabetes professionals to tailor an insulin regime that will enable you to do this. However, there are a few limitations on what sort of work you can do, for example it may not be possible to join the army or police force, be a pilot or (see "Choice of job or employment" on page 284).

Caring for your own diabetes

Goals for managing diabetes

A number of international authorities have put together recommended guidelines for the treatment of diabetes in young people. One of these is the International Society of Pediatric and Adolescent Diabetes (ISPAD, see page 291).[735] Other national and international programs for the treatment of diabetes in childhood and adolescents are to be found in the APEG Handbook on Childhood and Adolescent Diabetes from the Australasian Paediatric Endocrine Group,[701] the St. Vincent Declaration [151] the American Diabetes Association's Clinical Practice Recommendations,[19] and the Clinical Practice Guidelines of the Canadian Diabetes Association [541] among others.

An important goal of diabetes management is to reduce the number and severity of the symptoms and side effects you may experience. It is particularly important that young children grow and develop normally, and we ensure this by referring to standard weight and height development charts at every stage of treatment. In the past, insulin treatment plans were inadequate and prevented many children from grow-

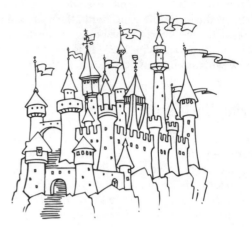

"My home is my castle", as the saying goes. Build yourself a castle of knowledge and motivation so you can feel safe and comfortable while dealing with your diabetes.

ing properly, but this is no longer acceptable. During puberty, insulin treatment plans need to be looked at and modified regularly.

Diabetes should not disrupt schooling or working patterns. It is difficult to study if your blood glucose is too high or too low, as this disturbs concentration. During puberty, your peer group becomes ever more important. Teaching teenagers how to balance an enjoyable social life with good diabetes management becomes a key goal at this time. As the young person matures into adulthood, having a family and children becomes increasingly important. In the long run, it is essential to prevent side effects and complications from diabetes.

How can you achieve these goals?

Traditionally there are three cornerstones of diabetes management: insulin, meal planning and exercise. The use of insulin is essential as this hormone is more or less missing from your

---

Goals of treatment

♠ No symptoms or discomfort in everyday life.

♠ Good general health and well-being.

♠ Normal growth and development.

♠ Normal puberty and peer-group relations.

♠ Normal schooling and professional life.

♠ Normal family life including the possibility of pregnancy.

♠ Prevention of long-term complications.

Diabetes today

Professor Johnny Ludvigsson, Sweden:

 Insulin
♥ Love
♥ Care

"It is no fun getting diabetes, but you must be able to have fun even if you have diabetes."

I would like to add a fourth cornerstone:

♥ Knowledge

Motivation of your own Self-care

If you want to manage well with diabetes you must:

① Become your own expert on diabetes.

② Have more knowledge about diabetes than the average doctor.

③ Accept your diabetes and learn to live with it.

body and it is essential for life. However, the other two cornerstones are being questioned by modern diabetes specialists, especially where children and teenagers are concerned. Eating sensibly is essential but meals that are appropriate for people with diabetes need not be very different from the sort of ordinary healthy meals that everyone can benefit from. Similarly, exercise is recommended for everyone and will help you achieve a good general level of fitness. In the past, exercise was an important part of diabetes treatment, however newer studies of diabetes and exercise do not indicate that it improves glucose control.[801] If your blood glucose levels are high with not enough insulin, it may not be a good idea to exercise. So exercise is no longer considered as a part of the actual diabetes treatment, although it is recommended for more general reasons.[349] See also the chapters on healthy eating and physical exercise.

Dr Johnny Ludvigsson, Professor in Pediatric Diabetology in Sweden, has re-defined the cornerstones of diabetes treatment as: insulin, love and care.[504] These goals coincide well with our clinic's view of diabetes treatment. Diabetes is a deficiency disease and it is natural to replace what is missing, i.e. insulin. Love and care are essential parts of every child's upbringing, and will be even more important for a child with a chronic illness.

I would like to introduce a fourth cornerstone in the treatment of diabetes, namely knowledge. A Chinese saying goes "Give a man a fish and he eats for a day. Teach him how to fish and he will eat for a lifetime".

Becoming your own expert

The more motivated you are, the better you will be able to manage your own diabetes. It is important you realize the treatment is for your own sake, not for your parents' or your family's, and certainly not to benefit your doctor or nurse. Your motivation for the best possible self treatment might be to be as good (or better...) at soccer as you were before, to achieve good grades in school without getting hypoglycemic, or to get the job you want and make it run smoothly despite irregular working hours. If you have diabetes you must become your own expert, learning to handle whatever life may throw at you in a satisfactory way.

The treatment of diabetes has changed a great deal in recent years, but public awareness has not necessarily caught up. So you are likely to come across a lot of people with out-of-date or fixed ideas, who think they know a great deal more than they actually do. But you need to be able to rely on your own knowledge. Indeed, to live your life in the way you want without too many unpleasant symptoms, you will actually need to know even more about diabetes than the average doctor does! To gain this knowledge you will have to ask questions and find out information if any aspect is less than crystal clear. Be sure to contact your consultant or diabetes nurse whenever you have questions on insulin dosages or other issues. If you save the question until your next visit, which might be three months away, you may simply forget all about it.

Becoming fully engaged with your diabetes and your own care is vitally important. Because you have to live with diabetes 24 hours a day, it is crucial that you decide as early as possible whether you are going to adjust your life around your diabetes, or whether you prefer to decide on a particular lifestyle and then adjust your diabetes treatment to enable you to achieve it. We encourage young people to be as active as possible in the management of their own diabetes from the start and aim to ensure that children have a good grasp of their diabetes by the time they reach puberty. This is important as there is so much else to occupy the mind of a young person during the teenage years. Children who have already come to grips with the basis of their own diabetes care before this stage will find they have more confidence to enjoy the increased freedom that adolescence should bring.

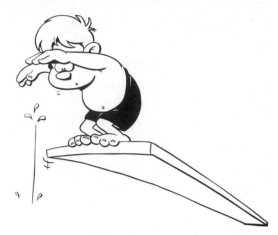

"To dare is to lose foothold for a short while — not to dare is to lose yourself."

Sören Kierkegaard, Danish philosopher 1813-55

It is not easy to take individual responsibility for your own diabetes. On the other hand you are the only one who can do it. Only you can be there 24 hours a day, and this is what it takes to make your diabetes function well both today and in the future.

Can you take "time off" from diabetes?

Well, this really isn't possible since your diabetes is with you 24 hours a day. But you can make a distinction between everyday life and having a good time on special occasions. Most people (with or without diabetes) will allow themselves something extra once in a while, even if they know that this little extra is not necessarily terribly healthy. If your usual lifestyle is appropriate for diabetes, you too can allow yourself to be a bit "more relaxed" with food if you are celebrating for example (see also "Party-time" on page 220).

If you go on vacation or a school trip, your routine is bound to differ from the one you have at home. The goal on these occasions should not be to have perfect control over your blood glucose. The important thing is that you feel well enough to participate in all activities. This may mean you have to accept having a slightly

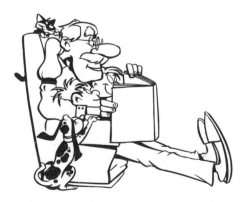

All children need love and care...

higher blood glucose level than usual, but of course you shouldn't let it get so high that it affects your well-being.

It is better to have 15 "bad" and 350 "good" days and feel happy about life, than 75 "half-bad" and 290 "good" days but feel miserable all the time. Many people with diabetes choose to have a slightly higher blood glucose level when they are about to do something important, such as an examination in school or an interview for a new job. And there are good reasons for this. In certain situations it is much more important to avoid hypoglycemia than to have a perfect blood glucose level.

Alternative and complementary therapies

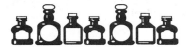

Sometimes we encounter questions about complementary or alternative treatment methods. In Sweden it is forbidden to treat children below the age of 8 with so called "alternative medicines" according to the law of quackery. Many parents have told us that despite this they have been informed about different types of treatment for children when they have consulted an alternative practitioner. In Finland, a 5 year old boy died in 1991 after his parents stopped giving him insulin and instead gave him different types of herbal and steam baths. Both the parents and the person responsible for the treatment were prosecuted for causing the death of the child.

Four cases have been reported in the United Kingdom of insulin doses being decreased or stopped completely and different types of alternative treatment being given instead (prayers, healing, special diet and treatment with vitamins and trace elements). Three of the people involved developed ketoacidosis, while the fourth suffered from high blood glucose levels and weight loss.[301]

Unlike an alternative therapy, which is used instead of a conventional one, complementary therapy means exactly what its name implies. It should be used in addition to medical treatment, to complement, rather than replace it. So, while a complementary therapy cannot be a substitute for insulin you may benefit from it in other ways, for example to help you to cope with the anger you feel at having to organize your life rather differently from your peers.

I have discussed this topic with parents on several occasions. In my opinion, three issues are especially important:

① We must talk frankly with each other about this subject. If you want to try an alternative or complementary treatment for your diabetes despite recommendations not to, it is better that you do this openly so that your doctor and diabetes nurse know about it.

② Children and adults with diabetes must continue taking their insulin and other medical treatment as prescribed by the doctor, otherwise their health will be in serious danger.

③ The alternative or complementary treatment must not be in any way dangerous or harmful to the person with diabetes.

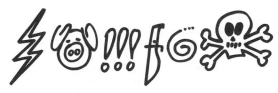

Sometimes you may feel like this when everything you have planned goes wrong and your blood glucose level ends up much too high or low. At a time like this, it might be a good idea to put your monitoring and adjustments "on hold" for a week and just take time off. Then, you can start afresh with renewed enthusiasm. Check your blood glucose only to avoid hypoglycemia. Most things in life are learned this way, in "waves". As you become more familiar with your diabetes, these moments of exasperation will occur less and less often.

Diabetes: some background

Diabetes mellitus, usually referred to simply as "diabetes", has been known to mankind since ancient times. Diabetes means "flowing through" and mellitus means "sweet as honey". Diabetes used to be described as either "insulin-dependent" (IDDM) or "non-insulin dependent" (NIDDM). Nowadays, you are more likely to hear the terms "*type 1 diabetes*" and "*type 2 diabetes*".

Egyptian hieroglyphic findings from 1550 BC illustrate the symptoms of diabetes. Some people believe that the type of diabetes depicted was type 2 and that type 1 diabetes is a relatively new disease, appearing within the last two centuries.[109]

In the past, diabetes was diagnosed by tasting the urine. No effective treatment was available. Before insulin was discovered, type 1 diabetes always resulted in death, usually quite quickly.

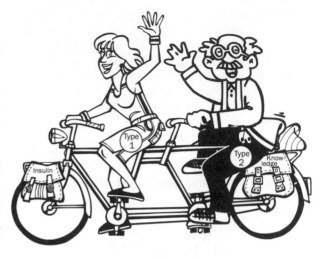

Insulin history

♠ The first human to be treated with insulin was a 14 year-old boy, Leonard Thomson, in Canada in the year 1922.

♠ James Havens was the first American treated with insulin in 1922.

♠ In the UK, insulin was first given as part of a research trial later the same year.

♠ In Sweden, the first insulin injections were given in 1923 to, among others, a 5 year-old boy who subsequently lived almost 70 years with his diabetes.

♠ In the early days, insulin was distributed as a powder or tablets which were mixed with water before being injected.

Type 1 diabetes

If you are going to get type 1 diabetes, you will probably know before your 35th birthday. Most people whose diabetes is diagnosed in childhood or the teenage years used to be type 1 diabetes, but now there is an alarming increase in type 2 diabetes in young people.

Type 1 diabetes is insulin-dependent, meaning that treatment with insulin is necessary from the time the disease is first diagnosed. In type 1 diabetes, the insulin-producing cells of the pancreas are destroyed by a process in the body known as "autoimmunity" (i.e. in which the body's cells attack each other, see page 322). This leads eventually to a total loss of insulin production. Without insulin, glucose remains in the bloodstream, so the blood glucose level increases, especially after eating meals. Glucose is then passed out of the body in the urine.

Type 2 diabetes

Type 2 diabetes is also called adult onset diabetes as the onset usually takes place after the age of 35. In type 2 diabetes, the ability to produce insulin does not disappear completely. But the body becomes increasingly resistant to insulin, so tablets are needed to balance this. The pills do not contain insulin, but act by increasing the body's sensitivity to insulin, or by increasing the release of insulin from the pancreas. It is rare for insulin injections to be necessary in the early stages of type 2 diabetes.

Although type 2 diabetes is also called non insulin-dependent diabetes, many people need treatment with insulin at a later stage in much the same way as people with type 1 diabetes.

A new generation of medication for type 2 diabetes (glitazones) is now being used in adults. These pills make the body more sensitive to insulin, and may also be helpful in other ways, for example by lowering the level of fats in the blood and reducing blood pressure. However, they are not yet approved for use in children.

An increasing number of reports from North America, Japan, the UK, and other parts of the industrialized world indicate that overweight teenagers are now beginning to develop type 2 diabetes. This appears to be more common in girls than in boys.[241,810] In North America, type 2 diabetes and heart disease among the young and middle-aged people from the members of the native American population is reaching epidemic proportions.[651]

In certain groups, the number of cases of type 2 diabetes as a proportion of the total number of newly diagnosed diabetes among children is extremely high. This proportion is nearly 100% in native Americans, 31% in Mexican Americans, and 70-75% in African Americans.[810] Type 2 diabetes is often diagnosed in African Americans after they become ill with the symptoms of ketoacidosis (see page 29).[810]

Other risk factors for type 2 diabetes in children and young people are low birth weight, type 2 diabetes in the family, ethnic origin (Canadian and American First Nation's people, Hispanic, African American, Japanese, Pacific Islander, Asian and Middle Eastern), high fat and low in fiber, lack of exercise, and signs of insulin resistance (such as high blood pressure and dark velvety discoloration of the skin (known as acanthosis nigricans).[241,651]

A possible reason for the increase in type 2 diabetes in young people may be that some people were "programmed" thousands of years ago to survive famine by conserving energy compared to periods when there was better access to food.[651] Today, when we have easy access to food, these "survival capacities" may cause problems instead. For example, the number of young people with type 2 diabetes is much higher in African Americans than among Africans still living in their home continent, although the genetic make-up of these two groups is very similar. This suggests that lifestyle and diet may be particularly important.[810]

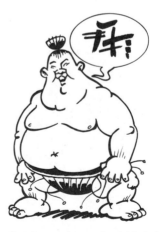

Being overweight will make you more vulnerable to type 2 diabetes as, in the long run, your body will not be able to produce the large amounts of insulin necessary to keep your blood sugar normal. Japanese sumo wrestlers with a body weight of 200-260 kg have an increased risk of type 2 diabetes when they stop their intensive training.

Other types of diabetes

LADA (Latent Autoimmune Diabetes in the Adult) is a form of type 1 diabetes that appears in adults and is caused by the body's own immune mechanisms. These persons are relatively thin and are very insulin sensitive. They usually produce insulin of their own for many years, much longer than the typical remission or "honeymoon" period seen in children and adolescents. Perhaps as many as 15% of people who are believed to have type 2 diabetes (and up to 50% of those who are not overweight) may have LADA.[826] One way of finding out whether someone actually does have LADA is to measure the level of certain antibodies that attack the insulin producing beta cells in the pancreas (ICA and GAD, see page 322).[826]

Some children and adolescents have a rare form of genetic diabetes (MODY, Maturity Onset Diabetes of the Young [779]). This is associated with a definite family history of diabetes.

How common is diabetes?

The number of individuals with diabetes varies enormously from country to country. In the US it is estimated that 20 million people have type 1 or type 2 diabetes, and in Canada over 2 million. The risk of a child developing type 1 diabetes before adulthood is approximately 0.3-0.5% in the Scandinavian countries,[452] 0.2% in the US and 0.3% in Canada.[212] This incidence varies between countries, and an estimated 430,000 children and adolescents aged 14 years or under are thought to have diabetes worldwide.[399] Each year, another 77,000 children in this age group are found to have diabetes, as are a further 119,000 aged 15 years or more.[399]

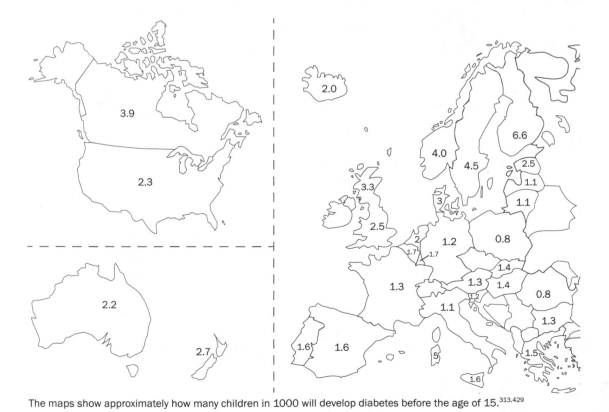

The maps show approximately how many children in 1000 will develop diabetes before the age of 15.[313,429]

In the US, approximately 13,000 new cases of diabetes are diagnosed in children every year.[23] Some 125,000 American individuals below the age of 19 years have diabetes, making this the second most common chronic disease in school-age children (the first being asthma).[23] In the UK there are at least 20,000 children under 15 year with diabetes.[405] In Sweden there are approximately 6,500 children and adolescents with type 1 diabetes and there are around 700 new cases of diabetes every year below the age of 18 years.[491]

There is a slow but steady increase in the number of cases diagnosed per year in most countries, especially in the younger age group.[168,293] The overall annual increase in Europe in the age group 0-14 years from 1989-1999 has been 3.2%.[314] However, in Sweden the incidence in the age group 15 - 34 years is decreasing,[624] which indicates that the same individuals are getting diabetes at an earlier age. The same trend of a continuing rise in number of new cases in the ages 0-14 years over the last 20 years (around 6% per year) but not for young adults aged 15-29 has been found in the UK.[266]

Finland has the highest incidence of childhood and adolescent diabetes in the world and Sweden comes in third after Sardinia. In Japan childhood and adolescent type 1 diabetes is very uncommon. Although 120 million people live in Japan (compared to Sweden's 8 million) the actual number of Japanese children and teenagers with diabetes does not exceed the number in Sweden.[441]

We don't know why there is such a difference from one country to another, but it depends at least partly on cultural and environmental differences. For example, diabetes is more common among Asian immigrants living in UK than in their relatives remaining in their countries of origin.[84] See also "What causes diabetes?" on page 321.

Can you catch diabetes?

Diabetes is not infectious. This may be obvious to adults but young children may be less confident. It is very important to get the message across to all friends, both at home and at school, that they cannot "catch" diabetes off you or anyone else. The best way may be to explain this to the whole class when going back to school. Ask the diabetes nurse to come to school and talk to friends and teachers about diabetes, and show them how injections and blood glucose tests are performed. Also tell them about the symptoms of hypoglycemia and what they can do to help. It is especially important for teenagers with newly diagnosed diabetes to tell their friends. If, for whatever reason, you don't do this shortly after you are diagnosed, it becomes increasingly likely you will not tell them at all. Telling other people is a very important part of accepting your own diabetes.

Principles of treatment for type 2 diabetes in young people [810]

➡ Change what you eat to include smaller portions with less fat and carbohydrate.

➡ Take up a form of regular exercise that involves your friends too. Walking, jogging and team sports can all be fun in groups.

➡ Get your school on board. Changing the type of food offered in the school cafeteria and regular physical exercise on the school timetable will help.

➡ You are likely to need insulin in the first week or so, especially if you had ketones or ketoacidosis when your diabetes was diagnosed.

➡ The use of oral anti-diabetic agents such as metformin can be effective for treating type 2 diabetes in young people.[416]

Does eating too much candy cause diabetes?

No! Eating candy will not influence your risk of getting type 1 diabetes in adolescence or childhood. If you are the parent of a young child, remember to tell this to your child's friends as younger children in particular often wonder whether sweet-eating will give them diabetes too. Parents can fall into the trap of thinking: "If we only had done this or that differently, perhaps our child wouldn't have diabetes". But they shouldn't blame themselves like this. Generally speaking, there is nothing a parent could have done differently to prevent his or her child from developing type 1 diabetes.

Type 2 diabetes is rather different however. While sweets do not in themselves cause type 2 diabetes, excess calories of any kind (candy, potatoes, sugary drinks) or just insufficient

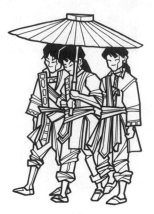

Juvenile diabetes is most common in the Nordic countries. In spite of having 15 times the population of Sweden, Japan has approximately the same number of children and teenagers with diabetes as Sweden.

physical exercise coupled with eating too much, is clearly related to obesity. And if you have a genetic susceptibility to type 2 diabetes, obesity will greatly increase your likelihood of developing it.

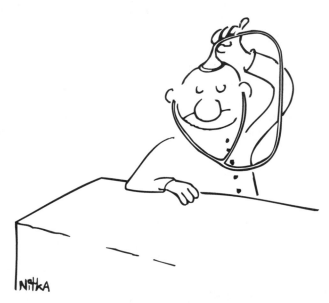

If you don't have diabetes, your body will automatically work the way it should. Before you developed diabetes, your pancreas produced insulin without you having to give it a thought. Now you must listen to your body's signals and give yourself insulin in a way that is suitable for the different situations you are faced with.

How your body works

It is important to understand how the body works in order to understand the difference in the way it works when you have diabetes. If you are not familiar with medical terms, or not interested in learning them, you can skip the terms in brackets. You do not need to know them to understand what is being said.

The three most important things making up the food we eat are sugar or starch (carbohydrates), fat and protein. When we eat, the digestion of starch (long chains of sugar, see page 204) begins immediately in the mouth with the help of a special enzyme (saliva amylase). An enzyme is a protein compound that breaks the bonds holding chemicals together. The food collects in the stomach, where it is mixed and broken down by the acidic gastric juice. The stomach then empties this mixture, a little at a time, into the small intestine through the lower opening of the stomach (pylorus, see illustration on page 21 and 64).

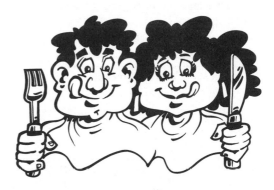

As soon as you see food your mouth will water and your body will begin to prepare to digest it.

Once the food is in the small intestine, it will be broken down even more by digestive enzymes from the pancreas and suspended in bile produced by the liver. If you eat sugar (for example, if you have hypoglycemia, see page 60) it cannot be absorbed into the blood until it has entered the small intestine. A study on adults indicates that glucose cannot be absorbed from the mouth (oral cavity) [321] or from the stomach.[277] In this sense the emptying rate of the stomach will have a considerable impact on how quickly the sugar you eat enters the bloodstream and increases your blood glucose level (see page 203).

The carbohydrates we eat are broken down into the simple sugars (mono-saccharides), glucose (dextrose, grape-sugar), fructose (fruit sugar) and galactose. Fructose must first be transformed into glucose in the liver before it can affect your blood glucose level. Food proteins are broken down into amino acids, and fat into very tiny droplets (known as chylomicrons, and composed mainly of triglycerides). Simple sugars and proteins are absorbed directly into the blood while the fat droplets are absorbed into the lymph system and enter the bloodstream through the lymph vessels.

Phases in glucose metabolism

① **Storing at meals:**
During a meal and for the following 2-3 hours glucose from the meal will be used as fuel by the cells. At the same time the stores of glycogen (glucose in long chains, see picture on page 204) fat and protein are rebuilt.

② **Fasting between meals**
After 3-5 hours the carbohydrate content of the meal is consumed and the blood glucose level starts to decrease. The glycogen stores in the liver will then be broken down to maintain a constant blood glucose level. The glucose produced in this way will be used by the brain while the body uses free fatty acids from fat tissue for its fuel.

The smallest building blocks in your body are called cells. All the cells in your body need glucose to function well. With the help of oxygen, glucose is broken down into carbon dioxide, water and the vital energy to make cells work throughout the body (see "A healthy cell" on page 24).

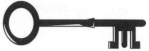

Insulin

Many of the different things your body does are controlled by hormones. Hormones act through the blood and work like keys, "opening doors" to different functions in the body. Insulin is a hormone that is produced in the pancreas in special types of cells called beta cells. The beta cells are found in a part of the pancreas known as "the Islets of Langerhans" which also contain alpha cells producing the hormone glucagon (see picture on page 23). Other hormones are also produced by the islets, and help the islet cells to communicate with each other. The pancreas has another very important function. It produces enzymes to help you digest your food. This part works quite well, even in a person with diabetes.

The venous blood draining the stomach and intestines passes through the liver before reaching the rest of the body. A large amount of glucose will be absorbed by the liver with the help of insulin, and then stored as a reservoir as glycogen (see page 32). These stores can be used between meals, during the night, and when a person is starving. Only glucose that is not absorbed by the liver can reach the peripheral bloodstream (reaching all over the body), and it is through this that glucose is delivered to the rest of the body. This glucose can be measured by a finger prick or a blood test from the vein.

The muscles can also store a certain amount of glucose as glycogen. Whereas the glycogen store in the liver can be used to raise the blood glucose level, the store in the muscles can only be used by the muscles themselves during exercise. The body's ability to store glucose is very limited. The glycogen stores are only sufficient for 24 hours without food for an adult and 12 hours for a child.[706]

The reason that insulin is so important is that it acts as the key that "opens the door" for glucose to enter the cells. As soon as you see or smell food, signals are delivered to the beta cells to increase insulin production.[253] Once the food has gone into your stomach and intestine, other special hormones send more signals to the beta cells to continue increasing their insulin production.

The glucose content of the blood is surprisingly constant during both day and night in a person without diabetes (approximately 70-120 mg/dl, 4-7 mmol/l). In adults, this blood glucose level corresponds to only about two teaspoons of sugar. If you think about it this way, you won't find it surprising that even a small amount of sugar, some candy for example, can disturb the balance of glucose in the body of a person with diabetes.

The beta cells contain a built-in "blood glucose meter" that registers when the level of glucose in your blood goes up and responds by sending the correct amount of insulin into your bloodstream. When a person without diabetes eats food, the insulin concentration in their blood increases rapidly (see figure on page 22) to take

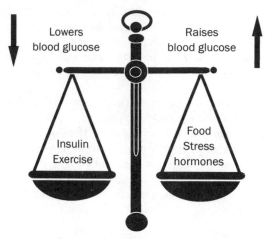

Lowers blood glucose

Raises blood glucose

Insulin
Exercise

Food
Stress
hormones

The blood glucose in your body is controlled by many different actions that balance each other to achieve an as even a level as possible throughout the day.

Not all cells require insulin to transport glucose into their interior. There are "insulin independent" cells that absorb glucose in direct proportion to the blood glucose level. Cells like this can be found in the brain cells, nerve fibres, retina, kidneys and adrenal glands, as well as in the blood vessels and the red blood cells.

It may seem illogical that certain cells can absorb glucose without insulin. However, in a situation where there is not enough glucose in the body, the insulin production will be stopped, reserving the glucose for the most important organs. If you have diabetes and your blood glucose level is high, the cells that don't need insulin will absorb large amounts of glucose. In the long run this will poison the cells, making those organs susceptible to long-term damage from having diabetes.

care of the glucose coming from the food, transporting it into the cells. This person's blood glucose level will normally not rise more than 20-25 mg/dl (1-2 mmol/l) after a meal.[253]

Insulin follows the bloodstream to the different cells of the body, sticking to the cell surface in special insulin receptors. This makes it possible for glucose to travel through the cell wall made penetrable to glucose. Insulin causes certain proteins inside the cell to come to the cell surface, collect glucose and then release it inside the cell. In this way, the blood glucose level is kept at a constant level.

The body needs a small amount of insulin, even between meals and during the night, to accommodate the glucose coming from the liver (see page 32). This is often referred to as the "basal insulin level" to distinguish between the need for insulin in the background between mealtimes, and the "boluses" of insulin needed to accommodate the eating of meals or snacks. Around 40-50% of the total amount of insulin produced by a person without diabetes, over any 24 hour period, will be secreted as basal insulin between meals.[86]

A large amount of carbohydrate from a meal will be stored in the liver (as glycogen, see page 32). If you eat more than you need, the excess carbohydrate is transformed into fat and stored in the fat tissue. The human body has an almost unlimited ability to store fat, so fat left over from a meal is stored in the same way. Proteins (amino acids) from the meal can be used by different body tissues. There is no specific way of storing amino acids. The liver can produce glucose from amino acids, for example, if you haven't eaten for some time. But this means that the body tissues themselves are broken down since the body has no way of storing amino acids.

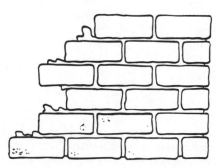

All the organs in the body are built of cells, which are like the bricks in a house. Each organ contains specialized cells to enable it to perform its function, so there are identifiable kidney cells, liver cells and muscle cells.

Your body doesn't realize it has diabetes

When you read about how your body functions if you have diabetes, remember that it always "thinks" and reacts as if it still was not having diabetes, that is to say, as if the insulin production was still working as well as it should. Your body doesn't understand why things go wrong when you become insulin deficient, because it doesn't realize what has happened. On the other hand your brain can help you by thinking through what will happen when your insulin

production stops working. It is very important therefore that you remember to stop and think about how your body reacts in particular situations, why it reacts like this, and how you can influence these reactions.

Your insulin doses will vary from day to day since you rarely conduct your life in the same way from one day to another. If you did not have diabetes, your beta cells would make automatic adjustments for this. But now it is up to you to notice how your body reacts on different days, and how much insulin you need in different situations.

What happens to the carbohydrates in the food?

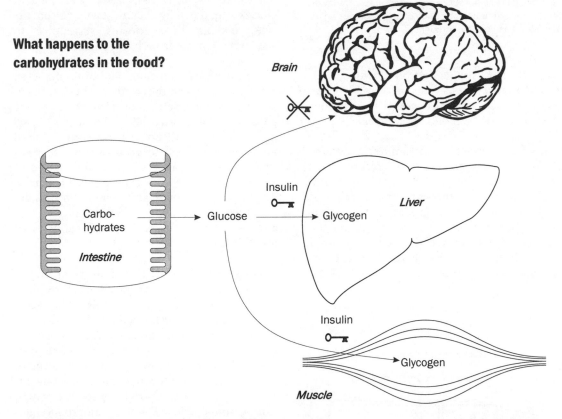

The complex carbohydrates in food are broken down to simple sugars in the intestine. Glucose is absorbed into the bloodstream and stored as glycogen in the liver and muscles. The key hormone insulin is needed to transport glucose into the cells of these organs. The brain cannot store glucose, so it has to depend upon a regular supply if it is to function well. The nervous system and some other cells (for example, those in the eyes and kidneys) can take up glucose without the help of insulin. There are advantages to this in the short term as the nervous system will not experience a lack of glucose, even if no insulin is present. However, in the long term, there are disadvantages for a person with diabetes, as the nervous system will be exposed to high levels of glucose inside the cells when the blood glucose level is high.

The anatomy of your body

When you eat, the food passes from your mouth through your gullet on its way down to your stomach. Sugar can not be absorbed into your blood until the food has passed the lower opening of your stomach (pylorus) and entered the intestine. In the intestine, it will be digested by enzymes from your pancreas and intestinal lining.

The small intestine is very long (3-5 metres or 9-15 feet in an adult) and is folded or coiled in order to fit comfortably inside your abdominal cavity or tummy. The first part of the small intestine, the duodenum, is 25-30 cm (10-12 inches) long.

After leaving the small intestine, the food passes into the large intestine (or colon) which is approximately 1½ meters (4-5 feet) long. The large intestine passes around the abdominal cavity before entering the rectum.

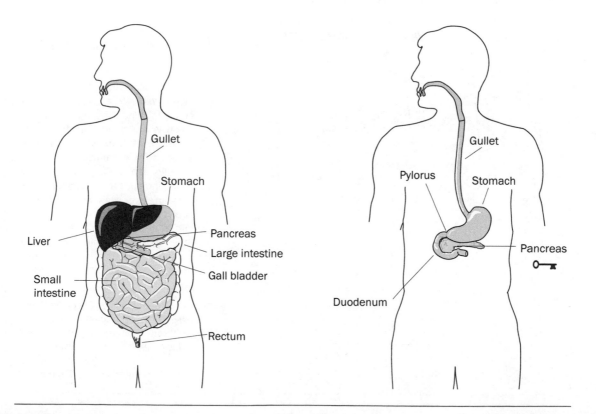

Pancreas

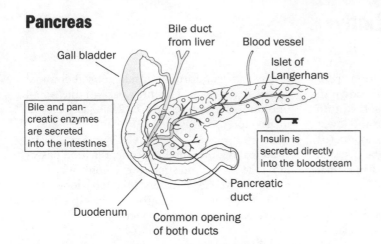

Gall bladder

Bile duct from liver

Blood vessel

Islet of Langerhans

Bile and pancreatic enzymes are secreted into the intestines

Insulin is secreted directly into the bloodstream

Duodenum

Common opening of both ducts

Pancreatic duct

"I am now your pancreas but one day, when you are older and learn to take care of yourself, your brain will become your pancreas."

The mother of Maria de Alva, former president of IDF (International Diabetes Federation).

Your pancreas is about the size of the palm of your hand. It is positioned under the left rib cage in the back of the abdominal cavity, close to the stomach. The pancreas has two main functions: it produces enzymes which help you digest food, and it produces insulin which helps control blood sugar. The digestive enzymes from the pancreas reach the intestine through the pancreatic duct. This drains into the duodenum together with the duct from the liver and gall bladder. There are approximately one million islets of Langerhans in the pancreas. Insulin produced in the beta cells of the islets is secreted directly into the small blood vessels passing through the pancreas.

Insulin and blood glucose

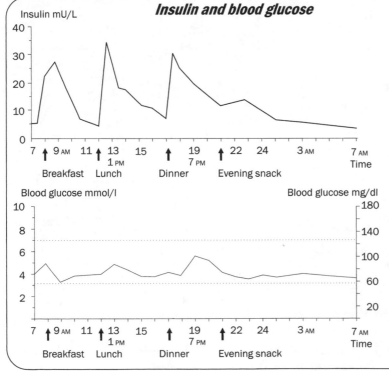

A person without diabetes

If a person doesn't have diabetes, the insulin concentration in the blood will increase rapidly after a meal.[583] When the glucose in the food is absorbed from the intestine, and the blood glucose has returned to normal levels, the insulin level will drop back to baseline once again. However, the insulin level will never go right down, as a low level of basal insulin is needed to take account of the glucose coming from the reserve stores in the liver between meals and during the night.

The resulting blood glucose level will be very stable in a person without diabetes as this graph illustrates.[523] The normal blood glucose level is between about 70 and 120 mg/dl (4 and 7 mmol/l).

Islets of Langerhans

If you look at an islet of Langerhans through a microscope, you will find it contains beta cells, which produce insulin, and alpha cells, which produce glucagon. Both of these hormones are secreted directly into the blood. The beta cells contain a sort of "built-in" blood glucose meter. If the blood glucose level is raised, insulin will be secreted. If it is lowered, the secretion of insulin stops. If it falls below the normal level, glucagon is secreted. Other hormones are also produced by the islets, and help the islet cells to communicate with each other.

The islets of Langerhans are very small, only 0.1 mm (four thousands of an inch) in diameter.

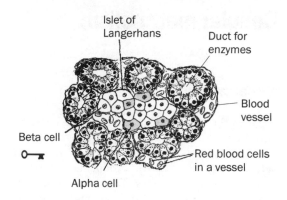

All the islets together contain approximately 200 units of insulin in an adult. The volume of them all combined is no larger than a finger-tip.

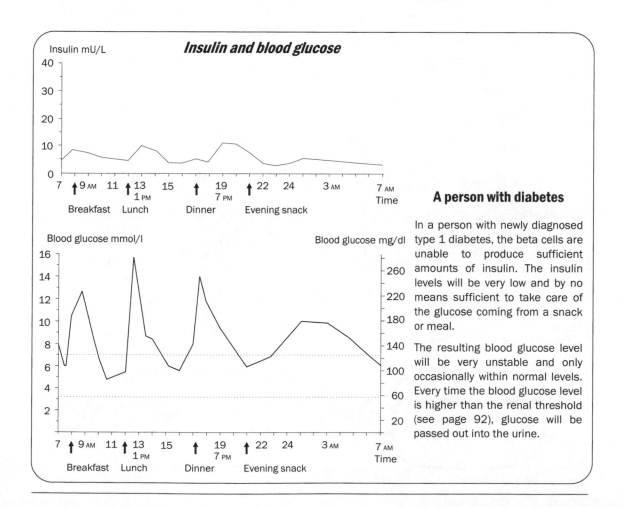

A person with diabetes

In a person with newly diagnosed type 1 diabetes, the beta cells are unable to produce sufficient amounts of insulin. The insulin levels will be very low and by no means sufficient to take care of the glucose coming from a snack or meal.

The resulting blood glucose level will be very unstable and only occasionally within normal levels. Every time the blood glucose level is higher than the renal threshold (see page 92), glucose will be passed out into the urine.

Cellular metabolism

A healthy cell

Sugar in the food is absorbed from the intestine into the blood in the form of glucose (dextrose) and fructose. Glucose must enter the cells before it can be used for producing energy or other metabolic processes. The hormone insulin is needed to "open the door", i.e. make it possible for glucose to penetrate the wall of the cell. Once it is inside the cell, glucose is metabolized with the help of oxygen into carbon dioxide, water and energy. The carbon dioxide travels to the lungs, where it is exchanged for oxygen.

Energy is vitally important to the cell if it is to function properly. In addition, glucose is stored (in the form of glycogen) in liver and muscle cells for future use. The brain, however, is not capable of storing glucose as glycogen. It is therefore dependent on an even and continuous supply of glucose from the blood.

Starvation

When no food is available, there is a shortage of glucose in the blood. In this case, opening the "cell door" with the help of insulin will not do any good. In a person who does not have diabetes, the production of insulin will be stopped almost completely when the blood glucose level goes down. The alpha cells in the pancreas recognize the lowered blood glucose level and

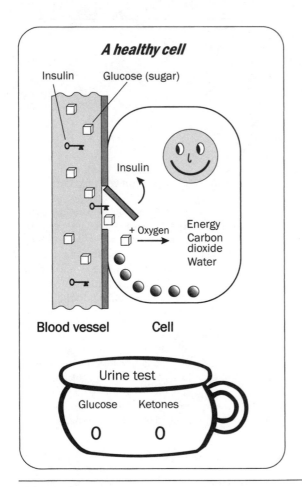

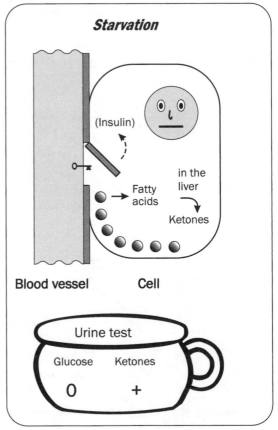

secrete the hormone glucagon into the blood-stream. Glucagon acts as a signal for the liver cells to release glucose from the reserve supply of glycogen. Adrenaline, cortisol and growth hormone are other hormones that are produced when the body is starving (see page 31).

If starvation continues, the body will use the next reserve system for glucose supply. Fat is broken down into fatty acids and glycerol with the help of the stress hormone adrenaline. The fatty acids are transformed into ketones in the liver (these are known as "starvation ketones")

and glycerol is changed into glucose. These reactions will take place if you are fasting or if you are too ill to eat, for example if you have gastroenteritis.

All the cells of the body (except the brain) can use fatty acids as fuel. Only the muscles, the heart, the kidneys, and the brain, however, can use ketones as fuel. The cells will retrieve some energy from this but less than when glucose is available. If the body is without food for too long, proteins from muscle tissue will start to break down too, so that they can be converted into glucose.

Diabetes and insulin deficiency

Type 1 diabetes is a "deficiency disease" in which the hormone insulin is missing. The result of this is that glucose is unable to enter the cells. The cells then act exactly as they would in the starvation situation described above. Your body will try to raise your blood glucose to even higher levels since it believes that the reason for the lack of glucose inside the cells is a low glucose level in the blood (see "Your body doesn't realize it has diabetes" on page 20). The hormones adrenaline and glucagon (see page 33) will give signals to the liver to release glucose from the glycogen stores.

In this situation, however, the starvation takes place in the midst of plenty. The bloodstream already contains an excess of glucose, which is being passed out into the urine. Inside the cells, fatty acids are being produced. These are then transformed into ketones in the liver ("diabetes ketones"), and the ketones are also passed out into the urine. When insulin is supplied, the cells can function properly again and this "vicious cycle" will be broken.

"Starvation ketones" and "diabetes ketones" are chemically identical but they are often referred to differently depending on how they originate (see page 99).

Diabetes and insulin deficiency

Glucose (sugar)

in the liver

Fatty acids

Ketones

Blood vessel   Cell

Urine test

Glucose   Ketones

+++   +++

High blood glucose levels

When your blood glucose level is high, glucose passes out of your body in the urine. This increased urine output is caused by the extra fluid excreted along with the glucose. So the first symptoms of diabetes are likely to be a raging thirst accompanied by a need to go to the toilet much more often. When you lose a lot of fluid, your skin and mucous membranes become dry. Women and girls often find this causes itching around their genitals. The itching can also be caused by a fungal infection which is more common if you have a high urine glucose level. In addition, your white blood cells, which play an important part in your body's defense against infection, will be less effective once your blood glucose level goes above about 250 mg/dl (14 mmol/l).[48]

Vomiting with diabetes is a warning sign, as it is often the first sign of insulin deficiency. A child who is unable to drink may go downhill very quickly and soon become seriously ill. Contact your diabetes healthcare team or the hospital if you are at all unsure as to how to handle the situation (see sick day rules on page 258).

What happens in the body when there is not enough insulin?

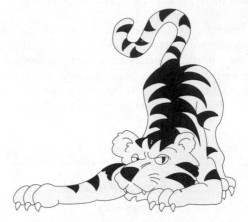

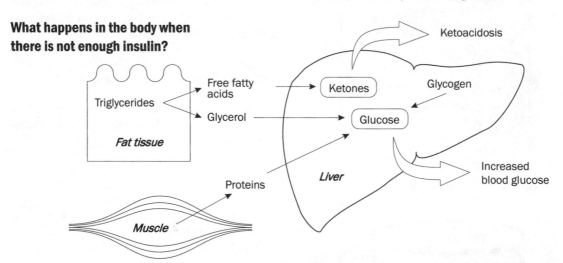

The reaction of a person's body without diabetes to shortage of insulin is quite logical if you remember that the levels of insulin are normally low only when the blood glucose is low too. So low insulin levels make the body "think" it must send more energy to the blood. This process in turn triggers the hormones adrenaline, cortisol, glucagon and growth hormone to stimulate the production of both glucose and ketones. Ketones can be used as fuel by your brain if you are starving. However, if you have diabetes which is untreated or undertreated, insulin levels will be low at the same time as your blood glucose level is high. Your body will be confused by this, and will respond by trying to increase the blood's supply of energy in the same way as it would have done before you developed diabetes. The amount of ketones in the blood will increase, which can lead to ketoacidosis. The blood glucose level will go right up, even if you don't eat anything.

If your blood glucose level rises temporarily (e.g. following a large meal), you may not even notice. Many people feel fine, even with a blood glucose level of 290-325 mg/dl (16-18 mmol/l). You may be a bit more tired and thirsty than usual, but the symptoms are not nearly as obvious as when your blood glucose level is low. One study of adults found no difference in neuro-psychological function (simple motor abilities, attention, reaction time, learning and memory) when comparing blood glucose levels of 160 and 380 mg/dl (8.9 and 21.1 mmol/l).[223] However, if the rise in your blood glucose level is caused by a lack of insulin, you are likely to feel unwell even if your blood glucose is not higher than 215-270 mg/dl (12-15 mmol/l) if your level of ketones is raised. It is the lack of insulin that makes you feel unwell, not the high blood glucose level as such.

Not enough insulin?

Insulin deficiency results in a lack of glucose inside the cells (see figures on page 25). This causes ketones to be produced, which can be used as fuel. If a lot of ketones are produced, however, they will have some very unpleasant effects. In smaller children, nausea and vomiting are often the first symptoms when the level of ketones in the blood increases. For example, if a child's bedtime insulin is forgotten, he or she may feel nauseous or vomit in the morning. If a child with diabetes vomits, you should **always** consider whether a lack of insulin may be to blame (for example forgotten injections). Alternatively, the sickness may indicate the start of an illness which will cause the child to need more insulin than usual. Either situation could rapidly become critical if the correct measures are not taken! See the chapter on illness on page 259 for further information.

Remember that your blood glucose level will rise when your insulin level is low, even if you don't eat anything. This is caused by an increased level of hormones stimulating the liver to release more glucose (see "Regulation of blood glucose" on page 31) to make up for the

---

Symptoms of insulin deficiency

These symptoms will develop more quickly if you take a smaller proportion of your daily insulin dose as intermediate or long-acting insulin. If you use an insulin pump you will be even more sensitive to insulin deficiency as the pump uses only rapid or short-acting insulin.

① **Production of ketones**

➟ Vomiting, feeling nauseous.

➟ Tiredness.

➟ Abdominal pain.

➟ Heavy breathing, the smell of acetone on the breath.

➟ Pain in the chest or stomach, difficulty breathing.

➟ Drowsiness.

➟ Diabetes coma (unconsciousness).

② **Depletion of energy stores, breakdown of muscle tissue**

➟ Weakness.

➟ Weight loss.

➟ Decreased growth (long-standing insulin deficiency).

---

lack of glucose inside these cells. This is logical if you remember that, before you had diabetes, there was a lack of glucose inside the cells only when your blood glucose level was low.

How to treat a high blood glucose level

A blood glucose level that is high only temporarily will not require any emergency treatment. However, if it is high on repeated monitoring, you should always check for ketones in your

Symptoms of high blood glucose

① Glucose in the urine:

➠ Needing to go to the toilet more frequently, including at night.

➠ Passing a lot of urine at a time.

➠ Fluid loss:
Very thirsty, dry mouth.
Dry skin, dry mucous membranes.

➠ Lack of energy.

② Weight loss, weakness.

③ Blurred eyesight.

④ Difficulty in concentrating, irritable behavior.[655]

When insulin levels are low, the blood glucose level will be high and blood and urine tests will show ketones. Once you have taken extra insulin, however, it will be more difficult to interpret your urine tests. Blood tests for ketones will give you more correct information in this situation. There are two types of ketones (beta-hydroxybutyric acid and acetoacetate) but only one type (acetoacetate) will show on the urine ketone strips. Often both types of ketones are increased when insulin levels are low. When extra insulin is given, further production of ketones is blocked. Early on in treatment, it may appear that there is a rise in ketones in the urine. This is because beta-hydroxybutyric acid is transformed into acetoacetate, giving the impression of an increase in ketones on the urine test strip.[469] Actually, however, the total amount of ketones in the blood has gone down (see also page 100).

blood or urine. If there are no ketones, it is unlikely that the cells are "starving" (see page 99). If you feel well, measure your blood glucose level once again before the next meal and, if necessary, add another 1-2 units of rapid (NovoLog/NovoRapid, Humalog, Apidra) or short-acting (Novolin R, Humulin R) insulin to your premeal dose if the level is still high (see page 131 for further advice).

If your blood glucose level continues high for several hours and you have ketones in your blood or urine, it is likely that your insulin level is low (see page 100). If the ketone level increases in spite of your taking extra insulin, you should always contact the hospital or your diabetes specialist. Blood levels of ketones above 3 mmol/l, or urine ketones increasing to large amounts, indicate that you are at risk of developing ketoacidosis.[794] See page 103 for more information on interpreting blood ketone tests. Don't hesitate to seek advice from your diabetes healthcare team if you feel unwell or are worried about your glucose or ketone levels. See also "What to do if your blood glucose level is high" on page 131.

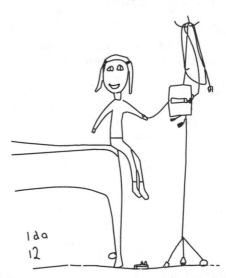

Ida
12

Ketoacidosis is treated with intravenous insulin and fluids. It is always caused by a deficiency in insulin and it is not uncommon to be in ketoacidosis if you have had symptoms of thirst and increased urine output for a longer period of time before the diagnosis is made. In some countries intravenous insulin is used at the onset of diabetes even if you are not in ketoacidosis, as it is thought to increase the beta cell restitution and the chance for sustained insulin production in the pancreas (see "Remission ("honeymoon") phase" on page 193).[696]

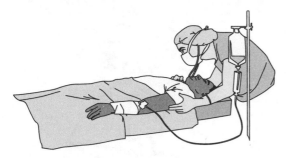

Ketoacidosis can rapidly develop into a life threatening condition. This must be treated adequately in a hospital with intravenous fluid and insulin.

Ketoacidosis

Ketones are produced when fat is broken down in the body for any reason. In normal circumstances, ketones are used as fuel by your muscles, heart, kidney and brain. If you have diabetes, ketones are produced in excess when there is a lack of insulin in your body, for example when insulin is omitted or not increased sufficiently during an illness or growth spurt. Too many ketones make your blood acidic, causing ketoacidosis.[206] Your body tries to get rid of these ketones by excreting them, either in the urine or in the form of acetone which is breathed out through the lungs, giving a fruity smell to the breath. Your breathing becomes faster (called Kussmaul breathing) as your body tries to get rid of as much acetone as possible.

General abdominal pain and tenderness may be caused by ketoacidosis, but these could have other causes (not related to diabetes), so it is important that other possible medical problems are not dismissed until they have been ruled out.[650] If you cannot increase the intake of fluid to compensate for the increased amount of urine you are passing, you will become dehydrated. If this continues without treatment, you will become unconscious and fall into a coma (diabetic coma).

Ketoacidosis is a life-threatening condition that must be treated with intravenous fluid and insulin in hospital.[482,650] Although effective treatment is now available, there are still people who die from ketoacidosis, ranging from less than 1% in developed countries[227] and 6-24% in developing countries.[482]

Ketoacidosis can occur at the onset of diabetes, though the likelihood of this happening varies considerably (between 15% and 67%) from one country to another.[227] It can also occur if you are unable to take your insulin for 12-24 hours, for some reason. Another situation which can cause ketoacidosis is if your body suddenly needs more insulin than usual, for example if you have an infection accompanied by a high temperature.

Insulin deficiency and ketoacidosis will develop more quickly if a smaller part of your daily insulin dosage consists of intermediate or long-acting insulin. The reason for this is that

Causes of diabetic ketoacidosis (DKA)

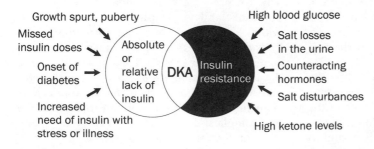

Growth spurt, puberty
Missed insulin doses
Onset of diabetes
Increased need of insulin with stress or illness

Absolute or relative lack of insulin

DKA

Insulin resistance

High blood glucose
Salt losses in the urine
Counteracting hormones
Salt disturbances
High ketone levels

Ketoacidosis is always caused by a relative or absolute deficiency of insulin. Relative insulin deficiency occurs if, for example, you don't increase your insulin doses when you are ill with fever, or during the growth spurt of puberty. The increased blood glucose level, along with other contributing factors, results in increased insulin resistance (i.e. a decreased sensitivity for insulin, see page 195). Much larger doses of insulin are needed to achieve the same blood glucose lowering effect as before the change.

Does ketoacidosis affect the brain?

♠ In an Australian study, the IQ in a group of children dropped approximately 10% when blood glucose levels were raised to 400-540 mg/dl (20-30 mmol/l).[186]

♠ When the blood glucose was normalized, the IQ also returned to the normal level. However, ketoacidosis seems to be able to damage intellectual function in a way that is not reversible.

♠ An American study found the IQ to be permanently lowered by approximately one point for every time a person needed hospital treatment for ketoacidosis.[278]

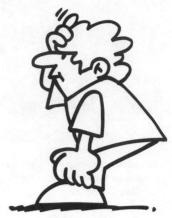

Symptoms of a low blood glucose level are usually fairly easy to recognize. However, when the blood glucose level is high many people won't have any symptoms at all. Try to train yourself to recognize the sensation of going into "autopilot", warning you when the blood glucose level is rising. If you can do this, you are less likely to need to rely on blood glucose tests. Thirst and the need to pass a lot of urine both occur when your blood glucose level goes above the renal threshold, but remember that this level can vary from one person to another (see page 92). Other common symptoms are apathy and a sense that everything is "slowing down". One study of children and adolescents aged 9-18 years found that higher blood glucose levels were reflected in impulsive behavior.[655] What signs can you see to indicate your own blood glucose level is high?

the insulin depot will be much smaller if you are using rapid or short-acting insulin, compared to when you use intermediate or long acting insulin. See "Depot effect" on page 79. With an insulin pump the depot is very small since the pump delivers only rapid or short-acting insulin. Some people, therefore, can feel nauseous or vomit after only one night without insulin if the pump fails (see page 172). With the use of rapid-acting insulin (Humalog, Novo-Log/NovoRapid) in pumps, the depot will be even smaller, resulting in even faster symptoms of insulin deficiency if the delivery is interrupted (see page 186).

Blurred eyesight and diabetes

Blurred eyesight can be a symptom of a high blood glucose level. This is caused by difference between the glucose content of the lens, compared to that of the blood. The lens contains no blood vessels (if it did they would block the passage of light into the eye). Glucose from the blood must therefore be transported into the lens through the surrounding fluid (aqueous humor, see figure on page 306). So, when the glucose content of the blood is changing rapidly, the glucose content of the lens is bound to

be different. If the glucose content of the lens is higher than that of the blood, the lens will try to absorb water, and this will make it swell. The lens will then refract the light differently, causing temporary shortsightedness. It affects your vision very much the same way as if you borrow someone else's glasses.

The eye itself won't be damaged by this phenomenon, and vision often returns to normal within a few hours. It is like borrowing somebody else's glasses — you can focus but it is tiresome for your eyes. This type of visual disturbance is common at the onset of diabetes and usually happens when the glucose level is changing rapidly. It has nothing to do with the eye complications that can occur after many years of diabetes. See also page 308.

Regulation of blood glucose

If you are not eating, the chances are your entire bloodstream will contain only about 5 g (1/5 ounce) of glucose (barely 2 teaspoons of sugar). If you are not fully grown, it will be even less. At the same time, your blood needs to deliver about 10 g (1/3 ounce) of glucose every hour to the tissues of the body.[4] Obviously, if something happens to the supply of glucose you will very quickly run out, resulting in a severe shortage of glucose in your blood within an hour.

Counter-regulation

In someone who does not have diabetes, the body is able to regulate its own blood glucose levels within narrow boundaries, normally between approximately 70-120 mg/dl (4 and 7 mmol/l). When your blood glucose falls below 65-70 mg/dl (3.5-4.0 mmol/l) you will feel unwell. A drop in your blood glucose level affects all your bodily reactions, as your body struggles to give your brain access to what little glucose is left. The body tries to get the remaining glucose moving, while the cells outside the brain attempt to economize by decreasing the amount of glucose they use. The brain is unable to store glucose, so it has to depend on an even and continuous supply from the blood. However, if no food has been eaten for a while, the

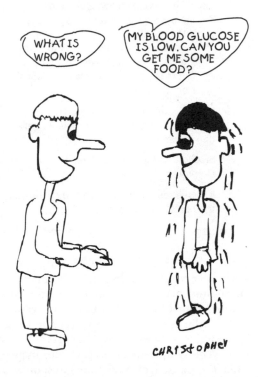

CHRISTOPHER

brain adapts and uses other types of fuel, mainly ketones.

While the hormone insulin lowers your blood glucose level, there are other hormones in your body which can raise it. The body reacts to low blood glucose with a defensive reaction known

---

Where does the glucose in your blood come from?

① From your food.

② From the breakdown of glucose stored as glycogen in the liver (called glycogenolysis).

③ From protein and fat used for production of glucose (called gluconeogenesis).

Counter-regulating hormones that increase blood glucose levels

① Adrenaline	}	Increases the blood glucose for 2-4 hours after hypoglycemia.[103]
② Glucagon		
③ Cortisol	}	The effect starts after 3-4 hours, and lasts for 5-12 hours after hypoglycemia.[103]
④ Growth hormone		

Effects of insulin

⮕ Insulin is produced in the beta-cells in the pancreas.

① Insulin decreases blood glucose by:
  ➡ increasing the uptake of glucose into the cells.
  ➡ Increasing the body's ability to store glucose as glycogen in liver and muscle.
  ➡ Decreasing the production of glucose from the liver.

② Insulin counteracts the production of ketones from the liver. It stimulates utilization of ketones in the cells.

③ Insulin also increases the production of muscle protein.

④ It increases the production and decreases the breakdown of body fat.

Body reserves during fasting and hypoglycemia

⮕ The store of glycogen in the liver is broken down to glucose.

⮕ Fat is broken down to free fatty acids that can be used as fuel. Fatty acids can be transformed into ketones in the liver. Ketones can also be used as fuel, mainly by the brain.

⮕ Proteins from the muscles are broken down to be used in the liver in order to produce glucose.

The liver

The liver functions as a bank for glucose. When times are good you deposit glucose in the liver, and when times are bad you will be able to withdraw it. The excess of glucose from a meal will be stored as a "reservoir" in the liver and muscle cells in the form of glycogen (see illustration on page 204). Insulin is needed to transport the glucose into both liver and muscle cells.

The liver can also produce glucose from fat and proteins to raise the blood glucose level (by a process called gluconeogenesis). The adult liver produces about 6 g (1/5 ounce) of glucose per hour in between meals.[706] The majority of this glucose will be consumed by the brain which can make use of glucose without the help of insulin. A smaller child's liver will produce up to six times as much glucose per kg body weight. The liver of a 5 year old will produce as much glucose in an hour as an adult. After a longer period without food, the kidneys can produce glucose in the same way as the liver does.[264] Recent research suggests that the kidneys can contribute as much as 20% of the body's total glucose production after a night without food.[133]

People with diabetes can also use the stores of glycogen when their blood glucose is low. If you have emptied your stores of glycogen, e.g. dur-

as counter-regulation. In counter-regulation, the autonomic nervous system cooperates with a number of different hormones to raise the blood glucose level. This defense against hypoglycemia is extremely important to your body. The symptoms associated with hypoglycemia are caused by the brain's response to a lack of glucose as well as by the direct effects of the counter-regulatory hormones.

Children are generally more sensitive to hypoglycemia than adults. In one study on healthy children and adolescents, hypoglycemic symptoms and adrenaline responses were evident when the blood glucose level was 68 mg/dl compared to 56 mg/dl (3.8 vs. 3.1 mmol/l) observed for adults.[417]

It may be difficult to understand the biochemistry of the hormones and which hormone is doing what. The figures on page 24 give you a short summary.

Liver and muscle stores

♠ Liver cells can release glucose into the blood from the store of glycogen.

♠ Muscle cells can only use the glucose released from the glycogen stores as fuel inside the cell.

♠ An adult has about 100-120 g (3.5-4.2 ounces) of glucose stored in the liver.[414]

♠ The glycogen store can be broken down to glucose when the blood glucose is low (glycogenolysis) and can compensate for about 24 hours without food in an adult.[706]

♠ In children, glycogen stores are smaller and can compensate for a shorter time without food.

♠ A pre-school child has enough glucose for about 12 hours without food, a smaller child even less.

♠ A child will use up glucose faster than an adult will, even when not very active. This is because a child's brain is larger in relation to body mass than an adult's brain.

ing a game of soccer when the body needs a lot of extra glucose, you will have smaller reserves for dealing with any hypoglycemic episode that might occur later, including during the night. This leads to an increased risk of hypoglycemia several hours after physical exercise (see page 245).

A healthy pancreas produces insulin. Since the blood flow from the pancreas goes to the liver first, this organ will have the quickest and highest concentration of insulin. When insulin is injected into the subcutaneous tissue, it will enter a superficial blood vessel and reach the liver only after the blood has passed through the heart. Because of this, people with diabetes have a much lower insulin concentration in the liver than people without diabetes.

Glucagon

During the day you tend to feel hungry at intervals of about 4 hours, whereas during the night you can do without food for up to 8 or even 10 hours. This is because glycogen from the liver is broken down into glucose during the night, with the help of the hormones glucagon and adrenaline Small children have small stores of glycogen, so they need to eat more often.

The glucagon production in the pancreas won't necessarily be affected in your early days with diabetes. However, once you have had diabetes for just a few years, your body's ability to secrete sufficient amounts of glucagon in response to hypoglycemia will usually disappear. This is something that happens in children

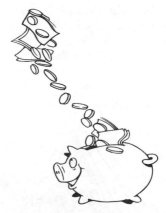

The liver acts like a bank for glucose in your body. When times are good, i.e. during the hours after a meal, glucose is deposited in the "liver bank" to be stored as glycogen.

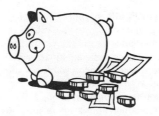

When times are bad, i.e. a couple of hours after the meal and during the night, glucose is withdrawn from the "liver bank" to keep the blood glucose level adequate.

as well as in adults.[15,30] It is probably not a long-term complication as such, but rather a reflection of the way your body adapts to repeated episodes of hypoglycemia.[160] Those individuals who still produce some of their own insulin appear to be better able to carry on secreting glucagon in response to hypoglycemia ("the glucagon defense").[15,160,592] Some research results suggest that the glucagon defense can be at least partly restored if you manage to avoid hypoglycemia[258,426] (see also "Hypoglycemia unawareness" on page 48).

In a person who doesn't have diabetes, the production of glucagon goes down when the blood glucose and insulin concentration rise after a meal. But this doesn't happen when a person has diabetes, even though their blood glucose level goes up. This is because insulin from injections into the subcutaneous tissue is less concentrated by the time it reaches the glucagon-producing alpha cells in the pancreas. In addition to the glucose derived from a meal, blood from the liver will contain glucose

> ### The effects of glucagon
>
> ⇒ Glucagon is produced in the alpha cells in the pancreas.
> ① Glucagon raises blood glucose by:
>   → Releasing glucose from the glycogen stores in the liver.
>   → Activating the production of glucose from proteins.
> ② Glucagon stimulates the production of ketones in the liver.

derived from glycogen, also contributing to an increase in blood glucose after a meal.[216]

Glucagon injections

If a person with diabetes is unconscious or unable to eat or drink, you can give an injection of glucagon to stimulate the breakdown of glycogen in the liver. This will raise the blood glucose level. Glucagon injections are not difficult to administer. It would be a good idea, for example, to encourage a teacher or counselor to learn how to do this before school outings or vacations.

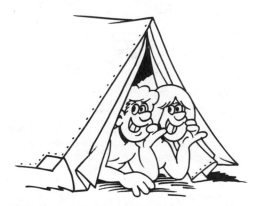

Glucagon directly affects your quality of life. Whenever you have a glucagon kit with you, you are armed with your own emergency treatment. You can go camping, hiking in the mountains or sailing with minimum danger. It is a good idea to take glucagon with you if you go on vacations, so you will not need to depend on local health care if you develop severe hypoglycemia. Make sure that your travelling companion knows where you store your glucagon, and how it should be used.

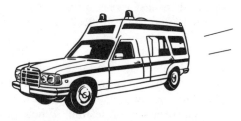

Give a glucagon injection if a person with diabetes develops severe hypoglycemia and becomes unconscious or has a seizure. If the person has not woken up within 10-15 minutes, call an ambulance. However, if he/she has woken up and has a normal blood glucose level by the time the ambulance arrives, it won't be necessary for him/her to go to hospital.

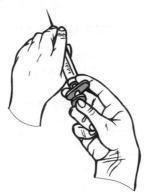

It may be difficult to mix glucagon for the first time in a situation where you really need it. In order to avoid panic at such a time, check the contents of the kit and read through the instructions as soon as you bring them home. Indicate the dose you would need on the syringe with a felt tip pen, so you will not have to worry about this when you are stressed. When the expiry date has passed and you have a new glucagon kit, you can use the old one for practicing the mixing and drawing up of glucagon. Write in your own words the directions for administering glucagon on a small piece of paper and put this with the kit.

Glucagon is given as a subcutaneous injection in the same way as insulin. If you are using an indwelling catheter (Insuflon) you should not use this for glucagon as the effect will be reduced if the catheter is not working properly. The dose of glucagon is 0.1-0.2 mg per10 kg (22 lb) body weight.[16,160] The blood glucose raising effect starts within 10 minutes and lasts for at least 30-60 minutes.[16] The effect will be just as good after a subcutaneous injection as after an intramuscular one, so it does not matter how deep you insert the needle.[16] The higher dose (0.2 mg/10 kg, 22 lb) will give a slightly higher rise in blood glucose, but it may also increase your risk of side effects.[16]

Everyone who has diabetes and is using insulin should have glucagon available.[373,735,508] Check the expiry date! When the expiry date has passed and you have picked up a new injection kit from the pharmacy you can use the old one for practicing and demonstrating mixing procedures. Don't eat anything for at least 30 min-

---

Glucagon

➡ Every person treated with insulin should have a glucagon kit and know how to use it.

➡ Give glucagon if a person with diabetes is unconscious, has seizures or cannot eat or drink.

➡ Dose: 0.1-0.2 mg per 10 kg (22 lb) body weight (1mg/ml solution). If in doubt, give more rather than less. Glucagon is not dangerous if you accidentally overdose.

➡ Glucagon takes effect within 10-15 minutes.

➡ The effect lasts for 30-60 minutes.
Eat something when you are feeling better to keep your blood glucose level up until the next meal. But don't eat too much at once.

➡ Nausea is a common side effect.
Wait at least 30 minutes before you eat to avoid this problem.

➡ Do *not* repeat the dose! One injection gives a sufficient level of glucagon in the blood.

➡ Loss of effect can be caused by:

Store of glycogen already depleted by	Glucagon counteracted by
1) Exercise	1) Alcohol [274]
2) Recent hypoglycemia	2) High dose of
3) Reduced food intake, e.g. through illness	insulin

➡ Always take glucagon with you, e.g. when going on a picnic, hiking trip, sailing trip or vacation abroad.

➡ Teach people close to you how to administer glucagon!

➡ Glucagon has the same effect whether injected into subcutaneous tissue or into the muscle.

---

utes after taking a glucagon injection, or you may feel nauseous or even vomit. This is a relatively common side effect, and usually occurs within 30-60 minutes. You will be more likely

Mini-dose glucagon

♠ A small dose of glucagon has been effective in treating mild or impending hypoglycemia associated with gastroenteritis or refusal to eat.

♠ In one study, children aged 2 years or under, received two "units" using a standard U-100 insulin syringe (= 20 μg), while those older than 2 years received one "unit" for each year of their life, up to 15 units (150 μg).[345] If, after 30 minutes, the blood glucose was essentially unchanged, the initial dose was doubled.

♠ The average increase in blood glucose was 60-90 mg/dl (3.3-5 mmol/l) within 30 minutes, and with a duration of effect of around one hour. Approximately 50% of the children needed more than one dose.

♠ Some children received up to 5 injections over a 25 hour period, without the glucagon losing its beneficial effect. They didn't suffer any more sickness or vomiting than before.

Glucagon, fatty acids and ketones

♠ Glucagon stimulates the transformation of fatty acids to ketones in the liver (see illustration on page 24).

♠ The fatty acids are formed from the breakdown of fat in the starving cells, caused by a lack of food or not enough insulin.

♠ The ketones contribute to nausea as a side effect after a glucagon injection.

♠ Ketones can easily be detected in blood or urine by self monitoring (see page 99). See also "After hypoglycemia" on page 65.

to suffer in this way if you eat large amounts of food. Don't repeat the glucagon injection either, as this will make nausea more likely without raising the blood glucose level any further.[16] If your blood glucose level does not go back to normal after a glucagon injection, this suggests your glucagon store has been completely emptied out, for example by heavy exercise or a recent hypoglycemic episode.

If you have to give glucagon, wait 10-15 minutes for the person to wake up. If they are still unconscious after this time, call an ambulance. However, if the person has revived, is feeling well and has a normal blood glucose when the ambulance arrives, it may not be necessary for them to go to hospital.

Glucagon is counteracted by insulin. This is logical given that people who don't have diabetes will never have high concentrations of both hormones at the same time. Insulin is secreted

when the blood glucose is high and glucagon when it is low. If hypoglycemia is caused by too large a dose of insulin, glucagon will have less effect than if the low blood glucose is caused by not eating enough (see also "Too little food or too much insulin?" on page 51).

Some people with diabetes, especially children and adolescents, feel nauseous after a difficult hypoglycemic episode, even if glucagon has not been injected. One explanation is that the production of glucagon from their own pancreas also can result in nausea as a side effect.

At present, glucagon can only be given as an injection, but recent experiments giving glucagon as a nasal spray have been encouraging.[720]

Adrenaline

Adrenaline is a stress hormone secreted by the adrenal glands. It raises the blood glucose primarily by breaking down the glycogen stores in the liver. The concentration of adrenaline rises when the body is exposed to stress, fever and acidosis (when the blood becomes acidic, e.g. in diabetic ketoacidosis).[463] Adrenaline also reduces the amount of glucose taken up by the cells of the body. This might strike you as odd until you remember that all bodily reactions

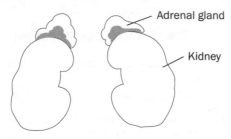

Adrenaline and cortisol are produced in the adrenal glands.

during hypoglycemia are aimed at reserving any available glucose for the brain.

The human body was originally designed for living in the Stone Age. If a person ran into a polar bear or a mammoth, the only alternatives were to fight or take flight. In both situations extra fuel, in the form of glucose, was needed by the body. The problem with our present way of life is that adrenaline is still secreted when we get excited or fearful, though this is more likely to be caused by a frightening TV program than by an activity which actually calls for extra strength. A healthy person, whose insulin production is working as it should, will not find this causes a problem. However, a person with diabetes will find their blood glucose level rises (see "Stress" on page 255).

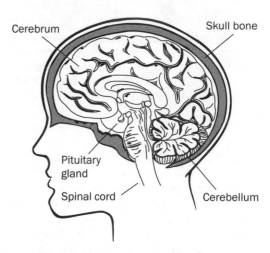

Cross-section of the brain. Growth hormone is produced in the pituitary gland.

When a person with diabetes becomes hypoglycemic, secretion of adrenaline can raise the blood glucose by stimulating the breakdown of the glycogen stores in the liver [706] and at the same time causing shakiness, anxiety, and a pounding heart. Adrenaline also stimulates the breakdown of body fat to fatty acids which can be converted into ketones in the liver. See illustration on page 24.

Cortisol

Cortisol is another important hormone which is secreted by the adrenal glands in response to stress and affects the body metabolism in many

---

Effects of adrenaline

➧ Adrenaline is produced in the adrenal glands.

① Adrenaline raises blood glucose by:
  → Releasing glucose from the glycogen stores in the liver.
  → Activating the production of glucose from proteins.
  → Reducing uptake of glucose into the cells.
  → Reducing insulin production (in people who don't have diabetes).

② Adrenaline causes symptoms of hypoglycemia, such as shakiness, rapid heartbeat and sweating.

③ It also stimulates the breakdown of body fat.

Effects of cortisol

➧ Cortisol is produced in the adrenal glands.

① Cortisol raises blood glucose by:
  → Reducing cellular uptake of glucose.
  → Breaking down proteins that can be used to produce glucose in the liver.

② It also stimulates breakdown of body fat.

ways. It increases the amount of glucose in the blood by producing glucose from proteins (gluconeogenesis) and by decreasing the amount of glucose that is absorbed and used by the cells. Cortisol also promotes the breakdown of body fat into fatty acids that can be converted into ketones.

Growth hormone

Growth hormone is produced in the pituitary gland, which is found just below the brain. Some of the body's most important hormones are produced in this gland. The most important effect of growth hormone is to stimulate growth. It has the effect of raising blood glucose by counteracting insulin on the cell surface, thereby reducing the uptake of glucose into the cells. Growth hormone increases muscle tissue and stimulates the breakdown of body fat.

During puberty, when a young person is growing quickly, large amounts of growth hormone are secreted. This results in the person needing more insulin.[226] Growth hormone is released in high concentrations during the night which explains why teenagers often need very high doses of bedtime insulin. The blood glucose raising effect of growth hormone will start after 3-5 hours.[103] This contributes to the problem of high morning blood glucose that is common among teenagers, especially if their A1C level is high [103] (see "Dawn phenomenon" on page 54).

Growth hormone also stimulates production of ketones, thereby increasing the risk of ketoacidosis in adolescents.[226]

> ### The effects of growth hormone
>
> ➠ Growth hormone is produced in the pituitary gland.
>
> ① It stimulates growth.
>
> ② It raises blood glucose by reducing the cellular uptake of glucose.
>
> ③ Growth hormone breaks down body fat.
>
> ④ It increases muscular mass.

Teenagers with diabetes have higher levels of growth hormone than their peers without diabetes. Despite this, their growth can be slower than it should be if their glucose control is not adequate. This is because the effect of growth hormone in the body is partly dependent on the protein IGF-1. IGF-1 is produced in the liver but insulin is necessary to stimulate this. Since the insulin concentration in the liver is lower in people with diabetes (see page 34) the levels of IGF-1 will also be lower.[226] IGF-1 has been given in a trial to children and adolescents with diabetes, and an improvement was seen in the levels of A1C (see page 104) in the blood. However, this improvement lasted for three months only.[2] A study of adults showed an improved A1C level, but also a worsening of retinopathy (eye damage) which has discouraged further research on IGF-I.[758]

Hypoglycemia

Hypoglycemia means "low blood glucose". Sometimes symptoms of hypoglycemia can be experienced when the blood glucose is not particularly low, or even when it is high (see "Blood glucose levels and symptoms of hypoglycemia" on page 43). It may be appropriate to refer to the symptoms of hypoglycemia as "sensations", warning of a particular blood glucose level, but not necessarily actually being proof of a low level.

The glucose level can be measured as whole blood glucose or plasma glucose. Most patient meters now display plasma glucose which is approximately 11% higher that whole blood glucose.[269] In this book the numbers refer mainly to plasma glucose, unless otherwise stated (in the previous edition whole blood glucose was used so the numbers were slightly lower).

Not everyone will have the same symptoms when they develop hypoglycemia. However, the symptoms usually follow the same pattern for each person.[160] You should check your blood glucose level whenever you have symptoms or simply feel strange. This is particularly important in the early days following diagnosis, when

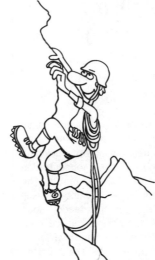

Avoid situations where hypoglycemia could have catastrophic consequences. This does not mean that it is impossible for people with diabetes to engage in risky sports such as mountain climbing, paragliding or scuba diving. What it does mean, however, is that they should prepare very carefully, think about the sorts of adverse situations that could arise, and not practice the activity alone. See the section on diving on page 252 for more information.

you are learning how to recognize your own individual reactions to hypoglycemia. When your diabetes is newly diagnosed it is important that the diabetes team at your hospital or outpatient clinic help you to understand what your individual symptoms mean. It is important that all family members know how to treat hypoglycemia in a safe and effective manner.

Usually symptoms of hypoglycemia are divided into two categories: symptoms caused by the body attempting to raise the blood glucose level by adrenaline for example (known as "autonomic" or "adrenergic" symptoms); and symptoms originating in the brain as a result of a deficiency of glucose in the central nervous system ("neuroglycopenic" symptoms). See the key fact boxes on page 40.

When a person with diabetes starts to become hypoglycemic, he or she is likely to notice bodily symptoms (e.g. shakiness, heart pounding) at first. However, observers are more likely

---

Hypoglycemic reactions

Hypoglycemic symptoms are usually divided into two types:

① Symptoms caused by the defense mechanisms in your body, such as adrenaline, attempting to raise the blood glucose (called adrenergic and autonomic symptoms).

② Symptoms from the brain due to low blood glucose (called neuroglycopenic symptoms).

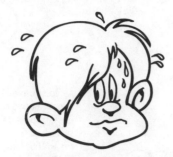

Symptoms of hypoglycemia from the body

Bodily symptoms (autonomic and adrenergic symptoms) are the result of both adrenaline secretion and the autonomic nervous system. They usually start when the blood glucose concentration dips below 65-70 mg/dl (3.5-4 mmol/l). The threshold for triggering these symptoms will change depending on the person's recent blood glucose concentrations (the "blood glucose thermostat", see page 43). In very young children, bodily symptoms of hypoglycemia are reported less frequently, if at all.[769]

⟹ Irritability.

⟹ Hunger, feeling nauseous.

⟹ Trembling.

⟹ Anxiety.

⟹ Heart palpitations.

⟹ Throbbing pulse in the chest and abdomen.

⟹ Numbness in the lips, fingers and tongue.

⟹ Looking pale.

⟹ Cold sweats.

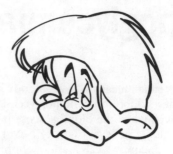

Symptoms of hypoglycemia from the brain

The blood glucose concentration at which your brain begins to show symptoms of dysfunction (neuroglycopenic symptoms) is lower than that for bodily symptoms, and largely independent of your recent blood glucose levels. [29,160]

⟹ Weakness, dizziness.

⟹ Difficulty concentrating.

⟹ Double or blurred vision.

⟹ Disturbed color vision (especially red-green colors).

⟹ Difficulties with hearing.[256]

⟹ Feeling warm or hot.

⟹ Headache.

⟹ Drowsiness.

⟹ Odd behavior, poor judgement.

⟹ Confusion.

⟹ Problems with short-term memory.

⟹ Slurred speech.

⟹ Unsteady walking, lack of coordination.

⟹ Lapses in consciousness.

⟹ Seizures.

to be aware of symptoms such as irritability, and behavioral changes, which indicate the brain is being affected. The brain's reaction to hypoglycemia is usually triggered at a slightly lower blood glucose level than the symptoms from the body.[33,160]

The brain is very sensitive to hypoglycemia so the body automatically reacts in such a way as to help avoid this. Both children and adolescents will find their mental agility and their

Different types of hypoglycemia

① **Mild hypoglycemia**
Self-treatment is possible and blood glucose levels are easily restored.

② **Moderate hypoglycemia**
Your body reacts with warning symptoms of hypoglycemia (autonomic symptoms) and you can take appropriate action. Self-treatment is possible.

③ **Hypoglycemia unawareness**
You experience symptoms from the brain (neuroglycopenic symptoms) without having had any bodily (autonomic) warning symptoms beforehand. However, it is obvious to people observing you that you are having symptoms.

④ **Severe hypoglycemia**
Severe symptoms of hypoglycemia disable you temporarily, requiring the assistance of another person to give you something to eat or a glucagon injection. Severe hypoglycemia can cause you to lose consciousness and have seizures.

The "glucostat"

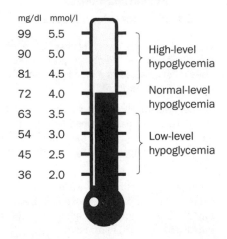

The blood glucose level at which you experience symptoms of hypoglycemia functions like a thermostat (the "glucostat"). Unfortunately this thermostat is adjusted up or down much too easily. When your blood glucose has been high for a couple of days you will have symptoms at a higher blood glucose level ("high-level hypoglycemia") and when it has been low for several days you will experience symptoms at a lower blood glucose level ("low-level hypoglycemia").

	Symptoms at mg/dl	mmol/l	Measure
High-level hypoglycemia	>70-80	4.0-4.5	Wait before eating
Normal-level hypoglycemia	65-70	3.5-4.0	Eat something with glucose
Low-level hypoglycemia	<65	< 3.5	Avoid all low blood glucose values

ability to plan, make decisions and pay attention to detail will be affected, as will the speed of their reactions. This will be evident when the blood glucose concentration is no lower than 60-65 mg/dl (3.3-3.6 mmol/l).[658] Adults seem to adjust slightly better to low blood glucose concentrations as they experience neuroglycopenic symptoms (i.e. symptoms from the brain, see above) at lower blood glucose concentrations (50-55 mg/dl, 2.8-3.0 mmol/l).[151,160]

Hypoglycemia is usually an unpleasant experience, involving loss of control over your body. This is indeed what happens as the brain does not function well without glucose. Some people become unusually irritable, while others may look pale, sick or sleepy. Fortunately, it is rare for people to do something uncharacteristically dangerous or stupid that may damage themselves or someone else. Traffic accidents on a bicycle or in a car can sometimes be caused by hypoglycemia (see page 286). Occasionally people do really strange things, for example one boy spread butter on a paper towel and tried to eat it. So it is very important that your family and friends understand that when you are hav-

Research findings:
Effects of low blood glucose

♠ In one study, tests involving associative learning, attention and mental flexibility were the ones most affected at a blood glucose level of 40 mg/dl (2.2 mmol/l).[223]

♠ Women were less affected than men in this study. This may be explained by women having lower levels of adrenaline and less pronounced symptoms of hypoglycemia than men.[31]

♠ Changes in EEG (brain wave) activity will occur when the blood glucose falls below 55 mg/dl (3.0 mmol/l) in children [75] and 40 mg/dl (2.2 mmol/l) in adults.[29]

♠ Unconsciousness occurs when the blood glucose level drops to approximately 20 mg/dl (1 mmol/l).[5]

♠ Symptoms of hypoglycemia can change over time, depending on your average blood glucose levels (see below).

What caused your hypoglycemia?

➟ Too little to eat or delayed meal.

➟ Skipped a meal?

➟ Neglecting to eat despite symptoms of hypoglycemia.

➟ Physical exercise?
The risk of hypoglycemia is increased during the rest of the day and also the night after heavy physical exercise.

➟ Too large a dose of insulin?

➟ New site for the injection?
e.g. from thigh to abdomen or to a site free of fatty lumps (lipohypertrophy).

➟ Recent hypoglycemia?
  ➟ glucose stores in the liver depleted.
  ➟ fewer warning symptoms of hypoglycemia (hypoglycemic unawareness).

➟ Very low A1C?(increased risk of hypoglycemic unawareness).

➟ Drinking alcohol?

➟ Not mixing the cloudy insulin thoroughly enough (see page 119).

➟ Variable insulin absorption (see "How accurate is your insulin dose?" on page 80).

➟ Gastroenteritis or tummy upset.

➟ Certain drugs used for the treatment of high blood pressure (so called non-selective beta blockers) can increase the risk of hypoglycemia (by diminishing the adrenergic symptoms of hypoglycemia).[748]

ing a hypoglycemic reaction you are not quite in control of yourself, and cannot help what you are doing.

Even if individuals with diabetes are aware of having symptoms of hypoglycemia, they may find it difficult to eat or drink. This can still be a problem if food is right in front of them. It might be difficult for parents to understand that their child can react so oddly, but adults with diabetes have described the feeling as follows: "You know you should drink the juice, but your body just does not obey the orders from the brain".

If the blood glucose is lowered quickly, even if it stays within the normal range, symptoms of hypoglycemia can be provoked in certain people. This type of reaction is more common in people with a high A1C[548] (see page 107) but there may be a difference between children and adults. In one study, the blood glucose level in a group of adults with diabetes with an A1C of 11% went down from 360-180 mg/dl (20 to 10 mmol/l) using intravenous insulin.[236] These subjects showed the same type of increased blood flow to the brain that both people in good control and people without diabetes had at a blood glucose of 40 mg/dl (2.2 mmol/l). However, in a group of children and adolescents with an average A1C of 10.8%, no symptoms of hypoglyc-

Symptoms of hypoglycemia in children and adolescents

Hypoglycemic symptoms in children and adolescents differ slightly from those experienced by adults in that behavior changes are more common. The table below is from a Scottish study in which parents were asked how often certain symptoms of hypoglycemia occurred in their children and teenagers, aged from 18 months to 16 years old.[535]

Pale skin	88%
Sweating	77%
Tearfulness	74%
Irritability	73%
Poor concentration	69%
Argumentativeness	69%
Hunger	69%
Tiredness	67%
Aggression	64%
Trembling	64%
Weakness	64%
Confusion	60%
Dizziness	51%
Headaches	47%
Abdominal / tummy pain	43%
Naughtiness	40%
Nausea	33%
Slurred speech	29%
Nightmares	20%
Blurred vision	19%
Seizures	16%
Double vision	11%
Bed wetting	10%

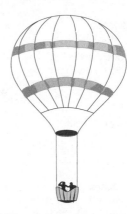

The level at which you start experiencing symptoms of hypoglycemia will change depending on how often your blood glucose level has been low in the last few days. Make it part of your routine to measure blood glucose as soon as you notice symptoms. If you usually become hypoglycemic when the level is 67 mg/dl (3.7 mmol/l, "normal-level hypoglycemia") and now have no symptoms until it falls to 58 mg/dl (3.2 mmol/l, "low-level hypoglycemia") you have probably had too many low blood glucose values recently. On the other hand, if you start experiencing symptoms of hypoglycemia with a blood glucose level of 72-81 mg/dl or higher (4.0-4.5 mmol/l, "high-level hypoglycemia") you have had too many high blood glucose values and your A1C is probably rising (see also page 57).

emia were noted when the blood glucose level was dropped from 380 mg/dl to 110 mg/dl (21 to 6 mmol/l).[319]

Blood glucose levels and symptoms of hypoglycemia

Symptoms of hypoglycemia may not be recognized by a person with diabetes, particularly when the focus of his or her attention is else-where. For example, some people report that they are less likely to recognize symptoms of hypoglycemia at work than when relaxing at home. Children may notice symptoms more readily when there is little distraction, compared to when they are playing with friends.

Your brain contains a kind of blood glucose meter that triggers defense reactions in your body and raises a low blood glucose level. It works in a similar way to a thermostat ("glucostat"), and is triggered at a certain blood glucose level. This reaction depends very much on where your blood glucose level has been during the last few days.[163,493] If your blood sugar has been high for some time, symptoms of hypoglycemia and release of counter-regulating hormones will appear at a higher blood glucose level than usual.[110,205] If your A1C is high, you may start having symptoms of hypoglycemia when your blood glucose level is 70-90 mg/dl (4-5 mmol/l).[110,369,417] However, this type of

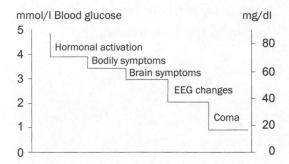

When your blood glucose is lowered, the reactions in your body and brain take place at different levels. These levels are in turn dependent on your recent blood glucose levels, i.e. if you recently have had higher blood glucose readings, the symptoms will occur at a slightly higher blood glucose level and if you recently have had lower blood glucose readings and hypoglycemia, the

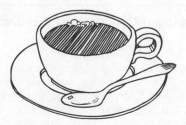

Caffeine in coffee and cola can increase your awareness of hypoglycemic symptoms.

reaction seems to occur less frequently in adults.[58]

When the "glucostat" adjusts to another blood glucose level, the effect will be most pronounced on your bodily (autonomic) symptoms (mediated by adrenaline or the autonomic nervous system). The blood glucose level where symptoms from the brain (neuroglycopenic symptoms) occur is influenced not so much by recent blood glucose levels as the bodily symptoms.[29,30,32,160] This may be due to the way in which the body's cells adjust to preserve as much glucose as possible for use by the brain when blood glucose levels are low.[111] The function of the brain is affected when the blood glucose falls below approximately (50-55 mg/dl, 2.8-3.0 mmol/l) in people who don't have diabetes.[780] A study of people whose glucose control was poor and whose A1C was high (9.2%) found their short-term memory was deteriorating by the time the blood glucose level had reached 70 mg/dl (3.9 mmol/l).[369] See also page 58.

To decrease the blood glucose level at which symptoms of hypoglycemia appear, you must keep yourself from eating until your blood glu-

cose level has come down to 65-70 mg/dl (3.5-4.0 mmol/l), even though you will have symptoms of hypoglycemia. Do everything you can to avoid high blood glucose levels during the two weeks that follow. The "glucostat" threshold will then automatically be lowered, until your symptoms of hypoglycemia appear at the appropriate level (see also "Insulin sensitivity and resistance" on page 195).

The opposite applies if your blood glucose has been low for some time or you have often been hypoglycemic. The "glucostat" will then change so that the defense mechanisms of hypoglycemia will not start until your blood glucose falls below 45 mg/dl (2.6 mmol/l).[29,368]

Coffee and cola contain caffeine which may cause the symptoms of hypoglycemia to be noticed at a slightly higher blood glucose level than usual.[202] This may be useful for individuals with "hypoglycemic unawareness" (see page 48) as caffeine enhances the intensity of the symptoms that warn of hypoglycemia.[802]

Some drugs used for treating high blood pressure (beta-blockers) can have the opposite effect and make symptoms of hypoglycemia less obvious. If you have diabetes and are taking beta-blockers, you should always check your blood glucose level if you start to sweat for no obvious reason, as this may be the only symptom of a very low blood glucose, 3.3 mmol/l (60 mg/dl) or below.[369] Some drugs for treating depression (so called SSRIs, for example Paroxetine/Paxil® and Sertraline/Zoloft®) have caused

> ## Research findings:
> ## Hypoglycemic symptoms
>
> ♠ In one study the threshold for symptoms of hypoglycemia changed, being 5 mg/dl (0.3 mmol/l) lower after only four days with low blood glucose values (42 mg/dl, 2.3 mmol/l) during one or a couple of hours per day.[809]
>
> ♠ In another study, a single episode of afternoon hypoglycemia (approximately 50 mg/dl, 2.8 mmol/l) caused fewer symptoms as well as a reduction of the hormonal defense when hypoglycemia occurred again the following morning.[163] The participants were also more than usually sensitive to insulin, i.e. the blood glucose was lower than the day before although the insulin level in the blood was the same.
>
> ♠ However, two days after a hypoglycemic episode, (2 hours of 50 mg/dl, 2.8 mmol/l) the ability to recognize symptoms of hypoglycemia was back to normal according to another study.[296]
>
> ♠ Night time hypoglycemia with an average blood glucose of 48 mg/dl (2.7 mmol/l) over a 3-hour period resulted in fewer bodily (adrenergic) symptoms but no significant difference in brain (neuroglycopenic) symptoms when having a new hypoglycemia with the same blood glucose level the next day.[260]
>
> ♠ However, the subjects in the study scored better during hypoglycemia on tests that measured memory, attention, and recognition after a night with hypoglycemia (compared to a control night with normal blood glucose). This indicates that the brain does have some ability to adjust to lower blood-glucose levels, thereby preserving brain function.

the symptoms of hypoglycemia to be lost in some people with diabetes.[676] Certain drugs (beta-stimulating agents) used to treat asthma increase the blood glucose level by stimulating adrenaline and have been successfully used to prevent night time hypoglycemia.[663]

Symptoms of hypoglycemia when the blood glucose level is high

Some children will experience the same symptoms when the blood glucose is high as when it is low. Younger children are particularly likely to find it difficult to differentiate between the two. They may feel hungry or hollow in the stomach when their blood glucose is high because the cells are starving due to a lack of insulin (see figure at the bottom of page 25 and "What to do if your blood glucose level is high" on page 131).

Severe hypoglycemia

Severe hypoglycemia is defined as a hypoglycemic reaction with documented low blood glucose (< 55 mg/dl, (3.1 mmol/l) or reversal of symptoms after intake of glucose, with symptoms sufficiently severe for the person to need help from another person or even admission to hospital.[194] In many cases, the person with diabetes will lose consciousness (either fully of partially) and may have seizures. Insulin coma involves severe hypoglycemia with loss of consciousness. In a review, 10-25% of individuals with type 1 diabetes were found to experience a severe hypoglycemic episode during a period of one year.[157] Severe hypoglycemia was more common in adults with long-term complications, alcohol use, a threshold for hypoglycemia symptoms of < 55 mg/dl (3 mmol/l) and use of certain medications (so called non-selective beta-blockers).[748] Other factors that will increase your risk of severe hypoglycemia include taking the wrong dose of insulin, missing a meal, or drinking alcohol after an unusual amount of activity such as energetic dancing. Some studies show severe hypoglycemia to be more common in younger children.[187] Others, however, do not.[336,768] It is rare in the first 12 months after diagnosis.[188]

Thresholds for reactions of hypoglycemia

	Without diabetes	With diabetes	
		A1C 9.0%	A1C 5.2%
mg/dl			
Symptoms start at	52	67	40
Adrenaline response	68	61	46
EEG-changes	~40	~40	~40
mmol/l		9.0%	5.2%
Symptoms start at	2.9	3.7	2.2*
Adrenaline response	3.4	3.3	2.6
EEG-changes	~2.2	~2.2	~2.2

With a low A1C you will get bodily (adrenergic) hypoglycemic symptoms and adrenaline responses at much lower blood glucose values than if your A1C is high.[29] However, the blood glucose level at which your brain starts showing symptoms is the same whether your A1C is high or low.

*Values have been recalculated to plasma glucose

An international study involving participants from 18 countries found that 20-30% of elementary school children and 15-20% of teenagers had severe hypoglycemia with unconsciousness or seizures in a year.[558] If this happens to you, you should immediately review your insulin doses with your diabetes team. Usually, you will be able to identify why it has happened, e.g. a dose of insulin that is too high, increased exercise, a missed meal, an incorrect dose administered, alcohol drunk after a lot of dancing or other activity. If you cannot identify a clear reason, you should decrease the "responsible" dose of insulin (see table on page 132). Anxiety about having another episode of severe hypoglycemia and the feeling of not being able to trust your body can be very frightening. If you have recurrent severe hypoglyc-

emia, you must discuss altering the insulin or food regimen with your diabetes team. Some people may find an insulin pump helpful in this situation.[370]

Seizures

A very low blood glucose, usually close to 20 mg/dl (1 mmol/l), can trigger seizures. Some very sensitive children may have muscle twitches when their blood glucose level is within the low normal range.[508] These children are likely to be conscious when the twitching starts. Some will be able to talk, and even maintain eye contact at this time.

Seizures are not usually dangerous, but can be very alarming for those who witness them. The child may even appear to be dying. However, breathing is seldom affected. Turn the child onto his or her side (recovery position), after making sure that the airways are free. This is the safest position for someone who might vomit. Prepare glucagon and give an injection (for doses see page 38). Call an ambulance if the child does not wake up within 10-15 minutes.

Insulin doses should always be looked at again after hypoglycemia with seizures, and the dose should be reduced if the cause of the blood glucose being so low cannot be identified. Anti-convulsive medicine can be considered for preventing repeated seizures, especially when these happen at a blood glucose level of 55-65 mg/dl (3.0-3.5 mmol/l), even if this is accompanied by a normal EEG (brain-wave trace).

We have seen several school children and teenagers who have had seizures when their blood glucose level has been around 55-70 mg/dl (3.0-4.0 mmol/l). After medication their blood glucose level can dip below 45 mg/dl (2.5 mmol/l) without seizures, while they treat their hypoglycemia by taking glucose.

Research findings:
Severe hypoglycemia

♠ The risk may be increased with lower A1C values. In an Australian study of children and adolescents on two insulin injections per day and an A1C of 9.1% the risk of having an episode of severe hypoglycemia with unconsciousness or seizures was 4.8%/year.[188]

♠ In a Finnish pediatric study using 3-4 doses/day and an A1C of 9% the risk was only 3.1%.[768] However, in a Swedish study using mostly 4-5 injections/day and an A1C of 8.1% the risk was 15%.[508] There was no correlation between A1C and the risk of severe hypoglycemia in this study.

♠ Compare this figure with the DCCT study (see page 314) where the 13-17 year old had a risk of 26.7% of unconsciousness or seizures in the intensively treated group (A1C of 8.1%) and 9.7% risk in the conventional group (A1C of 9.8%).[192]

Does severe hypoglycemia damage the brain?

It is not clear how or whether repeated severe hypoglycemia affects the physical or intellectual development of children with diabetes. Glucose is the most important source of energy for the brain. When the blood glucose is low, the blood flow to the brain can be increased to allow a larger supply of glucose.[236]

Small children (under the age of 5) are more vulnerable to severe hypoglycemia with seizures because their nervous systems are still developing.[71] Children under the age of 2 are especially vulnerable. Severe hypoglycemia should be avoided at all costs in this age group, even if it means having a higher A1C.[505]

Permanent neurological damage and EEG (brain-wave) changes have been described in exceptional cases where children have had such severe hypoglycemia that they have become unconscious, mostly with seizures.[713] One study of children and teenagers between the age of 10 and 19 years showed poorer results on neuro-psychological tests for those who developed diabetes before the age of 5, presumably having had more severe hypoglycemia.[657] However, when the same individuals were tested again as adults, their performance was no different from that of the control group, made up of people without diabetes. This indicated there had been no permanent neurological damage.[659] Another explanation for the lower test results in the teenage group may have been a long-standing poor diabetes control with high blood glucose levels.

In an Austrian study of children and adolescents aged 4-18 years, neurophysiological studies (so called auditory and visually evoked potentials) showed poorer results both in participants who had severe hypoglycemia (unconsciousness/seizures) and poor glucose control (A1C > ~10%) during the last two years.[693] In an Australian study, both recurrent severe hypoglycemia and chronically elevated blood glucose levels were associated with reduced memory and learning capacity in children two years after the onset of diabetes.[578] A Swiss study of children diagnosed with diabetes before the age of 10 found a decline in intellectual performance only in boys diagnosed before the age of 6.[686] This was attributed to long-term high A1C and ketoacidosis at the onset of diabetes, but not to severe hypoglycemia. A US study from 2003 did not find that severe hypoglycemia with seizures or coma in children aged 6-15 years had adverse effects on attention, planning or simultaneous processing when they were tested 18 months later.[818]

It seems as if children are especially vulnerable to seizures in combination with severe hypoglycemia. One study showed differences in the ability to concentrate in children who had experienced at least one severe hypoglycemic episode with seizures.[655] However, parents did not report any difference in the children's ability to concentrate, and their school work did not

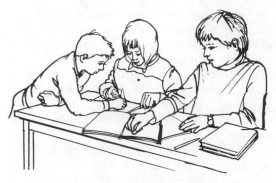

It is difficult to determine whether a child's development is affected by severe hypoglycemia. Single episodes will probably have no effect, but if the child has recurrent severe hypoglycemia with seizures during the first 2-3 years of life, some studies indicate that school performance will not be as good as it should be. If the child has been suffering from severe hypoglycemia, the insulin doses should always be adjusted to avoid another such episode. With young children, it may sometimes be necessary to accept a higher A1C in order to avoid severe hypoglycemia.

appear to suffer either. In the same study, children with high blood glucose levels at the time of the test appeared to be more impulsive in their behavior. An American study compared children with 1-2 vs. 3-4 injections per day.[359] The multiple injections group had more severe hypoglycemia (0.80 vs. 0.24 episodes per person per year) and tests revealed them to have reduced ability to recall past events. However, the rate of severe hypoglycemia when using multiple injections in this study was much higher than that reported from other centres.[336,575] Another study, of 55 children aged 5-10 years, found significant reduction in memory scores but only in the group that had experienced unconsciousness with seizures while severely hypoglycemic.[433]

Adults with diabetes seem to withstand severe hypoglycemia very well, even if they have been unconscious. Episodes of hypoglycemic coma were not found to be associated with any permanent brain damage in people who developed type 1 diabetes as adults.[462] Neither the DCCT [195] nor the Stockholm study [639] found

any impairment in neuro-psychological testing in people who had experienced repeated severe hypoglycemic episodes.

Hypoglycemia unawareness

Hypoglycemia unawareness is defined as a hypoglycemic episode that comes on without warning symptoms such as are usually associated with decreasing blood glucose. If you have frequent hypoglycemic episodes, the threshold at which you recognize symptoms will occur at a lower blood glucose level (see page 43). If the threshold for secreting counter-regulatory hormones falls below the blood glucose level that provokes a reaction in the brain, you will not have any physical warning symptoms. Because of this, you will not react in time (by eating, for example) so your hypoglycemia can rapidly become severe. Sometimes you will not even remember afterwards that you had hypoglycemia. This is a common phenomenon. In one study of children and adolescents 37% were

---

Research findings:
Hypoglycemia unawareness

⟫ In one study of adults, the ability to recognize symptoms of hypoglycemia had improved after only two days of careful avoidance of blood glucose levels less than 65 mg/dl (3.6 mmol/l).[493]

⟫ In a group of adults with an A1C of 6.3% and hypoglycemia unawareness, low blood glucose readings were carefully avoided.[258] These patients aimed instead for a slightly higher average blood glucose. After just two weeks, the patients found it easier to recognize their hypoglycemic episodes.

⟫ After three months, the threshold for triggering the counter-regulatory hormones (the defense against low blood glucose, see page 31) had changed from 42 to 56 mg/dl (2.3 to 3,1 mmol/l). At the same time A1C was raised to 7.4%.

unaware of some or all episodes of hypoglycemia.[54]

Hypoglycemic unawareness will increase substantially the risk of severe hypoglycemia in both children [54] and adults,[158] and is more common among those prone to severe hypoglycemia.[159] It should be part of your routine always to check your blood glucose as soon as you start getting symptoms that might indicate hypoglycemia. If your readings are below 65 mg/dl (3.5 mmol/l), this is a warning sign that your risk of becoming severely hypoglycemic may increase considerably.[748]

If you have hypoglycemia unawareness, you should aim for a slightly higher average blood glucose. Above all, you should avoid a blood glucose level that is lower than 65-70 mg/dl (3.5-4.0 mmol/l).[32] Within a fortnight, you are likely to find you can recognize symptoms of hypoglycemia more easily.[160,258] By training yourself to recognize subtle symptoms as your blood glucose is decreasing, you will increase your chances of treating your hypoglycemia in time.[30] See also page 58 and 108.

Many people with long-standing diabetes will have a reduced adrenaline response to low blood glucose, which will mean they have fewer warning symptoms from their autonomic nervous system. This contributes both to diminished symptoms and to less effective counter-regulation when the blood glucose is decreasing.[30] The change from porcine (pork) and bovine (beef) insulin to human insulin has been associated with an increase in hypoglycemia unawareness. Although several studies have looked at this issue, there has been no scientific evidence of such an increase.[30]

Rebound phenomenon

Your body will try to reverse hypoglycemia by using counter-regulatory responses (see "Regulation of blood glucose" on page 31). Sometimes this counter-regulation will be too effective and the blood glucose will rise to high

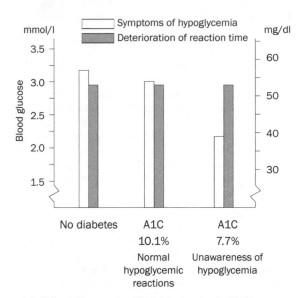

A British study compared individuals who did not have diabetes with two groups of people with type 1 diabetes having an A1C of 10.1% and 7.7% respectively.[525] Both diabetes groups had the same number of symptomatic hypoglycemic episodes while in the group with lower A1C all had recorded at least three blood glucose readings of less than 54 mg/dl (3.0 mmol/l) without symptoms of hypoglycemia (hypoglycemia unawareness) during the past two months. Most of them also had experienced one or more severe hypoglycemic episodes (where they needed help from another person) during the previous six months.

In the group with hypoglycemia unawareness, people had no symptoms of hypoglycemia until their blood glucose went down to 41 mg/dl (2.3 mmol/l). Despite this, their reaction times deteriorated at the same blood glucose level (52 mg/dl, 2.9 mmol/l) as those of the other groups. This means that if you have experienced hypoglycemia unawareness and drive a car with a blood glucose of 50 mg/dl (2.8 mmol/l), you may feel quite well but your reaction times will be slow, making you a danger on the roads.

levels during the hours following hypoglycemia. This is called "rebound phenomenon". During the hours when the levels of the counter-regulatory hormones are increased, your body will be resistant to insulin (see page 195), i.e. higher doses of insulin than usual are needed to lower the blood glucose to normal levels (for example when taking an injection before eating).

Two situations of hypoglycemia

▮▶ **Not enough food:**
Typical of this type is hypoglycemia before a meal. If you use premeal injections you will not yet have taken the insulin and the insulin level in the blood will not be so high. Adrenaline and glucagon, therefore, can easily release glucose from the liver and you may very well get a rebound effect with high blood glucose lasting several hours after hypoglycemia.

▮▶ **Too much insulin:**
Typical of this type is taking the insulin as usual but not eating enough (e.g. if you don't like the food). The blood glucose is low at the same time as the insulin level increases. The insulin then counteracts the production of glucose from the liver, resulting in more severe hypoglycemia. The high insulin level prevents the rebound phenomenon.

Many people, when experiencing hypoglycemia, have a tendency to eat too much, to compensate for the effect of low blood glucose. They are also likely to decrease the next insulin dose in order to avoid further hypoglycemia. Both these factors contribute to the rebound phenomenon, resulting in an even higher blood glucose level.

The rebound phenomenon will only develop if the insulin level in the blood is low during the hours following a hypoglycemic episode.[103] For example, it may occur if your hypoglycemia has been caused by exercise or skipping a snack. Your insulin level after night time hypoglycemia decreases as the night goes on if you are using NPH as your bedtime insulin. If hypoglycemia is caused by too large a dose of insulin, however, the high level of insulin will cause a smaller amount of the counter-regulating hormones to be secreted, making the rebound phenomenon much less likely to occur.

Children are more likely to experience rebound phenomenon, because their hormones react more strongly to hypoglycemia than those of adults.[30,417] The defense mechanisms are also triggered at higher blood glucose levels than those of adults.[417] The rebound phenomenon often lasts 12 hours or more in adults,[6] whereas in children the high blood glucose level usually lasts a few hours only (see the blood glucose graph on page 51). Sometimes a rebound phenomenon can keep the blood glucose level high for more than 24 hours.[649] As the hormone levels return to normal, so the blood glucose level too will gradually normalize.

If you take an extra insulin injection when your blood glucose is high due to a rebound phenomenon, your blood glucose may fall rapidly, causing you to become hypoglycemic again. The more sensitive your body is to insulin, the more likely this is to happen. You should therefore be careful about taking extra insulin after a rebound phenomenon. There are large individual differences in the tendency to develop rebound phenomena. If you are likely to have long-lasting rebound effects, you can try

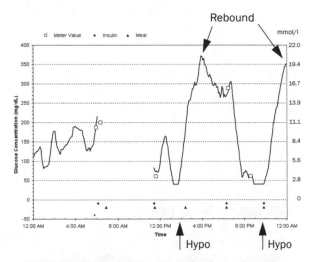

CGMS (Continuous Glucose Monitoring System, see page 97) chart showing two rebound phenomena in the same day in a 9-year old girl (arrows).

increasing your insulin injection at the meal following the hypoglycemic episode.[6]

Too little food or too much insulin?

Both can result in a low blood glucose level, but the body's way of handling the situation is different. The effect of glucagon in breaking down the stored glucose (glycogen) is counteracted by insulin. Insulin acts in the opposite direction, by transporting glucose into the liver cells to be stored as glycogen. From this it follows that the more insulin you have injected (resulting in a higher insulin level in the blood), the more difficult it will be to release glucose from the liver. This means that a low blood glucose caused by a large insulin dose (e.g. if you have taken extra insulin) will be more difficult to reverse than a low blood glucose due to inadequate food intake.

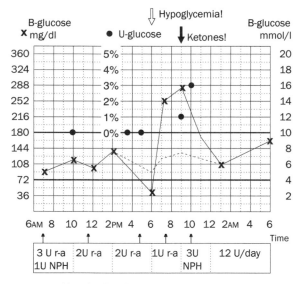

r-a = rapid-acting insulin

This 5 year old girl has recently been diagnosed with diabetes. She has a pronounced rebound phenomenon in the evening. Note the ketones in the urine after the hypoglycemic episodes, which are caused by her own production of glucagon (see also "Ketones" on page 99). The blood glucose may have followed the dashed line instead, if she had not experienced hypoglycemia and the resulting rebound effect.

Night time hypoglycemia

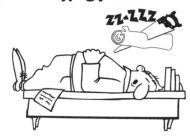

Night time hypoglycemia is more common than most people tend to believe. A number of studies have shown that as many as 30-40% of both children and adults have night time hypoglycemia.[518,530,620] Adrenaline responses are reduced during deep sleep which may contribute to the failure to wake up.[418] Symptoms of hypoglycemia may also be more difficult to recognize when you are lying down than when you are standing up.[371]

As many as 45% of children and adolescents using twice daily injections had night time hypoglycemia with blood glucose below 60-70 mg/dl (3.5-3.9 mmol/l) in two stud-

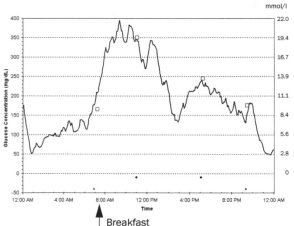

CGMS chart from a 13-year old boy, showing low glucose readings during the night. After breakfast there is a sharp rise in the glucose level, indicating that the insulin dose before breakfast needs to be increased. The glucose level falls again during the following night.

ies.[63,530] Half of the children did not show any symptoms of low blood glucose during the night. A negative effect on mood in the morning was observed in one of the studies.[530] When children using multiple injections or insulin pumps were studied on repeated occasions over a 6-month period, using continuous subcutaneous glucose monitoring (CGMS), every participant had at least one instance of a night time glucose level below 65 mg/dl (3.5 mmol/l).[511]

Often, a young person will not be woken by mild symptoms of hypoglycemia, and this provides the opportunity for the blood glucose level to drop even further. The only way to be certain whether your blood glucose level is low is to get up in the night and test it. It is a good idea to do this at least every second week. Sometimes children with diabetes wake up in the night on account of becoming hypoglycemic, and tell their parents. In other cases a parent will wake up to strange or unusual sounds. If your child has recently been diagnosed with diabetes, or if you have changed your bedtime insulin treatment, it would be a good idea to check the blood glucose once or twice during

the night. A baby alarm may be helpful for some families with young children. See page 91 and 149 for recommendations on when to test at night, depending on which bedtime insulin you use.

Night time hypoglycemia can be caused by too large a dose of bedtime insulin. Another cause can be too high a dose of short-acting insulin just before your evening snack which will result in hypoglycemia early in the night. There are several studies with NovoLog/NovoRapid and Humalog insulins which suggest that reducing the action time of the short-acting insulin (by the use of rapid-acting insulin) helps to decrease night time hypoglycemia.[384,612] Night time hypoglycemia can also be caused by vigorous afternoon or evening exercise (see page 245).

If you are injecting regular short-acting insulin in your thigh before the evening snack, the slow absorption of insulin can result in night time hypoglycemia.[355] If you inject your bedtime insulin holding the needle at right angles to the skin, or without lifting a skinfold, you might be injecting intramuscularly. The insulin will then be absorbed more quickly, putting you at risk of low blood glucose early in the night. [356]

A good basic rule for avoiding night time hypoglycemia is always to have something extra to eat if the blood glucose is below approximately 120-130 mg/dl (~7 mmol/l) before going to bed.[63,682] See also "Bedtime NPH insulin" on page 148. Remember that an extra sandwich

---

Night time hypoglycemia may be caused by:

➠ The dose of short-acting insulin before the evening snack being too high (hypoglycemia early in the night).

➠ The dose of bedtime insulin being too high (hypoglycemia around 2 AM or later with NPH-insulin).

➠ Short-acting insulin before dinner or the evening snack being given in the thigh (hypoglycemia early in the night is caused by a slower absorption from the thigh).

➠ Not enough to eat in the evening or an evening snack containing mostly "short-acting" foods being absorbed too quickly.

➠ Exercise in the afternoon or evening without decreasing the dose of bedtime insulin.

➠ Alcohol consumption in the evening.

Symptoms indicating night time hypoglycemia

➠ Nightmares.

➠ Sweating (damp sheets).

➠ Headache in the morning.

➠ Tiredness on waking.

➠ Bed-wetting (can also be caused by high blood glucose during the night).

before going to bed is never a guarantee that you will avoid night time hypoglycemia. If in doubt, the only way to be certain is to get up in the middle of the night to check your blood glucose level.

You can also experiment with the evening snack to find something that gives a slower rise in blood glucose over a longer period of time. Try, for instance, bread with cheese or nut butter on it. Your stomach will empty more slowly, resulting in sustained glucose absorption. High fat ice cream may have the same effect. However, extra fat will not be a good idea if you are prone to weight problems.

The most "long-acting" carbohydrate available for an evening snack is raw corn starch, which gives a rise in blood glucose over about 6 hours and is effective in preventing night time hypoglycemia. It is given to children with diseases other than diabetes who experience problems maintaining their blood glucose during the night. However, one drawback is the taste. It cannot be heated or prepared in any way or the carbohydrates will become more "short-acting". Younger children can usually get used to the taste of corn starch formula. Older individuals may find the taste of a corn starch bar (Nite Bite) more acceptable.

Another possibility worth trying, if you are having problems with night time hypoglycemias, is to eat ordinary (not "light") potato chips as an extra late snack before going to sleep (unless you have weight problems). The manufacturing process and the high fat content result in the

---

Research findings:
Corn starch and hypoglycemia

♠ In a study of children and adolescents, the number of hypoglycemic episodes (< 65 mg/dl, 3.7 mmol/l) at 2 AM and before breakfast were reduced from approximately one per week to 0.3 per week when 25-50% of the carbohydrate in the evening snack was given as uncooked corn starch in milk.[432]

♠ In children aged 2.5-6 years, 0.3 g/kg (0.6g/lb) of corn starch reduced the number of night time blood glucose readings < 100 mg/dl (5.6 mmol/l) by 64%.[211] Extra pancreatic enzymes were not being given.

♠ Unheated corn starch (0.3 g/kg, 0.6g/lb) given to adults at the time of the bedtime injection over a 4-week period increased the blood glucose level at 3 AM by, on average, 35 mg/dl (2 mmol/l) in adults with diabetes.[46]

♠ The number of night time hypoglycemic episodes < 60 mg/dl (3.4 mmol/l) were reduced by 70% without changing the A1C.

In these studies, patient meters showing whole blood glucose readings were used. Values have been recalculated to plasma glucose.

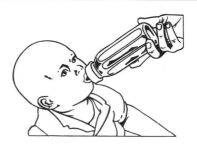

Corn flour mix when going to bed

Mix 2 tablespoons of corn flour with 100 ml (~½ cup) of water. This mixture contains 14 g of very slow-acting carbohydrates. It should be mixed cold and heated up as little as possible. Heat breaks down the cells of the corn flour making the carbohydrates faster-acting.

If the child has a meal of formula at bedtime you can replace parts of it with corn flour mix. Begin with a small part and increase gradually it as the child accepts it. Try to lower the temperature a little each day so that the child comes to accept drinking the mixture at room-temperature.

If the child is less than 3 years old, it might be necessary to add pancreatic enzymes for breaking down the corn starch. Ask your pediatrician about this.

Some older people find the taste of corn starch bars acceptable, so these may be useful.

glucose from potato chips being absorbed very slowly. The blood glucose will still not have reached its peak after 3 hours (see graph on page 234).[132] Twenty-five grams of potato chips have the same content of both fat (8 g, 0.3 ounces) and carbohydrates (15 g, 0.5 ounces) as an open cheese sandwich. This is often an attractive alternative to minimize the risk of night time hypoglycemia for youngsters and teenagers who play demanding sports.

A late evening snack with high protein content has been recommended to avoid night time hypoglycemia. However, according to one study the addition of protein (bread with meat) did not give better protection against hypoglycemia three hours after the snack.[312] A fiber-enriched bedtime snack (with beta-glucan) did not help to prevent children developing hypoglycemia at around 2 AM.[629]

Dawn phenomenon

Blood glucose levels rise early in the morning because of the so called "dawn phenomenon" which occurs in 80-100% of adults with type 1 diabetes.[103] This effect is caused by an increased secretion of growth hormone raising the blood glucose late in the night and early in the morning.[6,102,226] The dawn phenomenon increases the morning blood glucose by approximately 25-35 mg/dl (1.5-2 mmol/l) compared to the blood glucose levels at midnight when adequate amounts of insulin are supplied throughout the night.[103] A high morning blood glucose is a common problem for growing children, especially during the later part of puberty when the growth spurt is at its peak.[226] It may be difficult to tailor the insulin regimen to match the an increasing insulin blood glucose level in the morning. Lantus or an insulin pump can be good alternatives in this case. Younger children (who go to bed early) tend to have their highest need for basal insulin earlier in the night (often before midnight).[150].

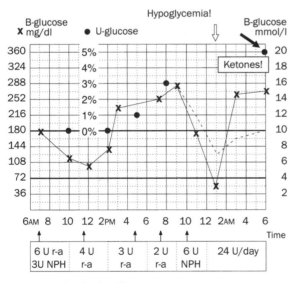

r-a = rapid-acting insulin

Night time hypoglycemia with rebound phenomenon. Without a blood glucose test at 1 AM, this 6-year old girl would appear to have had a high blood glucose all night long. An increase in her bedtime insulin would have led to an even lower blood glucose the following night (the Somogyi phenomenon). Note the presence of both ketones and glucose in the morning urine. Without the night time hypoglycemia, her blood glucose may have followed the dashed line.

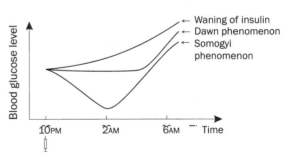

Different factors influence the blood glucose level during the night and in the morning. The dawn phenomenon depends on the night time secretion of growth hormone and the Somogyi phenomenon is a night time rebound phenomenon. The insulin waning effect depends on the pharmacological properties of the intermediate-acting insulins used for bedtime injections. Long-acting insulins (Lantus, Ultralente, Humulin U) do not have this disadvantage. In one study looking at adolescents, the risk of night time hypoglycemia decreased by 43% after switching to once-daily Lantus at bedtime.[566]

Somogyi phenomenon

If your blood glucose level is low at night, you are likely to continue sleeping without noticing it. However, the secretion of counter-regulating hormones in your body can result in a rebound phenomenon with a rise in blood glucose to high levels in the morning if the level of insulin in the blood is low. If you haven't recorded a low blood glucose value in the middle of the night, you may believe that your bedtime insulin needs to be increased. A higher dose of bedtime insulin the next night will give an even lower blood glucose level and a more intense rebound effect, resulting in an even higher blood glucose level the following morning. You can easily end up in a vicious cycle. This type of night time rebound phenomenon is called the Somogyi phenomenon after the chemist who first described it.[457,714]

If your morning blood glucose is sometimes low and sometimes high, it may be because you have problems with the Somogyi phenomenon. Some nights your blood glucose might be low enough to start the rebound phenomenon, causing the morning blood glucose to be high. On other nights, the blood glucose will not be low enough to trigger the rebound phenomenon and the morning blood glucose will subsequently be lower.

The Somogyi phenomenon has been questioned over the years, but consensus today is that it is mainly seen in individuals using less intermediate and long-acting insulin (such as multiple injection therapy and insulin pumps) resulting in a lower level of insulin in the blood in the morning before waking up.[103,156] These people also have a higher than normal rise in blood glucose after breakfast following night time hypoglycemia.[457]

If you are using twice-daily injections, the proportion of intermediate-acting insulin is higher, and the amount of insulin your body will be able to store is larger (see page 79). Insulin can be released from this store (or "depot") during the night, resulting in a level of insulin that is unlikely to be low enough to allow a night time rebound phenomenon. [103]

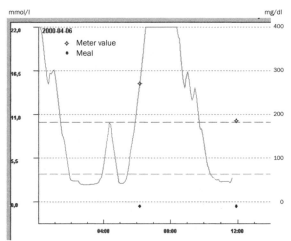

CGMS chart from a 16-year old girl, showing a dawn phenomenon with considerable increase in glucose levels from the middle of the night until waking-up time.

CGMS chart from a 17-year old boy, showing a pronounced Somogyi phenomenon with high glucose level early in the night, very low readings in the middle of the night, and further high levels on waking. Had he relied on his high morning reading alone, he might very well have increased his bedtime dose, resulting in even lower night time levels.

A urine test in the morning may be difficult to interpret in this situation. It can show both ketones (caused by a low blood glucose early in the night or by insulin deficiency later in the night when the blood glucose was high) and glucose (from the later part of the night). You can have the same urine test result (ketones and glucose) if your blood glucose has been high all night without hypoglycemia (see page 154).

Will low blood glucose levels return to normal if the child doesn't wake up?

The intermediate-acting insulin that was given during the afternoon or at bedtime will have lost most of its action by morning, and blood glucose levels will rise even if a hypoglycemic child does not wake up. Long-acting insulin will still be having effect in the morning but the body will then try to raise the blood glucose level by different defense mechanisms (see "Regulation of blood glucose" on page 31).

Can you die from hypoglycemia?

All parents are worried about night time hypoglycemia and wonder if their child might die from this. However, this almost never happens and we always try to prevent night time

> ### Research findings:
> ### Hypoglycemia and death
>
> ♠ Between the years 1977-1990, 2653 boys and 2341 girls were diagnosed with diabetes in Sweden. Nine of these (aged 15-23) were found dead in their beds. Hypoglycemia may be a possible cause as none had signs of alcohol in their blood.[672]
>
> ♠ During the same period, seven children and adolescents died because of ketoacidosis. The total risk of dying was increased by 2-3 times for children and adolescents with diabetes compared to their peers without diabetes.[672]
>
> ♠ In 1989, 22 such cases (aged 12-43 years) were recorded in England.[744]
>
> ♠ In another British study all deaths under 20 years of age were recorded from 1990 to 1996.[240] Ketoacidosis caused 69 deaths and hypoglycemia 7. In three cases there was no evident explanation for the deaths, defining them as "dead-in-bed".

hypoglycemia by advising an evening or bedtime snack. On very rare occasions, otherwise healthy individuals with type 1 diabetes have been found dead in their bed in the morning. This extremely rare phenomenon has been called the "Dead-in-bed" syndrome.[717]

A possible explanation for such night time deaths could be an erroneous injection of short or rapid-acting insulin at bedtime instead of the usual intermediate or long-acting insulin.[333] Teenagers and young adults often have high doses of bedtime insulin and it is not uncommon to take insulin from the wrong vial or pen when administering the bedtime insulin. For example, this happened twice to the same 13 year-old during one of our diabetes summer camps. Lantus can be confused with rapid-acting insulin if syringes are used for both types of injection as both are clear solutions. In one case, this resulted in hypoglycemia that needed

> ### Taking the wrong type of insulin
>
> ☞ Be careful not to mix up different bottles or types of insulin when using syringes.
>
> ☞ Make sure that the pens you use for day time and night time insulin are so different that you cannot accidentally use the wrong pen, even if it is completely dark.
>
> ☞ Often only the color coding will differ between pens from the same company. You may want to consider using disposable pens for one type of insulin and a regular pen for the other or use pens from two different manufactorers.

treatment with intravenous fluids containing glucose.

Another explanation is that nerve damage after many years of diabetes can result in the body's response to hypoglycemia being blunted or absent. This is more likely to be the case in people who have had diabetes for more than 20-30 years.

Adults with type 1 diabetes have died from hypoglycemia after drinking alcohol (which prevents the liver from producing glucose). Such cases are more likely when the individual has been suffering from another disease (such as a heart disorder) that worsens the effects of a severe hypoglycemic attack.[581,744]

Hypoglycemia and other diseases

People with diabetes are at increased risk of other auto-immune diseases (see page 300). If you encounter an increased number of hypoglycemic episodes, in spite of lowering your insulin doses, you may need to be investigated for the following diseases:

➠ Celiac disease.

➠ Hypothyroidism (underactive thyroid gland).

➠ Adrenal insufficiency (deficiency of cortisol).

Why does the blood glucose level vary, at which hypoglycemia is noticed?

The hot air balloon

A hot air balloon can be used to illustrate the variations in the level where hypoglycemia is first noticed. The height of the balloon corresponds to your average blood glucose level during the day. The basket under the balloon corresponds to the blood glucose level where you first notice symptoms of hypoglycemia. With an average glucose level of 180 mg/dl (10 mmol/l) symptoms are usually noticed when the level is around 65 mg/dl (3.5 mmol/l).

The A1C scale on the right corresponds to the average blood glucose level over a 2-3 month period, which is presented on the left side of the scale. An average blood glucose of 180 mg/dl (10 mmol/l) will give an A1C of approximately 8% (DCCT equivalent numbers, see page 104).

The illustrations on the next page show what will happen when the blood glucose level changes. However, illustrating the level of hypoglycemia with only one basket is really a

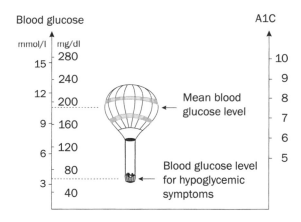

simplification. The level at which you recognize hypoglycemia will change depending on your recent blood glucose levels but the level where clear thinking and reaction times are impaired is less dependent your recent blood glucose.[32,525] This implies that while the body can adjust to a low blood glucose level, brain function cannot adjust so much. See also page 43.

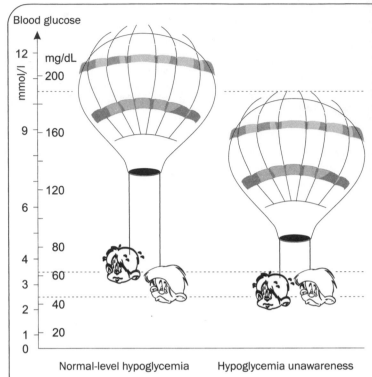

Normal-level hypoglycemia   Hypoglycemia unawareness

Bodily symptoms of
hypoglycemia

Thinking ability and reaction
times are impaired due to
hypoglycemia in the brain

Normally you will notice bodily symptoms (such as shaking and cold sweats) at slightly higher blood glucose levels than symptoms from the brain (such as difficulty in concentrating). This enables you to continue to think clearly and to take appropriate action promptly.

If you have many low blood glucose readings (less than 45-55 mg/dl, 2.5-3.0 mmol/l) you will risk having hypoglycemic unawareness (see page 48). The hypoglycemia may then go unnoticed until the blood glucose level is so low that it affects the brain. By then, you will find it difficult to think clearly and your reaction times will have slowed down. Bodily symptoms begin to occur when your blood glucose level drops even lower, but by this time you will have problems taking appropriate action.

It would be much better if your bodily symptoms could appear before the symptoms from the brain, warning you in time to do something about your low blood glucose level in an effective way.

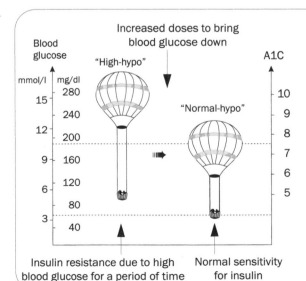

Increased doses to bring
blood glucose down

Insulin resistance due to high
blood glucose for a period of time

Normal sensitivity
for insulin

High blood glucose levels

If your blood glucose has been high for a period of time the "glucostat" (see page 41) in your body will readjust and you will notice symptoms of hypoglycemia at higher blood glucose levels ("high-level hypoglycemia"). If you have had an average blood glucose level of 270 mg/dl (15 mmol/l) for a week or two (sometimes even less) you may even be noticing symptoms of hypoglycemia when your blood glucose is 80-100 mg/dl (4.5-5.5 mmol/l). When you tighten your blood glucose levels the level at which you will notice hypoglycemic symptoms will fall. It will then be very important to measure your blood glucose when you experience symptoms of hypoglycemia and not to eat until it comes close to 65-70 mg/dl (3.5-4 mmol/l). After 1-2 weeks of "suffering" your sensitivity for insulin will again be normal, and you will recognize symptoms of hypoglycemia at a lower glucose level ("normal-level hypoglycemia").

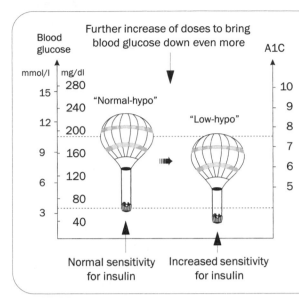

Blood glucose / mmol/l / mg/dl axis; Further increase of doses to bring blood glucose down even more; A1C axis (10, 9, 8, 7, 6, 5). "Normal-hypo", "Low-hypo". Normal sensitivity for insulin / Increased sensitivity for insulin.

Low blood glucose levels

If you continue with the increased insulin doses, your blood glucose level will fall even more after a week or two since your sensitivity to insulin now increases (less insulin resistance). With a lower average blood glucose, the level where bodily symptoms of hypoglycemia appear will also go down. If your average blood glucose level is 125-145 mg/dl (7-8 mmol/l) you will probably not notice symptoms of hypoglycemia until your glucose level falls as low as 55-65 mg/dl (3.0-3.5 mmol/l) ("low-level hypoglycemia"). The risk of having hypoglycemia unawareness will increase.

When your average blood glucose level decreases, your sensitivity to insulin will increase, so you will need to lower your insulin doses to avoid hypoglycemia. See the graphs on page 198 and 199 for further explanation of how the insulin resistance is affected by your recent blood glucose level.

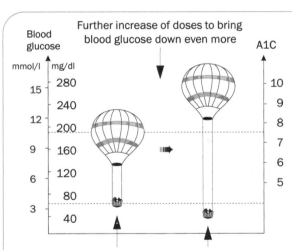

Blood glucose / mmol/l / mg/dl axis; Further increase of doses to bring blood glucose down even more; A1C axis (10, 9, 8, 7, 6, 5). Normal sensitivity to insulin / Insulin resistance due to multiple high blood glucose peaks *and* hypoglycemia unawareness due to frequent episodes of low blood glucose.

Very variable blood glucose levels

Sometimes it may be difficult to manage your insulin doses in that when you increase them you will indeed have many low blood glucose readings but also many high values (often caused by rebound phenomena). The high values will make you resistant to insulin and raise your A1C. At the same time, these low values cause your body to adapt to low blood glucose levels, resulting in a loss of warning symptoms until your blood glucose drops below 55-65 mg/dl (3.0-3.5 mmol/l).

This problem can be difficult to resolve. Start by decreasing insulin doses to avoid blood glucose levels less than 65-70 mg/dl (3.5-4 mmol/l). When your hypoglycemic symptoms start coming at levels of 65-70 mg/dl (3.5-4 mmol/l) again, you can carefully increase those doses that are needed to cut off the high blood glucose peaks.

Treating hypoglycemia

Although giving pure glucose may be the pre-ferred treatment for hypoglycemia, any form of carbohydrate that contains glucose will raise blood glucose levels.[274] Ten grams of glucose will raise the blood glucose of an adult by about 35 mg/dl (2 mmol/l) after 15 minutes.[116,160] The blood glucose will rise over 45-60 minutes and then start to fall. Smaller children can be given a smaller amount of glucose. For instance 1.5 g of glucose/10 kg (1.5 g/20 lb) body weight will raise the blood glucose by approximately 35 mg/dl (2 mmol/l) (see table on page 62). It is important not to take too much glucose "just to be on the safe side" since the blood glucose will then rise too steeply. If you tend to eat too much when your blood sugar is low, you will put on weight.

The glucose from food can only be absorbed into the blood after it has passed from the stom-ach into the intestine. Glucose can not be absorbed from inside of the mouth [321] or the stomach.[277] Glucose given rectally (as a supposi-tory) will not raise blood glucose levels in children [14] or adults.[42]

Always take glucose tablets with you wherever you go. Older children can keep them in their pockets. Younger children may find some kind of small bag that can be attached to their wrist or belt useful. Make sure that your friends know where you keep your glucose tablets in case you need help finding them after becoming hypoglycemic. It may also be useful to ensure you always have a small amount of cash available in case you need to buy yourself something to eat.

Practical instructions:

① Test your blood glucose. The sensations of a hypoglycemic reaction do not necessarily imply that your blood glucose is actually low. If your symptoms are so intense that it is difficult to measure the blood glucose you should of course eat something con-taining glucose or sugar as soon as possi-ble. If your blood glucose happens to be high, a little extra glucose will not make much difference. This will outweigh the risk of having a more severe hypoglycemia if you had not started reversing it right away.

② If your blood glucose is low (less than 65-70 mg/dl, 3.5-4.0 mmol/l), have some-thing sweet to eat, preferably glucose tab-lets. Start with a lower dose according to the table on next page and wait 10-15 min-utes for the glucose to take effect. If you don't feel better after 15-20 minutes and your blood glucose has not risen, you can take a repeat dose of the same amount of glucose.

Glucose will give a quicker rise in blood glucose than other types of carbohy-drate.[116] Avoid food and drink containing fat (e.g. chocolate, cookies, milk or choco-late milk) if you want a quick increase in blood glucose. Fat causes the stomach to

Which dose of insulin contributed to your hypoglycemia?

① *Multiple injection therapy*

premeal *rapid-acting* insulin and 2 doses of basal insulin per day

Time of hypoglycemia	"Responsible" insulin dose Time of inj.	Type
After breakfast	Breakfast	Rapid-acting
Before lunch	Breakfast	Basal insulin
After lunch	Lunch	Rapid-acting*
After dinner	Dinner	Rapid-acting
After evening snack	Evening snack	Rapid-acting
Before midnight	Evening snack	Rapid-acting
After midnight	Bedtime	Basal insulin

Basal insulin can be intermediate-acting (NPH) or long-acting (Lantus, Ultralente, Humulin U).

With rapid-acting insulin (NovoLog/NovoRapid, Humalog) the premeal dose will be "responsible" for hypoglycemia during 2-3 hours after the injection. After that, the basal insulin is more likely to contribute to hypoglycemia.

* NPH for breakfast can contribute to hypoglycemia after lunch.

Premeal *short-acting* insulin and NPH-insulin at bedtime

Time of hypoglycemia	Time of inj.	Type
Before lunch	Breakfast	Short-acting
In the afternoon	Lunch	Short-acting
In the evening	Dinner	Short-acting
After evening snack/ Before midnight	Evening snack	Short-acting
After midnight	Bedtime	NPH insulin

② *2-dose treatment*

Short-acting and NPH-insulin before both breakfast and dinner

Time of hypoglycemia	"Responsible" insulin dose Time of inj.	Type
Before lunch	Breakfast	Short-acting
In the afternoon	Breakfast	NPH insulin
Early evening	Dinner	Short-acting
After evening snack/ Before midnight	Dinner	NPH insulin
After midnight	Dinner	NPH insulin

empty more slowly, so that the glucose reaches the bloodstream later (see page 206).

A blood glucose level of 65-80 mg/dl (3.5-4.5 mmol/l) may require a management decision such as eating some carbohydrate, postponing exercise, or change in insulin dosage.[274] In this situation, a glass of juice or a piece of fruit may be appropriate.

③ If the person is conscious but has difficulty in chewing, give glucose gel (HypoStop®, Insta-Glucose®) or honey. Gels are very useful for infants and toddlers since no chewing is required.

④ If the person is unconscious or has seizures, give a glucagon injection (for dosage, see page 38). Never give an unconscious person food or drink because it might be accidentally inhaled and cause suffocation or subsequent pneumonia.

⑤ Don't take any physical exercise until all symptoms of hypoglycemia have vanished. Wait at least 15 minutes before you do anything that demands your full attention or quick understanding, such as driving, operating a machine or taking an exam in school.

⑥ Don't leave a child alone after a hypoglycemic reaction. If this happens in school, make sure someone who knows how to cope with the situation will be able to look after the child at home. Smaller children need someone to take them home if their parents cannot come to the school.

⑦ If eating something containing glucose or sugar doesn't bring the blood glucose level back to normal, it may be because the stomach isn't emptying its contents into the intestine (where the glucose is absorbed). If your blood glucose doesn't increase sufficiently within 30-60 minutes, try drinking

How many glucose tablets (4 g) are needed to treat hypoglycemia? [160]

Body weight		Approximate rise in blood glucose	
		50 mg/dl	100 mg/dl
Kg	lb	2.7 mmol/l	5.5 mmol/l
10	22	½ tablet	1 tablet (4 g)
20	45	1 tablet (4 g)	2 tablets
30	65	1½ tablet	3 tablets
40	90	2 tablets	4 tablets
50	110	1½ tablets	3 tablets
60	125	3 tablets	6 tablets
70	155	3½ tablets	7 tablets
Glucose /10 kg		2 g	4 g
" /10 lb		1 g	2 g

"Rule of thumb"

1 tablet (4 g) of glucose/10 kg (½ tablet/10 lb) body weight will raise the blood glucose approximately 110 mg/dl (6 mmol/l), i.e. your blood glucose will be approximately 110 mg/dl higher after 15-30 minutes than it would be without extra glucose. Usually, an increase of 35 mg/dl (2 mmol/l) will be enough, but if you have recently taken insulin and your blood glucose level is falling, you may need more glucose. Check the type of glucose tablets you use as they are likely to contain 4-5 g of glucose.

some carbonated lemonade to encourage the relaxation of the muscle (pyloric sphincter) that controls the exit of food from the stomach to the intestines.

⑧ Occasionally, there may be additional problems and hypoglycemia will carry on for hours unless some other measure is taken (for example, if you have gastroenteritis). The most effective of these is likely to be injecting a small dose of glucagon, which may need to be repeated (see page 36).

⑨ If there is no apparent explanation for hypoglycemia to have occurred, you should decrease the "responsible" dose of insulin the next day. For more information, see the chapter on adjusting insulin, page 132.

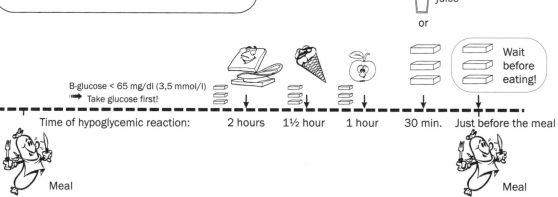

It is important to consider how much time there is before your next meal when you have hypoglycemia. Don't eat more than you will need to get you through to your next meal. It is all too easy to have too much to eat since it takes a while before the blood glucose rises and makes you feel better. If your blood glucose is below 65 mg/dl (3,5 mmol/l) or the symptoms of hypoglycemia are troublesome, it is best to take only glucose, then wait 10-15 minutes before eating anything else to cure the hypoglycemia as soon as possible. If you become hypoglycemic while sitting with a meal in front of you, it may be quite a while before you feel better again if you eat immediately. It is better to eat something with a higher sugar/glucose content (e.g. glucose tablets), wait 10-15 minutes or until you feel better, and then enjoy your meal.

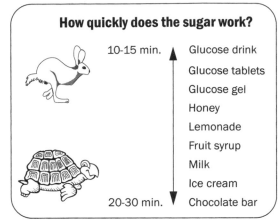

How quickly does the sugar work?

10-15 min.
Glucose drink
Glucose tablets
Glucose gel
Honey
Lemonade
Fruit syrup
Milk
Ice cream
20-30 min.
Chocolate bar

Should you always eat when you feel hypoglycemic?

① Measure your blood glucose.

② If it is < 65 mg/dl (3,5 mmol/l), eat something sweet, preferably glucose.

③ If it is 65-70 mg/dl (3.5-4 mmol/l), eat something if your next meal is more than ½-1 hour off or if you know that your blood glucose is decreasing, e.g. after physical exercise.

④ If it is > 70-80 mg/dl (4.0-4.5 mmol/l), you may be having hypoglycemic symptoms at too high a blood glucose level. Wait a short while and test yourself again. Don't eat until the blood glucose has fallen below 70 mg/dl (4.0 mmol/l), see point ③. See also the text on page 44 and 57.

Timing and hypoglycemia

The time interval between the bout of hypoglycemia and your next meal will determine which response is appropriate.

Hypoglycemia just before you eat

Take glucose and wait 10-15 minutes before starting to eat. If you eat straightaway, your food will mix with the glucose in your stomach. Since it normally takes about 20 minutes for solid food to be digested (sufficiently to be emptied into the intestines) an increase in your blood glucose will take at least this long. Remember that glucose from the food must reach the intestines before it can be absorbed into the blood.

Hypoglycemia 45-90 minutes before your next meal

The same advice applies as in the example above for a rapid reversal of your hypoglycemia. Afterwards you will need something to eat (a piece of fruit, for example) to keep your blood glucose level up until the next meal.

Hypoglycemia 1-2 hours before your next meal

Take glucose and wait 10-15 minutes before you eat anything else in order to reverse your hypoglycemia quickly. Since it will be a while until your next meal, it is important to eat something that contains more "long-acting" carbohydrates. If the hypoglycemia develops slowly, you can skip the glucose and have a glass of milk and/or a sandwich instead. An alternative approach is to take fast acting sugar only, and repeat if necessary. This has the advantage of helping to avoid unwanted weight gain. Try to find out what works best for you and discuss with your diabetes team.

Helping someone with diabetes who is not feeling well

If you find yourself in the situation of helping someone else with hypoglycemia, it is very unlikely you will know what the person's blood

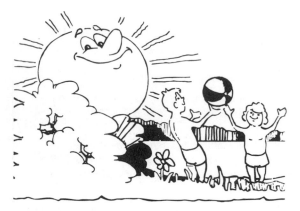

Younger children often run around a lot while playing and so get a certain degree of exercise in a natural way. Glucose gel may come in handy if a child develops hypoglycemia while at the park or the beach. Glucose tablets will easily become wet and sticky.

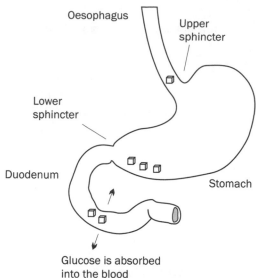

Glucose is absorbed into the blood

Sugar must reach the intestine to be able to be absorbed into the bloodstream so that it can raise the blood glucose level. Glucose cannot be absorbed through the lining of the mouth (oral mucosa),[321] or from the stomach.[277] The lower sphincter (pylorus) regulates the emptying of the stomach. Different factors influence how quickly the stomach empties (see page 203) and this will have a direct effect on the speed with which glucose can be absorbed into the blood to correct hypoglycemia.

glucose level is, and you may lose precious time trying to measure it. The best course of action is to give something containing sugar as quickly as possible and then call for help. Make sure that people (e.g. teachers, sports coaches etc.) who may need to help, know this simple advice.

Remember that the little packets of sugar available in cafes and fast food restaurants will be very effective in this situation, as will fruit juice or fizzy drinks such as lemonade or cola (as long as it is not the "diet" variety).

If a high blood glucose is making the person feel ill, the extra glucose will not have any adverse effects. It is not the high blood glucose as such which causes the unpleasant sensations, but the lack of insulin that also causes the high blood glucose. If the blood glucose is low, it is essential the person in question gets sugar as quickly as possible.

Glucose

Pure glucose has the quickest effect when correcting hypoglycemia.[116] Emergency glucose is available in tablets and gel form (for example InstaGlucose®). It is important to think of glu-

cose as a medicine for hypoglycemia and not as a "sweet". Everyone with diabetes should always have glucose handy and must know when they need to take it. Friends must also know in which pocket the glucose tablets are kept. A wrist bag or waist bag for carrying glucose is useful.

Sports drinks contain different mixtures of sugars and give a quick increase in blood glucose. Pure fruit juice contains mostly fructose, which gives a slower increase in blood glucose. A glass of juice containing 20g (2/3 ounce) of carbohydrate gives a slower increase in blood glucose than glucose tablets containing the same amount of carbohydrate.[116] Ordinary sugar is sucrose (also called saccharose) which is composed of both glucose and fructose (see illustration on page 204). It will therefore not give the same increase in blood glucose as an equal amount of pure glucose, but it is useful if glucose is not available.[297]

It is extremely important that everyone understands why children with diabetes must carry glucose tablets with them everywhere they go. Those who do not understand might otherwise think that the child is "cheating", eating the tablets as candy instead of taking them as a medication for hypoglycemia.

Fructose

Fructose has a sweeter taste than ordinary sugar. Fructose is absorbed more slowly from the intestine and is not as effective as glucose in raising the blood glucose level. [264] Fructose does not affect the blood glucose directly. It is mainly taken up by the liver cells (without the help of insulin) where it is converted into glucose or triglycerides. A high intake of fructose will increase the body fat.[264] Fructose can also raise the blood glucose by stimulating glucose production in the liver.[264] Honey contains 35-40% glucose and the same amount of fructose. Sorbitol, found in many candies, is converted in the liver to fructose (see also page 225 and 225).

Candy and hypoglycemia

Candy containing only pure sugar (caramels) will raise the blood glucose quickly. However, it is not a good idea to reserve candy so you only give them to children when they are hypoglycemic. This strategy can encourage children to try to make themselves hypoglycemic so that they will getcandies. It is best to reserve glucose tablets as "medicine" for low blood glucose. Medicine is not for treating your friends so glucose tablets will not be regarded as candy. Giving a child candy for treating hypoglycemia involves a risk of them being shared out among friends, leaving none for when they are really

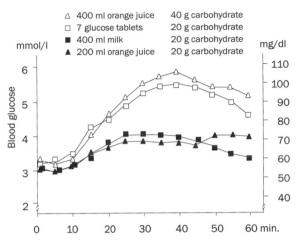

The graph shows results from a study where 13 adults with type 1 diabetes were given different types of sugar to reverse hypoglycemia.[116] Four hundred ml (2/3 pint) of water was given with the glucose tablets. Milk contains fat and gives a slower rise in blood glucose, as fat leads to a slower emptying of the stomach.

needed. Another advantage with emergency glucose tablets is that they deliver a precise dose, allowing better control when it is most needed. If your child has hypoglycemia at school, this will also make it easier for the teacher to know how much to treat with. An alternative may be to give candy for hypoglycemia only when the child is engaged in sports.

Candy containing chocolate and chocolate bars raise the blood glucose very slowly and should not be used to treat hypoglycemia (see graph on page 234). This is particularly important when blood glucose levels are below 65 mg/dl (3.5 mmol/l) as you then will risk a rebound phenomenon (see page 49).

After hypoglycemia

Usually you will feel better within 10-15 minutes after you have eaten something containing glucose. However, it will often take one or two hours after the blood glucose has normalized before returning to a level of maximum performance again, necessary for example for an exam at school. It is difficult to state a time limit, but one study tested children at a diabetes camp following recovery from hypoglycemia (the time intervals varied between 10 and 45 minutes). These children were found to score less well on neuro-psychological tests that measured memory and concentration.[623] A study of adults with diabetes, however, found that reaction times returned to normal 10-40 minutes after the blood glucose had risen to a level above 3.3 mmol/l (60 mg/dl).[358]

Headaches are common after recovering from hypoglycemia, particularly if your blood glucose level was very low. Although they are less common, you may also experience transient neurological symptoms such as a temporary paralysis or difficulties of speech caused by some degree of brain edema (swelling).[617,698] If you find yourself suffering any of these, you should contact your doctor.

If you are caring for a child with diabetes who doesn't wake up or return to full consciousness within 15-30 minutes after being severely hypoglycemic, even though his or her blood glucose has returned to normal, this may indicate swelling of the brain (brain edema).[517] It may take many hours before the child is awake and behaving in the usual way again. *This is an acute condition that requires immediate treatment in hospital!*

Sometimes people feel nauseous or vomit after hypoglycemia, especially if the blood glucose has been low for some time. This will often be associated with raised levels of ketones in the blood and urine. Both ketones and nausea are caused by the hormone glucagon, which is secreted from the pancreas during hypoglycemia. This is the same type of side effect that can be experienced after a glucagon injection. If the vomiting continues you should contact the hospital. Since the glucagon secretion from a person's body usually decreases after several

---

Research findings:
Recovery from hypoglycemia

♠ In one study of adults without diabetes, hypoglycemia was induced using insulin (blood glucose 50 mg/dl, 2.7 mmol/l, for 70 minutes). The reaction time was decreased for 1½ hours and only returned to normal 4 hours after the blood glucose had normalized.[237]

♠ Another study of adults found cognitive functions (short-term memory, attention and concentration) to be normal in the morning after a night with hypoglycemia (blood glucose < 40 mg/dl, < 2.2 mmol/l, for 1 hour).[60]

♠ A British study of adults shows their capacity for exercise was unchanged after an episode of night time hypoglycemia (45-55 mg/dl, 2.6-3.0 mmol/l for 1 hour) even though participants complained of more fatigue, less well-being and felt that they had experienced a bad night's sleep.[445]

♠ In children, cognitive testing (coordination, memory, attention and creative thinking) was not affected after a night time hypoglycemia (< 70 mg/dl, 3.9 mmol/l) but their mood was influenced negatively.[530]

In these studies, patient meters showing whole blood glucose readings were used. Values have been recalculated to plasma glucose.

---

years with diabetes, this reaction is more common in people who have had diabetes for a few years only.

Learning to recognize the symptoms of hypoglycemia

Every time your blood glucose measures less than 65-70 mg/dl (3.5-4.0 mmol/l) you should ask yourself: "Exactly what symptoms caused me to take the blood test now? Did I experience

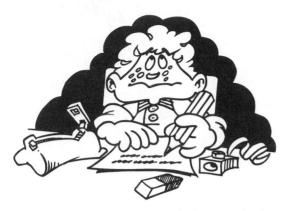

It will be difficult to achieve top results in an examination if you have hypoglycemia, or have had it recently. Usually it will take a couple of hours after a difficult hypoglycemic episode before you are back on top form.

changes in their behavior and how they feel while hypoglycemia is developing. Such programs include the use of simple cognitive tests, and their success has been demonstrated.[154] To test for bodily symptoms, stand up and walk around. Move your outstretched arm in a circle or hold a pen between your fingers to test for shakiness. To test for symptoms from your brain, repeat your mother's or brother's age and birthday, your friends' phone numbers or the combination for your locker or bike lock. Younger children may try counting backwards from 100. Whatever test you set yourself should be sufficiently difficult when your blood glucose level is normal, for you to notice the difference when doing the same thing while your blood glucose is low.

any symptoms 10 or 20 minutes earlier that might have warned me my blood glucose was falling?" If your blood glucose is below 55-65 mg/dl (3.0-3.5 mmol/l) and you have not experienced any symptoms, you should always ask yourself: "Were there really no symptoms at all warning me that my blood glucose was low?" Ask your friends if they have noticed any change in your behavior that could have been caused by a drop in your blood glucose.

There are now programs that train people with diabetes to recognize subtle and variable

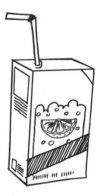

A carton of juice can come in handy when a child has low blood glucose. It is easy to carry with you and if the child does not want to eat anything it is often easier to give a sip of juice than to use glucose tablets or gel.

Insulin treatment

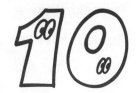

The pancreas of a person without diabetes will always be secreting a small amount of insulin into the bloodstream, constantly throughout the day and night (called basal secretion). After a meal, a larger amount of insulin is secreted to deal with the glucose coming from the food (called bolus secretion, see graphs on page 22). The goal of all insulin treatment is to mimic this function and provide insulin to the bloodstream.

In the past, bovine (beef) and porcine (pork) insulin were used for all people with diabetes. Nowadays, mostly human insulin is used, i.e. insulin with a chemical structure identical to the insulin produced by the human pancreas. Human insulin is produced using gene technology or by semi-synthetic methods. Genetic engineering involves the insertion of human insulin-producing genes into a yeast cell or bacteria. In this way the yeast cells or bacteria are tricked into producing insulin instead of their own proteins.

Short and rapid-acting insulins are pure insulin without any additives. They are in the form of a clear liquid and don't require stirring or mixing before use. Different additives are used to make

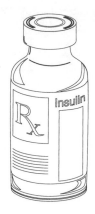

the insulin longer-acting, and these are what make it cloudy. The cloudy part of the contents will collect as sediment at the bottom of the vial or cartridge. This sediment must be mingled again with the rest of the contents by turning over or rolling (but not shaking) the vial 20 times before use.[406] The newer basal insulins such as Lantus and Levemir are clear because they are both solutions rather than suspensions. These types of insulin have an extended effect because of changes to the molecular structure which slow down their absorption, rather than added molecules such as zinc or protamine.

Production of human insulin

① **Semi-synthetic method:**

Porcine insulin is engineered enzymatically	Older method of making human insulin.

② **Biosynthetic DNA-technology method:**

Production from baker's yeast	Novo-Nordisk insulins.
Production from coli-bacteria	Eli-Lilly insulins. Sanofi-Aventis insulins.

Methods of postponing the action of insulin

①	NPH insulin	Binds to a protein from salmon (protamin).
②	Lente insulin	Excess of free zinc.
③	Lantus	Clear solution but precipitates (gets cloudy) after injection due to a higher pH in the subcutaneous tissue.
④	Levemir	Binds to a protein in the bloodstream (albumin).

Regular short-acting insulin

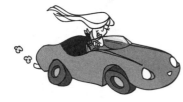

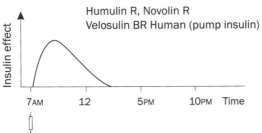

Humulin R, Novolin R
Velosulin BR Human (pump insulin)

Regular short-acting insulin (also called soluble insulin) is given as a bolus injection before meals. The listed brand names are examples of insulins. Ask your diabetes healthcare team to find out which insulins are available where you live.

Long-acting insulin

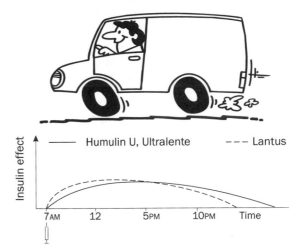

——— Humulin U, Ultralente   – – – Lantus

Long-acting insulin has effect over up to 24 hours. Humulin U and Ultralente are usually injected twice daily to give a basal insulin level between meals and during the night. The new long-acting insulin Lantus gives a more stable insulin effect and is injected once or twice daily.

Intermediate-acting insulin

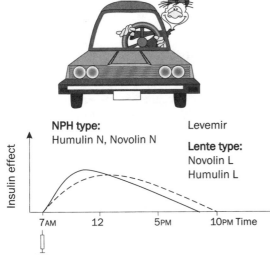

NPH type: Levemir
Humulin N, Novolin N

                         Lente type:
                         Novolin L
                         Humulin L

Intermediate-acting insulin is used as basal (background) insulin when injecting twice-daily and once or more daily in a multiple daily injection regimen. There are different types: NPH insulin (———) and lente (zinc-depot) insulin (– – –). The new basal insulin Levemir has an action profile similar to (– – –) but with less day to day variation.

Intravenous insulin

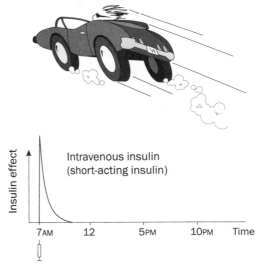

Intravenous insulin
(short-acting insulin)

Short-acting insulin given intravenously has an extremely rapid action with a half-life (length of time when half of the insulin is broken down) of only 3-5 minutes.[716]

In intravenous insulin therapy, short-acting insulin is given directly into the bloodstream. This is the most effective way to treat diabetic ketoacidosis. It is given only in hospitals as an intravenous drip or in a motorized syringe. There is no advantage in giving rapid-acting insulin intravenously, since the blood glucose lowering effect is not quicker than for regular short-acting insulin.[723] Since the half-life of insulin is very short, only about 4 minutes,[270] the blood glucose will increase sharply if intravenous insulin is stopped. If intravenous insulin is being used, the blood glucose must be checked every hour (even during the night) to monitor the correct dosage.

Intravenous insulin is often used during surgery or if a patient is suffering for any length of time from diarrhea and vomiting. It also gives us a practical way of working out how much insulin the patient needs over a 24 hour period, for example when starting treatment with an insulin pump.

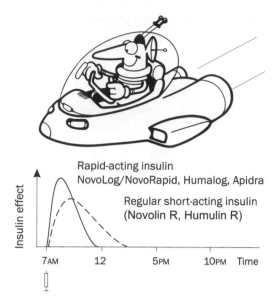

The new rapid-acting insulin analogs (NovoLog/ NovoRapid, Humalog, Apidra) have a much more rapid action than regular short-acting insulin. You can inject them just before a meal and still get a good insulin effect at the time when the glucose from the food reaches the bloodstream. However, the insulin effect wanes after 2-3 hours,[378] causing the blood glucose to rise before the next meal. Because of this, a basal insulin that takes effect during the day is usually given (see page 129).

Rapid-acting insulin

Normally, insulin molecules stick together in groups of six (so called hexamer formation, see illustration). These groups must be broken up before the insulin can be absorbed into the blood. If the insulin molecules could be injected in a solution of single molecules (monomeric insulin), the action would be much quicker. Due to the shorter action span, it would also be possible to achieve more normal insulin levels between meals, lessening the need for snacks.[253] Regular short-acting insulin is actually a bit too slow in action. The insulin level in your blood is not high enough during the meal. Rather, it is higher than necessary a couple of hours later, which is what causes you to need a snack.

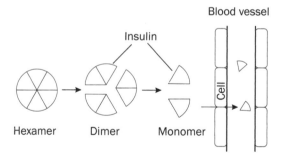

Insulin is always in a so called hexamer form when it is injected. It must then divide into dimers and monomers before it can pass between the cells of the blood vessel to enter the bloodstream. The new rapid-acting insulin analogs (NovoLog/NovoRapid or Humalog) dissolve much faster than regular short-acting insulin, thus making the time of action much faster.[393] Massage of the injection site can also enhance the dissociation, into monomers causing a faster absorption of the injected insulin.[490] The addition of zinc (as in lente insulins) stabilizes the hexamer, delaying the absorption.

By changing the protein building blocks in the insulin molecule, the problems of hexamer formation are considerably reduced. The rapid-acting insulin analog (Lispro or Humalog), which was introduced to the market around the world in 1996, takes effect very quickly.[393] Today, it is used by many children and adults with diabetes.

NPL is a new intermediate-acting insulin originating from Humalog. The longer effect is achieved by adding protamin, in the same way as for ordinary NPH insulin. NPL has the advantage of being stable for at least a year if mixed with Humalog. It has the same action profile as ordinary NPH insulin.[404]

Another rapid-acting insulin analog that is being used successfully both in adults [383] and children [559] was introduced in 1999 (Aspart or NovoLog, NovoRapid in most countries). A double-blind study of people with type 1 diabetes showed that the two analogues, Humalog and NovoLog/NovoRapid gave very similar levels of insulin in the blood and had identical action on the blood glucose profiles.[616] A third rapid-acting insulin analog called Apidra (glulisine) will be introduced soon.

Basal insulin

People without diabetes always have a low level of insulin in their body between meals and even during the night (see graphs on page 22). This steady release of insulin from the pancreas takes care of the glucose that is released between meals from the store in the liver. This constant low level of insulin is known as basal insulin or background insulin. The basal insulin dose given to people with diabetes in whom this natural supply is not available, will be either intermediate-acting or long-acting.

New basal insulins

Once a day injections of existing intermediate or long-acting insulin preparations do not provide an appropriate 24 hour basal insulin level

(between meals and during the night) in most people with diabetes.[654] The long-acting analog Lantus (Glargine) was introduced in 2000. By altering the insulin molecule, the blood-glucose lowering effect has been spread more evenly over up to 24 hours,[588] resembling the background insulin secretion in a healthy person. The subcutaneous uptake of insulin is more stable from day to day with Lantus, compared to NPH insulin.[484]

Occasionally, people report a burning sensation when injecting Lantus,[633] which may be a disadvantage for children in particular. However, this seems to be a minor problem, as the vast majority of children for whom Lantus is prescribed feel no pain when injecting.

Levemir (Detemir) is another new basal insulin which was introduced in 2004. A 6-month study of adults using NovoLog/NovoRapid as premeal insulin showed that with Levemir the same A1C levels (7.6%) as with NPH insulin (Novolin N, Humulin N) were obtained, but with a lower risk of hypoglycemia, especially during the night.[777] Overnight glucose profiles were more even with Levemir, and body weight was significantly lower after 6 months in the Levemir group. In another study the variability

---

Research findings: Lantus

♠ Lantus has been shown to give similar levels of basal insulin over 24 hours as an insulin pump.[484]

♠ In one study, researchers found both lower morning blood glucose and less night time hypoglycemia.[613]

♠ In another study, adults compared Lantus (given once at bedtime) with NPH (given once or twice daily).[653] Fasting glucose was 40 mg/dl (2.2 mmol/l) lower when using Lantus.

♠ In the group using NPH once a day, the doses of Lantus were similar. But Lantus doses for the group using NPH twice daily were 6-7 units lower than the sum of the NPH doses.

of insulin effect between different days was smaller with Levemir, compared to NPH and Lantus.[350]

Pre-mixed insulin

The cartridges of pre-mixed insulin that are available for insulin pens contain different proportions of short-acting and intermediate-acting insulin of NPH type. You can also find cartridges containing mixtures of rapid-acting and intermediate-acting insulins. With pre-mixed insulins the proportions of the two insulins cannot be adjusted. If you change the dose you will get more or less of both types of insulin. It is important to assess the use of different mixtures depending on your meal schedule. For example, the prolonged effect of the intermediate-acting part in a 30-50% mix with rapid-acting may be useful if you have a long wait between lunch and dinner.

A larger dose lasts longer

A larger insulin dose will give a stronger insulin effect which also lasts a longer time.[344,477] An exception to this rule is the rapid-acting insulin Humalog which lasts for the same period of time even when the dose is increased.[815]

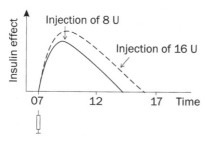

A larger insulin dose (dashed line) gives both a stronger and longer-lasting insulin effect.

Units and insulin concentrations

Insulin is measured in units, abbreviated U (international units, previously abbreviated IU). One unit of insulin was defined as the amount of insulin that will lower the blood glucose of a healthy 2 kg (4.4 lb) rabbit that has fasted for 24 hours to 45 mg/dl (2.5 mmol/l) within 2,5 hours.[774] Quite a complicated definition, don't you think? With better analytical methods, one unit has been defined as 6 nmol or 29 mg of insulin.[382] See also "How much does insulin lower the blood glucose level?" on page 130.

Today, the most common insulin concentration around the world is 100 units/ml (U-100). In many countries other concentrations are used, mostly 40 U/ml (U-40).

Some standard pens for insulin 100 U/ml can be used for giving half-units and there is a pen that

Disposable syringes

♠ Disposable syringes can be practical to use if you need to change the insulin dose in very small increments.

♠ In one study, syringes for 30 units (100 U/ml) were found to be accurate for adjusting doses of ± 0.25 units in the interval between 2.5 and 3.5 units.[702] However, they may be difficult to use for very small doses of only 0.5 - 1 unit.

♠ Another study found an error rate of 10% when doses of less than 5 units were given by syringe.[502] When a pen injector was used, the error was only 5%.

♠ In a study where parents were supposed to deliver 1.0 units of insulin, the actual dose varied between 0.6 and 1.3 units.[130] The variability was even greater when the dose was administered by pediatric nurses.

♠ Syringes for U-100 insulin must not be used with U-40 insulin (risk of under-dosage), nor should syringes for U-40 insulin be used with U-100 insulin (risk of over-dosage).

has half-unit increments on the scale (NovoPen ®Junior). Insulin 40 U/ml or 50 U/ml can be used for low doses (less than 2-3 units) when giving insulin to young children. For the youngest children, insulin can be diluted to 10 units/ml to make small insulin dose adjustments possible.

Insulin units are counted in the same way, regardless of the concentration. A weaker insulin will be absorbed more quickly.[282] Insulin of 40 U/ml gives approximately 20% higher insulin levels 30-40 minutes after injection compared to the same number of units of 100 U/ml.[704] People taking insulin need to be aware that it will take effect more quickly if they switch from 100 U/ml to 40 U/ml.

Twice-daily treatment

Twice-daily injections are still the standard treatment for some people with type 1 diabetes today. This may be advantageous when the person has a low total daily insulin requirement, for example during the honeymoon phase. It is also useful if the person, for whatever reason, finds it difficult to take multiple injections. A twice-daily injection regimen usually means that there is less flexibility for planning mealtimes. The afternoon dose of intermediate-acting insulin may not last long enough, especially in adolescents, to cover insulin requirements during the night, so morning hyperglycemia may result. A large amount of intermediate-acting insulin during the day will increase the need for snacks between meals.

Three-dose treatment

If the insulin given with dinner with a 2-dose treatment does not last until morning, you can take only the short-acting component (Novolin R, Humulin R) for dinner and postpone the injection of intermediate-acting NPH (Novolin N, Humulin N) or Lente insulin until bedtime.

This regimen decreases the risk of night time hypoglycemia compared to a 2-dose treatment.

Multiple injection treatment

Multiple injection treatment implies taking rapid-acting insulin (NovoLog/NovoRapid, Humalog, Apidra) or short-acting (Novolin R, Humulin R) before each main meal, and one or two doses of intermediate-acting (Novolin N, Humulin N) or long-acting insulin (Lantus, Ultralente, Humulin U) to cover the need for insulin between meals and during the night.

Multiple injection treatment has been used since 1984 and the first insulin pen was introduced in 1985. Studies in both children [684,761] and adults [191,342,681] have shown that it is possible to improve glucose control with this regimen. Using multiple injection treatment will not necessarily give you a better A1C,[220,390] but you may well find you are happier and have a better quality of life [391] as well as more freedom to choose a lifestyle you enjoy and greater flexibility over meal planning.[740]

With multiple injection treatment it is fairly easy for people with diabetes, along with the rest of their family, to understand how their insulin affects blood glucose at any given time of day. This is particularly important as the goal of the diabetes education is to enable the person with diabetes (and where appropriate, the family) to take an increasing responsibility for their treatment, so that they eventually become experts on their own diabetes.

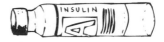

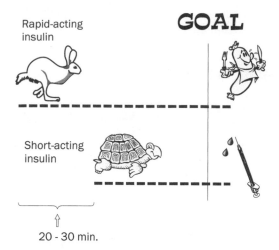

Rapid-acting insulin

GOAL

Short-acting insulin

20 - 30 min.

The rapid-acting insulins (NovoLog/NovoRapid and Humalog) are very quick to take effect, and can be given immediately before the meal. However, since it takes 20-30 minutes for regular short-acting insulin (Novolin R, Humulin R) to begin its action, you must give the insulin a head start or the race will be very uneven.[661] The carbohydrates from your meal will enter the bloodstream first and raise your blood glucose level. The insulin will enter your bloodstream later, putting you at risk of a low blood glucose before your next meal. Taking your injection 30 minutes before the meal is particularly important at breakfast time but if you recognize these problems you should take your injection 20-30 minutes before all meals.

Injections before meals (bolus insulin)

Bolus insulin is the rapid or short-acting insulin that you take before a meal. Rapid-acting insulin begins to act after 10 minutes and is at its most effective after just one hour. If you are using rapid-acting insulin, you will not have to be as strict about mealtimes if you have a dose of basal insulin as well in the morning (see page 140). Short-acting regular insulin (Novolin R, Humulin R) begins to act 20-30 minutes after a subcutaneous injection and begins its maximal effect after 1.5-2 hours. The blood glucose lowering effect lasts for about 5 hours. This means that with a multiple injection regimen there

should not be more than 5 hours between your main meals and injections of regular short-acting insulin. Children and teenagers having a late evening snack will need a fourth injection of premeal insulin, otherwise they will run short of insulin late in the evening before the bedtime injection begins to take effect.

One big difference between rapid and short-acting insulins for multiple injections is that with short-acting insulin you need to take snacks between main meals to avoid hypoglycemia. With rapid-acting insulin, the opposite is the case. If you eat a large afternoon snack, you will often need another injection of analog insulin, unless you are playing a vigorous sport or being otherwise very active. Check your blood glucose level to help you decide what dose you need.

If, for whatever reason, you prefer only four injections per day, one alternative is to take a combination of rapid or short-acting and intermediate-acting insulin at the time of the evening snack. Mixing these insulins in one syringe or taking them as pre-mixed insulin is not an ideal method however. If you inject yourself in the thigh, there is a risk of hypoglycemia early in the night from the short-acting component. But if you inject yourself in the abdomen, there is a risk that the intermediate acting insulin will not last until morning.

When should you take your premeal dose?

Rapid-acting insulin

The rapid-acting insulin analogs (NovoLog/NovoRapid and Humalog) can be injected just before a meal and still give a good insulin effect at the time when glucose from the meal enters the bloodstream. You must then adjust the above mentioned time tables. If your blood glucose is high before the meal, you can try waiting 15-30 minutes before eating.[631] If it is low, you can try waiting for your insulin until after you have eaten. NovoLog/NovoRapid [119,183] and Humalog [678,204] can also be given after the meal with good effect if you are not sure exactly how much you or your child are going to eat when you start the meal. NovoLog/NovoRapid and Humalog are usually combined with once or twice-daily injections of basal insulin (intermediate or long-acting, see page 140).

Short-acting insulin

There is no difference in effect between different brands of regular short-acting insulin. Rapid-acting insulins (NovoLog/NovoRapid and Humalog) start working sooner than regular short-acting insulin. The abdomen or tummy is the most common injection site for premeal injections (see page 113). If you take regular premeal insulin in the thigh (or buttocks) you will probably need to add another 15-30 minutes to these time limits. The time limits given in this chapter refer to abdominal injections of regular short-acting insulin if not otherwise stated. If you use rapid-acting insulin you must adjust the time intervals as indicated above.

Your insulin store from the bedtime injection will be almost gone by the morning. You should therefore have your morning injection of regular insulin at least 30 minutes before breakfast. Wait for longer if your blood glucose is high,

---

Research findings: Multiple injections

♠ Studies indicate that more than 90% of participants have found multiple injections acceptable.[392]

♠ In a French pediatric study of 5-19 year olds, 77% experienced an improvement in their quality of life when switching from a 2-3 dose regimen with syringes to a 4-5 dose regimen with pen injectors.[761] No significant change in glucose control was observed in the group as a whole, but the sub-group with poor control improved their A1C significantly.

♠ In the DCCT study (see page 314), the majority of participants on intensive treatment used multiple injections with syringes if they were not on insulin pumps.

♠ Results from the DCCT study show that starting an intensive treatment regimen at an early stage sustains the insulin production in your own pancreas, reducing the risk both of severe hypoglycemia and the development of diabetic complications.[199]

♠ In 1987 we switched all patients in our clinic (aged 2-20 years) from twice-daily injections with syringes to multiple injection treatment with insulin pens. Only one person was dissatisfied with this new regimen and switched back to twice-daily injections.

♠ Today our policy is to use multiple injections from the onset of diabetes. Most children use rapid-acting insulin and take two injections of basal insulin per day. This regimen mimics the insulin secretion of the pancreas better than a twice-daily regimen (see graphs on page 22, 128 and 129).

When should I take my premeal insulin? (abdominal injections)

Meal	Rapid-acting insulins*	Regular short-acting insulin
Breakfast	Just before the meal	At least 30 min. before
Other meals	Just before the meal	0-30 min. before (see text)
Hypoglycemia at mealtime	After the meal	Just before you eat
High blood-glucose at mealtime	Wait 15-30 min. before eating	Wait 30-60 min. before eating

*NovoLog/NovoRapid, Humalog, Apidra

and for less time if it's low. NovoLog/ NovoRapid and Humalog can be given just before the meal unless your blood glucose is high. See the table on page 139 for recommended times of injections at breakfast.

Ideally, regular short-acting insulin should be administered 20-30 minutes before all meals since the blood glucose is not affected immediately.[678] However, at lunchtime some of the short-acting breakfast insulin still remains in your body and the same holds true for the other meals. Because of this, the 30 minute insulin "head start" is not as essential with other meals as it is with breakfast.

Children using small doses will absorb the insulin faster than adults, especially if they do not have much subcutaneous fat. Because of this, they rarely need to wait 30 minutes before they eat [505] (provided the premeal blood-glucose isn't high). Taking insulin 30 minutes before each meal can be very difficult for younger children as it causes so many interruptions to their daily routine. So younger children are recommended to take their insulin just before meals (except breakfast). Some children, however, will absorb the insulin slowly and individual advice on this point is necessary. Older children and teenagers

are unlikely to experience problems taking the insulin 30 minutes before meals.

If you inject regular insulin just before your meal, it is important that the food is not absorbed too quickly from the intestine. Otherwise, the blood glucose will increase before the insulin reaches the bloodstream. Any fat content of the meal will slow down the gastric emptying rate. For example, ice cream made with milk products has a higher fat content and will therefore give a slower rise in blood glucose than a popsicle. See the nutrition chapter, page 200.

The blood glucose reading before a meal will indicate when it is appropriate to take the injection. If your blood glucose is high, you can wait 45-60 minutes before eating, if this is convenient. If you have a low blood glucose, you should leave the injection until it is time to eat or wait 15 minutes at the most (see the table on page 135).

Remember that it takes at least 2 hours for the bedtime injection of NPH type insulin to have any significant effect (even longer in the case of

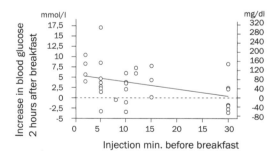

It is important to give regular short-acting insulin 30 minutes before breakfast. In this study, the blood glucose increased about 90 mg/dl (5 mmol/l) when the children took their insulin immediately before breakfast, compared to less than 20 mg/dl (1 mmol/l) when taking insulin 30 minutes before the meal.[661]

Can regular insulin injections be taken just before a meal?

To find out, take the injection just before your meal and measure your blood glucose before and 1½-2 hours after the meal. The blood glucose should have risen 55-70 mg/dl (3.0-4.0 mmol/l) at the most. If it has risen more, the effect of your regular insulin is too slow.

Try the same thing when you take your insulin 15 and 30 minutes before eating, to find out which suits you the best. If the blood glucose is too high, even when you have taken the insulin 30 minutes before the meal, you will probably need a higher dose.

If you use rapid-acting insulin (NovoLog/ NovoRapid or Humalog) it should normally be injected just before the meal.

Lantus). This means that the time span between the last dose of regular insulin and the bedtime injection should not be more than 3-4 hours. With rapid-acting Humalog, this interval should be shorter since there is a risk of a rise in blood glucose and ketones if the interval is longer than 2-3 hours.[9]

For younger children who can get their bedtime NPH dose while asleep, there is often a longer interval as they go to bed early. It may then be a good idea to use regular short-acting insulin (Novolin R, Humulin R) for the evening snack to get a longer insulin effect that lasts until the bedtime insulin effect can take over. If the last dose of NPH is given at dinner time, this advice will not apply.

Insulin pump

If you are using an insulin pump, you will take the premeal doses (called bolus doses) by pressing some buttons on the pump. In addition to this, the pump will deliver small doses of insulin continuously to cover your body's need of a low insulin level in the blood between meals and during the night. See the pump chapter on page 160.

Can I skip a meal?

Your body needs to have some insulin in the blood, even between meals, to take care of the glucose produced by the liver. If you use Novo-Log/NovoRapid or Humalog and take basal insulin as well in the morning (or one daily dose of Lantus), you may try to skip both the meal and the corresponding NovoLog/NovoRapid or Humalog dose. If your blood glucose is high, you may need a corrective dose of a few units of rapid-acting insulin. Increase the dose of Novo-Log/NovoRapid or Humalog, if necessary, the next time you eat.

If your blood glucose is above around 270 mg/dl (15 mmol/l) and you want to skip a meal, you still need to take some insulin to bring your blood glucose level down. You can compensate by eating more at snack-time or at the next meal when the insulin has lowered the blood glucose (also see "Temporary changes of the premeal dose, e.g. during illness (see p. 131 if you use a correction factor)" on page 135).

If you are using multiple injection treatment with regular short-acting insulin (Novolin R, Humulin R), you must take a low dose of insulin even if you skip a meal as the mealtime dose of short-acting insulin also covers the need of basal insulin between meals. Half the ordinary insulin dose will usually be enough, but you will need to try this out yourself. Intervals between meals and injections of regular insulin should not exceed 5 hours. Listen to your hunger signals and you will know when you must eat. You cannot skip a meal and also skip the snack a couple of hours later. And if your blood glucose is low, you must eat something immediately.

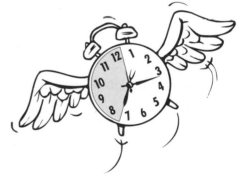

Can I change my meal times?

You can usually adjust your timetable for meals and injections by one hour in either direction. If you are using rapid-acting insulin (NovoLog/NovoRapid or Humalog) you won't need to be as strict about meal times if you take basal NPH insulin in the morning too (see page 140) or if you use long-acting insulin (Lantus, Ultralente, Humulin U) as your basal insulin. Just remember not to go for more than 5 hours between meals and injections of regular short-acting insulin if you don't use a basal insulin during the day. If you wait more than 5 hours between injections of regular insulin, you will be at risk of insulin deficiency.

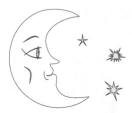

Bedtime insulin

The bedtime insulin injection is the most difficult dose to adjust. Although we do not eat during the night, our bodies need a continuous low level of insulin to take care of the glucose being produced by the liver. The most common bedtime insulin with multiple injection treatment used to be intermediate acting insulin of NPH type. An insulin with longer effect (Lantus, Ultralente, Humulin U) may be a better alternative for some people. The use of Lantus that has a more even effect is increasing, in children as well as in adults. Another alternative is the new basal insulin Levemir.

The bedtime insulin covers one third of a 24 hour day, so is likely to be the dose that has the greatest effect on your A1C (see page 104). High blood glucose readings during the night can give you a high A1C even if your glucose level during the daytime is normal.

When should bedtime insulin of NPH type be taken?

It is important to take your bedtime injection at the same time every night on week days. If you change the time from one day to another, it will be difficult to see a pattern in your blood glucose readings. Since the most important thing is to get the bedtime insulin to last until morning (see graphs on page 149), it is a good idea to take your bedtime injection as late as possible, i.e. shortly before your usual bedtime. There is no point your sitting up late, waiting to take your injection. While 11 PM might be fine for adults, older children will usually find 10 PM more appropriate. Parents should be aware that many young children will sleep through a late night injection with only the smallest disturbance, if they give this just before they themselves go to bed at around 11 PM. An indwelling catheter (Insuflon, see page 122) can make this easier if the child wakes up when the parents use regular syringes or pens.

The dose of NPH insulin (Novolin N, Humulin N) taken in the evening will take effect after 2-4 hours and will usually give effect on your blood glucose for a good 8-9 hours of sleep. Lente insulins (Monotard, Humutard) are a bit more long acting and at their most effective after the first 4 or 5 hours. Remember that smaller doses of insulin not only have less effect but also last for a shorter period.

If you use pen injectors, it is very important to turn over or roll the NPH pen cartridge carefully at least 20 times before injecting for thorough mixing.[406] The cartridge with NPH insulin contains a small glass or steel ball that will help to mix the insulin with the clear liquid.

When should the long-acting injection be taken?

The new long-acting insulin analog Lantus, can be taken at the evening snack, at bedtime or even in the morning. The injection of Lantus will be effective after 3-4 hours so if you need more insulin effect around midnight, it may be best to take it at the time of the evening meal (7-8 PM). Most people find one daily dose of Lantus is sufficient, but some may need to split the dose and give part of it in the morning (see page 155).

Since long-acting insulins act for up to 24 hours, sometimes even longer, it is important not to change the dose more often than 2 (or 3) times/week.

The ultralente type insulins (Humulin U, Ultralente) are made long-acting by binding the insulin to large crystals and an excess of free zinc. They begin to take effect 2-4 hours after the injection, are at their most powerful between 6-12 hours and may still be having some effect after 24 hours.[279] Because of this very long action you should take the injection earlier in the evening, e.g. at the evening snack or even at dinner (if you eat four meals a day, see graph on page 128). The timing is very individual and you will need to experiment to find out what suits you best so that you wake up with a good blood glucose level before breakfast. You should take at least 40-50% of the total 24 hour insulin dose as long-acting insulin to get a good basal insulin effect (30-40% if you are using short-acting insulin). Remember that these long-acting insulins continue to have an effect even into the next day.

With high doses of long-acting insulin, it is often advisable to divide the dose and take half in the morning and half before dinner, the evening or bedtime meal. If you use rapid-acting insulin (NovoLog/NovoRapid or Humalog) for premeal injections, you will probably need to divide the long-acting basal insulin into two daily injections.

Lente insulins are not available in cartridges for insulin pens. The reason for this is that the insulin is in crystal form and the crystals will break if a glass ball is used in the cartridge for mixing. Lantus is a clear solution and is usually given with a pen injector but can also be given with a syringe.

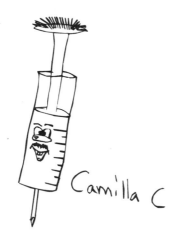

Camilla C

Mixing insulins

Insulin of NPH type (Novolin N, Humulin N) can be mixed with both rapid-acting Novo-Log/NovoRapid [325] and Humalog [420] and regular short-acting insulin.[348] If, however, you mix insulin of Lente type (Humulin L, Novolin L, Humulin U, Ultralente or similar) with short-acting insulin, you will lose part of the short-acting effect. This is due to an excess of zinc in the Lente insulin that binds to the short-acting insulin and flattens the peak of action, making it more long-acting.[72,348] If you prepare the mixture from vials stored in the refrigerator and inject immediately after mixing in the syringe, this problem seems to be less pronounced.[601] If you use long-acting insulin lente insulins (Humulin U, Ultralente) together with short-acting insulin in a multiple injection treatment these should preferably be taken as separate injections. It is also not a good idea to use lente insulins in indwelling catheters (Insuflon) for the same reason. However, rapid-acting Humalog seems to be an exception to this rule. Mixing Humalog and Ultralente did not change the peak action when injected within 5 minutes of mixing.[56] Although the recommendation is not to mix the long-acting insulin Lantus with any other insulin,[104] one study shows that it can be mixed with both NovoLog/NovoRapid and Humalog without any negative effect on blood glucose.[427]

Depot effect

If only intermediate or long-acting insulin is used, a depot (store) of insulin is formed in the subcutaneous fat tissue, corresponding to about 24 hours of insulin requirements.[79] The smaller the share of intermediate or long-acting insulin you use, the smaller the depot will be. If you are using a multiple injection treatment you will be using less intermediate or long-acting insulin and the depot will correspond to only about 12 hours of insulin requirements.[79] If the dose of bedtime insulin is changed, the size of the insulin depot makes it necessary to allow 2-3 days for your body to adjust until you see the full effect of the change (see "Basic rules" on page 137).

The disadvantage of a large insulin depot is that the insulin effect will vary from day to day. The disadvantage of a small insulin depot is that little or no extra insulin is stored in your body. The depot functions like a "spare tank" in that the extra insulin stored in your body can be used if you run short of insulin, for example if you forget an injection. If your insulin needs are increased (e.g. when you get an infection) or if you forget an insulin injection, you are more susceptible to insulin deficiency (elevated levels of ketones, nausea or vomiting). With pump therapy only rapid or short-acting insulin is used, resulting in a very small depot of insulin. If the insulin supply is stopped or blocked, symptoms of insulin deficiency will develop within as little as 4-6 hours (see page 172).

How accurate is your insulin dose?

A correctly used insulin pen will give a very accurate insulin dose with an error of only a few per cent. However, the effect of a given insulin dose also depends on a number of other factors. The effect of an identical dose of insulin, given to an individual at the same site, can vary by as much as 25%. It can vary by nearly 50% when the same dose is given to two different individuals.[344,368] This is the explanation for the often very frustrating fact that you can eat the same food, do exactly the same things and give identical doses of insulin for two days in a row, but may get quite different blood glucose results.

Insulin absorption

The absorption of insulin from the injection site can be influenced by a number of factors. Heat will increase the absorption. If the room temperature increases from 20° to 35° C (68- 95° F), the speed of absorption of short-acting insulin

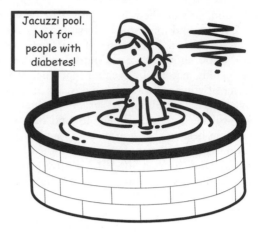

You may feel sad and disappointed when you see a sign like this, maybe even feel as if you have the plague. The reason for the warning is that insulin will be absorbed faster when the skin is heated by the hot water. This might cause hypoglycemia If you are aware of this phenomenon and have taken proper precautions, you can spend time in a spa bath or jacuzzi without worrying. When using rapid-acting insulin (NovoLog/NovoRapid, Humalog) the absorption will be less affected by the skin temperature.

Adults with diabetic foot ulcers or nerve damage have to talk this over with their doctor or podiatrist before using a spa bath, since hot water softens the skin on the feet and increases the risk of infection.

will increase by 50-60%.[454] Taking a bath or a sauna at a temperature of 85° C (185° F) may increase the absorption by as much as 110%! In other words, you could be at risk of hypoglycemia if you inject short-acting insulin shortly before taking a hot bath. A temperature of just 42° C (108° F) in a shower, spa bath or jacuzzi may double the insulin level in your blood, while a cold bath (22° C, 72° F) will decrease the absorption of insulin.[67] Massage of the injection site for 30 minutes has been found to give higher insulin levels and lower blood glucose, with both short-acting,[490] and long-acting insulins.[67]

The skin temperature is also important. In one study, the same insulin injection gave twice the

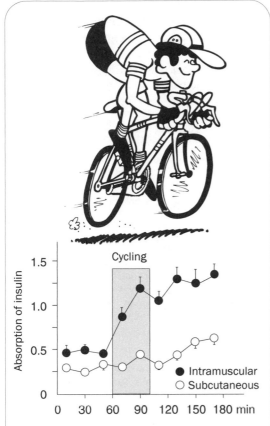

After an injection in your thigh muscle, the absorption rate will increase considerably when you exercise the muscles in your legs. Short-acting insulin (10 U) was given at 0 minutes. After an injection in the subcutaneous fat you will only see a slight increase in the absorption rate, probably due to the subcutaneous insulin depot being "massaged" by the moving muscles.[281]

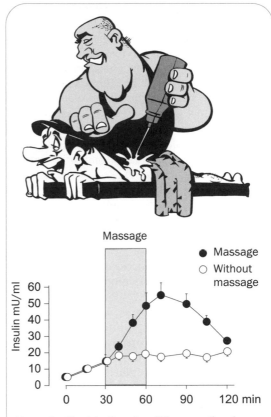

Massaging the injection site will increase the absorption of insulin considerably.[490] Short-acting insulin (10 U) was given at 0 minutes. You can utilize this if you want your short-acting insulin to take particularly rapid effect, for example if you have a high blood glucose level and increased levels of ketones in blood or urine. Give the injection site a thorough rubbing for 15-30 minutes and you will find that the insulin takes effect much faster.

concentration in blood after 45 minutes when a skin temperature of 37° C was compared to that of 30° C (same room temperature).[704] In the same study, individuals with a thicker subcutaneous fat layer (10 mm) had lower insulin levels than those with a thin subcutaneous fat layer (2 mm). Also see "Where do I inject the insulin?" on page 111.

What happens if a child won't finish a meal?

If it is your child who has diabetes, you will be only too aware as a parent how much your child will eat of any particular dish. If lunch is served at school, it may be helpful, if possible, to read through the school menu in advance and discuss what your child does and doesn't like, and what can be eaten instead. Smaller children are especially unpredictable as to how much they will eat at the time when the insulin is given. If the child eats less than anticipated there will be a risk of hypoglycemia. It is not ideal to give insulin after the meal, but in this situation it might be the best alternative when you use rapid-acting insulin. (NovoLog/ NovoRapid [183] or Humalog [204]). You can also try giving insulin corresponding to a smaller meal first and then give the rest of the insulin if the child eats a normal sized meal after all. If the child uses pump or indwelling catheters (Insuflon), the extra dose will not create a problem.

A child with good glucose control will often have a well balanced opinion of how much he or she needs to eat. If the blood glucose is high, the child will often not be as hungry as usual and will not need to eat as much but may need a bigger snack later on to balance the insulin level. (see "Hungry or full?" on page 215). Even adults often feel more fullness when the blood glucose level is high.[415]

A practical rule is to always offer bread to eat after a cooked meal so that the child can eat enough even if he or she does not like the food that has been served.

If a child has more or less than usual to eat, you can compensate when it is time for the next snack. If the child has had a small lunch, schedule the snack a bit earlier and give him or her a little more at this time, perhaps something extra tasty if appetite has been a problem. If you use rapid-acting insulin (NovoLog/NovoRapid, Humalog), you will probably need to give extra insulin for a larger than usual snack.

If the child eats less while using twice-daily injections, it may be possible to decrease the dose of short-acting (Novolin R, Humulin R) or rapid-acting (NovoLog/NovoRapid, Humalog) insulin but give the same dose of intermediate-acting insulin (Novolin N, Humulin N).

Factors influencing the insulin effect

① Subcutaneous blood flow (increased blood flow will give a faster insulin absorption).

Increased by	Heat, e.g. sauna, jacuzzi, hot shower, hot bath or fever.[344,755]
Decreased by	Cold, e.g. a cold bath.[67] Smoking (constriction of the blood vessels).[451,454] Dehydration.[344]

② Injection depth — Faster absorption after an intramuscular injection.[282,775]

③ Injection site See page 113 — An abdominal injection of short-acting insulin will be absorbed faster than a thigh injection. The absorption from the buttocks is slower than from the abdomen but slightly faster than from the thigh.

④ Insulin antibodies — Can bind the insulin resulting in a slower and less predictable effect.

⑤ Exercise — Increases the absorption of short-acting insulin even after you have finished exercising, particularly if the injection is given intramuscularly.[280,454]

⑥ Massage of the injection site — Increased absorption of short-acting insulin, probably due to a faster breakdown of the insulin.[490]

⑦ Subcutaneous fat thickness — A thicker layer of subcutaneous fat gives a slower absorption of insulin.[362,704]

⑧ Injection in fatty lumps (lipohypertrophies) — Slower [824] and more erratic absorption of insulin.

⑨ Concentration of the insulin. — 40 U/ml is absorbed faster than 100 U/ml.[282]

What if you forget to take your insulin?

You can try the following suggestions if you have had diabetes for some time and are confident about how the insulin you inject works. *If you are even slightly unsure you should contact the hospital or diabetes clinic.*

Forgotten premeal injection (multiple injection treatment)

Take the same dose of regular short-acting or rapid-acting insulin or decrease it by a unit or two, if you remember immediately after you have eaten. If one or two hours have passed, you can try taking about half the dose of regular short-acting insulin or, even better, rapid-acting insulin (NovoLog/NovoRapid or Humalog). If a longer time has passed, add a few units to your next meal injection, but not until you have measured your blood glucose level.

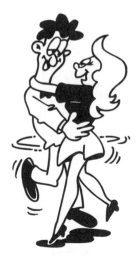

If you are out clubbing, remember that dancing is exercise too. Don't forget to eat something during the evening. Because of the exercise you will probably not need an extra meal injection, that is if you are not planning on staying up very late. You may also need to decrease your bedtime injection by 2-4 units to avoid hypoglycemia if you have been dancing a great deal.

Forgotten bedtime injection (multiple injection treatment)

If you wake up before 2 AM you can still take your bedtime insulin, but you should decrease the dose by 25-30% or 1-2 units for every hour that has passed since the normal time of injection. If there are less than five hours before your usual waking time, measure your blood glucose and take an injection of regular short-acting insulin (*not* NovoLog/NovoRapid or Humalog which have too short an insulin action in this situation). You can try a dose of regular insulin with half the number of units of your normal bedtime injection of intermediate-acting insulin. However, never inject more than 0.1 U/kg (0.5 U/10 lb) of body weight at one time.

If you wake up with high blood sugar, nausea and elevated levels of ketones in your blood or urine, you have symptoms of insulin deficiency. Take 0.1 U/kg (0.5 U/10 lb) body weight of short-acting insulin (even better, NovoLog/NovoRapid or Humalog) and measure your blood glucose again after 2-3 hours. If your glucose level has not decreased, take another dose of 0.1 U/kg (0.5 U/10 lb) body weight. *If you still are feeling nauseous or if you vomit, you should contact your doctor immediately.*

Forgotten injection with twice-daily treatment

If, for example, you forget the morning dose, take the same dose or decrease the regular short-acting (or rapid-acting) part by 1 or 2 units if you remember immediately after having eaten (but take the same NPH dose). If you remember after an hour or two, you can try decreasing the rapid or short-acting part by about half and the intermediate part by about 25%. If you remember your injection even later, measure your blood glucose before the next meal and take only rapid or short-acting insulin at this meal. If you are using pre-mixed insulin, it won't be possible to decrease only one of the components. Give a smaller dose of this insulin when you remember, or use only rapid or short-acting insulin until it is time for the afternoon injection.

If you have forgotten your evening injection and remembered at night, you must take a smaller dose of intermediate acting insulin before going to bed. A little more than half should be enough but you must test this with blood glucose controls. You will probably also need an injection of rapid or short-acting insulin at your evening snack. Try the same dose (or a few units less) than the short-acting part of your evening injection. You should check your blood glucose at night to avoid hypoglycemia

What if you take the wrong type of insulin?

At bedtime

Taking your premeal insulin instead of the bedtime insulin by mistake when going to bed is not uncommon. This may happen if your day and night pen injectors are very similar. Long-acting Lantus insulin is a clear solution so it can be easy to mistake short-acting or rapid-acting insulin for the long-acting variety if both are drawn from vials and given with syringes.[7]

Don't worry, this is not a catastrophe! However, you may have problems with low blood glucose for a couple of hours and you will have a rather sleepless night as you will need to check your blood glucose levels at frequent intervals during it. Make sure you are not alone at home, as you will need somebody awake and ready to help you throughout the night. If you are alone in this situation, you would be best off going to hospital.

You need to have glucose and food close at hand. Start by checking your blood glucose values at least every hour, and more frequently if your blood glucose falls below 110 mg/dl (6

mmol/l). Eat one or more extra meals during the night, preferably food that is rich in carbohydrates but contains as little fat as possible. If you need to take glucose to counter hypoglycemia, the effect will be much slower if you have a fat-rich meal in your stomach. If you happen to take a large dose of NovoLog/NovoRapid or Humalog instead of bedtime insulin, you should expect a very rapid insulin effect. In this situation, it is even more important that what you eat is rich in carbohydrates and low in fat.

Taking the wrong type of insulin will only be dangerous if you take short or rapid-acting insulin at bedtime without noticing it. If you are used to low blood glucose levels, your body might not give any warning symptoms until the blood glucose is dangerously low (see "Hypoglycemia unawareness" on page 48). See also page 56.

Remember that the effect of short-acting insulin usually diminishes after 5 hours (a little later if you have taken a dose larger than 10 units). Because of this, you need to take your bedtime dose of intermediate or long-acting insulin as well, but lower it to approximately half the dose and wait a few hours after taking the accidental injection. In the morning you can take your breakfast insulin as usual, adjusting it according to your morning blood glucose reading.

During the day

If you happen to take a dose of intermediate-acting instead of rapid or short-acting insulin during the day, it will not give you much of a blood glucose lowering effect for that meal. The effect will come some hours later. If, for example, you have taken intermediate-acting insulin for breakfast (on a multiple injection treatment), you can try taking a small dose (roughly half your ordinary dose) of short-acting or even better, rapid-acting insulin, to help take care of your breakfast. Measure your blood glucose before lunch and if it is high (more than 180 mg/dl, 10 mmol/l), take half your ordinary lunchtime dose.

Sleeping in weekends

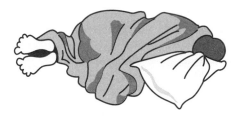

You can sleep a little longer at weekends without problems. One hour more is rarely a problem and usually you can even extend your sleeping in for two hours. Some people with diabetes experience problems with high morning blood glucose (see page 152), and they will find it difficult to sleep longer since their glucose level can rise rapidly during the early hours. Switching to the long-acting insulin Lantus usually solves the problem, but in some families it may be solved by parents giving an early morning injection. The child or teenager can then sleep in for an hour while their blood glucose starts to decrease before having breakfast.

If you stay up late at night and plan to sleep in late in the morning, you should take your bedtime insulin when you go to bed. It will then last the duration of a normal night's sleep, including the extra hours in the morning.

If you are planning on having an early breakfast, however, you should decrease the bedtime dose as the night will then be shorter than usual. Otherwise there is a risk of hypoglycemia when your breakfast insulin starts working.

If you have a late breakfast, your lunch will usually be a little late too, since you will not be as hungry by your normal lunchtime. In this way your whole day will be shifted and you will usually have no problem spreading your meals evenly over the day. Just remember that the time between the injections of regular short-acting insulin should not exceed five hours. With rapid-acting insulin analogs, this time interval is less important since the need for insulin between the meals is covered by the basal insulin. If you use an insulin pump, having a sleeping in will not cause a problem as long as you have adjusted the basal rate to keep your blood glucose levels at the same level in the morning even if you don't have breakfast (see page 184).

When switching time with daylight savings at summertime and wintertime, you need only adjust your watch. You do not need to gradually adjust the time for meals and insulin injections.

Staying awake all night

Being up all night is not common practice, but it is sometimes unavoidable for teenagers or young adults. One of our patients, an 18 year

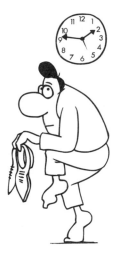

If you stay awake very late (2-3 AM), you will need another injection of premeal insulin (and food) late at night. Remember to give the injections of regular short-acting insulin not more than five hours apart. With rapid-acting insulin (NovoLog/NovoRapid and Humalog) you can have a longer interval between meals if your basal need for insulin between meals is covered by long-acting insulin (Lantus, Ultralente, Humulin U) or twice daily intermediate-acting insulin (Novolin N, Humulin N).

old boy, worked as a travel guide and was required to stay awake all night in the bus on the way to a ski resort. During intercontinental flights, people often have to stay awake for long periods (see "Passing through time zones" on page 297).

If you stay awake all night you should not take your bedtime insulin. Instead, you inject regular premeal insulin when you eat every fourth or fifth hour. Adjust the dose according to how much you eat (compare the size of your meal with your usual lunch, dinner or evening snack). You should not use the amount of insulin taken at breakfast for comparison because more insulin is commonly needed for breakfast (see "Starting insulin treatment" on page 127). If you use rapid-acting insulin (NovoLog/ NovoRapid or Humalog), and twice daily intermediate acting basal insulin (Novolin N, Humulin N), you may need to take half the night time dose to cover your basal need of insulin during a long-distance flight. If you use long-acting insulin (Lantus, Ultralente, Humulin U), this will probably give sufficient basal effect throughout the flight.

Shift work

It may be difficult to combine diabetes with shift work. When you come back home after a night shift you will need to take insulin to cover both the meal you will eat and the background insulin you will need while you sleep during the day. Rapid-acting insulin (NovoLog/ NovoRapid or Humalog) will probably be a better mealtime insulin in this situation as its effect will have declined before the basal insulin has reached a higher effect. With regular short-acting insulin there will be a risk of overlapping effects, which could cause hypoglycemia after 3-4 hours. An insulin pump may be easier to use in this situation, since you can easily adapt the basal rates to your shift hours.

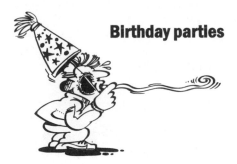

Birthday parties

It is very important for children with diabetes to be able to take part in birthday parties or school parties without being embarrassed about having diabetes. We believe people with diabetes should learn how to handle whatever food is served at a party instead of bringing their own "diabetes food". It is often a good idea to call the parents giving the party beforehand and ask them to provide drinks containing artificial sweeteners (preferably the same for all children so that a child with diabetes will not feel singled out). You can also request that not too many "goodies" be served. At many parties, the children receive a bag of candies at the end to take home rather than eating sweets all through the party, which works particularly well for a child with diabetes.

Food served at birthday parties these days tends not to be as sweet as it used to be. There may be cake or ice cream on the menu, but preceded by pizza, hamburgers or hot dogs. Try giving an extra unit of insulin with the birthday cake, depending on the size of the cake slices and also on the amount of activity (running around, dancing and so on) that is likely to happen at the party (see extra doses on page 133). If the party is a very active one, the child may not need any extra insulin at all! It is a good idea to check your child's blood glucose level once the party is over and make a note of the result in your logbook. This will help you plan ahead for the next party.

If your child is at day care or preschool, the best time to celebrate a birthday may well be during break time. Make sure that all drinks for your child (and preferably for the other children as well) contain artificial sweeteners. Staff are usually very obliging for the small extra arrangements needed to accommodate a child with diabetes. Sometimes you might need to give an extra unit of insulin if birthday cake or other sweet foods are served. In the US, federal laws against discrimination apply to those with diabetes in the public schools, but not in religious or private school settings (see page 236).

If you are taking your child to an adult party, you are likely to find cookies, cakes and other sweet things being served. Your child will need extra insulin to be able to pick and choose from all that is on offer. Try to find some kind of compromise here, for example only a few cookies or a small piece of cake (and, if needed, one or two extra units of insulin). It is generally not a good idea to eat too much of everything offered at a party. And do tell grandparents (who have only their grandchild's best interests at heart) that so called "sugar free" cookies or "diabetes cookies" are not a very good alternative. They are often not sugar free at all and, anyway, many children find their taste disgusting.

Of course, how you manage will depend on how often you or your child go to parties. Once in a while, a person with diabetes can certainly make an exception and accept some candy or a piece of cake if it is offered. But if exceptions are being made every week, they cease to be exceptions. Eating too many sweet things too often will affect both your weight and your long term blood glucose levels.

Insulin at school and day care centers

Sometimes it is difficult to get help with insulin injections at a day care center or nursery, or to get the teacher to remind the child to take their insulin at school. The staff have no formal obligation to give injections when needed, but some schools have a nurse or teacher's assistant who will help. At some larger schools where several pupils have diabetes, they might meet at lunchtime, to eat together, and a staff member may be able to be on hand to help them if necessary. The Canadian Diabetes Association can provide an excellent resource for teachers entitled "Kids with Diabetes in Your Care. A Practical Guide". See also page 281.

Sleeping away from home

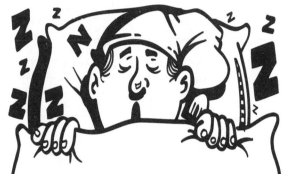

Many children thoroughly enjoy having "sleepovers" at friends' homes. This often means late night talking or playing games. It is advisable for the child to have a "midnight snack" to prevent hypoglycemia. However, it is quite natural for parents of children with diabetes to be worried when faced with this situation. It is easy to be overprotective if you don't feel confident about how to deal with it. It is important that the friend's parents are familiar with how and when a child should take his or her insulin, and what to do if the child develops hypoglycemia. A good idea is to write down a list of instructions for the child with when and how much insulin should be taken depending on blood glucose measurements. Don't forget to leave your telephone number if you will be out for the night or have your mobile phone available.

Monitoring

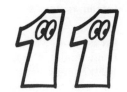

"Everyone is like a child when starting something new." This saying is particularly relevant to the adjusting of insulin dosages. It is difficult, if not impossible, to manage your diabetes without monitoring it at home. Trying to manage your diabetes without home monitoring is like driving a car without a speedometer, fuel gauge, or temperature gauge. Without these instruments, your car may run for a little while, but you will probably end up in the wrong place or have a breakdown.

Home monitoring tests can be divided into:

① Immediate tests   Tests that you can perform at any given moment, in order to find out what your blood glucose level is, or whether your ketone level is raised.

② Routine tests   Tests that you perform regularly, and which help you to make long-term adjustments in your insulin doses, eating habits and other activities.

③ Long-range tests   Tests that reflect your diabetes control over a long period of time. These include such tests as fructosamine and A1C.

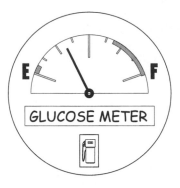

Measuring your blood glucose level is like checking the fuel gauge in your car. The difference is that you don't just need to be careful to avoid running out of gas (sugar), you need to make sure the level doesn't go too high either.

How many tests should I take?

Blood tests

It is recommended practice to take a 24 hour glucose profile at least every other week, even for very young children.[509] This means measuring your blood glucose before and 1½-2 hours after each meal (including the evening snack) as well as once during the night, preferably between 2 and 3 AM. It is also a good idea to take certain tests every day, as a matter of routine, to help you adjust your daily dosages. Monitoring on other occasions should serve to answer a specific question such as: "Is this the beginning of a hypoglycemic reaction?" or "Can I get through the night without eating something extra?", "How much insulin should I take in the morning?" There is no point in taking tests unless you are going to respond to the results.

Timetable of monitoring	
Test	**Reflects the blood glucose levels over:**
Blood glucose	Minutes
Urine glucose	Hours
Fructosamine	2-3 weeks
A1C	2-3 months

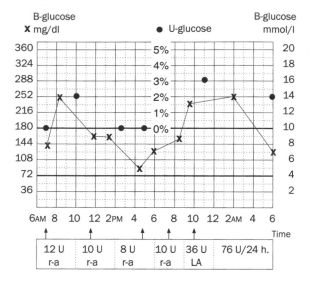

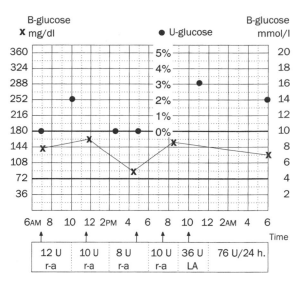

r-a = rapid-acting insulin, LA = Lantus

A 24 hour glucose profile can look like this when you take blood glucose tests before and 1½ hours after meals. It is a good idea to combine the individual readings by drawing a line to link them if the readings are not more than 3-4 hours apart, which also makes it easier to read the chart. You will gather more information if you test the urine passed first thing in the morning for glucose and ketones frequently on the same day you perform the 24 hour glucose profile. Today, most blood glucose meters have a memory but still it is very valuable to record every test and insulin dose in a logbook to be able to recognize patterns after meals and other daily events.

Remember that you will not know anything about your blood glucose levels in between the times when you have performed tests. From the test results this chart may appear reassuring, but it covers the same day as the chart on the left, except with fewer readings. It is easy to fool yourself into believing that the lines also reflect the blood glucose levels in between the individual readings. But look at the urine test results. They show that glucose has been excreted into the urine, which indicates that the blood glucose must have been high somewhere in between the blood glucose measuring tests.

Four or more blood glucose tests per day (before each main meal and before going to bed) are generally necessary to give the information needed to adjust your insulin doses from day to day in order to give you an acceptable level of control over your diabetes.[703] More frequent monitoring is needed in situations when you change your diet or other habits. After a while you will be more familiar with how much insulin is needed in different situations and you will then be able to get away with fewer tests.

You will need to test more frequently at times when your insulin requirements are changing.

These include, for example, periods when you are under stress, if you have an infection, when you are exercising vigorously or playing sports, or if you are eating out or going to a party. At such times, it is a good idea to take a blood glucose test before and 1½-2 hours after each meal and, if necessary, to change the dose accordingly. If you want to see what effect "quick-acting" carbohydrates (like candies) have on your blood glucose, you should test this about 30 minutes after eating them. With slower carbohydrates, like chocolate or ice cream, measure your blood glucose level after 1-1½ hours.

Urine tests

Although urine glucose monitoring is no longer recommended as the primary method of glucose monitoring,[25] it does have its advantages. Urine glucose monitoring can be particularly useful in situations where blood glucose monitoring is difficult or impractical, provided that the level of renal threshold is known. In the case of a small child who is still in diapers, it will usually be possible to squeeze a drop of urine out of the diaper for testing.

Measuring urine glucose is a "screening method" in that it enables you to determine when during the day glucose is excreted. When you have established this, you can follow up with blood glucose tests. This can be practical in periods when your diabetes is very stable, for example during the "honeymoon" phase. A urine glucose test can add information to the blood glucose test in the morning about the night time glucose levels (see page 154).

Ketones could earlier only be measured in urine tests but there are now good methods available for measuring ketones in the blood at home. The blood strips for ketones are much more expensive in many countries, however, and this can make using urine strips more practical. Urine strips may be better to use for screening

mmol/l and mg/dl			
mmol/l	mg/dl	mg/dl	mmol/l
1	18	20	1.1
2	36	40	2.2
3	54	60	3.3
4	72	80	4.4
5	90	100	5.6
6	108	120	6.7
7	126	140	7.8
8	144	160	8.9
9	162	180	10.0
10	180	200	11.1
12	216	220	12.2
14	252	250	13.9
16	288	300	16.7
18	324	350	19.4
20	360	400	22.2
22	396	450	25.0

The numbers in this book refer to plasma glucose unless otherwise stated, as this is what most new patient meters display (the previous 1998 edition had whole blood glucose numbers). Plasma glucose levels are also used by doctors to diagnose diabetes, and in most studies. Plasma glucose is approximately 11% higher than whole blood glucose.[269]

for ketones, but once detected, following the blood ketones gives you more accurate guidance (see page 103).

"Good" or "bad" tests?

It is common to refer to normal blood glucose readings as "good" and high readings as "bad". A young person who hears these terms used frequently may begin to look upon him or herself as "bad". "High blood glucose" sounds more neutral and is a more appropriate term. Test results are just pieces of information, and do not reflect on the quality of the person with diabetes.

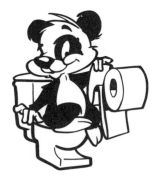

It is a good idea for younger children to get into the habit of taking a urine test every time they go to the toilet.

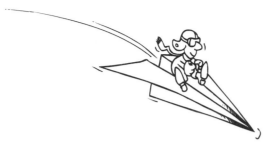

Send your blood glucose charts by mail or fax to your diabetes healthcare team and you can discuss them over the telephone. It may even be possible to send them by e-mail. Check this with your clinic.

Diabetes or not?

In a person who does not have diabetes, the blood glucose level will be regulated within close limits (normally between 60 and 125 mg/dl, 3.3-7 mmol/l). This is despite the fact that intake and expenditure of food varies enormously throughout the day from one person to another. In the fasting state, the blood glucose level is normally below 100 mg/dl (5.6 mmol/l). Higher values indicate that the person's body is not able to handle glucose in the way that it should (impaired glucose tolerance). A fasting plasma glucose level greater than 126 mg/dl (7.0 mmol/l), or a non-fasting casual plasma glucose level higher than 200 mg/dl (11.1 mmol/l) with symptoms of diabetes (thirst, unexplained weight loss and needing to urinate a lot more than usual) indicates that a person has diabetes.[20] The diagnosis should be confirmed by repeat testing on a different day unless the blood glucose is very high or ketones are present.

You should not rely on home blood glucose meters in order to diagnose diabetes. If a person without diabetes has recorded a high reading, you should never announce to the person "you probably have diabetes". Instead, ask them to

check their fasting blood glucose with their doctor.

Are some things forbidden?

We are often asked whether you are allowed to do this or that when you have diabetes. The best answer is that nothing is totally forbidden. It is important, however, to experiment in order to find out what you as an individual can and cannot do. It is a good idea to experiment with both food and insulin, provided this is done in conjunction with blood glucose monitoring. The only risk you are running is of having a temporarily high or low blood glucose.

Always write in your logbook the results of your tests along with details of the activity you were participating in. Next time you play soccer, or go for a pizza or to a party, you will find your notes really valuable.

---

24 hour profile tests

Blood tests:

(1) Before each meal.

(2) 1½-2 hours after each meal.

(3) One test during the night depending on which bedtime insulin you use:
2-3 AM - NPH insulin
(Novolin N, Humulin N, Insuman NPH)
3-4 AM - Lente insulin (Monotard, Humutard) and Levemir
4-6 AM - Long-acting insulin
(Lantus, Ultralente, Humulin U)

(4) In many cases more intensive monitoring may be needed at times, with premeal and pre-snack blood glucose values along with tests every 2-3 hours during the night.

Urine glucose

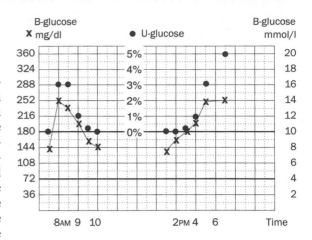

All the urine produced by your kidneys is collected in your bladder. This means that when you measure urine glucose, it will reflect an average blood glucose level since the last time you passed urine. It is also important to remember that urine glucose concentration is measured as a percentage. This means that 5% will represent much less glucose when you have small amounts of urine than if you have large amounts of urine with 5% glucose. A negative glucose reading says nothing about how low the blood glucose is or has been, only that is has not been above the renal threshold since the last time you went to the toilet.

You can determine your renal threshold by checking your blood glucose every 30 minutes, while watching for glucose to be shown in the urine. You can test this either as the blood glucose is going up or as it is going down. In this chart, the test taken in the morning contained glucose until the blood glucose dropped to between 200 and 160 mg/dl (11 and 9 mmol/l). In the afternoon, glucose was noted in the urine when the blood glucose rose from 160 to 180 mg/dl (9 to 10 mmol/l). This implies the person's renal threshold is between 160 and 180 mg/dl (9 and10 mmol/l).

Renal threshold

The kidneys produce urine. They also try to reabsorb as much glucose as possible, so there is normally no glucose in the urine. When the blood glucose is above a certain level, the kidneys' "glucose absorption pump" becomes saturated and glucose will be passed out with the urine instead. The level where this happens is called the renal threshold and is usually between 145-180 mg/dl (8-10 mmol/l) in children,[505] and 125-215 mg/dl (7-12 mmol/l) in adults. The renal threshold usually increases

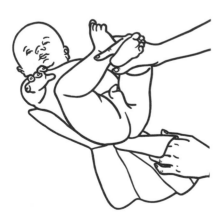

It may be difficult to attain urine samples from modern diapers, which often absorb urine very effectively. Try putting a piece of a cloth inside the diaper to absorb some urine. It is easier to squeeze a couple of drops of urine out of an older-style disposable diaper (with a plastic covering), or a towelling diaper.

Urine tests		
Glucose	Ketones	Interpretation
0	0	OK (can have been low).
+	0	Too much glucose (or more insulin needed).
+	+	Not enough insulin ("diabetes ketones").
0	+	Not enough food ("starvation ketones").

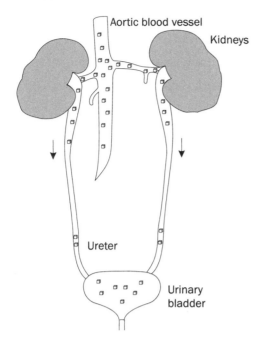

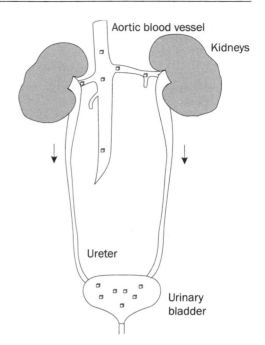

When the blood glucose level is higher than the renal threshold (usually 145-180 mg/dl (8-10 mmol/l) glucose will appear in the urine. The urine from the kidneys collects in the bladder before urination.

When the blood glucose level has returned to normal values, glucose will stop leaking from the kidneys. However, there will still be glucose from the urine held in the bladder, as the fresh urine takes some time to clear from the body. So, when you take your next urine test you will find a high urine glucose, although by this time, your blood glucose level will be registering as normal (see also the charts on page 154).

with age. Certain individuals have a very low renal threshold, down to 90 mg/dl (5 mmol/l), while others have a high threshold of up to 270 mg/dl (15 mmol/l). It is important to know your renal threshold when interpreting urine tests.

You can determine your renal threshold by checking your blood glucose and passing urine once every 30 minutes. If there is glucose in the urine and your blood glucose is decreasing, your renal threshold will be the level at which the urine is negative for glucose. If the blood

glucose is increasing and your urine tests are negative for glucose, the renal threshold will be at a level where glucose is first noted in the urine (see chart). The renal threshold does not affect kidney function, but if your renal threshold is either very high or very low, you will find urine tests less reliable.

Blood glucose

When you take a blood test it will reflect your blood glucose level at that moment. However, the blood glucose can go up or down very quickly, and you may have quite a different reading 15 or 30 minutes later. Always check your blood glucose level when you are not feeling well so that you can avoid eating extra just to be on the safe side when you suspect hypoglycemia. This is especially important in the early days of being diagnosed with diabetes, when you are not yet fully familiar with all the symptoms of hypoglycemia. Later on, you will become more confident about these. (See also "Symptoms of hypoglycemia when the blood glucose level is high" on page 45.)

Recognizing symptoms of high blood glucose is usually more difficult. However, teenagers often seem to learn how their body reacts when their blood glucose is high. Some develop a kind of "auto-pilot" which enables them to adjust insulin doses and food portions without as many blood tests as might be expected. Always try to guess your blood glucose level before checking it, and you will eventually become familiar with the way your body reacts when your blood glucose level is low or high.

How do I take blood tests?

Wash your hands with soap and water before taking a blood test. This is not just to ensure hygiene (though of course that is important), but to ensure there is no sugar on your fingers giving a false high reading, for example from glucose tablets, candy or fruit. Use warm water if your fingers are cold. Do not use alcohol for cleaning your hands as this will make your skin dry. The risk of an infection from a finger prick is minimal.

There are a variety of different finger-pricking devices for taking blood glucose tests. With

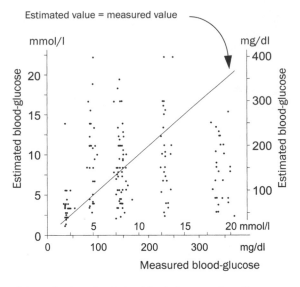

It is easier to estimate low blood glucose values than high ones. In an American study of adults with diabetes, individuals were asked to estimate their blood glucose values.[803] Potentially serious errors (dangerous failure to treat high/low blood glucose or erroneous treatment) were made by 17% when their blood glucose was 34 mg/dl (1.9 mmol/l) but by as many as 66% when the blood glucose was 330 mg/dl (18.4 mmol/l).

some you can adjust the pricking depth. Pricking devices and lancets can vary considerably in size and the way they puncture the skin. Try different types to find out which suits you best. From the point of view of hygiene, you can use the same lancet for a day's blood tests assuming that your fingers are clean. However, the lancet will be very slightly blunted every time you use it, so the pricks might become more painful with repeated usage.

If you prick the sides of your fingertips, your sensitivity will be less affected, which may be important if you play the piano or guitar, for example. Don't use your thumbs and right index finger (or left if you are left-handed) for finger pricking. You need the sensation of touch most in these places and sometimes you will even feel pain the day after a finger prick.

Most blood glucose meters have memories for storing test results and can show the average of your readings over 2-4 weeks which will give you a good picture of how your blood glucose levels have been during this time. The stored information can be transferred to a computer to view, analyze and print. This may be a very useful tool for young people with diabetes who may be interested, as well as for their parents and members of the diabetes team. Some newer meters have built-in blood glucose graphing programs for summarizing patterns of blood glucose control.

Borrowing someone else's finger-pricking device

Borrowing another person's device for pricking your fingers is not a good idea. This is because one small drop of blood left on the device can cause contamination if it is infected. For example, an epidemic of hepatitis B in a hospital ward was caused by using the same pricking

Lancets for blood glucose tests

Brand	Diameter of needle	Fits to device
B-D Ultra-Fine 33	0.20 mm	Standard
B-D Ultra-Fine II	0.30 mm	Standard
Monolet Thin	0.36 mm	Standard
Surelite	0.66 mm	Standard
ComforTouch	0.45 mm	Standard
Unilet G Ultralite	0.36 mm	Standard
Medisense Lancet	0.36 mm	Standard
Softclix II	0.36 mm	Softclix
Soft Touch	0.36mm	Standard
Cleanlet Fine	0.36 mm	Standard
Microlet	0.50 mm	Standard

Standard = Autoclix P, B-D Lancer-5, Glucolet, Microlet, Monojector, Penlet II among others.

All lancets can be used for finger-pricking without using them in a device.

All the names mentioned above are ® or ™ of respective company. Other lancets may be available in your country.

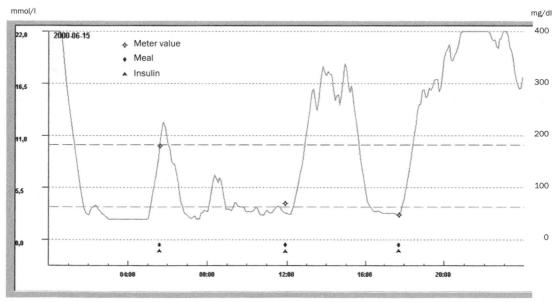

Minimed CGMS chart showing wide fluctuations of glucose levels during the day and night in a 16-year old boy with an A1C of 7.2%. The three tests that the boy took (¤) are not sufficient to detect patterns that can lead to appropriate changes in insulin dosages. The dashed lines represent 55 and 180mg/dl (3.0 and 10 mmol/l).

Why take blood tests?

☞ *Advantages*

⟹ You can take a test instead of eating "just to be on the safe side".

⟹ Helps you learn about hypoglycemia and the symptoms of it.

⟹ Lets you know when you need to change insulin doses, e.g. with infections, stress, physical exercise, or going to a party.

⟹ The only way to find out if you have night time hypoglycemia.

⟹ Blood glucose monitoring is necessary to get good glucose control and in the long run lessen the risk of complications as much as possible.

☞ *Disadvantages*

⟹ Pricking your finger can be painful.

⟹ Monitoring takes time and extra effort.

Sources of error when measuring blood glucose

False high reading	False low reading
Glucose on fingers	Drop applied too late
	Finger removed too quickly
	Not enough blood on the strip
	Water or saliva on finger

Regular use of the control strip or control solution provided with your meter for calibration is very important to get and maintain reliable values.

device (Autolet®) despite switching lancets between each test.[222]

Does the meter show the correct value?

The margin of error in a correctly used blood glucose meter is approximately 10%. This means that with a blood glucose level of 360 mg/dl (20 mmol/l), the meter can show 36 mg/dl (2 mmol/l) above or below the correct value. However, at a blood glucose of 55 mg/dl (3 mmol/l) the error should not exceed 5 mg/dl (0.3 mmol/l). It is very important to apply enough blood to the strip. Too small a drop will give a false low reading. Don't rub the blood onto the strip. If you have sugar on your fingers

when you take the test, this will cause a false high reading.

Ask your diabetes nurse for advice about the available meters and their prices. Often you can get a discount on the cost of a new meter if you hand in your old one at the time of purchase.

Comparing different meters can be confusing as they often show different readings. For example, one may show a blood glucose level of 215 mg/dl (12 mmol/l), while another (used at the same time on the same patient) shows a level of 250 mg/dl (14 mmol/l). However, this difference is well within the error margins stated by the manufacturers of the meters. It is advisable to stick to one meter that works well, as the difference of 10 or 20 mg/dl is not particularly significant at high readings. Bring the meter with you when you come to clinic, and ask your diabetes nurse to check your meter with glucose control solution at regular intervals.

In hospital, blood for glucose monitoring is often taken through an intravenous needle to lessen the pain. In people without diabetes, venous blood tested after a meal has about 10% less glucose than capillary blood. This is logical if you remember that venous blood has already delivered some of the glucose it contains to the body tissues. However, in people with diabetes, the difference was only 2 mg/dl (0.1 mmol/l).[473] This can probably be explained by the lack of fine-tuned insulin release in response to the blood glucose level.

Continuous glucose monitoring

The Medtronic MiniMed CGMS (Continuous Glucose Monitoring System®) is a device that monitors glucose levels (40-400 mg/dl, 2.2-22 mmol/l) every 10 seconds and records an average value every 5 minutes. It measures through a thin plastic tube in subcutaneous tissue, and can be worn for up to 3 days. The current design does not allow you to read the glucose values in real-time. When the monitor is connected to a computer, the data can be downloaded and viewed on screen. Using this method has made it easier to see patterns of glucose fluctuation, which has in turn led to changes in treatment and improved glucose control, in children [436,511] and in adults.[89]

The GlucoWatch Biographer® looks like a watch and monitors blood glucose through the skin on the wrist 3 times/hour for 12 hours (after a 2 hour warm up) using a method called iontophoresis. It has alarms for high, low and rapidly falling glucose levels and you can download the information for pattern analysis.[233]

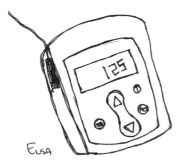

The CGMS monitor measures glucose continuously for up to 3 days through a small cannula that is inserted into your subcutaneous tissue.

Alternative site testing

♠ Some new meters are used for testing blood glucose at alternative sites. This may be helpful if you play the piano, for example, and do not want to keep pricking your fingers.

♠ In the fasting state, the glucose readings from the forearm are similar to the fingertip.[422]

♠ After an intake of 75g of glucose, the rise in blood glucose in adults was 47-137 mg/dl (2.6-7.6 mmol/l) lower on samples taken from the forearm compared to the fingertip.[422]

♠ When blood glucose fell quickly after an insulin injection, the values from the fingertip were 61-119 mg/dl (3.4-6.6 mmol/l) lower than the forearm.[422]

♠ Blood glucose changes appeared in average 35 minutes later in forearm tests compared to the fingertip. By rubbing the skin vigorously for 5-10 seconds before pricking, the accuracy from a forearm test was improved considerably, but with large individual differences.[422]

♠ In another study where tests were taken after a meal, lower glucose readings were produced from the forearm and thigh compared to the fingertip, in spite of vigorous skin rubbing.[249]

♠ The differences are caused by a greatly increased blood flow in the fingertip. To be on the safe side, it seems best to rely on fingertip tests when checking for hypoglycemia, (for example when driving a car or after exercise).

Children and blood glucose tests

Small children think of their body as a balloon. If you puncture a balloon it will burst and the contents will pour out. A child may think, quite logically, "If I have a lot of jabs for blood tests, won't all the blood go out of my body?" The Band-Aid that is put over the puncture wound

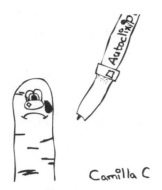

You can try to anesthetize the fingertip with a piece of ice before pricking it. A topical anesthetic cream (EMLA®, ELA-Max®) will not work on your fingertips as the skin is too thick. Sticking slightly on the side of the fingertip is preferable since it bleeds well and hurts less.

has an added significance: it can be seen as stopping the body contents from being poured out. Even those children who don't ask what will happen to their body need to be reassured that the doctors and nurses will take only a tiny amount of blood for the test and the body will quickly produce new blood again. The red blood cells are produced in the bone marrow, and live for only about 120 days. This means that there is a continuous production of new red blood cells going on in the body.

At times, it may be difficult to make your own child agree to giving a drop of blood for monitoring if the pricking hurts. If a small child struggles, the whole procedure will be more painful for everyone involved. Child psychologists recommend that, in this situation, the parents (preferably both together) hold the child tightly in order to get the pricking done as quickly and efficiently as possible. After it is done, it is important to comfort the child. Remind the child that struggling makes the test more painful, especially as they are likely to need several jabs rather than just one if they are wriggling and fighting. It is also a good idea to let young children watch their parents and members of the diabetes team take blood tests from themselves, so they can see that is doesn't hurt too much if they remain calm. Remember

that the goal is to get your child to accept blood glucose monitoring in the long run, not only for the time being.

If the child is feeling unwell it is important to emphasize that after taking a blood glucose test you will be able to do something to make the symptoms better. When children have experienced actually feeling better after testing and taking the necessary measures, they are often more willing to take the test the next time it is necessary.

Some young children are upset by the sight of blood coming from their fingers. If this applies to your child, you can try pricking the ear lobe instead.

Does continuous finger pricking cause loss of feeling?

A lot of people are afraid that constantly pricking their fingers to test blood will cause them to lose all feeling in them. Fortunately, all the evidence suggests that this won't happen. When fingers that had been pricked an average of 1000 times were compared to control fingers not used for pricking, it was only pressure sensitivity that was affected (due to an increased skin

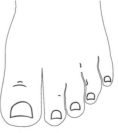

Taking blood glucose tests from your toes in the evening, during the night or in the morning will spare your fingertips. Young people with healthy feet can usually do this without problems.[39] However, if you have reduced feeling in your feet, or any type of sores on them, you should avoid taking blood from the toes.

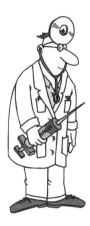

A question of conscience: "Do you take the tests for your own sake or do you take them to have something to show your doctor or diabetes nurse / educator when you come to the clinic?"

Ketones

➡ Can be measured with both urine and blood tests.

➡ Common symptoms: Hunger (!)
　　　　　　　　　　　Nausea
　　　　　　　　　　　Vomiting.

☞ *Always check for ketones when you are feeling unwell!*

---

thickness). There were no signs of decreased sensitivity to heat or touch.[288]

Ketones

Ketones are produced by the body when the cells do not have enough glucose energy. The body then breaks down fat to produce energy and the breakdown products are called ketones. Ketones can be used as fuel by the muscles, heart, kidneys and brain.

If a person has diabetes, ketones are produced in excess when there is a lack of insulin and the blood glucose levels are usually high. Diabetes ketones therefore indicate high blood glucose levels and the need for extra doses of insulin (see page 133).

Ketones can be measured both in blood and urine. Blood ketone monitoring (see page 101) for home use is a new method. It is not available in all countries, however, so some people have to rely on urine tests to find out how high their body's ketone levels are. Positive urine ketone readings are found in anyone who is fasting (regardless of whether or not they have diabetes) and in up to 30% of first morning urine samples from pregnant women.[25]

It is particularly important to check for ketones if you are ill, if you are under a lot of stress, or if you are feeling nauseous or vomiting, as well as when your blood glucose level is consistently high (above 300 mg/dl, 16 mmol/l).[25]

Ketones in the blood or urine indicate that the cells are starving. Check the key fact box on page 92 for information on how to interpret urine tests. The ketones produced when the body is starving, or when there is a deficiency of insulin, are chemically the same. But they are often described differently as "starvation ketones" or "diabetes ketones" respectively, since they are produced in different situations. (See also the section on "Cellular metabolism" on page 24.)

Starvation ketones

Starvation ketones are produced when the blood glucose level is low. The urine glucose concentration will then be low too. The reason the cells are starving is because there is not enough food and glucose in the blood, which happens when you haven't been eating enough, when you have been vomiting, or if you have gastroenteritis. If low blood glucose is caused by a high dose of insulin, the production of ketones will be stopped as insulin counteracts the transformation of fat and fatty acids to ketones.

When to check for ketones

⫸ When you are acutely ill, for example suffering from a common cold with fever.

⫸ When your blood glucose has been higher than 250-270 mg/dl (14-15 mmol/l) for more than a couple of hours.

⫸ If you are having symptoms of insulin deficiency (nausea, vomiting, abdominal pain, rapid breathing, fruity smell on your breath).

⫸ Regularly during pregnancy (see page 273).

Diabetes ketones

If you are deficient in insulin, the available glucose will be in the wrong place, i.e. in the bloodstream outside the cell instead of inside the cell. Both the blood glucose level and the urine glucose concentration will then be high.

If your body is producing a lot of ketones, your blood will become acidic and you will be at risk of developing ketoacidosis (see page 29). Passing ketones into the urine is the body's way of getting rid of these excess ketones. High blood glucose level at the same time as ketones and high urine glucose concentration (3-5%) always suggests a shortage of insulin, as long as the urine test is taken during the day and you have not suffered from hypoglycemia recently (see the blood glucose chart on page 51).

Ketones in the morning urine

When you wake up in the morning, urine has been in your bladder for so long that it is difficult to say exactly when during the night the glucose or ketones entered the urine. A urine test might show both glucose and ketones if you had hypoglycemia early in the night, followed by a rebound effect in the morning (see page 49) with high blood glucose resulting in both glucose and ketones in the urine. The same results

will be seen if your blood glucose has been high all night and the cells have been starved of sugar by a shortage of insulin (see chart on page 54). In this case, the ketones may make you feel nauseous when you wake up in the morning. Ketones without glucose in the urine indicate that you did not eat enough before going to bed (see page 154).

Will ketones make you feel ill?

It is the increased level of ketones that makes you feel ill, not the high blood glucose level as such. If you have a high blood glucose and ketones in your blood or urine, you are likely to feel nauseous and generally unwell (see "Symptoms of insulin deficiency" on page 27). However, if your blood glucose level is temporarily high, but without raised ketone levels, you will often feel fine. You may not even notice your body isn't working as well as it should if you have had high blood glucose levels for some time and a high A1C. But when your blood glucose has returned to normal levels again, you will almost certainly be aware of the difference. "Is this how alert I should really feel?" is a frequent comment.

If your blood glucose level is normally below 180 mg/dl (10 mmol/l), you will be more likely to notice an increase. Even if you don't recognize this clearly yourself, somebody else (such as a teacher, parent or friend) will certainly notice that you are tired and irritable when your blood glucose level is high.

Vomiting and ketones

If you are the parent of a child with diabetes, you should always suspect an insulin deficiency if your child starts vomiting. Keep suspecting this until the opposite has been proven! *Vomiting and diarrhea may be caused by gastroenteritis, but vomiting alone is very likely to be caused by ketones produced as a result of insulin deficiency.* The blood glucose level will then be high and you will find that ketone levels are raised. It is important to stress this point firmly if, for example, you need to contact a doctor while on vacation. It is all too easy for vomiting to be misinterpreted as gastroenteritis by non-specialist doctors or those who are unfamiliar with a particular patient. If this happens, they are then likely to advise, wrongly, that you lower the insulin dose. In fact, a child or young person in this situation needs more insulin, not less. (See also "Nausea and vomiting" on page 259.)

Blood ketones

New meters (Precision Xceed, Bioscanner Ketone) for measuring the levels of ketones in the blood were introduced in 2001.[124] These measure a different type of ketone (beta-hydroxybuturic acid) from that measured by the urine strips (acetoacetate). In a US study of young people aged between 3 and 23 years, there was a 60% reduction in hospital admissions and a 38% reduction in emergency room visits among the group checking blood ketones, as compared with the group checking urine ketones during a 6 month follow-up.[470] Among patients/families using blood ketone measurements, 70% reported they would check blood ketones more often than urine ketones.

The advantage of measuring ketones in the blood is that an increased level can be detected earlier, for example when the level of insulin is insufficient because of an infection. Occasionally, only the level of beta-hydroxybuturic acid is increased when the body becomes insulin deficient, and urine strips will then not give any reaction.[469] Ketones produced if a person is not eating enough ("starvation ketones") also show up on a blood test. Ketone levels of 0.1-0.2 mmol/l are common in adults with diabetes if the test is taken before breakfast.[9] Among children with diabetes aged between 1 and 10, 12% had a morning blood ketone of 0.2 mmol/l or above.[667] People without diabetes who have not eaten overnight, usually do not have levels above 0.5 mmol/l.[662] Mild infections associated with vomiting and diarrhea in children without diabetes commonly cause ketone levels to rise to above 1.0 mmol/l.[469]

It may be difficult to interpret a morning urine test showing ketones as you will not know at what time during the night the ketones were produced. However, if the level of ketones in the blood is raised, you can interpret the results like this:

Ketones + high glucose level = lack of insulin.
Ketones + low glucose level = lack of food.

If you, or your child with diabetes, feels nauseous or vomits, you should test for ketones. This is because nausea and vomiting are common signs of insulin deficiency. Measuring ketones in the blood is more effective than urine tests for following progress and making sure that the level is decreasing when extra insulin is given. This is very important because if the level continues to rise, there is a risk of developing ketoacidosis. In such a case you should always contact your diabetes team.

After you have taken extra insulin, your body will stop producing ketones. Measuring blood ketones will give you accurate readings of a decreasing level. However, ketones will still continue to be passed into the urine for several hours and can sometimes be measured 1-2 days after ketoacidosis (see page 29).[206,308] The reason for this is that ketones are partly transformed into acetone which is stored in fat tissue. Acetone is slowly released to the blood and excreted via the urine and lungs, giving the breath a fruity smell. [206]

The measuring of ketones in the blood is particularly helpful for people using an insulin pump, as the risk of insulin deficiency goes up when the continuous supply of insulin is interrupted. If your blood glucose is high (>250 mg/dl, 14 mmol/l) for a few hours, and giving extra insulin via the pump does not decrease it, you should check for ketones. An increased level indicates problems with the pump and you should take an extra dose of insulin with a pen or syringe (see page 173). If the ketone level is above 3 mmol/l this indicates that you have ketoacidosis. You should contact your doctor for further advice as soon as possible.[794] Pregnant women should check for ketones each morning, and more often if they feel nauseous, vomit or have an infection with a raised temperature (see page 276).

Comparison of blood and ketone readings [470]

Blood ketones (mmol/l)	Urine ketones
0-0.5	Negative - trace
0.6-1.0	Trace - low
1.1-1.5	Moderate - large
1.5-3.0	Large

If blood ketones are 3.0 mmol/l or above you should contact your doctor or go directly to the E.R.

Interpreting blood ketones (adapted from [470,667])

Blood ketones mmol/l	Blood glucose			
	< 180 mg/dl < 10 mmol/l	180-250 mg/dl 10-14 mmol/l	250-400 mg/dl 14-22 mmol/l	> 400 mg/dl > 22 mmol/l
< 0.5	No need to worry.		Measure again after 1 - 2 h.	
0.5 - 0.9	Measure again after 1 - 2 hours.	May need extra insulin, for example before exercising.	Take 0.05 U/kg (0.25U/10 lb).	Take 0.1 U/kg (0.5U/10 lb). Repeat if needed.
1.0 - 1.4	"Starvation ketones" Eat something rich in carbohydrates.	Eat and take 0.05 U/kg (0.25 U/10 lb).	Take 0.1 U/kg (0.5 U/10 lb).	Take 0.1 U/kg (0.5 U/10 lb). Repeat if necessary.
1.5 - 2.9	"Starvation ketones". Eat, then take insulin when blood glucose has risen. Risk of developing ketoacidosis. Contact your diabetes team!	Eat and take 0.1 U/kg (0.5 U/10 lb).	Take extra insulin (0.1 U/kg, 0.5 U/10 lb). Repeat dose if ketones do not decrease.	
3.0 or above	"	"	"	
	There is an immediate risk for ketoacidosis if the ketone level is 3.0 mmol/l or above - treatment is needed urgently! Contact your doctor or go to nearest E.R..			

Check for ketones when your blood glucose is repeatedly above 250 mg/dl (14 mmol/l) and during days when you are unwell. High blood glucose and elevated ketones indicate a lack of insulin. "Starvation ketones" are usually below 3,0 mmol/l. If you have nausea or vomit, you must try to drink sugar-containing fluids in small portions to keep your blood glucose up in order to give extra insulin. Always contact your diabetes team/the emergency department in this situation. When your ketone levels are raised, the number one priority is to give extra insulin. Never mind if your blood glucose doesn't decrease as much, the important thing is that the ketone level decreases after you have taken extra insulin. The ketone level may increase slightly within the first hour after taking extra insulin but after that, it should go down. If you use an insulin pump, you should remember to take extra insulin with a pen or syringe, *not* with the pump, and to change out the insulin/tubing/infusion set.

The A1C test

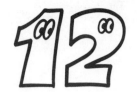

A1C (HbA_{1c}) is the name for the test used to measure average glucose control over a longer period of time. It is named after a subgroup of adult hemoglobin, the red pigment in blood cells, (compared to fetal hemoglobin, HbF) in which glucose molecules are hooked to the hemoglobin molecules in the red blood cells. Hemoglobin binds and transports oxygen in the red blood cells. The A1C test is based on red blood cells living approximately 120 days. They are produced in the bone marrow and are normally destroyed and recycled in the spleen. During the red blood cell's life span, glucose is bound to its hemoglobin depending on how high or low the blood glucose level is.[308]

A1C is a measure of the percentage of the hemoglobin in the red blood cells that has glucose bound to it. This reflects an average measurement of the blood glucose levels during the last 2-3 months.[25,494,739] The blood glucose levels from the week prior to testing will not be included in the reading as this fraction of A1C is not stable. If A1C is monitored at regular intervals (at least every three months) at the diabetes clinic, the results will provide a good summary of how your glucose control has been throughout the year.

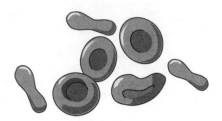

Hemoglobin in the red blood cells takes up oxygen in the lungs and transport it to the cells. They take carbon dioxide from the cells back to the lungs. During their lifetime in the blood circulation, glucose also sticks to hemoglobin, which can be measured by A1C.

It is important to remember that A1C reflects an average of your blood glucose levels. You can get an acceptable A1C reading with a combination of high and low blood glucose values. More often than not, you will feel better when your blood glucose level is relatively even. However, there is no scientific evidence that you will have more complications as a result of your diabetes if your blood glucose level is unstable than if your blood glucose readings are all the same, assuming that A1C is unchanged too. On the contrary, some recent data indicate that it might be the other way around (see page 315).[193]

It is more difficult to obtain an acceptable A1C value during puberty, since the secretion of growth hormone will raise your blood glucose levels.[226] During puberty it is not uncommon to have an increase in A1C of up to 1% (for example from 7 to 8%), even if you are as careful with your diabetes as you were before puberty.[558]

What level should A1C be?

It is difficult to state an interval within which your A1C should be because different laborato-

---

A1C

⟫ Glucose is bound to hemoglobin in the red blood cells.

⟫ The level of A1C depends on the blood glucose levels during the life span of the red blood cells.

⟫ A red blood cell lives for about 120 days.

⟫ A1C reflects the average blood glucose during the previous 2-3 months.[739]

A1C and blood glucose

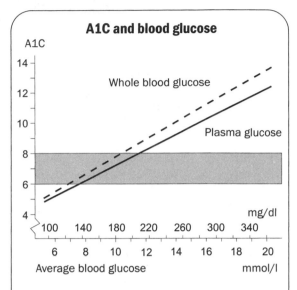

Your A1C value depends on the average blood glucose levels during the last 2-3 months. A 1% increase in A1C (measured with DCCT-equivalent method) means that you have had an average increase of approximately 35 mg/dl (2 mmol/l) in blood glucose levels compared to when your last test was taken.[646] The graph shows readings from the American DCCT study and is redrawn from reference [646]. The solid line shows the relationship between A1C and plasma glucose (11% higher than blood glucose in this study [269]). Aim at having an A1C value of 7% or below if possible.[25] If it is above 8%, you and your diabetes team have some work to do together, assessing and revising your diabetes care.[25]

A1C	Plasma glucose		Whole blood glucose	
%	mmol/l	mg/dl	mmol/l	mg/dl
5	5.6	103	5.1	92
6	7.6	138	6.9	124
7	9.6	173	8.6	156
8	11.5	208	10.4	188
9	13.5	243	12.2	219
10	15.5	278	13.9	251
11	17.5	314	15.7	283
12	19.5	349	17.4	314

This table from reference [646] shows the mean glucose values that a certain A1C value represents. Most meters used nowadays display plasma glucose.

A1C in different studies

A1C, % (average of all studies)	6.0	8.0	10.0
Linköping, Sweden [97]	5.4	7.4	9.5
Stockholm, Sweden [637]	5.0	7.1	9.2
Oslo, Norway [175]	6.6	8.3	10.1
Steno, Denmark [263]	6.7	8.7	10.8
DCCT, US [191]	6.3	8.4	10.5

Unfortunately A1C values are not the same when measured at different laboratories. Remember this when you compare your own A1C with the results of studies you find, for example on Internet. The table is from reference [465].

ries have different reference values. Many laboratories have the reference values of their methods at the same level as the DCCT reference laboratory,[190] and this is the recommended standard in Canada,[127] US and UK.[528] The American Diabetes Association recommends that the goal of therapy in adults and adolescents should be an A1C below 7% and that the treatment regimen should be re-evaluated in patients with repeated A1C above goals.[25] The Canadian Diabetes Association recommends that adolescents should aim for an A1C below 7%; that children 5 to 12 years old should aim for an A1C below 8%; and that in children under 5 years, an A1C below 9% is acceptable.[127]

Many studies have shown that with an A1C value of less than 8% the risk of long-term blood vessel complications will be considerably less.[191,638] If your A1C is above 9% we feel that this is unfair to your body since we know that in the long run it will sustain damage from this (see "Lowering the risk of complications" on page 314).

As of today there is no international standard for measuring A1C but a true reference laboratory method is under development.[374,453] A given blood test can have values ranging from 8% to almost 15% in different laboratories.[82]

To know what your A1C value really means you should compare it with the results of one of the long-term studies (see page 316). The NGSP (National Glycohemoglobin Standardization Program) has developed a standardization allowing laboratories to relate their results to those of the DCCT and a majority of laboratories in the US, Canada and UK already give their answers in DCCT numbers. Many other countries are also standardizing their A1C methods to show DCCT equivalent numbers, enabling centers and patients in different countries to compare their results. A1C methods calibrated to give the same values as the DCCT study are most useful since you can compare your own value directly with the results of the study. If you have 7% with this method, you know that the risk of long-term complications is low while an A1C of 9% is a warning signal of considerably increased risks. In Sweden the readings are approximately 1% lower than the DCCT numbers.[507]

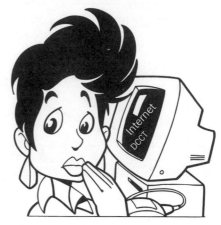

Many countries (US, Australia, UK, Denmark, France, Netherlands among others) have standardized their A1C monitoring methods to show DCCT-equivalent numbers. In times of increased international communication it is very important to check the level of the A1C method if you read about the results of studies from different countries.

Studies of adults have shown that those with a lower A1C experience better levels of psychological well-being. This includes less anxiety and depression, improved self-confidence and a better quality of life.[368] This has also been confirmed in children and adolescents (see page 348).[375]

The occurrence of severe hypoglycemia will limit how low an A1C the individual person can achieve. An A1C within the range for individuals without diabetes usually means they are at high risk of severe hypoglycemia and/or hypoglycemia unawareness. In the DCCT study, patients with low A1C had a significantly higher risk for severe hypoglycemia.[194] However, the risk decreased during the years of the study. At centers where intensive insulin treatment has been routinely implemented for a longer time, the relationship between the A1C value and severe hypoglycemia is not as pronounced.[575,782]

Is checking your A1C worthwhile? For whose benefit is the A1C test being done? Many

patients feel as if they are visiting a "control station", and being examined by health professionals to see how well they have "behaved themselves". From the professional point of view, however, the A1C test is most valuable to individuals with diabetes themselves. When you see the reading, you will know if your way of life over the last three months has allowed you to achieve the average blood glucose level you want for the future. It may be difficult to manage this every time but we often see teenagers taking such a degree of responsibility for their own health that it seems natural for them to say: "Oh, now my A1C has increased again. I will have to do something about it." And without anything more being said at the clinic, the A1C value comes right down by the next visit.

When the A1C method was introduced, 240 adults with diabetes measured it every third month without otherwise changing their diabetes treatment otherwise.[475] After one year, the average A1C value was unchanged but it turned out that those with very low values had increased them and those with high values now

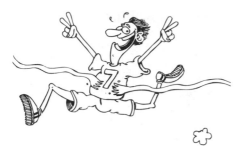

Set up your own personal goal for your A1C in collaboration with your diabetes team. This goal will be different for different people and perhaps also different during different times of your life. It may be more difficult to achieve the same A1C level for example at times when you are having problems at home or at work. By competing with yourself and setting a reasonable goal you will have a fair chance of winning your race.

had lower, showing the benefit of knowing your A1C level.

How often should you check your A1C?

A1C should be checked regularly every third month in all people with insulin-dependent diabetes.[25] A high level (> 8-9% with DCCT numbers or an equivalent method) is not acceptable, considering the risk of future complications. If your A1C is this high, it is a good idea to check it every month until it has gone back to an acceptable level. In children and adolescents, the A1C value is usually slightly higher (~0.4%) in the autumn and winter than in the spring or summer.[576]

After a visit to your diabetes healthcare team you may feel more motivated to "get your act together", and keep your blood glucose readings low. However, after a few weeks this determination can slip to the back of your mind, as daily life gets back in the way again. It is important to remember that it was not only insulin treatment that was intensive in the DCCT study. A1C was taken at every visit with monthly intervals, and telephone contact was

A1C goals by age

	DCCT method and equivalent
Normal value, person without diabetes	4.1-6.1%
Toddlers and preschoolers (<6 years)[703]	<8.5 (but > 7.5%)
School age (6-12 years)[703]	<8.0%
Adolescents and young adults [703]	< 7.5%*
Needs improving and re-evaluation of treatment [25]	8-9%
Not acceptable High risk of complications	> 9%
High risk of severe hypoglycemia (if not in "honeymoon" phase)	< 6%

There may be individual differences in the A1C value it is realistic to achieve. Discuss with your diabetes team what value may be realistic for you.

* A lower goal (<7.0%) is reasonable if it can be achieved without excessive hypoglycemia.

made between the visits. So get into a routine of visiting your diabetes healthcare team every month to check A1C until it has come down below 8%, preferably to 7.5% or lower.

Some clinics send their A1C tests to the laboratory, so it may be some days before you get the result while others ask you to send in a blood sample a week before the clinic. Others use a desktop method (such as DCA-2000®) that gives a result after a few minutes.

Even if your blood glucose control is improving and your tests are showing lower readings, it will still take some time for this to show in your A1C. Half the change will show after about one month, and three quarters of the change after two months.[739] If you start with a very high A1C (12-13%) and normalize your blood glucose levels completely (as often happens at diagnosis) it will go down by approximately 1% every tenth day.[738]

Can my A1C be "too good"?

If you have a very low A1C your average blood glucose is low and you may have a high risk of developing serious hypoglycemia without any warning symptoms ("hypoglycemic unawareness", see page 48), unless you are in the remission phase (see page 193). If you have a low A1C (< 6-7%) and problems with severe hypoglycemia or hypoglycemia unawareness, it may be a good idea to aim for a slightly higher blood glucose level.

In very young children (under 2 years of age) the brain is still developing and repeated severe hypoglycemic episodes and seizures can damage the brain (see page 47). In pre-school children, avoiding severe hypoglycemia should have the highest priority and it may be necessary to accept a slightly higher A1C.

A1C when travelling

Sometimes you will want to know your A1C but for one reason or another, it may be difficult to visit a diabetes clinic. For example, you may want to test your A1C at shorter intervals after a change in your insulin dose. A home test for monitoring A1C may then be practical (Metrika A1C Now). Another way is to put a few drops of blood on a filter paper and send it to the laboratory. This might be particularly useful if you are travelling, and cannot get hold of a doctor who knows enough about you or your diabetes. If you have well-controlled diabetes, sending an A1C test every three months may be fine. You can call your diabetes team to discuss the result.

If your healthcare team uses "A1C by mail" for routine testing, make sure you have taken the test long enough in advance to have the results ready in time for the visit.

Is it worth taking tests?

A Belgian study of children and young adults with an average A1C of 6.9% found that A1C was affected both by the actual number of tests taken (on average up to 77 blood glucose tests per month) and the number of visits to the dia-

---

For how long do blood glucose levels affect A1C?

Your recent blood glucose level affects A1C much more than that from 2-3 months ago. However, your values during the last week will not show on most methods since this fraction of A1C is very unstable. Of a given A1C value, the contribution of the blood glucose is (counting backwards): [739]

Day	1-6	very low
Day	7-30	50%
Day	31-60	25%
Day	61-90	15%
Day	91-120	10%

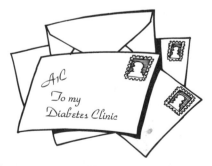

Send an A1C test by mail to your diabetes healthcare team if you are away from home for any length of time, or bring along a A1C home test kit.

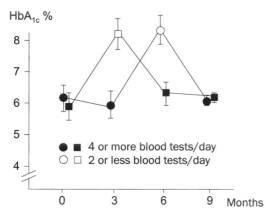

HbA$_{1c}$ %

● ■ 4 or more blood tests/day
○ □ 2 or less blood tests/day

In this study, 2 groups of patients took 2 or 4 blood glucose tests/day during 3 month periods. The glucose control was significantly better in both groups when they were taking four tests a day. [681] The A1C values are recalculated from HbA$_1$, an older method of analysis.

betes healthcare team (on average 6.6 visits/patient/ year).[220]

It is important to reflect on the reasons for your blood glucose values and, if necessary, to take action and change your insulin doses after having evaluated the tests. The blood glucose level will not improve by merely measuring it. Remember that the tests are for your own sake, not just to show your diabetes nurse or doctor. (See also "Lowering the risk of complications" on page 314.)

Fructosamine

Monitoring fructosamine is a method of measuring the amount of glucose that is bound to proteins in the blood. The value reflects the blood glucose level during the last 2-3 weeks. Fructosamine can be good indicator during times of rapid changes in glucose control, for example when you start with a new method of treatment. However, if you only take a fructosamine test every third month you will not get a representative measurement of your glucose control over a longer period of time. This method, therefore, is not recommended for routine monitoring of long-term glucose control.[25]

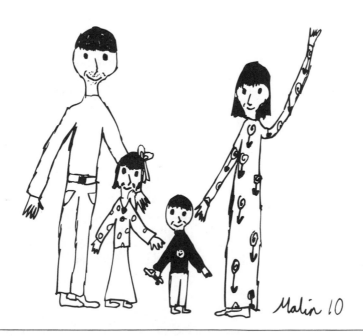

Injection technique

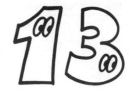

The only way insulin can work on the cells is by binding to the receptors on the cell surface. Because of this, insulin will take effect only when it has entered the bloodstream and the bloodstream has supplied it to the cells. Today, the only practical method of administration is by injection or infusion. However, a great deal of research is currently being carried out to explore alternative ways of administration (see page 329).

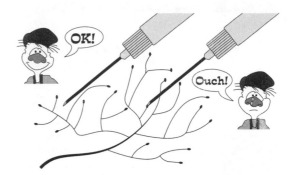

Nerve fibers look like thin branches of a tree. If you hit a nerve you will feel more pain than if you inject between the nerve fibers.

Getting used to injections

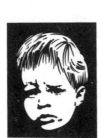

Having an injection is never going to be pleasurable. It is an annoyance at best, and at worst it can be painful, certainly at the beginning. But most people can adapt to most things, if they are allowed to take them at the right pace. Most school-age children learn quickly how to give themselves injections. The average age for learning this is 8 years.[817] However, there are a few children and adolescents who find them close to unbearable even after many years of diabetes.[331] The use of indwelling catheters (Insuflon®, see page 122) may help to decrease the injection pain for someone who is new to injections, especially if they use multiple injections from the start.[337]

Injections for parents

How do you teach yourself or your child to take or give insulin injections? It helps if the child can play with the pen or syringe and inject in teddy bears or dolls. The first step is usually to practice injecting oranges and then to inject a nurse or parent. After this, they may be ready to try an ordinary injection on their own. It is very important for adults to show the children in their care that giving themselves injections is not such a big deal. If mom and dad can overcome their fear of needles, the child will find it a lot easier to learn how to self-inject. Let small children try injections (giving saline, not insulin) and blood glucose monitoring on their parents (and perhaps also on a brave brother, sister or grandparent) as often as they want to, as this will demonstrate that injections are not dangerous. But remember that needles should not be shared! Use a new needle for each person. If you are the parent of a young child with diabetes, try to put yourself in the child's situation and think how it would appear if your parents appeared to be scared of having injections. "I am supposed to take several injections every day the rest of my life and yet my mom doesn't want to have one. Nor does dad, but they are grown up and can do just about anything... Having an injection must be something terrible!"

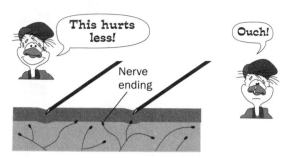

Try to find an injection site that hurts less when you press the needle against your skin!

Don't tell younger children too far ahead when it's time for an injection or blood glucose test. Many children will become anxious if they know something unpleasant will happen too far in advance. Other children want to know exactly and in plenty of time what will happen and when. Try to find out which approach suits your child best.

Taking the pain out of injections

Pain is generated by thin nerves and their endings. The nerves spread like the branches of a tree. If you hit a nerve directly, this will be painful. You can test out the position of nerves by pressing the needle carefully against your skin, and feeling where it hurts more and where it hurts less. Remember to hold the needle so that the sharp end of the needle will penetrate the skin (see picture on page 112). Certain areas on your abdomen and thighs will probably hurt less than others. However, the disadvantage of always using the same places for injections is that you will soon start to develop fatty lumps (lipohypertrophy, see page 189). Insulin will be absorbed more slowly from such lumps.[824] If you insert the needle quickly with thrust, you will feel less pricking. However, some people prefer to push the needle slowly and carefully through the skin.

Where do I inject the insulin?

In the fat or in the muscle?

The recommendations for how to inject insulin have changed considerably over the years. With old (25 mm, 1 inch) needles it was natural to use a raised skin fold when injecting. When the 12-13 mm (½ inch) needles were introduced, it was thought that a perpendicular injection would deposit the insulin within the subcutaneous (fatty) tissue. However, as mentioned below, you risk injecting into muscle when using this technique, and people are now being advised again to inject at an angle into a raised skin fold,[756] except when using the very short 5 or 6 mm needles.

Insulin should be given by subcutaneous injection, i.e. into the fat beneath the skin, not into the muscle. To avoid injecting into the muscle, it

---

**Research findings:
Injection technique**

♠ In a British study, the distance from the skin to the muscle was measured using ultrasound. The conclusion was that most boys and some girls who used the perpendicular injection technique risked injecting into muscle or even into the abdominal cavity.[711]

♠ In a French study, 31% of children who used a whole-hand skin fold with perpendicular injection technique performed the injection intramuscularly. The figure was as high as 50% in young slim boys.[618]

♠ Even with an 8 mm needle there is a considerable risk of injecting into the muscle when using a perpendicular injection technique (despite lifting a skin pinch-up with a correct two-finger technique).[764]

♠ The safest way to inject with the 5-6 mm needles is to lift a skin fold with two fingers and inject at a 45° angle.[376]

is important to lift a skin fold with the thumb and index finger ("two-finger pinch-up") and insert the needle at a 45° angle (see illustration on page 114).[280,756] Lifting a skin fold is important, even if you are using an 8 mm (1/3 inch) needle. With 5-6 mm needles, injections can be given without lifting a skin fold if there is enough subcutaneous fat (at least 8 mm as skin layers may be compressed when injecting perpendicularly[74]). Lean boys, however, usually have less fat, especially on the thigh.[74,711]

Wiggle the needle slightly before injecting. If the tip feels "stuck" you have probably reached the muscle. If this is the case, withdraw the needle a little before injecting. You can also inject insulin into your buttocks where there is usually a layer of subcutaneous fat that is thick enough to insert the needle perpendicularly without lifting a skin fold. The speed of injection (varied between 3 and 30 seconds) does not affect how rapidly the insulin is absorbed according to a Danish study.[360]

Some research has found that injecting into the muscle is not necessarily more painful,[355,816] but the insulin is absorbed more quickly. An injection into the muscle can be experienced as

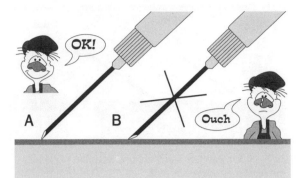

Look closely at the needle tip before pushing it through the skin. The tip of the needle is cut very sharp so that it will pierce the skin easily. If you prick the skin with the eye of the needle facing towards the skin (B) you will feel more pain than if you prick the skin with the sharp tip pointing towards the skin (A).

uncomfortable, even if it is not particularly painful. The uptake of short-acting[280] and intermediate-acting[775] insulin is increased by at least 50% from an intramuscular injection compared to a subcutaneous injection in the thigh. However, the insulin absorption is the same when comparing intramuscular and subcutaneous injections in the abdomen.[280]

The thicker the layer of subcutaneous fat, the smaller the blood flow. This results in a slower absorption of insulin. In one study, short-acting insulin (8 units were injected into the abdomen) was absorbed twice as fast from a subcutaneous fat layer of 10 mm (3/8 inch) compared to 20 mm (3/4 inch).[362] The same result was found in patients using insulin pumps. You can take advantage of this phenomenon by injecting where the subcutaneous fat is thinner, if you wish the insulin to take effect more quickly. Also, insulin that is injected above the navel will be absorbed slightly more quickly than insulin injected below or beside the navel.[283]

Some people find it more convenient to inject themselves through clothing. Although this can cause unpleasant skin reactions, these seem to be unusual.[268] However, it is more difficult to get hold of a proper skin fold through clothing,

---

Recommended injections sites

Rapid-acting insulin	Abdomen (belly)
Short-acting insulin	Abdomen (belly)
Intermediate-acting insulin	Thighs or buttocks
Long-acting (Ultralente, Humulin U)	Thighs or buttocks
Long-acting Lantus	Abdomen, Thighs or buttocks

The buttocks are the preferred injection site for intermediate and long-acting insulin in children with thin subcutaneous fat on the thigh.[161] They may also be used for injecting short and rapid-acting insulin to spread the injection sites and lessen the development of fatty lumps (lipohypertrophies). The buttocks may be a better injection site for pregnant women, especially once the abdomen has become large and tight.

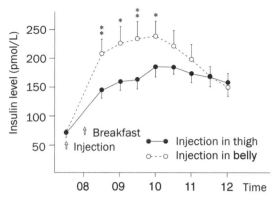

In an American study, adults took the same dose of short-acting insulin before breakfast in the abdomen one day and in the thigh one day.[51] The injection in the belly gave both a faster onset of insulin action and a higher peak level of insulin in the blood.

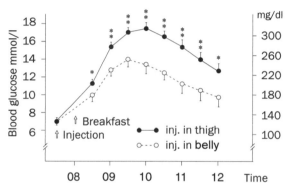

Blood glucose values from the same study as above. Because insulin enters the blood more quickly after an injection in the belly, this will cause the glucose content from breakfast to enter the cells more effectively, resulting in a lower blood glucose level.

and this increases the risk of accidentally injecting into muscle. There is also a risk of blood staining your clothes.

In the belly or the thigh?

In adults, insulin is absorbed more rapidly after a subcutaneous injection in the abdomen (belly) compared to an injection in the thigh, and the blood glucose lowering effect is also in-

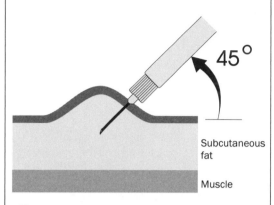

Subcutaneous injection technique 8-13 mm needle

45°

Subcutaneous fat

Muscle

① Eject a tiny amount of insulin (½-1 unit with a pen) in the air to ensure that the tip of the needle is filled with insulin.

② Lift the skin with your thumb and index finger ("two-finger pinch-up").

③ Penetrate the skin at an angle of 45° (but 90° to the skin surface).

④ Hold the skin fold and inject the insulin.

⑤ Count to 10 slowly or 20 quickly (about 15 seconds).[304] When using a syringe it is enough to wait for only a few seconds.

⑥ Withdraw the needle.

⑦ Let go of the skin fold.

⑧ If you have problems with leakage you can press a finger over the hole in the skin after the needle is withdrawn or consider using a longer needle.

When injecting into the buttocks the subcutaneous fat layer is usually thick enough to inject even with 8 and 13 mm needles without lifting a skin fold.

Disinfection of the skin before injection is not necessary as the infection risk is negligible.

creased[51,280] (see figures, page 113). The absorption from a subcutaneous injection in the belly is comparable to that of an intramuscular injection in the thigh.[280] This is caused by an

Subcutaneous injection technique
5-6 mm needle

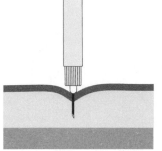

Subcutaneous
fat

Muscle

① Eject a tiny amount of insulin (½-1 unit with a pen) in the air to ensure that the tip of the needle is filled with insulin.

② The 5-6 mm needle can be used for perpendicular injections if the subcutaneous tissue is at least 8 mm thick,[74] otherwise you need to pinch a skinfold.

③ Penetrate the skin at an angle of 90°.

④ Inject the insulin.

⑤ Count to 10 slowly or 20 quickly (about 15 seconds).[304] When using a syringe it is enough to wait for only a few seconds.

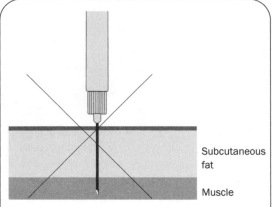

Subcutaneous
fat

Muscle

If you inject at a 90° angle with a 12-13 mm needle, there is a considerable risk of accidental intramuscular injection. This risk is substantial even with the shorter 8 mm needle if you inject in areas with a thin subcutaneous layer, such as the outside of the thigh, the upper arm or the sides of your body.[764] Insulin from an intramuscular injection is absorbed more quickly into the bloodstream and this will give you a stronger but shorter effect from the insulin dose. However, you can take advantage of this type of injection in the thigh if you want your insulin to start working more quickly, or if you have problems with lipohypertrophies (see page 189).

If you inject with the needle held at right angles to the body with an 8 or 13 mm needle, into the abdomen or belly, you run a considerable risk of injecting the insulin directly into your abdominal cavity.[282]

increased blood flow in the subcutaneous fat in the belly compared to that in the thigh.[51] The insulin uptake from the buttocks is quicker than from the thigh but not as quick as from the belly.[582] In some countries, the upper and outer area of the arm is used for subcutaneous injections as well, the uptake being similar to that in the thigh.[747] This injection site is not recommended in other countries (like Sweden) since the subcutaneous layer is very thin and it is difficult to lift a skin fold at the same time as injecting at an angle of 45°.

The absorption of intermediate-acting insulin (NPH-insulin) is better balanced after an injection in the thigh and will give a lower insulin effect early in the night and a higher insulin effect later in the night, compared to an abdominal injection.[356]

As insulin is absorbed faster from the belly than from the thigh, we recommend giving the pre-meal doses of rapid-acting (or short-acting) insulin in the belly and the bedtime injection of intermediate or long-acting insulin in the thigh (or in the buttocks). It is not recommend changing the site of injection between the thigh and the belly from day to day as this will vary the effect of the insulin.[50] A young child has a smaller area on the abdomen or belly that is suitable for injections, so it is advisable to use the buttocks for rapid and short-acting insulin as well.

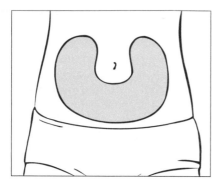

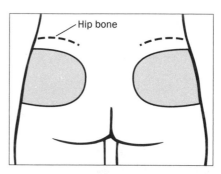

The abdomen is usually used for injections of short-acting and rapid-acting insulin (NovoLog/NovoRapid or Humalog). It will be absorbed slightly faster above the bellybutton compared to other areas of the abdomen.[283] Always use the same area for a given type of insulin, e.g. the belly (or buttocks for small children) for short-acting insulin and the thigh for bedtime insulin. It is important to rotate the injection sites within each area to avoid the development of fatty lumps (lipohypertrophies, see page 189).

You can also use your buttocks for injections. Inject a few centimeters below the edge of the hip bone. The buttocks can be used for injections in small children who have a thin subcutaneous fat layer on the abdomen or a tendency to develop fatty lumps (lipohypertrophies). The absorption of insulin is slightly slower from the buttocks than from the belly. The illustrations are from reference [707].

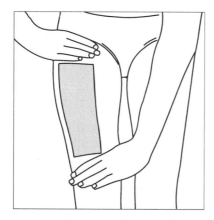

Put one hand above the knee and one below your groin. The area between your hands is suitable for injections in the thigh. Remember that insulin will be absorbed more slowly from the thigh than from the belly.

A small child using indwelling catheters for injecting short-acting insulin can try using this device for the bedtime insulin as well if it is NPH-type insulin. However, if you encounter problems with night time hypoglycemia or high blood glucose readings in the morning, it is better to give the bedtime insulin in the thigh as a separate injection (see also page 122).

Don't give short-acting insulin in the thigh late in the day. The slower uptake may result in hypoglycemia early in the night.[355]

Rapid-acting insulin

The difference in uptake between injection sites is not as pronounced when using rapid-acting insulin. If you are using NovoLog/NovoRapid,[562] or Humalog[747] the uptake is only slightly faster from the abdomen than the thigh. There was no difference in absorption between subcutaneous and intramuscular injections when using Humalog for thigh injections in a German study.[634]

New long-acting insulin

The new long-acting analog Lantus (glargine) gives the same effect when injected in the belly, thigh or arm.[588]

The absorption of insulin is affected by many other factors as well (see page 82).

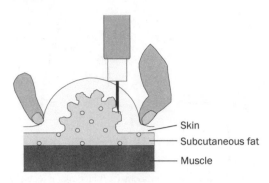

The safest way to inject with the 5-6 mm needles is to lift a skin fold with two fingers and to inject at a 45° angle.[376] However, if you inject slightly to one side with a 5-6 mm needle, there is a risk of an injection into the superficial skin (intracutaneous injection, see figure) from which the insulin may be absorbed more slowly.[726] With 5-6 mm needles, the injections can be given perpendicularly without lifting a skin fold to avoid intracutaneous injections [726] if there is enough subcutaneous fat which often is the case in girls (at least 8 mm as the skin layers often are compressed when injecting perpendicularly [74]). Lean boys, however, have a thinner subcutaneous fat layer, especially on the thigh.[74,711] When injecting into the buttocks, the subcutaneous fat layer is usually thick enough to inject without lifting a skin fold.

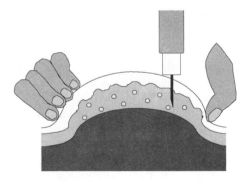

If you lift the skin with a whole-hand grip there is less risk of a superficial injection with a 5-6 mm needle. This technique, however, should not be used with the longer 8 and 13 mm needles since the muscle will be lifted as well resulting in a risk of intramuscular injection.[618]

Is it necessary to disinfect the skin?

There is no need to disinfect your skin with alcohol before injecting with an insulin pen or syringe. The risk of skin infection is negligible [534] and alcohol disinfection often causes a stinging pain when the needle is inserted. Good hygiene and careful hand-washing are more important.

If you use an insulin pump or indwelling catheter you should wash the skin with an antiseptic solution or use chlorhexidine in alcohol or a similar disinfectant if you have problems with skin infections. Some skin disinfectants contain skin moisturizers which may cause the adhesive to loosen more easily.

Storage of insulin

Insulin withstands room temperature well. Most manufacturers recommend that insulin in use should be discarded after 4 weeks at room temperature (not above 25-30° C, 77-86° F).[310] Check the package leaflet for the type of insulin you are using and the expiry date on the bottle or cartridge. At room temperature, insulin will lose less than 1.0% of its potency every month.[310] According to one study, regular, Lente and NPH insulin used for up to 110 days kept the insulin concentration at 100 U/ml.[632] Even after a year or more of being stored at room temperature, as long as it is kept in darkness, the insulin will lose only 10% of its effect.[585] Check the expiry date on the bottle or cartridge.

A practical routine is to have your spare insulin supplies stored in the refrigerator (4-8° C, 39-46° F) and the bottle or cartridge that is currently in use, stored at room temperature. Storing it at room temperature makes the preservatives more effective in killing any bacteria that may have contaminated the vial during repeated use for injections.[632] Humalog that is diluted (with sterile NPH medium) to 50 U/ml (U-50) and 10 U/ml (U-10) is stable for one month when stored at 5° C and 30° C.[722]

Don't put your insulin too close to the freezer compartment in the fridge as it cannot withstand temperatures below 2° C (36° F). Don't expose insulin to strong light or heat, such as the sunlight in a car or the heat of a sauna. Insulin loses its effect when it is stored at temperatures above 25-30° C (77° F). Above 35° C (95° F) it will be inactivated four times as fast as it is at room temperature.[315] A practical way on vacation is to store insulin in a cooled thermos flask or wrapped in moist flannel to keep it cool.

In very hot climates where there is no refrigerator available, insulin vials and cartridges can be stored in a box that is floating in an earthenware pitcher (matka) filled halfway with water without losing in activity. The pot should be kept in the shade. An Indian study showed that insulin stored in this way did not lose any of its effectiveness after 60 days with temperatures up to 40° C (104° F).[630]

You need not store human insulin in the dark as it keeps just as well in daylight (but not sunlight).[315] However, beef insulin degrades more rapidly in daylight.[315] Human insulin carried in a shirt pocket for 6 months did not deteriorate significantly more quickly than when it was stored at room temperature.[315] Never use

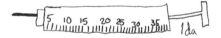

Insulin is sensitive to heat and sunlight, so don't leave it in the sun or a hot car.

short-acting regular insulin that has become cloudy. Intermediate or long-acting insulin that contains clumps or that has a frosty coating on the inside of the vial should not be used either.[654]

If you mix Lente-type insulins (Novolin N, Humulin N, Novolin L, Humulin L) with short-acting insulin in the same syringe before injecting, the insulin will start acting more rapidly if you inject yourself immediately after mixing insulin from refrigerated vials [601] (see also page 79).

Syringes

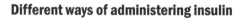

Disposable syringes have been used since the 1960s and are still the standard injection device in many countries. They are graded in units for U-100 insulin, containing 30, 50 or 100 units. Syringes are used when mixing two types of insulin into the same injection or for types of insulin that are not available in pen cartridges. You will need to be careful when travelling, especially if you are visiting countries that use a different concentration of insulin. It is particularly important not to use U-40 insulin in a U-100 syringe or vice versa. In countries where pen injectors are less common, syringes are used for multiple injection therapy. In many countries with lower economic standards, non-disposable glass syringes with needles that require manual sharpening are still used.

Different ways of administering insulin

♠	Syringes	1-5 injections/day.
♠	Insulin pen	4-6 injections/day.
♠	Insuflon®	Indwelling teflon catheter. Can be used if injection pain is a problem.
♠	Insulin pump	Delivers a basal rate over 24 hours and bolus doses at meal times.
♠	Jet injector	Injection without a needle. A thin jet stream of insulin is shot through the skin.

Mixing insulins in a syringe

➡ Start by injecting air into the bottle of inter-mediate-acting insulin (cloudy insulin).

➡ Take the syringe out of first bottle.

➡ Inject air into the bottle of the short or rapid-acting insulin (clear insulin).

➡ Draw up the short or rapid-acting insulin (clear insulin).

➡ Take out the syringe of the second bottle.

➡ Carefully insert the needle into the bottle of intermediate-acting insulin (cloudy insulin).

➡ Draw up the correct dose (without injecting into the bottle).

➡ Take the syringe out of the first bottle.

➡ It is best to draw up the insulins in this order as it matters less if a drop of short-acting insulin enters the bottle of intermediate-act-ing insulin than the other way around.

Injections with syringes

Cloudy insulin (intermediate and long-acting) needs to be mixed before use. This is done by gently turning or rolling the bottle between the hands (10 -) 20 times.[406] Do not shake the vial as this will lead to problems with air bubbles in the syringe. Start the injection by drawing air into the syringe corresponding to the dose of insulin you will inject. Then inject the air into the insulin vial, turn it upside down and then draw up the correct dose of insulin. Hold the syringe with the needle upwards, then tap on it a couple of times to get rid of the air bubbles.

Pen injectors

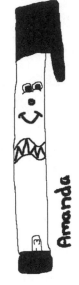

A pen injector (insulin pen) is a practical tool that is loaded with a cartridge of insulin for repeated injections. The stan-dard cartridges contain 300 units (3 ml). Pen injectors will give a more accurate dosage compared to syringes, espe-cially in the low doses.[243,392] Some pens can be adjusted to half units (NovoPen® Junior). Children will need a pen which can give single or half unit incre-ments but many teenagers and even adults find that they also appreciate being able to adjust the doses in half unit incre-ments. When you use a pen injector, start by holding the pen with the needle upwards and eject 1-2 units into the air to ensure insulin flow (an "air shot", see also page 121). Insulin pens are usually made for insulin U-100 but there are

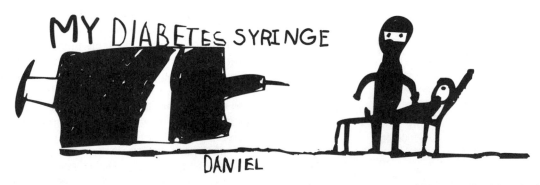

A small syringe can be experienced as a huge, frightening thing by someone who is afraid of injections. Daniel made this drawing of his insulin syringe on one of the first days in the hospital.

Needles for insulin pens

Brand	Diameter of needle	Size of needle	Length
B-D Ultra-Fine III	0.25 mm	31G	5 mm
NovoFine	0.25 mm	31G	6 mm
Penfine	0.25 mm	31G	6 mm
Unifine	0.30 mm	30G	6 mm
B-D Ultra-Fine III	0.25 mm	31G	8 mm
Penfine	0.25 mm	31G	8 mm
Unifine	0.30 mm	30G	8 mm
NovoFine	0.30 mm	30G	8 mm
Omnican mini	0.30 mm	30G	8 mm
Penfine	0.33 mm	29G	10 mm
Penfine	0.33 mm	29G	12 mm
Omnican fine	0.33 mm	29G	12 mm
Unifine	0.33 mm	29G	12 mm
B-D Ultra-Fine	0.33 mm	29G	13 mm
NovoFine	0.36 mm	28G	12 mm
Optipen	0.36 mm	28G	12 mm

pens available for U-40 as well (see page 72).

Disposable pens are also available for most insulins. They are a practical alternative for carrying spare insulin, for example when you are travelling. Make sure that you have an extra disposable insulin pen at school, at work, with your grandparents or anywhere else you visit often.

Why aren't all insulins available for pens?

Most intermediate and long-acting insulins are cloudy and the bottle must be turned or rolled (not shaken!) at least 20 times before the insulin is injected to mix it up well.[406] The pen cartridge contains a small glass or steel marble that will help stir the insulin when the pen is turned. Ultralente-type insulins (Humulin U, Ultralente) are in crystal form and the crystals will break if a glass marble is present. Therefore, no pens are available for this insulin.

Replacing pen needles

Sterile, disposable pen needles and syringes are designed for single use only. However, many patients reuse them for several injections. The risk of infected injection sites when reusing disposable needles seems to be negligible.[145,690] However, the injections may hurt more [136] since the needle becomes blunted due to tip damage after repeated use [501] and the silicon lubricant wears off. There is also some evidence that reusing needles with damaged tips causes repeated small injuries to the tissue when injecting. This can cause a release of certain growth factors that may lead to the development of fatty lumps (lipohypertrophy) which may affect the amount of insulin required and its absorption.[725]

You should replace the needle of intermediate-acting insulin after every injection, because of the risk of leakage of fluid from the cartridge or air entry (see page 121) if the needle is left on.[392] The needle may also be blocked by insulin that has crystallized inside the barrel. Remove the needle directly after the injection and put the new one on immediately before the

Needle choice guidelines [724]

Sex and age	Body type	Needle recommended
Children < 12	All	5-8 mm
Males 12-18	All	5-8 mm
Females 12-18	Normal	5-8 mm
Females 12-18	Overweight	5-8 or 13 mm
Adult males	Normal	5-8 mm
Adult males	Overweight	8 or 13 mm
Adult females	Normal	5-8 or 13 mm
Adult females	Overweight	13 mm

All injections should be given with a lifted skin fold ("two-finger pinch-up") at a 45° angle regardless of the needle used, except for injections in the buttocks where perpendicular injections without pinch-up can be used. Injections with 5-6 mm needles can be done without pinch-up if the subcutaneous fat layer is at least 8 mm.[74]

next injection. Eject a unit or two into the air with each new pen needle (the "air shot") to make sure that the tip of the needle is filled with insulin.

Different pens for day and night time insulin

It is easy to take the wrong pen injector by mistake if the pens for day time and night time insulin are similar.

To avoid taking the wrong type of insulin we recommend that you always use two completely different pens for day time and bedtime insulin, so that you can feel the difference even if it is completely dark. If you have experienced taking the wrong type of insulin even once, having two completely different pens can start to look like a cheap form of life insurance.

Air in the cartridge or syringe

When the cartridge warms up with the needle attached (e.g. when you carry it in an inner pocket), the liquid in the cartridge will expand and a few drops will leak out through the needle. When the temperature falls again, air will be sucked in. In one study the surrounding temperature was lowered from 27° to 15° C (81° to 59° F). This caused air corresponding to 4 units of insulin to be sucked into the cartridge.[135]

A particular problem will occur with intermediate-acting insulin when the temperature is lowered. As the insulin is in the cloudy substance that sinks to the bottom of the cartridge, only the inactive solution will leak out through the needle. The result will be that the remaining insulin will become more potent, up to a concentration of 120 or 140 U/ml. If the pen is stored upside down the problem will be reversed. The insulin crystals will then be closest to the needle and leak out when the temperature increases and the liquid expands. The remaining insulin will then be diluted. In one

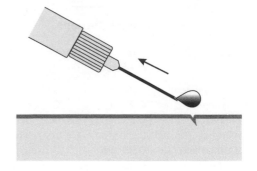

If there is air inside the pen cartridge, you may see a drop of liquid coming out from the needle-tip after your have withdrawn the needle from your skin.

study the insulin concentration in used vials and cartridges of NPH insulin that had not been mixed thoroughly varied between 5 and 200 units/ml.[406]

The problem of altered concentration will not occur with clear insulins as the insulin is completely dissolved in the liquid. However, the air as such can cause problems of accuracy. You will be less likely to have problems if you remove the needle after each injection and store

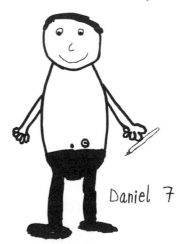

Daniel made this drawing before he was discharged from the hospital. The giant syringe is now a small insulin pen and on his stomach he has placed a small indwelling catheter. The initial fear of needles has been substituted by a more realistic view of the modern injecting equipment that is now available.

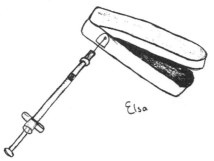

B-D Safe-Clip® can be used to cut off the needle point from both syringes and pen needles.

the pen with the needle pointing upwards, for example in the pocket of your jacket.

It is possible, on occasion, to accidentally inject a bubble of air from the syringe or cartridge along with the insulin. Subcutaneously placed air is quite harmless to the body and will soon be absorbed by the tissue. The real problem is that you will have missed out on a certain amount of insulin (as much as was displaced by the air). You may need to take a unit or two extra to compensate for this. The same also applies if you are using an insulin pump. Air injected through the tubing is completely harmless but you will have missed a certain amount of insulin at the same time which may cause problems.

Insulin on the pen needle

Sometimes a drop of insulin will leak from the tip of the needle after it has been withdrawn from the skin. The drop contains up to 1 unit of insulin and is caused by air in the cartridge which is compressed when you press the pen mechanism.[304] You can avoid this problem by waiting about 15 seconds for the air to expand before withdrawing the pen needle.[304] You can also remove the needle after each injection which will prevent air from being sucked into the cartridge. This problem will not occur when you are using a syringe because you inject all the insulin it contains. Remove the air in the pen cartridge according to the figure on page

121. Even if all air is removed, it is a good idea to hold the needle in for 10 seconds to prevent insulin dripping from the tip of the needle.[37]

Used needles and syringes

Discard used syringes, pen needles and finger pricking lancets in an empty jar or milk bottle so that no one will be pricked by mistake. You can get a special cutter to remove needle points (B-D Safe-Clip®).

How to get rid of the air in the insulin cartridge

When you replace the needle you can get rid of the air by following these steps:

① When the needle is removed, depress the pen mechanism a few times so that the pressure inside the cartridge will be increased. Tap on the cartridge to make the air rise.

② Slowly push the needle through the membrane on the cartridge.

③ Air will leak out as soon as the needle penetrates the membrane. If you push the needle through the membrane too quickly an air pocket will remain in neck of the cartridge (see illustration).

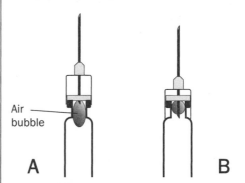

Push the needle slowly through the membrane when you replace it to allow air to leak out (A). When the needle is pushed quickly all the way in, a small pocket of air is formed in the neck of the cartridge (B).

Injection aids

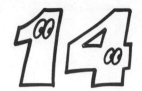

The development of thinner needles means that injections for adults are now less painful than they used to be.[516] However, in a double-blind study, children and adolescents did not appear to feel a difference in the amount of pain experienced from 0.30-0.40 mm needles.[335] "Placebo injections" (no needle was attached to some pen injectors, but the people in the study were not aware if this was the case) caused significantly less pain. This contradicts the common belief that the needles of today are so thin that most of the experienced pain is psychological in origin.

Automatic injectors

An automatic injector will thrust the needle very quickly through the skin, and this keeps pain to a minimum. With one type (Injecto-matic®, Inject-Ease®) the syringe needle is pushed through the skin automatically, but you have to push the insulin in yourself. A similar device (PenMate™) is available for the pen injectors from NovoNordisk. With another type (Autoject®) the syringe needle is pushed in and the insulin is injected automatically. The Dia-pen® both inserts the needle and injects the insulin automatically. The Autopen® is a pen injector that injects the insulin automatically after you have pricked the skin yourself with the needle.

Jet injectors

A jet injector uses very high pressure to form a thin jet stream (thinner than a needle) of insulin that penetrates the skin. The insulin is absorbed quickly and the glucose control can be as good as it is with an insulin pump.[142,392] Some find the device less painful while others experience the pain of a jet injector to be comparable to that of an ordinary injection needle. Bleeding, bruising, and delayed pain after the injection have been described.[389] A jet injector might be a good alternative for patients with pronounced nee-dle-phobia if the person is not helped by using Insuflon. However, some children may find the device very noisy when the insulin mechanism is triggered.

Insuflon

We like to make the introduction of injections at the onset of diabetes as painless as possible. Our present policy is to give all pre-school children their injections by means of indwelling catheters (such as Insuflon®) when their diabetes is newly diagnosed. Older children and adolescents are also given the chance to try this method during their first week of subcutaneous

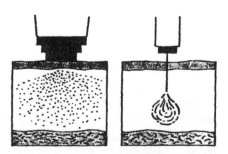

With a jet injector, the insulin is pressed through the skin by using a very high pressure. Once inside, it will spread more widely (left picture), compared with the depot from a regular injection with a pen or syringe (right picture).

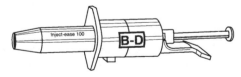

The Inject-Ease will insert the syringe needle automatically when you press the spring.

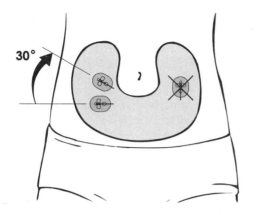

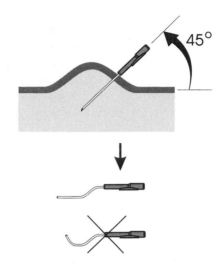

Use the shaded area of the abdomen for insertion of the indwelling catheter (or pump needle). Insert it in a horizontal position or up to 30° from a horizontal line. Otherwise there is a risk of bending the catheter when you lean forwards. If you have problems with fatty lumps (lipohypertrophies) you can insert the indwelling catheter in the buttocks as well.

Aim at an angle of 45° to the skin when you are inserting Insuflon or a pump needle/catheter. After removal, you can check the catheter profile to see how it was inserted. A "fish-hook" appearance (lower picture) indicates that it was inserted too superficially.

injections after diagnosis. We take all the blood glucose tests by means of an intravenous cannula. These procedures ensure as little pain as possible in the early stages of what will be a life-long relationship with diabetes. After a week or so, the child has had time to adjust psychologically and learn the correct injection techniques. When this has been mastered, he or she can start to try regular injections. Children are given a choice of which injection method to use when they are discharged from hospital. Some 20-25% continue with indwelling catheters while the others choose to start giving themselves regular injections. Insuflon is even used by many adults who find the injections painful

or uncomfortable. In children and adolescents, the use of indwelling catheters from the onset of diabetes has decreased pre-injection anxiety, injection pain and other injection problems significantly.[339]

The use of indwelling catheters makes multiple injection treatment for small children much easier. It is also helpful for people who are not used to giving insulin by injection. Such people may include grandparents, babysitters or day-care staff. In addition, an indwelling catheter also makes it easier to give extra injections if they

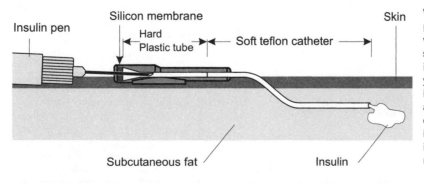

When using Insuflon you pierce a silicon membrane with the needle instead of the skin. The soft teflon catheter is placed under the skin, and you inject the insulin through it. The catheter is replaced on average every 4-5 days. This can easily be done at home. If it is painful, you can use a topical anesthetic cream before replacement.

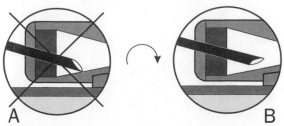

A   B

Insert the needle with the opening of the tip directed towards your skin and it will slide in more easily (picture B). Wiggle the needle sideways and rotate it if it still gets stuck.

are needed, as an additional injection will not involve the child in any extra pain. This can be particularly useful in situations such as, for example, choosing to give a child half an insulin dose before a meal even though you cannot be sure just how much that child will eat. This leaves you with the option of giving the child some extra insulin after the meal depending on how much he or she actually has eaten.

Children using indwelling catheters are probably at less risk of developing needle-phobia through having been spared traumatic injections during their early experience of diabetes.[339] One study showed that, in particular, the younger patients using indwelling catheters and multiple injection treatment would have found this method more difficult to accept if indwelling catheters had not been available.[331]

When should the catheter be replaced?

The average time between replacements is 4-5 days.[329] Some patients will be quite comfortable replacing their catheter once a week while others may need to replace it twice a week. If you disinfect the site with alcohol before inserting the catheter, you will cut the risk of infection.

Which insulin can be given in the catheter?

Small children usually use the same indwelling catheter both for short or rapid-acting insulin at

mealtimes and for bed-time insulin of NPH-type (Novolin N, Humulin N, Insuman NPH). However, if the bedtime insulin needs a longer-acting time, it is better to give it as a separate injection in the thigh. Older children usually accept this easily. It is not advisable to mix insulins of lente-type (Monotard, Humulin L, Ultralente) with short (Novolin R, Humulin R) or rapid-acting insulin (NovoLog/NovoRapid, Humalog) to give in the catheter since part of the short or rapid-acting effect will vanish (see "Mixing insulins" on page 79). However, if the person is already coping well with mixing these types of insulin, there should be no disadvan-

---

Tips for using indwelling catheters

➡ Use topical anesthetic cream (EMLA®, ELA-Max®) when inserting the catheter in small children and when new to the technique. Apply it for 1½ -2 hours before insertion.

➡ Lift a skin fold and insert Insuflon at a 45° angle (see figure on next page). Lift the skin with three or four fingers if the subcutaneous tissue is thin, as is likely to be the case in small children.

➡ Insert with a slight thrust and there will be less risk of "peel-back".

➡ Apply end of the adhesive that covers the insertion site first. Never try to remove an adhesive that is already stuck to the skin.

➡ Insert the injection needle with the opening turned towards the skin and it will not get stuck on the plastic wall. Rotate the needle gently. (See figure on page 124.)

➡ Use an adhesive of stoma-type (such as Compeed™) if you experience itching or eczema from the enclosed adhesive.

➡ Use an 8-10 mm needle for both pens and syringes and there will be no risk of piercing the teflon catheter by pushing the needle too far in. With the new Insuflon design that will be introduced soon, different needle lengths may be used. Check this with the inserted instructions.

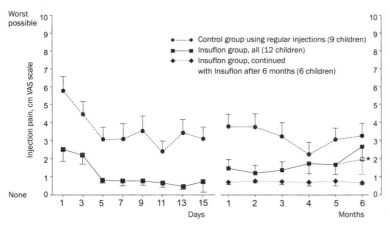

Injection pain in children younger than 8 years using indwelling catheters for introducing insulin injections at the onset of diabetes.[339] This study demonstrated a reduction in pre-injection anxiety, injection pain and other injection problems over a six-month period. Those children who continued to use Insuflon throughout the whole study scored the pain even lower.

(*Data from two children were excluded; one skipped Insuflon for a week due to eczema problems, one had pneumonia).

tage giving them through an indwelling catheter. Mixing Lantus and rapid-acting analog insulin in a syringe before injection did not affect the 24 hour glucose values in one study.[427] If Lantus is to be given via Insuflon, one should give this insulin first.

Dead space

The dead space of the catheter (the hollow inside that will be filled with insulin with the first injection) is approximately half a unit of insulin, measured in a clinical setting.[338] If the doses are very small, one can add 0.5 extra unit with the first injection after replacing an indwelling catheter.

When you give yourself your bedtime insulin, the catheter will already be filled with short or rapid-acting insulin. This will partly be exchanged for intermediate-acting insulin during the injection. Remaining in Insuflon will be a mixture of approximately 0.3 units of bedtime insulin and 0.2 units of short or rapid-acting insulin.[338] In practice, these tiny amounts of insulin are usually insignificant.

Infection and redness

A very small number of patients develop infections requiring antibiotic treatment (one out of 140 patient months or one out of 850 used catheters). If you develop an infection of the catheter canal in the subcutaneous tissue, it is likely to cause redness and/or pain around the insertion site. If you have problems with redness or infections at the insertion site, we recommend you to use chlorhexidine in alcohol (Hibiclens™ or similar disinfectant) for skin disinfection and hand washing. Don't use products containing a skin moistener since this causes the adhesive to come loose more easily.

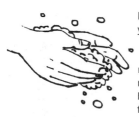

Hygiene is more important if you use an insulin pump or indwelling catheter. Always wash your hands before replacing the catheter. We recommend using chlorhexidine in alcohol for disinfection of the insertion site.

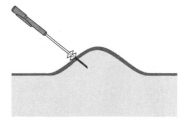

The catheter can peel backwards on the metal needle (called "peel-back") if you penetrate the skin too slowly. This is a typical beginner's problem.

Research findings: Insulin absorption and Insuflon

♠ A1C test results, blood glucose levels, and insulin were all unaltered when using Insuflon during a two-month so called cross-over study.[330]

♠ Studies of insulin pump users have shown both an unchanged insulin absorption during five days' use [583] and an increased absorption after three days of using the same injection site.[496]

♠ Studies from Finland with indwelling catheters show no change in insulin absorption during five days of use.[423]

♠ A Swedish study using radio-actively labelled insulin did not show any change in absorption during four days of using indwelling catheters.[332]

Problems with indwelling catheters?

Problem	What to do about it
Adhesive comes off	Wash the **anesthetic** cream (EMLA®, ELA-Max®) off carefully with water. Apply Skin-Prep™, Mastisol™ or Tincture of Benzoin™ that leave a sticky film when drying. Warm the adhesive with your hand after application. Apply extra tape if necessary.
Itching, eczema from adhesive	Apply Hydrocortisone cream. Use a stoma type adhesive (e.g. Compeed®).
Sticky traces of adhesive	Wipe off with remover such as Detachol™ or Uni-Solve™.
Infection/irritation at the injection site	Wash hands and skin with chlorhexidine in alcohol (Hibiscrub™). Replace the catheter more frequently.
Leakage of insulin	An increased pressure when injecting indicates a bent catheter. Replace it! Use 8-10 mm needles.
Sore skin from plastic wings	Apply a piece of tape beneath the wings.
Scars in the skin from old catheters	Caused by an infection of the injection site. Replace Insuflon more frequently. See infection advice above.

Redness and/or itching can be caused by an allergic reaction to the adhesive. Application of 1% hydrocortisone cream usually helps. If the

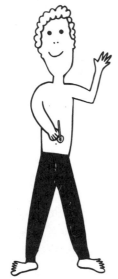

RoBERT 8 years

An eight-year old boy made this drawing of himself using an indwelling catheter. Before he started using this, his father had to come home from work twice a day to help his mother hold him, so they could give him his insulin injections.

problem continues, we have successfully used a stoma type adhesive (such as Compeed® or Duoderm®). Cut a hole for the catheter hood before applying it. Another alternative is to apply a skin film (for example Tegaderm®) first, and insert Insuflon through it, putting the regular adhesive on top of the skin film. Itching can also be caused by perspiration in hot weather or during sports activities. The itching usually disappears when the person stops sweating.

Adjusting insulin doses

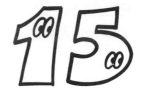

Starting insulin treatment

When type 1 diabetes is first diagnosed, treatment with subcutaneous insulin is started without delay. The total dose may be as high as 1.5-2 units/kg/day (0.7-0.9 units/lb/day) in the period immediately after diagnosis, but it soon goes down. Smaller children are more sensitive to insulin and usually need fewer units/kg. However, insulin dosages are very individual and two children of the same age often need quite different amounts.

2-dose treatment

In the UK and many other countries, most children are started on 2 injections/day. Many children will use combinations or mixtures of short (Novolin R, Humulin R) or rapid-acting insulin (NovoLog, Humalog) and intermediate-acting insulins (Novolin N, Humulin N) before breakfast and before dinner. These doses and mixtures are adapted to the size of meals and usual activity levels. With a 2-dose treatment it is essential that the last meal of the day is taken immediately before going to bed (bedtime snack) to prevent night time hypoglycemia.

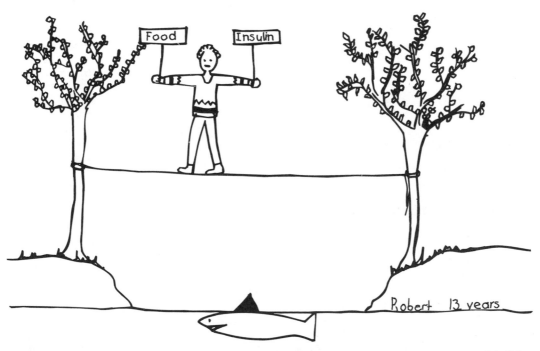

Many things need to be balanced in your body to keep the blood glucose level steady. It isn't easy to make all the pieces fit, and it can often be difficult to work out exactly what went wrong. Sometimes, we just have to accept that there is no obvious explanation for why the blood glucose level was high or low at a given time. In this drawing, Robert uses a shark to illustrate how it feels when his body loses this balance.

3-dose treatment

A 3-dose insulin treatment usually consists of a combination of rapid or short-acting and intermediate-acting insulin for breakfast, rapid or short-acting insulin for dinner and intermediate-acting insulin at bedtime. This may be a suitable regimen for a smaller child, especially if it is difficult to find someone who can give the lunchtime dose at school or in the day center. A combination of rapid or short-acting and intermediate-acting insulin at breakfast may also be a good solution for the teenager who tends to forget lunchtime insulin doses when at school or out with their peer group. In situations like this, pre-mixed insulin that can be administered with a pen may be an alternative choice.

Multiple injection treatment

In Sweden, the US, and other countries, it is common to use a multiple injection treatment with premeal doses of rapid-acting insulin from the onset of diabetes, even for younger children and toddlers. In some places children are started on insulin pumps from the onset of diabetes but usually this form of therapy is started later. With multiple injections, premeal injections will be given for the main meals breakfast, lunch, dinner, and evening snack. An extra bedtime snack will usually be given only if the blood glucose level is low with this type of insulin regimen.

Insulin is adjusted in relation to the carbohydrate content of the meal. Before breakfast,

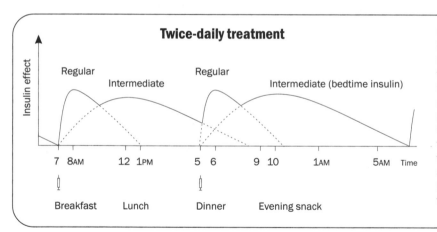

Before the introduction of the insulin pen in 1985, the usual regime was twice-daily injections, mixing short-acting and intermediate-acting insulin. The advantage was fewer injections per day. But the disadvantage was difficulty in adjusting doses to take account of changes in food intake or physical activity, and problems with night time hypoglycemia when the dinner time dose was increased.

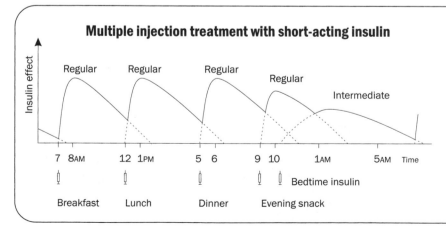

Five daily insulin doses (4 doses of short-acting insulin and 1 dose of intermediate-acting) will better mimic the body's normal meal time insulin secretion. The system is easy to understand as each insulin dose affects only one meal. Today, rapid-acting insulin is more often used for multiple injection therapy (see page 140).

higher doses of insulin are needed in relation to the size of the meal. This is due partly to increased levels of growth hormone (the dawn phenomenon) and partly to a reduction over time in the effect of the bedtime insulin dose. In addition, breakfast usually contains a greater proportion of carbohydrates than other meals (e.g. from juice, bread, cereals).

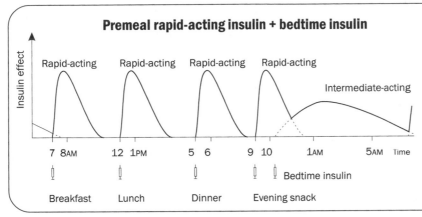

Premeal rapid-acting insulin + bedtime insulin

If you use rapid-acting insulin (NovoLog/NovoRapid or Humalog) for the premeal bolus doses you will have a better effect with that meal. However, you are likely to be short of insulin by the time of the next meal as rapid-acting insulin will not last for more than 3-4 hours at the most.

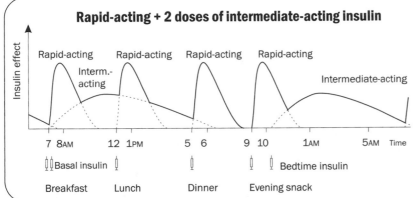

Rapid-acting + 2 doses of intermediate-acting insulin

You can take a dose of intermediate-acting NPH insulin (Novolin N, Humulin N) for breakfast to attain a better insulin effect before lunch and dinner. However, it is difficult to get this dose to last until the evening snack without risking too strong an insulin effect at lunchtime, especially in children and adolescents. A third dose of intermediate-acting insulin at lunchtime may solve the problem.

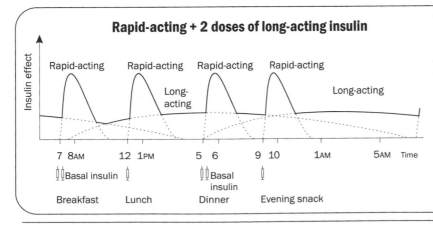

Rapid-acting + 2 doses of long-acting insulin

With long-acting insulin you will have a level of basal insulin in between meals. Previously, Ultratard and Humulin Zn were used this way, but today Lantus is more common. It gives a more even effect and is usually given only once daily, in the evening, morning or for dinner. When using small doses you may need to give it twice daily. Compare this insulin curve with the curve of a person without diabetes on page 22.

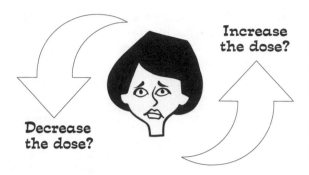

Increase the dose?

Decrease the dose?

The instructions for adjusting insulin doses in this chapter apply mainly to multiple injection treatment. However, many of the principles can be applied even if you are using a 2- or 3-dose treatment. If you are in the remission (honeymoon) phase and produce insulin of your own, you should reduce the recommended doses (see page 157).

How much does insulin lower the blood glucose level?

The actual blood glucose lowering effect of a given insulin dose depends on many factors; the meal size, the amount of insulin taken earlier in the day, the amount of exercise and even the level of stress. A dose of 0.1 unit/kg (0.5

Questions before taking insulin

① What is my blood glucose level?

② What am I going to eat?
More or less food than usual? Food with a higher or a lower carbohydrate content?

③ What am I going to do after the meal? Physical activity, normal work or school, relaxation?

④ What happened last time I was in the same situation? (Check your logbook!)

Different types of insulin treatment

Multiple injection treatment with rapid-acting insulin
(Humalog, NovoLog/NovoRapid, see page 140)

Meal	Type of insulin	% of 24 h. dose
Breakfast	Rapid-acting	15-20
	Basal insulin	15-20
Lunch	Rapid-acting	10-15
Dinner	Rapid-acting	10-15
Evening snack	Rapid-acting	10-15
Bedtime	Basal insulin	25-30

With Lantus as basal insulin ~50% is given as one dose in the evening or morning but some may need 2 doses of this insulin (see page 155).

Multiple injection treatment with short-acting insulin
(Novolin R, Humulin R)

Meal	Type of insulin	% of 24 h. dose
Breakfast	Short-acting	20-25
Lunch	"	15-20
Dinner	"	15-20
Evening snack	"	10-15
Bedtime	Intermediate-acting	25-30 (-40)

2-dose treatment

Meal	Type of insulin	% of 24 h. dose
Breakfast	Rapid-acting or short-acting	20 - 25
	Intermediate-acting	35 - 40
Dinner	Rapid-acting or short-acting	10 - 15
	Intermediate-acting	25 - 30

The pre-dinner intermediate-acting insulin can be given with the evening snack or before bedtime if a 3-dose treatment is preferred.

How much does one unit lower blood glucose?

Units/24 hours	Rapid-acting analog	Short-acting regular
20	90 mg/dl	75 mg/dl
30	60 mg/dl	50 mg/dl
40	45 mg/dl	38 mg/dl
50	36 mg/dl	30 mg/dl
60	30 mg/dl	25 mg/dl
70	26 mg/dl	21 mg/dl
80	23 mg/dl	19 mg/dl
90	20 mg/dl	17 mg/dl

The figures are from the "1800 Rule" for rapid-acting insulin [797] (divide 1800 by daily insulin dose for mg/dl, 100 for mmol/l) and "1500 Rule" for regular short-acting insulin [185,209] (divide 1500 by daily insulin dose for mg/dl, 83 for mmol/l). This method is widely used to calculate "the correction factor" or "insulin sensitivity factor", i.e. the glucose-lowering effect of one unit of insulin.[800]

If a person takes 40 units/day and has a blood glucose of 250 mg/dl (14 mmol/l) before the meal, an extra dose of 2 units will lower the blood glucose level by an additional 90 mg/dl (5.0 mmol/l) with NovoLog/Rapid or Humalog, 76 mg/dl (4.2 mmol/l) with short-acting insulin. In the same way you can subtract units from the premeal dose if the blood glucose level is low.

Units/24 hours	Rapid-acting analog	Short-acting regular
20	5.0 mmol/l	4.2 mmol/l
30	3.3 mmol/l	2.8 mmol/l
40	2.5 mmol/l	2.1 mmol/l
50	2.0 mmol/l	1.7 mmol/l
60	1.7 mmol/l	1.4 mmol/l
70	1.4 mmol/l	1.2 mmol/l
80	1.3 mmol/l	1.0 mmol/l
90	1.1 mmol/l	0.9 mmol/l

The actual blood glucose lowering effect of an extra unit is of course dependent upon many factors including food intake, insulin dose, exercise, variable absorption etc. For this reason, the tables must not be used to predict the exact lowering of blood sugar in any individual. They only show the average effect. These rules are determined for adults and the doses may be too high for children or for people who have had diabetes for a shorter period of time. By experimenting, you can find out how well they work for you. During the night, a correction dose will usually have a higher effect so you can try by giving half the above mentioned doses.

units/10 lb) body weight will give a substantial blood glucose lowering effect and extra doses in the home should rarely exceed this amount as it will only increase the risk of hypoglycemia after a couple of hours (although the newer rapid-acting insulins will be safer in this respect).

One unit of insulin given between meals will lower your blood glucose by about 20 mg/dl if you weigh 150-170 lb and 35 mg/dl if you weigh 65-90 lb (1 mmol/l if you weigh 70-80 kg and about 2 mmol/l if you weigh 30-40 kg). A more specific way of counting, is to divide 1800 (1500 for short-acting insulin) by your daily insulin dose in units and you will have the blood glucose lowering effect of one unit in mg/d/l (100 for rapid-acting and 83 for short-acting insulin to get the results in mmol/l).[209] See key fact box on page 131.

What to do if your blood glucose level is high

Don't go looking for high blood glucose readings. If you change your ordinary insulin doses on a daily basis in line with every individual blood glucose reading, you will soon find it impossible to identify which dose actually does what. The blood glucose can swing up and down like a roller coaster, resulting in frequent, and often difficult, hypoglycemic episodes without your understanding why.[59] While you may often know the reason for a temporary high or low blood glucose reading, sometimes things go wrong with no obvious explanation.

Your blood glucose is high but you are feeling perfectly well

A temporary high blood glucose level from time to time is impossible to avoid in everyday life. A person with diabetes, whether child or adult, will not necessarily feel at all unwell when this happens, nor will it affect long-term diabetes control. A temporarily very high blood glucose level (>450-550 mg/dl, 25-30 mmol/l) can often be caused by not drinking enough. If the person is able to pass plenty of urine, the blood glucose level can go down to approximately 360 mg/dl (20 mmol/l) without extra insulin.[515] If you find your blood glucose reading is very high when you are feeling fine, therefore, it may be a good idea to drink plenty of extra water or sugar-free drinks. You should also check your blood or urine for ketones (see below).

Don't take extra insulin immediately if the ketones are negative — this could cause you to become hypoglycemic after a while. A temporary high glucose will usually come down without extra measures. Wait until the next meal and then increase your insulin dose by 1-2 units (or use your correction factor, see below) *if the blood glucose level still is high.* An alternative is to have a little less to eat or to skip your snack.

When does the insulin dose have the most effect?

Time of injection	Effect when?
Rapid-acting: (NovoLog/NovoRapid, Humalog, Apidra)	
Before meal	For that meal
Short-acting: (Novolin R, Humulin R)	
Before breakfast	Until lunch
Before lunch	Until dinner
Before dinner	Until the evening snack
Before evening snack	Until midnight
Intermediate-acting: (Novolin N, Humulin N, Levemir)	
At bedtime 10 PM (multiple inj. treatment)	During the night until breakfast
2-dose treatment: Morning	Lunch and afternoon
Dinner	Evening and night
Long-acting: (Lantus, Ultralente, Humulin U)	
At dinner-time	During the night and the morning thereafter

Your blood glucose is high before a meal

This can be addressed in different ways. If you are using a correction factor based on your insulin sensitivity (see table on page 131), add the amount of insulin needed to lower your blood glucose to your target level. In other cases, increase your premeal rapid or short-acting dose by 1-2 units if you are eating a standard meal. Instead of increasing the insulin dose you can decrease the carbohydrate content of the meal if you are using multiple injection therapy (see page 135). You are usually not as hungry when the blood glucose level is high (see "Hungry or full?" on page 215). Drink water instead of milk or juice with your meal. If your blood glucose is high (> 215-270 mg/dl, 12-15 mmol/l) at snack-time, you will probably not need the snack at all.

Your blood glucose is high at bedtime

If you need to give yourself extra insulin in this situation, it is better to give rapid-acting insulin (NovoLog/ NovoRapid or Humalog), as the effect of this will usually disappear before the bedtime insulin has begun to act. There is always a risk of night time hypoglycemia when you take additional short-acting insulin before going to bed. If your blood glucose level is high (more than about 215 mg/dl, 12 mmol/l) you can increase the dose of bedtime insulin by 1-2 units or according to your correction factor. (see the algorithm on page 133 if you are using a 2-dose therapy). Check your blood glucose at 2-3 AM if you have taken extra insulin at bedtime or changed the dose.

You are feeling unwell

If you are feeling unwell, nauseous or vomiting you should check for ketones in your blood or urine. **The presence of ketones is a sign of insulin deficiency!** (See page 99.)

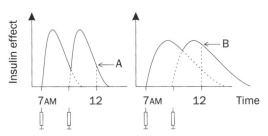

Rapid-acting insulin   Ordinary short-acting insulin

Rapid-acting insulin is preferable when the blood glucose level is high. You can give an extra dose at snack-time without risking dose overlapping and hypoglycemia, since much of the effect is gone after 2-3 hours. Compare the insulin effect at noon (arrow A) with the right chart illustrating ordinary short-acting insulin (arrow B). When taking an extra dose of rapid-acting insulin before going to bed, the effect of this dose will have waned before the effect of the bedtime dose starts.

If your blood glucose is high (>250 mg/dl, 14 mmol/l) and if ketones are present, give yourself an extra dose of insulin, (0.1 U/kg, 0.5 U/10 lb) to lower your blood glucose and block the production of ketones in the liver (see page 36). Extra insulin should not be administered more often than every second (rapid-acting) or third (short-acting) hour in case the insulin effects accumulate and cause hypoglycemia. Rapid-acting insulin (NovoLog/NovoRapid or Humalog) is the best type to use in this situation. Its quick effect means there is less risk of the doses overlapping.

If you are caring for a child with diabetes, and he or she is hungry, some chewing gum may be a good idea as it will give them something to hold in their mouth until the insulin begins to work. Also, encourage the child to drink some water or diet pop, as high blood glucose causes people to pass a lot of urine.

High blood glucose and ketones

If your blood glucose level repeatedly tests high (270-360 mg/dl, 15-20 mmol/l) and particularly if you have ketones in your blood or urine (as a sign of insulin deficiency), you need extra insulin.

① Give 0.1 units/kg (0.5 units/10 lb) of short-acting insulin or preferably rapid-acting insulin (NovoLog/NovoRapid or Humalog). See algorithm on page 133 if you are using a 2-dose treatment.

② Test your blood glucose level again after 2-3 hours.

③ Give another 0.1 units/kg (0.5 units/10 lb) if your blood glucose level has not gone down.

Do not give extra rapid-acting insulin more often than every second hour, or you will risk dose overlap resulting in hypoglycemia after a couple of hours.

Contact your diabetes team or doctor if you vomit or are in the least unsure about what you should do. This is equally, if not more, important if you are looking after a child with diabetes.

Your blood glucose level is high at the same time of the day, several days in a row

Take a blood test ~2 hours after the meal several days in a row, first ensuring that on each day the meal has a similar carbohydrate content:

Extra doses when using 2-dose treatment

When you are using a 2-dose treatment, this table can be used for extra doses of rapid-acting insulin (NovoLog/NovoRapid, Humalog) that can be given any time up to 10 or 11 PM depending on age.[736]

Blood glucose

Age, years	270-305 15-17	305-360 17-20	>360 >20	mg/dl mmol/l
0-6	0.5-1U	1-2U	2-3U	
7-11	1-2U	2-3U	3-5U	
12-15	2-3U	3-4U	4-8U	
16+	3-4U	4-6U	6-12U	

If it is > 180 mg/dl (10 mmol/l),
increase your usual dose by 1-2 units.

Change the present premeal dose of rapid or short-acting insulin. If you are using an insulin:carb ratio for calculating the dose, this needs to be adjusted to a higher amount of insulin. However, it is important that you wait a couple of days between each dose increase otherwise it will be difficult to see which change led to what.

Different ways of adjusting insulin doses

There are many different ways of adjusting insulin doses. Check with your diabetes team which method they recommend for you.

Fixed insulin doses

With this system you eat your meals and snacks at the same time of the day each day. The meal plan emphasizes having the same amount of carbohydrates for a given meal each day. A 2-dose treatment usually works along this line.

Varied insulin doses but not counting grams of carbohydrate

With this system you take premeal insulin for each meal and vary the size of the dose according to the carbohydrate content, but without

---

Important

Never decrease the amount of food to regulate your blood glucose level if you are ill. Drink sugar containing drinks if your appetite is poor!

Don't adjust insulin doses in relation to food quantities "by eye" or carbohydrate counting when you are ill. See the chapter on illness, page 258.

---

counting the exact grams of carbohydrate in each meal

Counting grams of carbohydrate to determine insulin doses

With this system you need to determine the grams of carbohydrate in each meal and you use the so called insulin-to-carbohydrate (insulin:carb) ratio to determine you insulin dose (see page 216). A correction dose for high or low blood glucose is calculated using your insulin sensitivity factor (see table on page 131).

What about the food you eat?

Once you have learnt about the way the carbohydrate content of a meal relates to your individual insulin dose, it is often possible to determine the effect of your meal on blood glucose levels just by looking. If you eat a little more carbohydrate (for example, an extra potato or some more pasta) than usual, you can take (½-)1-2 units of rapid or short-acting insulin extra if you are on a multiple injection or pump therapy. If you eat a little less, you can decrease the dose by (½-)1-2 units. If you are counting carbs, correct the dose according to your insulin:carb ratio. Measure your glucose level after ~2 hours to determine whether the dose was correct. However, if you eat some more meat, chicken or fish, you need not increase your insulin dose since this type of food does not contain carbohydrates. Make a note in your logbook for future reference in case you are confronted with a similar situation another time.

A useful "rule of thumb" is that 1 unit of insulin takes care of approximately 10 grams of carbohydrate. This applies if you eat something extra between meals which contains mainly sugar (such as cake or ice cream at a party). When eating a mixed meal, many other factors influence the blood glucose response. See also page 202. For a description of how to count

Temporary changes of the premeal dose, e.g. during illness (see p. 131 if you use a correction factor)

1-2 U implies changing the rapid or short-acting dose by 1 unit for a premeal dose of < 10 U and 2 units for a premeal dose of > 10 U. If the dose is < 3 units, change by only ½ U. The table is modified from reference [368].

Blood test before meal	Measure / Change in dose
< 60-70 mg/dl < 3.5-4 mmol/l	1) Take 10 g of glucose (3 dextrose tablets) or 1 glass of sweet juice (see table on page 62). 2) Wait 10-15 minutes before eating anything else to allow glucose to pass into the bloodstream. 3) Take the insulin after eating (just before, with short-acting). 4) You may need to decrease your dose by 1-2 units.
70-145 mg/dl 4-8 mmol/l	Take your ordinary dose.
145-200 mg/dl 8-11 mmol/l	1) Increase the dose by 1-2 U or drink water with the meal.* 2) Take the insulin just before you eat (at least 30 min. before with short-acting).
200-250 mg/dl 11-14 mmol/l	1) Increase the dose by 2-3 U or drink water with the meal.* 2) Take the insulin 10 min. before you eat. (45 min. before with short-acting)
250-360 mg/dl 14-20 mmol/l	1) Increase the dose by 2-4 U and drink water with the meal.* 2) Take the insulin 20 min. before you eat (60 min. before with short-acting), or wait until the blood glucose level returns to normal before you eat.
> 360 mg/dl > 20 mmol/l	1) Increase the dose by 0.1 U/kg (0.5 U/10 lb) body weight. 2) Same as 250-360 mg/dl.
Consider for a moment...	Why the blood glucose might be high? Missed insulin dose? Other illness or fever? Have you eaten more than usual?
Ketones?	Contact your diabetes staff, clinic/ward or emergency department if you vomit or feel generally unwell.

* if you normally drink something containing carbohydrates with the meal.

carbohydrates in a more exact manner, see page 216.

Changing the content of the meal to affect blood glucose

At times it may be an option to change the size of the meal depending on the actual blood glucose level. The feeling of fullness after a meal is often increased when the blood glucose level is high.[415] If the blood glucose before the meal is increased (145-250 mg/dl, 8-14 mmol/l) you can drink water instead of milk with the meal or decrease the carbohydrate content of the meal. If the blood glucose is more than 270-360 mg/dl, 15-20 mmol/l, it may be a good idea to wait a while after taking the insulin to let the glucose level begin to decrease before eating. The carbohydrate content can be decreased by eating less pasta, potato, rice or bread.

Reduction in food should be used very cautiously with growing children. Children themselves should be involved in discussions and any decisions about this. They should also be offered increased amounts of food later in the day to compensate. In general, witholding food or having a child eat consistently without being hungry, in an effort to control blood glucose, should be discouraged.[274] But it can be a practical solution on occasions when a child whose blood glucose is high, does not feel hungry. The feeling of fullness can be the same if the amount of non carbohydrate food is increased although the decreased amount of carbohydrate contributes to a lower glucose level after the meal.[274]

The stomach empties more slowly when the blood glucose level is high.[692] This makes it much more likely that food will still remain in your stomach from the previous meal if you have a high blood glucose level. Food will then continue to empty into the intestine (where glucose can be absorbed into the blood) even though you have not necessarily eaten recently.

What if your blood glucose level wasn't what you expected it to be?

➠ Had you eaten the usual amount of food?

➠ Was the timing between your meal and the injection correct?

➠ Had you been more active physically than usual?

➠ Were you feeling ill, with a cold or fever?

➠ Could you have had hypoglycemia with rebound phenomenon?

➠ Was your injection technique different from usual? Did you change the injection site for your premeal injection (e.g. from abdomen to thigh)?

➠ Did you inject into muscle rather than fat?

➠ Did you inject into a fatty lump (lipohypertrophy)?

➠ The variability in effect of injected insulin doses is huge, even when 2 identical doses are given under the same conditions. This variation lies outside the "human factor" and may explain much of the frustration of trying to find correct doses.

By how much at a time should the dose be changed?

If you need to change the rapid or short-acting insulin dose, for instance when you are running a temperature, while you are exercising, or when you are eating more or less food than usual (unless you are counting grams of carbohydrate), we recommend the following changes to start out with:

If your usual insulin dose is	Change the dose by
1 - 3 units	½ unit
4 - 9 units	1 unit
> 10 units	2 units

Fluids are emptied from the stomach more quickly than solid food.[778] Drink early in the course of the meal if your blood glucose is low. If it is high, it is better to wait until the end of the meal before drinking as your stomach will be more slow to empty. See also "Emptying the stomach" on page 203.

You may feel hungry even if your blood glucose level is high. This is due to a lack of glucose inside the cells which signals hunger. If you eat as usual (without taking extra insulin) despite a high blood glucose level, your blood glucose will remain high. If this continues for some time it will result in increased insulin resistance, e.g. a given insulin dose will be less effective than usual (see page 195).

Feeling ill, especially with fever, is likely to depress your appetite. In spite of this, the blood glucose level will often be high, due to an increased need for insulin during illness. You should then increase the insulin doses and try to eat the usual amount of carbohydrate. Do not attempt to reduce the carbohydrate content in the meal to compensate for a high blood glucose level if you are ill! If your appetite is poor, it is important to drink plenty and eat food with a high carbohydrate content, e.g. bread, potatoes, rice, pasta, or cereal. This will give the insulin "something to work with" (see page 258 for further advice on insulin treatment when ill).

Changing insulin doses

Check your blood glucose before and ~2 hours after meals and during the night. (See the key fact box on page 91). Aim for blood glucose values not below 70 mg/dl (4.0 mmol/l) and not above 180 mg/dl (10 mmol/l) when adjusting insulin doses. See key fact box for recommended levels before and after meals. If there are difficulties in finding a pattern in regular blood glucose monitoring, a continuous glucose measurement will give much more information (CGMS, see page 97).

Basic rules

① You cannot interpret a 24-hour glucose profile correctly if you have had hypoglycemic episodes. A high blood glucose level could be the result of a rebound phenomenon following a hypoglycemic episode. Begin by decreasing the doses to avoid hypoglycemia before attempting long-term adjustments. If you have a hypoglycemic reaction without an apparent reason (such as exercise or too little food) you should decrease the "responsible" insulin dose the following day (see table on page 61).

② Symptoms of hypoglycemia should appear at a normal level, i.e. at 65-70 mg/dl (3.5-4.0 mmol/l). If they first appear when your blood glucose has fallen below 65 mg/dl (3.5 mmol/l), you should take great care to avoid all low blood glucose levels for the next 1-2 weeks. This will help improve the situation. If you have hypoglycemic symptoms at levels above 70-80 mg/dl (4.0-4.5 mmol/l), you should resist the temptation to eat until the blood glucose has fallen to 65-70 mg/dl (3.5-4.0 mmol/l). After a couple of days, the symptoms will appear at a lower blood glucose level (see pages 43 and 58).

③ It is a good idea to try and keep the carbohydrate content of the meals and amount of physical activity as consistent as possible when you are calculating insulin:carb ratios and adjusting insulin doses.[800] The total carbohydrate content of meals and snacks is more important for the premeal insulin dosage than the type or source.[274]

④ Don't change more than one dose at a time. It is otherwise easy to end up in a vicious cycle where you don't know what has caused what.

⑤ Don't make large changes in your doses all at once. Change doses of less than 3 U by ½ U at a time, 3-10 U by 1 unit, and those more than 10 U by 2 units at a time or use your insulin:carb ratio.

⑥ Wait a couple of days between insulin changes so that you can see clearly what the outcome is. There is always a depot of insulin in your body and it will take a couple of days before this has reached equilibrium (see "Depot effect" on page 79). Intermediate-acting insulin (Novolin N, Humulin N) should not be changed more often than every 2 or 3 days. When using long-acting insulin (Lantus, Ultralente, Humulin U) you should not change the dose more often than 2 (or 3) times per week.

What is the best blood glucose level to have?

Ideally, your blood glucose readings during the day should be between 70 and 180 mg/dl (4.0-10.0 mmol/l).[32,151] If you have problems with hypoglycemic unawareness you should be careful to avoid all readings below 65-70 mg/dl (3.5-4 mmol/l, see page 48).

Blood glucose	Before meal	2 h. after meal
Ideal	70-110 mg/dl 4-6 mmol/l	90-140 mg/dl 5-8 mmol/l
Acceptable	90-130 mg/dl 5-7 mmol/l	145-180 mg/dl 8-10 mmol/l
Hypoglycemic unawareness	90-160 mg/dl 5-9 mmol/l	145-200mg/dl 8-11 mmol/l

⑦ Review blood glucose readings and insulin doses once a day when you have time to sit down and plan preliminary doses for the following day in your logbook. If you do this, you will be much less likely to make rash decisions.

⑧ Be careful about extra insulin on days when you are making adjustments to the longer acting insulins. You will otherwise distort all the information you have built up relating to the usual doses. If you feel that you need to give yourself extra insulin (if you are ill, for example) it is better to stop your blood glucose monitoring for the 24 hour profile. Start over again after a couple of days or a week when you are back to normal doses again.

For the same reason, you should not eat anything extra if you measure a low blood glucose level, between 65 and 80 mg/dl (3.5-4.5 mmol/l), but feel well when doing a 24 hour chart. This applies also to the 2-3 AM blood glucose test (but be sure to check again after ½-1 hour). You want to know the blood glucose values during a night with normal sleep, not when you have been eating. As you have no symptoms you would have slept on without eating if you had not been taking the test. If you have hypoglycemic symptoms, you may get a rebound effect which will make it difficult to interpret the blood glucose levels and then it is better to restart the 24 hour testing another day.

⑨ If you don't understand why your blood glucose reading turned out the way it did, try keeping to the same doses for another day or two. You will often see the pattern better then.

Keeping good records

Register all blood glucose readings in your logbook, otherwise you can never make an adequate judgement. If you have difficulties remembering to write them down, an electronic logbook can be a good alternative. Most blood glucose meters have memories and can be connected to a computer to be read. In an American study, patients who recorded their blood glucose readings in a logbook had lower A1C values (7.1% compared to 7.9%) than those who did not record their tests.[85]

Blood glucose goals by age group [703]

The American Diabetes Association recommends that blood glucose goals should be individualized and lower goals may be reasonable on benefit-risk assessment. Goals should be higher in children with frequent hypoglycemia or hypoglycemia unawareness.[703]

Blood glucose	Before meal	Bedtime/ overnight
Toddlers < 6 years	100-180 mg/dl 5.5-10mmol/l	110-200 mg/dl 6-11 mmol/l
School age 6-12 years	90-180 mg/dl 5-10 mmol/l	100-180 mg/dl 6-10 mmol/l
Adolescents 13-19 years	90-130 mg/dl 5-7 mmol/l	90-150mg/dl 5-8 mmol/l

---

What is the best order for changing the doses?

(multiple injection treatment)

① Lower the doses to avoid hypoglycemia. Then concentrate on one dose at a time for a couple of days.

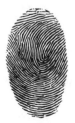

Just as all fingerprints are different all insulin doses are different and unfortunately they often seem to work differently every day. This is perfectly logical if you think about it — we are all very different as individuals and insulin must be adjusted to fit the individual lifestyle.

When should you take your pre-breakfast insulin?

Timing the breakfast dose will be easier if you are using NovoLog/NovoRapid or Humalog. This may be difficult to accomplish as part of a stressed morning routine if you use regular short-acting insulin, since it is then more important to take the insulin some time before breakfast. Measure your blood glucose as soon as you wake up, then adjust the time of your breakfast accordingly. Use this as a baseline for experimenting with different times:

Blood glucose level		Insulin at breakfast	
mg/dl	mmol/l	Rapid-acting insulin	Ordinary short-acting insulin
< 55	< 3	after the meal	just before
55-90	3-5	just before	15 min. before
90-180	5-10	just before	30 min. before
180-250	10-14	10 min. before	45 min. before
> 250	> 14	20 min. before	60 min. before

② Start by adjusting the dose for the evening snack if you are on multiple injections so that you will have an appropriate blood glucose level when going to bed.

③ Adjust the bedtime insulin dose (dinner dose if on 2-dose therapy) to obtain good overnight and pre-breakfast blood glucose levels.

④ Adjust the breakfast insulin dose.

⑤ Adjust the doses for lunch and dinner (if on multiple injections).

Premeal bolus doses

Insulin for breakfast

It is more difficult to obtain a good blood glucose level during the night than during the day.

Ideally, you want to start the morning with a normal blood glucose level. If you have problems with your blood glucose early in the morning when using NPH as bedtime insulin, you may be better off with Lantus as your basal insulin. The premeal insulin dose for breakfast will usually need to be slightly higher in relation to the amount of carbohydrates (see "Starting insulin treatment" on page 127). Since breakfast generally contains more carbohydrates than other meals, the breakfast injection is likely to contain the largest premeal dose of the day.

Insulin for lunch and dinner

Measure your blood glucose level before and 2 hours after the meal. The same strategy applies for lunch and dinner doses as for breakfast. If lunch at school is very early, the dose can be divided into two, where one dose is taken with the early lunch and one with a larger snack in the afternoon.

Insulin for evening snack

When using multiple injections, premeal insulin is usually given with the evening snack. Aim to start the night with an appropriate blood glucose level by monitoring it shortly before the evening snack and adjusting food and the dose of rapid or short-acting insulin thereafter. This system works especially well for younger children and for those going to bed fairly early, as long as they do not have too much physical exercise after eating.

Two units of rapid or short-acting insulin per open sandwich is usually an appropriate dose if you have a glass of milk along with the sandwiches for the evening snack. For advice on gram carbohydrate counting, see page 216.

When using a 2-dose treatment, no insulin is given at bedtime. A bedtime snack is usually essential to avoid night time hypoglycemia with this type of insulin regimen.

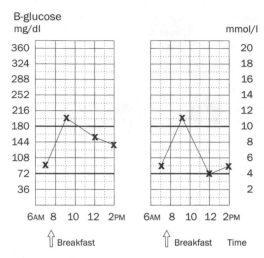

B-glucose
mg/dl   mmol/l

6AM 8 10 12 2PM   6AM 8 10 12 2PM

⇡ Breakfast   ⇡ Breakfast   Time

If you use rapid-acting insulin (NovoLog/NovoRapid, Humalog) you can try increasing the breakfast dose by 1-2 units in both examples above or change your insulin:carb ratio to a lower number of carbs. If you are using regular short-acting insulin and your blood glucose readings look like the chart on the left, you can try increasing the breakfast dose by 1-2 units. If the blood glucose level decreases before lunch (as on the chart on the right) you will have problems with hypoglycemia if you increase the pre-breakfast insulin dose of short-acting insulin. It is then better to take it earlier, i.e. 45 minutes before breakfast, if you usually have a 30 minute interval.

Blood glucose before lunch

The pre-breakfast dose of regular short-acting insulin can be adjusted by referring to the results of tests taken before lunch. With rapid-acting insulin you can use readings taken ~2 hours after breakfast. See the chart on page 140. If you are using a correction factor, see table on page 131.

Blood glucose	Measure
< 70 mg/dl < 4 mmol/l	Decrease the breakfast dose by 1-2 units.
> 145 mg/dl > 8 mmol/l	Increase the breakfast dose by 1-2 units.
> 220-360 mg/dl > 12-20 mmol/l	Think! Is there any particular reason for your blood glucose level to be high just now? Did you miss your breakfast dose? Are you unwell?
Hypoglycemia between breakfast and lunch?	Decrease the breakfast dose by 1-2 units.

Weekend or weekday?

Your physical activity level can vary a great deal depending on whether you are at school, working or enjoying the weekend. It is normal, and relaxing, to sleep in at the weekend, and the time-table for meals may be different. Factors such as these may make it appropriate to have different insulin doses for weekdays and weekends. Make notes in your logbook and try to find a schedule that works well for you.

Physical exercise or relaxation?

If you will be exercising within a few hours of a meal, you may need to eat a little extra or decrease your short or rapid-acting premeal dose by 1-2 units (see also the chapter on physical exercise, page 242). If you will be resting more than usual, you may need to increase the dose by 1-2 units.

Using rapid-acting insulin analogs

The rapid-acting insulins NovoLog/NovoRapid and Humalog have led to major improvements in the treatment of diabetes. Another rapid-acting insulin, Apidra, will be introduced shortly. These insulins more closely resemble the insulin release of a healthy pancreas during the eating of a meal (see page 22). The rapid effect is caused by the splitting of the insulin into smaller parts directly after the injection, allowing it to be absorbed into the bloodstream very quickly (see page 70). The two rapid-acting in-

Blood glucose before evening snack

When taking the rapid or short-acting dose before the evening snack when using multiple injections, you should aim to have a blood glucose level of around 110-145 mg/dl (6-8 mmol/l), up to 180 mg/dl (10 mmol/l) for children, at bedtime. If you are using a correction factor, see table on page 131.

Test before evening snack	Measure
< 90 mg/dl < 5 mmol/l	Decrease the dose by 1-2 units.
>180-215 mg/dl >10-12 mmol/l	Increase the dose by 1-2 units or eat less for your evening snack.
> 325-360 mg/dl >18-20 mmol/l	Give 1-2 units extra and eat less for your evening snack. You can also try taking your regular dose if you eat a very small meal (or skip the meal completely) but then you must check your blood glucose level again before going to bed.

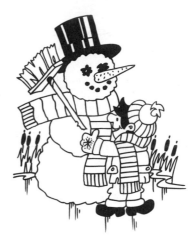

In winter, most children will rush outside to play if they see snow fall. However, the extra exercise often makes it necessary to lower the doses by a unit or two at dinner and the evening snack to avoid hypoglycemia. If children have been out playing for many hours, it is advisable to lower the bedtime dose as well.

sulins NovoLog/NovoRapid (aspart) and Humalog (lispro) have identical effects on blood glucose control, whether they are given as injections [616] or via an insulin pump.[92]

At the present time, we in Sweden give almost all those children and adolescents with newly diagnosed diabetes an intensive insulin treatment with multiple premeal doses. This regimen consists of NovoLog/NovoRapid or Humalog before meals (3-4 doses) and basal insulin (intermediate twice daily or long-acting once or twice daily).

NovoLog/NovoRapid [119] and Humalog [678] take effect so quickly that even taking the injection after a meal can produce a good insulin effect on the carbohydrates in that meal. While this approach is not really recommended as a rou-

tine for older children or adults, it can be a very practical strategy for younger children if you are not sure how much they are going to eat.

Rapid-acting insulin works well during the remission phase (honeymoon phase, see page 193) for premeal doses as you are likely to be producing enough of your own insulin to provide the basal requirement during the day. A study of adults in the remission phase found a fall in the numbers of low blood glucose readings some hours after the meal, when this type of insulin treatment was being used.[590]

When using rapid-acting insulin for meals, you will also need another insulin to ensure that your need for basal insulin between meals is met. Without basal insulin, your blood glucose will begin to rise 3-4 hours after an injection of rapid-acting insulin.[393,492] If you are using Lantus, one dose per day may cover your need for basal insulin. Younger children using small doses often need to take Lantus twice daily to be sure it is effective round the clock. See page 155 for further advice on using Lantus.

When can rapid-acting insulin be used for premeal injections?

Since the effect of rapid-acting insulin is too short to cover the periods between meals, you will need to take a basal insulin (i.e. another type of insulin that covers the basal need of insulin between meals) as well. You can try using rapid-acting insulin (NovoLog/NovoRapid or Humalog) in the following situations:

➥ If you take two injections of intermediate NPH (Novolin N, Humulin N) or one to two of long-acting (Lantus, Ultralente, Humulin U) insulin as basal insulin (see page 129).

➥ If you use NPH as basal insulin only for bedtime, NovoLog/NovoRapid or Humalog may still be a good alternative if you eat frequent, regular meals (not more than 3-4 hours apart). However, you will need to be more strict with your meal times.

➥ If you are in the remission phase (honeymoon phase), your pancreas may produce enough insulin on its own to cover the basal needs between meals.

➥ NovoLog/NovoRapid and Humalog are very good alternatives if you use an insulin pump since the pump will supply the basal insulin (see page 186).

➥ If you have insulin antibodies (see page 190) you will produce your own long-acting insulin by binding insulin to the antibodies. One sign of having insulin antibodies is that you get redness in the skin after injections. If you are using regular short-acting insulin you can try replacing it with rapid-acting insulin. The chemical structure of this insulin is slightly different and it may give you fewer problems with antibodies and redness after insulin injections.

Achieving a better A1C with rapid-acting insulin

Rapid-acting insulins have a very quick but fairly short span of action. This may result in a lack of insulin in your body by the time of the next meal, especially if your meals are widely spaced. Many research studies do not show any significant improvement in A1C when switching to Humalog unless this change is combined with other measures. Below are some alternatives that have been tried with good results:

➥ Need of basal insulin between meals.
1) Intermediate-acting (NPH) or long-acting insulin (Humulin U, Ultralente) also in the morning.[235,647]

2) 10-40% intermediate-acting insulin (NPH) mixed with the rapid-acting insulin for all main meals.[207,235]

3) Use Lantus as a basal insulin.[402]

➥ Adjust your diet to the action profile of the rapid-acting insulin (smaller snacks [647] or no snacks at all [459] and larger main meals).

Many teenagers appreciate the possibilities of increased mealtime flexibility, which may be a reason for the change to rapid-acting insulin.[104] In a US study, teenagers using Humalog found coping with diabetes less difficult and reported less negative impact of diabetes on quality of life and fewer worries about diabetes.[316]

When using other types of basal insulin you will probably need to take an injection of intermediate-acting (Novolin N, Humulin N) or long-acting insulin (Humulin U, Ultralente) also in the morning to avoid lack of insulin and rise in blood glucose before the next meal. If you take basal insulin in the morning, you will have more freedom to adjust your mealtimes, even if your meals are irregular with up to 6-7 hours between them.

Adults may try using only one dose of NPH basal insulin to start with. In a US study, only 20% of the adults needed to be switched to twice daily basal insulin.[828] This study also found that patients using Ultralente as twice daily basal insulin had a slightly higher A1C than the NPH group (8.2% vs. 7.7%). In an Australian follow-up of 100 adults transferred to Humalog, 54% required an additional NPH dose in the morning.[147]

NovoLog/NovoRapid or Humalog may be good alternatives if you work shifts (see page 86).

Adjusting the basal insulin

The basal insulin should give a steady level of insulin between meals during the day. Check the blood glucose before meals and, if necessary, change the dose of basal insulin (see the graph on page 143). See page 148 for advice on NPH insulin and page 155 for Lantus. It may be a bit difficult to decide how to adjust the doses of basal insulin. Ask your diabetes team for advice, especially when you are new to using rapid-acting insulin.

High blood glucose levels

NovoLog/NovoRapid and Humalog are well suited as "emergency insulins" in a situation when you need to lower a high blood glucose level fast (e.g. if you have nausea and ketones). You rarely need to take more than 0.1 unit/kg (0.5 unit/10 lb) body weight as an extra dose at one time. Test your blood glucose level again after two hours. Give another 0.1 units/kg (0.5 units/10 lb) if the level has not gone down. Some people need to take more than 0.1 unit/kg in this situation. Increase the dose slightly if you need to, as you work out what is appropriate for you.

You can take an extra injection of rapid-acting insulin at snack-time, and the effect of this injection will be almost over by the time you are ready for your next meal 2-3 hours later.[378] If you inject yourself with short-acting insulin at regular 2 hour intervals, you run the risk of the effects of these injections overlapping. This would make you more likely to experience hypoglycemia later on (see figure on page 133). If your blood-glucose level is high at bedtime, you can take a small dose of rapid-acting insulin and have less risk of hypoglycemia later in the night compared to short-acting insulin.

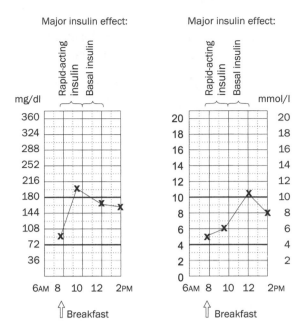

When adjusting your premeal doses of NovoLog/NovoRapid or Humalog, it is a good idea to check your blood glucose before and 2 hours after the meal. If the blood glucose readings are like the graph on the left, you should try increasing your breakfast dose of rapid-acting insulin by 1-2 units or adjust your insulin:carb ratio to a smaller carb number if you are counting carbohydrates. The dose of basal insulin (intermediate or long-acting) or basal rate (if you are using an insulin pump) seems to be correct since the glucose level doesn't change much more until lunchtime.

On the right graph, the blood glucose doesn't rise until two hours after breakfast. The breakfast dose is correct but the dose of basal NPH insulin in the morning needs to be increased by a unit or two. If you are taking one dose of Lantus in the evening, you can try increasing this dose. However, if increasing Lantus in the evening results in morning hypoglycemia, you may be better off dividing the Lantus dose and taking part of it in the morning.

Hypoglycemia

If you are using rapid-acting insulin, your premeal dose will be "responsible" for hypoglycemia that occurs within 2-3 hours of the meal (see key fact box on page 61). Due to the very short time action of rapid-acting insulin, you

Do you need regular short-acting insulin while using rapid acting insulin for meals?

Short-acting insulin (Novolin R, Humulin R) will give you a longer insulin effect (around 4-5 hours compared with 2-3 hours for NovoLog, Humalog) and may be better in certain situations (sometimes we call it the "party-insulin"):

⟹ A meal with 2-3 courses that takes longer than usual to eat.

⟹ A birthday party where food will be served several times within a couple of hours.

⟹ A meal rich in fat (such as pizza) or protein (such as a large steak).

Rapid-acting insulin can be mixed with short-acting insulin to give a slightly prolonged insulin effect for example:

⟹ To cover a mid-morning snack.

⟹ When the interval between meals is longer.

⟹ When eating a meal with high fat content.

If you have a pump you can use a prolonged bolus dose to achieve a longer insulin effect for meals like this. The only way to find out what works best for you is to experiment while checking your blood glucose.

who injected Humalog immediately before the meal compared to those who took regular short-acting insulin 30-45 minutes before.[35] The risk of hypoglycemia has also been shown to decrease among people using Novo-Log/NovoRapid.[383] In a clinical follow-up of 100 adults switching to Humalog, 86% reduced their A1C and 57% reduced the frequency of hypoglycemia.[147] 47% managed to reduce both A1C and the hypoglycemia frequency.

In several studies, the frequency of hypoglycemia decreases even during the night when using NovoLog/NovoRapid[384] or Humalog.[35,118,354,612] This may be because a dose of regular short-acting insulin for the last meal of the day gives a long enough effect to last into the night.

Exercise

If you take a dose of Humalog within 1-2 hours before exercising, you may often need to lower the dose (see page 249).[767] If you have exercised late in the evening you may need to decrease your breakfast dose of rapid-acting insulin. Remember to decrease your bedtime insulin by 2-4 units after strenuous exercise.

Pre-mixed insulin

Pre-filled mixtures of rapid-acting and intermediate-acting insulin are available (Novo-Log/NovoRapid Mix 70/30 and Humalog Mix 75/25). If you have a long wait (4-5 hours or more) between lunch and dinner, you may have problems with rising blood glucose before the next meal. This is caused by the waning of the breakfast intermediate-acting insulin. In such a situation, it may be a good idea to take a pre-mixed insulin (e.g. 50/50) at lunchtime or add some NPH insulin in the syringe. When you calculate the doses, try to think in terms of half-quantity NovoLog/NovoRapid or Humalog and half-quantity intermediate-acting insulin. A mixture of 70% rapid-acting and 30% NPH insulin has shown good results in adults, but is

will need to rely more upon carbohydrates with a high glucose content (glucose, honey, sugar) to treat hypoglycemia. If hypoglycemia occurs later, the basal insulin usually contributes more. Due to the rapid decline of the insulin effect after 2-3 hours, hypoglycemia caused by Novo-Log/NovoRapid and Humalog will resolve more quickly than those caused by regular short-acting insulin.

A meta-analysis (analysis of many studies) suggests that people who use rapid-acting insulin are at lower risk of hypoglycemia than those who use short-acting insulins.[118] In a study where the participants were free to adjust their premeal doses, the number of hypoglycemic episodes decreased by 11% among those people

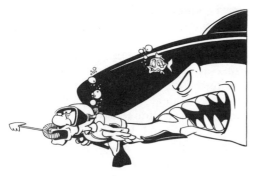

Sometimes people can feel burdened by so many tests and changes in insulin doses. If this applies to you, take a break for a week or two, taking blood glucose tests only when necessary to avoid hypoglycemia. Make sure that you concentrate instead on having as good a time as possible. (The same principle applies to parents monitoring their children.) You can then come back to monitoring again afterwards with renewed commitment and enthusiasm.

not yet commercially available.[759] In children, it is generally preferable to mix insulins in a syringe rather than using premixed insulin (see page 72).

Switching to rapid-acting analogs

If you are using rapid-acting insulin, you can inject yourself immediately before your meal, then you will not have to worry about the time interval before eating. In practice, many individuals using short-acting insulin end up taking their premeal doses shortly before eating (perhaps feeling guilty about ignoring their diabetes team's advice to wait 20-30 minutes before eating). This sort of "bending the rules" can often pass without problem, but on occasions, the person can find their blood glucose level rising sharply after the meal, only to be followed by a low blood glucose some hours later when the effectiveness of the short-acting insulin has passed its peak.

When more than 2-3 hours have passed since the last meal, the liver will supply glucose to prevent the blood glucose level from falling too low. A low basal level of insulin is necessary to keep the blood glucose level stable. If there is no insulin available at all, the counter-regulatory hormones (adrenaline and glucagon, see page 33) will raise the blood glucose level by increasing the output of glucose from the liver even more. Regular short-acting insulin, when used for premeal injections, covers both the carbohydrate contents of the meal and the need for basal insulin until the next meal.

The action of rapid-acting insulin will begin much more quickly than regular short-acting insulin when given as an abdominal injection, almost as quickly as the insulin that is produced in the beta cells of a healthy pancreas. This means you can administer it just before meals and still get a good insulin effect when your blood glucose level starts rising. Because this insulin better matches the blood glucose profile after a meal, you will probably have to reduce your premeal doses by about 10% when starting with Humalog.[590] Otherwise there will be a risk of hypoglycemia 2-3 hours after the meal,[459] especially if it contains pasta (giving a slow rise in blood glucose) or fewer carbohydrates and more fat, e.g. meat with a cream sauce.[122]

Adjust the premeal doses for rapid-acting insulin in the same way as for regular short-acting insulin, depending on the carbohydrate content of the meal and your actual blood glucose level. If you are using NPH insulin (Novolin N, Humulin N) for basal insulin, you should adjust the bedtime dose as you did before. Long-acting insulin (Humulin U, Ultralente) takes effect so slowly that you should probably take it around 5-7 PM to get the benefit during the night.

However, long-acting Lantus can be given later in the evening.

In a Finnish study, patients were advised to transfer at least half of their snack carbohydrates to the previous main meals, when starting with Humalog.[647] This resulted in a 0.25% decrease of A1C (for those who followed the dietary advice) and less hypoglycemia, even during the night.

Examples of doses when switching to rapid-acting insulin

Beware! These doses are only suggestions for your first doses when switching to rapid-acting insulin. In the early days you must test your blood glucose before and after every meal as well as during the night.
You must not change insulin types on your own before discussing them with your doctor or diabetes nurse. See action profile graphs on page 129:

Example 1: 8 year old weighing 32 kg (70 lb)

		Breakfast	Lunch	Dinner	Evening	Bedtime	U/24h.
Previous dose	2-dose treatment	18 U Mix 70/30 (=5 Reg. + 13 NPH)	–	14 U Mix 70/30 (=4 Reg. + 10 NPH)	–		32
	Multiple injections with Reg.	6 U Reg.	5 U Reg.	5 U Reg.	4 U Reg.	12 U NPH	32
New dose	Rapid-acting and NPH	6 U HL/N 5 U NPH	4 U HL/N	5 U HL/N	4 U HL/N	– 8 U NPH	32 (40% basal)
	Rapid-acting and Lantus	6 U HL/N 6 U LA	5 U HL/N	4 U HL/N	3 U HL/N 8 U LA	–	32 (42% basal)

Example 2: teenager (50-60 kg, 110-130 lb) or young adult (70-80 kg, 150-190 lb)

		Breakfast	Lunch	Dinner	Evening	Bedtime	U/24h.
Previous dose	2-dose treatment	14 U Reg. 18 U NPH	–	10 U Reg. 26 U NPH	–		68
	Multiple injections with Reg.	14 U Reg.	12 U Reg.	10 U Reg.	8 U Reg.	24U NPH	68
New dose	Rapid-acting and NPH	12 U HL/N 10 U NPH	9 U HL/N	8 U HL/N	7 U HL/N	22 U NPH	68 (47% basal)
	Rapid-acting and Lantus	12 U HL/N	10 U HL/N	7 U HL/N	7 U HL/N 32 U LA	–	68 (47% basal)

Reg. = regular short-acting insulin, NPH = NPH insulin, NL = NovoLog/NovoRapid, HL = Humalog, LA = Lantus. (With smaller doses of Lantus, it is sometimes necessary to give it twice daily.)

The difference in rapid-acting doses with Lantus or NPH as basal insulin is caused by different insulin profiles:
Breakfast ➟ a higher level of basal insulin with Lantus ➟ a slightly lower NovoLog/Rapid or Humalog dose
Lunch ➟ 　　　"　　　　"　　　　NPH ➟ 　　　"　　　　　"
Dinner and evening snack ➟ 　"　　　　Lantus ➟ 　　"　　　　　"

Switching from short to rapid-acting insulin

Always talk to your diabetes team if you are interested in changing type of insulin. A rule of thumb is that the total number of units/day should be about the same with the new type of insulin. However, when using Lantus you may need a slight reduction. It is very important to take frequent tests, especially when you are new to a certain type of insulin.

① Premeal doses

A - You are on multiple injections:
Decrease the premeal doses by 1-2 units and add these units as an extra injection of basal insulin for breakfast. If you will be using NPH insulin (Novolin N, Humulin N) you can continue taking the same number of units of bedtime insulin as before. If you plan to use long-acting basal insulin (Lantus, Ultralente, Humulin U) you will probably need to decrease the premeal doses by 2-3 units.

B - You are on 2 doses/day:
You already take basal insulin twice daily as NPH or Lente insulin (alone or in a mix). Begin by distributing 50-60% of your total number of units/24 hours as rapid-acting insulin on the number of main meals you eat (usually 3-4 depending if you eat an evening or bedtime snack). The breakfast dose usually needs to be slightly larger than the dose for other meals.

Divide the remaining number of units/day as shown below:

② Distribution of basal insulin:

Begin with approximately 40-50% of your daily dose as basal insulin. You will probably end up with 40-60%, often slightly higher for adults than for children or teenagers.

NPH:

Begin with approximately 40% of your daily dose as basal insulin, one third in the morning and two thirds at bedtime.

Lantus:

Begin with 50% of your daily dose as a single dose at your evening snack or at bedtime. Young children may be better off taking Lantus in the morning to avoid low glucose levels in the night. When using small doses, it may be better to split the dose into two and to take around half the dose in the morning and half in the evening.

Ultralente (Humulin U, Ultralente):

Begin with approximately 50% of your daily dose as basal insulin, slightly less than half in the morning (often 2-4 U more at dinner time).

With regular short-acting insulin, the dose for the last meal of the day will also contribute to the insulin levels during the early part of the night. Adults who switched to Humalog found that a 20% decrease of the evening snack dose combined with a 25% increase in the bedtime NPH dose resulted in a better glucose levels after the meal and unchanged glucose levels overnight.[10] In our experience, younger children using rapid-acting insulin often have their blood glucose level rise shortly after falling asleep. One way of compensating for this is to give short-acting insulin (Novolin R, Humulin R) for the evening snack, and increase the dose until the right balance is achieved.

Can you eat the same things as before?

To avoid a lack of insulin between meals when using premeal doses of regular short-acting insulin, the gap between major meals preceded with insulin injections should not be more than five hours. If you are using rapid-acting insulin you need not be so strict about timing if you have a sufficient supply of basal insulin.

You may need to think again about the make-up of some of your meals. Cereals with milk for breakfast will now be fine, but food that is absorbed slowly such as pasta or beans (with a low glycemic index, see page 209), which had previously been covered well by regular short-acting insulin, may give you problems now. This also applies to meals rich in fat, since fat causes the stomach to empty more slowly. With rapid-acting insulin the result may be a lowering of the blood glucose level within one hour after the meal, before the glucose in the food has been absorbed into the blood. If your blood glucose is low (below 70 mg/dl, 4.0 mmol/l) before such a meal, it is a good idea to take your injection of rapid-acting insulin after the meal to stop your blood glucose from dropping even lower before the carbohydrates in the meal have time to enter your bloodstream.[397]

If you start the meal by drinking something containing sugar, such as a glass of juice, your blood glucose may be prevented from falling. You could also take an injection of regular short-acting insulin with this type of meal while using rapid-acting insulin for the other meals.

Many parents find it difficult to estimate how much food their toddlers will eat at a meal. In this situation it is an advantage to be able to give the injection after the meal when they know how much the child has actually eaten. Rapid-acting insulin is effective early enough, even if it is taken after the meal.[119,656,678]

Snacks become less necessary if you use rapid-acting insulin. This is because the insulin effect coincides better with the blood glucose raising effect of a meal. As a result, insulin levels between meals are lowered. So if you do have a substantial snack between meals, you will probably need an extra dose of insulin to be sure you avoid an increase in blood glucose.

Rapid-acting insulin has a quick effect that fits well with sugary candy. However, for treats containing fat, such as ice cream and chocolate, the effect may be too quick. A dose of regular short-acting insulin may then be more appropriate. The alternative is to inject Novo-Log/NovoRapid or Humalog after a treat of this type.

Rapid-acting insulin may be a good alternative if you have irregular eating habits. Some people find they can even manage to skip a meal (and the dose of NovoLog/NovoRapid or Humalog), especially if they use a basal insulin regimen with Lantus. Check your blood glucose more frequently if you try this. However, if you eat very slowly, or eat many small meals (rather than main meals) during the day, regular short-acting insulin may be a better alternative.[95] If you are having a dinner with a lot of courses, you can try to divide your meal dose of rapid-acting insulin and take part of it for the appetizer and part for the main course. An alternative is to take regular short-acting insulin for

meals when you are sitting still for longer than usual, or a prolonged bolus when using a pump.

Bedtime NPH insulin

During the day, it is fairly easy to observe reactions and watch for signs of hypoglycemia. At night however, when everyone is asleep, it is much more difficult. Besides, the night is long and high blood glucose levels during the night can have a substantial effect on your A1C. It is often difficult to ensure that bedtime insulin of

---

Tests to take when adjusting the bedtime NPH dose

The tests will be more representative if your day has been routine, without heavy physical exercise or hypoglycemia. The blood glucose level should be about 110-145 mg/dl (6-8 mmol/l), up to 180 mg/dl (10 mmol/l) for children when you take the bedtime dose to ensure a "normal" night. It is advisable to take a test in the middle of the night every 1-2 weeks to make sure that you are not at risk of night time hypoglycemia.

☞ Blood tests: Before evening snack
Evening at 10 PM
Night at 2-3 AM
Morning

☞ Urine tests: Morning (ketones?)

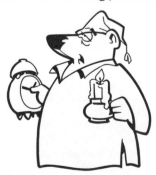

Getting up in the middle of the night to take a test is not much fun. Try to take tests during "normal" nights when you will obtain most information.

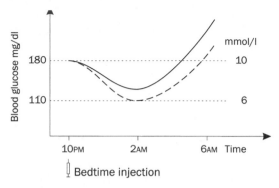

Bedtime injection

The blood glucose level during the night usually assumes a "hammock-like" curve when you use insulin of NPH type for bedtime injections (Novolin N, Humulin N) in a multiple injection therapy. This insulin will have its greatest effect 4-6 hours after the injection.[663] If you increase the dose, the morning blood glucose will be lower (dashed line) but the risk of night time hypoglycemia will increase. The blood glucose level at 2-3 AM (approximately four hours after injection) can therefore be used as an indicator when adjusting the bedtime insulin dose.[103] Ideally, you should aim for a blood glucose of about 180 mg/dl (10 mmol/l) when you take the bedtime insulin and then let it fall about 70 mg/dl (4.0 mmol/l) to reach 110 mg/dl (6 mmol/l) at 2-3 AM (which usually is the lowest point during the night).

If your blood glucose level is below 125-145 mg/dl (7-8 mmol/l) at the time of taking the bedtime insulin, you may need a bedtime snack to prevent night time hypoglycemia.

intermediate NPH type will last till morning. A smaller dose is not only less effective, it also lasts for a shorter period of time.

Many different factors contribute to a high blood glucose level in the morning. The most widely used bedtime NPH insulins (Novolin N, Humulin N) have their greatest effect in the middle of the night. At the same time, the body's insulin sensitivity is increased between midnight and 2 AM compared to 6-8 AM,[103] (the night time secretion of growth hormone increases the blood glucose early in the morning, see "Dawn phenomenon" on page 54). When combined, these factors result in an increased risk of hypoglycemia early in the night. See page 155 if you are using Lantus as your long-acting insulin.

It is difficult to state the best blood glucose to go to bed on. Studies have shown that blood glucose levels of more than approximately 120-130 mg/dl (7 mmol/l) when going to bed,[63,682] or at midnight,[530] decrease the risk for night time hypoglycemia. It is a good idea, therefore, to start the night with a slightly higher blood glucose level, preferably 145-180 mg/dl (8-10 mmol/l) if you use intermediate-acting insulin (Novolin N, Humulin N) at bedtime. You will then have "more glucose to draw from" and you can give a higher dose of bedtime insulin without risk. A higher dose will last longer, and thus have a better effect on the morning blood glucose level (see page 72).

Blood glucose monitoring before bedtime insulin

Younger children will usually allow blood tests and injection of bedtime insulin to be done while they are asleep. On the other hand, giving food to a newly awakened child can be very tricky, especially when the blood glucose level is low. It is often more practical to test before eating the evening snack. You can then adjust the amount of food and insulin dose, in order to start the night with the best possible blood glucose level.

Test before bedtime insulin	Measure
< 110 mg/dl < 6 mmol/l	Give a sandwich and milk
110-215 mg/dl 6-12 mmol/l	Give the ordinary dose
> 215 mg/dl > 12 mmol/l	Increase the bedtime dose by 1-2 U or give a small dose of NovoLog/NovoRapid or Humalog

Giving an extra dose of insulin along with the bedtime insulin may increase the risk of a hypoglycemia early in the night. It is best to use rapid-acting insulin (NovoLog/NovoRapid or Humalog) as the peak effect of this insulin will decline before the bedtime insulin of NPH type begins to act. With Lantus there will be less risk of night time hypoglycemia in this situation.

Later in the night, the effect of the bedtime insulin decreases at the same time as the insulin sensitivity also decreases due to the dawn phenomenon (see page 54). This causes a morning rise in the blood glucose level. Night time hypoglycemia followed by rebound phenomenon (so called Somogyi phenomenon) can occur if the insulin levels are low during the later part of the night and can further contribute to a high morning glucose (see charts on page 54 and 151).

In adults on multiple injection treatment, the risk of night time hypoglycemia seems to follow a different pattern, probably due to a lower degree of hormonal activity. In one study,[61] only 30% of the night time hypoglycemia would have been detected by a 3 AM blood glucose test. In another study,[783] 29% of the patients

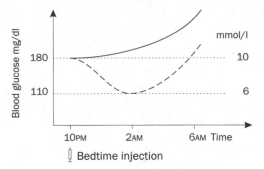

⬇ Bedtime injection

A small difference in insulin dose can cause a large difference in the blood glucose level due to an either/or effect. The insulin sensitivity increases (decreased insulin resistance) early in the night, causing the blood glucose to fall, but only if the blood glucose is within normal levels for people without diabetes, below about 125 mg/dl (7 mmol/l, dashed line). If the blood glucose increases after midnight, the insulin resistance will increase as well and the bedtime insulin dose will not be able to lower the blood glucose level sufficiently (solid line).

Night time glucose monitoring

Test your blood glucose levels at the time when you expect them to be at their lowest. This may differ from person to person. See page 91 for suggestions on times for monitoring.

① **Monitoring for a 24 hour chart**
If you have something to eat in the night, the entire night's blood glucose values will be affected and the chart will be difficult to interpret. Eat only if the blood glucose level is less than about 70-90 mg/dl (4-5 mmol/l) or you are feeling unwell. The same applies if you are caring for a child. If the level is above 70-90 mg/dl (4-5 mmol/l) it is better to take another test ½-1 hour later to see in which direction the level is heading.

② **Monitoring because of actual risk of night time hypoglycemia**
If you (or your child) have not eaten well or have exercised more than usual during the afternoon/evening, you should take precautions to avoid hypoglycemia during the night. Eat something if your blood glucose level is < 110-125 mg/dl (6-7 mmol/l), and you will be able to sleep on safely.

had night time hypoglycemia (< 54 mg/dl, 3 mmol/l) but none of these occurred between 1.30 and 3.30 AM. This suggests a longer time to peak action of the bedtime insulin (of NPH type) which was taken at 11 PM. The conclusion from this study was that after midnight (e.g. 1-2 AM) hypoglycemia always was preceded by a bedtime glucose reading of < 135 mg/dl (7.5 mmol/l) and that early morning hypoglycemia did not occur if the blood glucose level on waking was > 100 mg/dl (5.6 mmol/l).

If the blood glucose level early in the night is higher than it would be in a person without diabetes (about 125 mg/dl, 7 mmol/l) the blood glucose level as such will cause insulin sensitivity to decrease (increased insulin resistance). The result will be that increased insulin sensitivity, present at a normal blood glucose level, will not occur.[103] This is an important part of the explanation why it is so difficult to adjust the bedtime insulin dose. You will have a sort of either/or situation when it will be practically impossible to find "the correct" insulin dose.

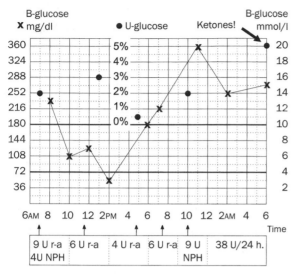

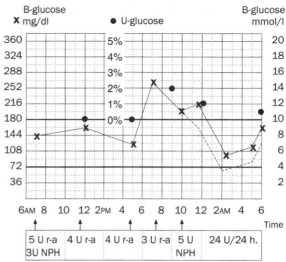

r-a = rapid-acting insulin

r-a = rapid-acting insulin

The blood glucose level rises early in the night and is still high in the morning after a night with high values. With a large insulin dose for breakfast, the blood glucose level will fall before lunch, but you will risk hypoglycemia in the afternoon.

Start by decreasing the lunchtime dose to avoid the afternoon hypoglycemia. Then increase the pre-evening snack insulin dose, (or perhaps eat slightly less), and increase the bedtime insulin (remember to check the blood glucose at 2-3 AM!). Then you can adjust the dose before breakfast when you have obtained a better blood glucose level during the night.

This person used NPH insulin as basal insulin. The dawn phenomenon (see page 54) contributes to a rising blood glucose level during the later part of the night. If you increase the insulin dose for bedtime you will have a lower morning blood glucose level (dashed line) but you will also increase the risk of night time hypoglycemia. You must therefore check the blood glucose at 2-3 AM when adjusting your bedtime insulin dose. Compare with the graphs on the top of page 149.

This will result in even higher blood glucose later in the night and in the morning.

In practice, the blood glucose level will vary a great deal from morning to morning due to this either/or effect. The dawn phenomenon on the other hand is mostly constant from night to night. The large and often frustrating variability in morning blood glucose, despite the same insulin dose, is caused by variations in the speed of absorption of the injected dose of bedtime NPH insulin, in combination with a waning insulin effect early in the morning.[103] Levemir may be a better alternative in this case, since it gives a more predictable effect with a considerably smaller the day to day variation in absorption.[350]

The long-acting insulin Lantus gives a more even insulin level during the night, resulting in

Either:

If the insulin dose is high enough to bring the blood glucose down to about 125 mg/dl (7.0 mmol/l) or less early in the night, the insulin sensitivity increases and there will be a risk of night time hypoglycemia.

Or:

If the insulin dose is too small causing the blood glucose to increase above 125 mg/dl (7.0 mmol/l), the insulin sensitivity will decrease.

both a decreased risk of night time hypoglycemia and less rise in the early morning blood
glucose level.[633] See page 155.

What should you do next?

Increase the bedtime NPH dose by 1-2 units at a
time until the blood glucose level at 2-3 AM
approaches 110-145 mg/dl (6-8 mmol/l). The
blood glucose level should be at least 110 mg/dl
(5-6 mmol/l) when you take the 2-3 AM test to
avoid night time hypoglycemia. A level of 110
mg/dl (6 mmol/l) as such is not disturbingly low
but you should have some leeway as the blood
glucose level another night might very well be
20-40 mg/dl (1-2 mmol/l) lower, even if you
take the same insulin doses.

Try giving the bedtime insulin of NPH type
(Novolin N, Humulin N) as late as possible to
ensure that it lasts until morning. Giving it at
10 PM usually works well for most people. You
must of course consider your family routines,
particularly if the family member with diabetes
is a young child. It is not a good idea to sit up
late in order to give the bedtime dose. For many

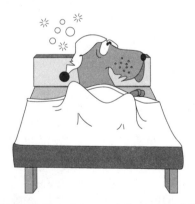

The only way to know for sure what your blood glucose
level is in the middle of the night is to take a test. Take it
at 2-3 AM if you use NPH insulin (Novolin N, Humulin N),
at 3-4 AM when using intermediate-acting Levemir or
Lente insulin like Monotard or Humutard and at 4-6 AM
when using long-acting insulin (Lantus, Ultralente,
Humulin U).

High blood glucose levels in the morning: what can you do?

If the bedtime injection uses NPH type insulin
(Novolin N, Humulin N) it may cause problems
because its effectiveness can cease before the
morning. In order to make it last longer, you will
need to increase the dose (see page 72). However,
if you are to do this without risking night time
hypoglycemia, you may need to start the night with
a slightly higher blood glucose than usual, tenta-
tively 180-215 mg/dl (10-12 mmol/l). Try following
these steps:

① Lower your evening premeal dose by 1-2
units at a time, until your blood glucose level
is 180-215 mg/dl (10-12 mmol/l) at the time
you take your bedtime insulin.

② Increase your bedtime insulin dose slowly.
However, your blood glucose should always
be at least 110 mg/dl (5-6 mmol/l) at 2-3
AM.

③ You might have to accept a rather high morning blood glucose level. This will be OK as
long as you feel well and your A1C is acceptable.

④ You can also try using another insulin that is
slightly longer lasting like Levemir or a lente
insulin (Novolin L, Humulin L). With these
insulins the lowest blood glucose level will
usually be slightly later, often around 3-4 AM.

Long-acting insulins (Ultralente, Humulin U)
have a much longer duration. They can sometimes cause problems with hypoglycemia the
next morning, or even the following afternoon. So long-acting insulins often need to
be injected much earlier, preferably at the
same time as the pre-dinner dose (at 4-5
PM), if they are to have a good effect during
the night. If the dose is large, it is often best
to split it into two: one dose before breakfast
and one before dinner. See page 155 for
details on Lantus.

The difficult, often impossible, balance of NPH bedtime insulin

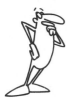 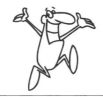

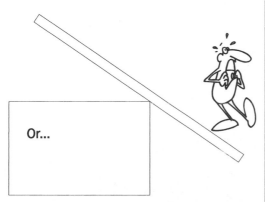

Either...

You must increase the bedtime insulin dose to lower the blood glucose level in the morning...

Or...

... but if you increase it too much, the insulin sensitivity early in the night will increase when the blood glucose is lowered and you will be at risk of hypoglycemia. This will happen not only if you increase the bedtime dose too much, but also if you forget to decrease the bedtime insulin when needed, e.g. after a game of soccer or when you have had less to eat for your evening snack than usual. See the text for a strategy to address this "either/or" dilemma. The very variable absorption of injected insulin further adds to the frustration of finding a correct bedtime dose. If you recognize these problems you may be better off trying Levemir, as its effect varies less from night to night, or Lantus which has an effect that is longer and more even.

children, it may be possible to administer a late (11 PM) bedtime insulin dose without them waking, or even stirring. If the child has an indwelling catheter (Insuflon, see page 122), it will be easy to give the late night dose while he or she is sleeping.

If you still have a high morning blood glucose level (more than 180 mg/dl, 10 mmol/l), you might need to try another bedtime insulin with a slightly longer like Levemir or lente (Novolin L, Humulin L) or much longer duration (Lantus, Ultralente, Humulin U). See key fact box on page 152. Discuss this with your doctor or diabetes nurse. If you are using rapid-acting insulin (NovoLog/NovoRapid or Humalog) you can administer a small extra dose along with the bedtime insulin if your blood glucose level is high. This is because this insulin will have ceased to be effective before the intermediate-acting insulin kicks in. We don't recommend giving extra short-acting insulin at bedtime to decrease a high blood glucose level, not even if you inject it in the abdomen. The effect of such a dose will overlap with the bedtime injection, putting you at risk of hypoglycemia around 2-3 AM.

Blood glucose levels at night

If you are taking tests from a child for a 24 hour profile, you should not give anything to eat if the blood glucose is low in the middle of the night (70-90 mg/dl (4-5 mmol/l) and the child is not showing any symptoms of hypoglycemia. After all, the child would not have woken up if you had not taken the test — and what you are interested in is what happens during an ordinary night. Instead of giving the child food, check the blood glucose once again after ½-1 hour and don't forget to check the morning blood glucose as well. This will be a tiresome night but you will learn a lot about how your child's diabetes works. An adult with diabetes may find it more difficult to reset the clock and go back to sleep. It is therefore best to eat something in this situation. Don't forget to record all test results in your logbook.

Morning tests

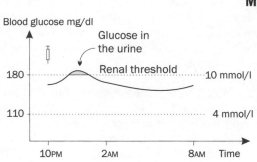

Morning tests: Blood glucose   145 mg/dl (8 mmol/l)
                Urine glucose   0.1%
                Ketones   0

When the blood glucose level rises above the renal threshold, glucose passes into the urine. Since the blood glucose level is not so high in the morning you know that it has been higher sometime earlier in the night. You will need to know what your renal threshold is if you are to interpret urine tests correctly (see page 92).

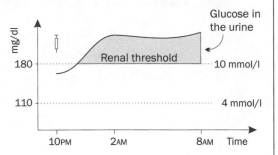

Morning tests: Blood glucose   250 mg/dl (14 mmol/l)
                Urine glucose   5%
                Ketones   ++

The blood glucose level has been high during most of the night due to a lack of insulin. This has caused a large amount of glucose to pass into the urine. The ketones in the urine are caused by a lack of glucose inside the cells.
.

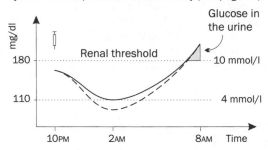

Morning tests: Blood glucose   215 mg/dl (12 mmol/l)
                Urine glucose   0.5%
                Ketones   0 (or +)

The blood glucose level has been adequate during most of the night since the urine glucose concentration is low. Only blood glucose monitoring during the night can determine how low the blood glucose level actually has been. What you do know from the urine test is that the blood glucose level only has been above the renal threshold for a short while, since the urine glucose concentration is low. If ketones are present when urine glucose during the night is low, this indicates that the blood glucose has been low as well ("starvation ketones", dashed line).

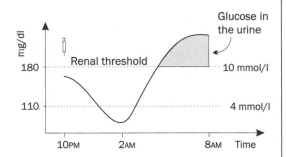

Morning tests: Blood glucose   250 mg/dl (14 mmol/l)
                Urine glucose   5%
                Ketones   ++

There has been a rebound phenomenon after hypoglycemia in the night. Ketones were passed into the urine during hypoglycemia (starvation ketones) and glucose was passed into the urine when the blood glucose level was high. The morning tests are exactly the same as in the example above. If you misread this, believing that the blood glucose has been high all night, you may very well increase the insulin dose instead. The blood glucose level would then fall even lower the following night, giving an even more pronounced rebound phenomenon. This type of reaction is called the Somogyi phenomenon (see page 55). The only way to distinguish it from the pattern in the upper right example is to check your blood glucose at 2-3 AM.

Possible causes for high blood glucose in the morning

① Insufficient insulin effect late at night due to the dawn phenomenon (see page 54) or too low a dose of bedtime insulin?

② Rebound phenomenon after night time hypoglycemia?

③ Not enough insulin to cover the evening snack or bedtime snack?

④ Too high a blood glucose level in the evening?

⑤ Forgot to mix the bedtime insulin thoroughly when using cloudy insulin? (Levemir and Lantus don't need mixing.)

Night time hypoglycemia

The first thing to do is to decrease the bedtime insulin dose and/or make sure that a reasonable bedtime snack is eaten every night. See page 51 for further instructions. If you practice competitive sports or do hard physical training some days or evenings every week, you will probably need less insulin before your evening snack and at bedtime on these days (see "Physical exercise" on page 242).

Using long-acting Lantus

When switching to the long-acting insulin analog Lantus from intermediate-acting NPH insulin (Novolin N, Humulin N) you can begin with the same number of units if you take NPH at bedtime only.[633] If you take NPH twice a day, it is advisable to decrease the total NPH dose slightly (by around 20%) and give it as one dose of Lantus.[229] You can give the Lantus dose at bedtime or at dinner depending on the individual effect of the insulin.[326] Use your morning blood glucose to adjust the dose but make sure that you also check some night time glucose lev-

els (for example at 4-5 AM) especially when you just have started with Lantus. Lower the dose if your morning glucose level is low (< approximately 70 mg/dl, 4.0 mmol/l). Since the effect of Lantus lasts for up to 24 hours [588] it is best not to change the dose more often than 2 (or 3) times in any week.[588] In clinical practice, the effect of Lantus in doses given to adults decreases after around 20 hours.[326] For younger children on one dose of Lantus/day, it often works better to give it in the morning. A smaller dose of Lantus will last for a shorter time, meaning that some children will need two injections every day.

If you find that you have a tendency towards lower glucose levels before lunch than when you wake up, you could try taking Lantus earlier in the evening (perhaps even at dinnertime). Aim for an ideal blood glucose of 70-110 mg/dl (4-6 mmol/l) on waking but 125-160 mg/dl (7-9 mmol/l) is also acceptable.[633,685] If you have problems with night time hypoglycemia, Lantus can be given in a single dose in the morning.[326] Several children divide their Lantus dose, injecting between half and one third in the

---

Research findings: Lantus

♠ When compared to NPH insulin given once or twice daily, one dose of Lantus at bedtime results in a lower fasting blood glucose, and less hypoglycemia but unchanged A1C. This is the case for children from age 5,[460,685] adolescents,[460,685] and adults.[633]

♠ Lantus has been used in children as young as 2 years.[597]

♠ Overnight profiles when Lantus has been given at 8-10 PM have shown lower levels of insulin and a smaller drop in night time blood glucose compared to NPH.[551]

♠ When Lantus was given as a supervised injection at lunchtime in school to children with an A1C of > 8%, there was a drop in average A1C from 10.1% to 8.9%.[402]

Switching to Lantus

Example of doses:

Morning NPH	Bedtime NPH	Lantus
-	12 U	12 U
-	36 U	32 U
8 U	14 U	18 U
12 U	26 U	30 U

If you take Intermediate-acting NPH insulin once daily, you can begin by taking the same number of Lantus units in the evening. With twice daily NPH, it is best to decrease the combined doses by approximately 20% and give it as one dose of Lantus. If you are taking large doses of NPH, it is a good idea to lower the dose even more to reduce the risk of hypoglycemia. You can then increase the Lantus dose, aiming at a wake-up blood glucose of 80-160 mg/dl (4.5-9 mmol/l).

morning. In such cases, the basal insulin effect between meals has been too low in the afternoon, but increasing the evening dose has led to morning glucose levels that are too low.

If you eat an afternoon snack after school you often need a premeal injection when using a single dose of Lantus as basal insulin. If the afternoon snack is small, it may work without a premeal dose if you split the Lantus dose and take part of it in the morning. Another solution is to add a small amount of NPH insulin to the lunchtime dose of rapid-acting insulin or to take an injection of NPH in the morning as additional basal insulin.

After extra exercise in the afternoon you may need to reduce the Lantus dose in the evening by 2-4 units to avoid night time hypoglycemia, although this may give you less basal insulin effect during the next day. You can also try reducing the evening Lantus before a daytime exercise session that will last more than 2-3 hours. Due to its prolonged action, Lantus has been used successfully in people who are being fed continuously by means of a stomach tube.[625]

Puberty

During the teen years and puberty, when the body is developing quickly, the need for insulin is increased and young people are likely to find they must increase their doses considerably. Girls grow fastest the year before their first menstruation, while boys have their growth spurt later on in the teen years. During puberty the levels of growth hormone (see page 38) in the body increase, increasing the blood glucose level.[226] This leads to a decreased sensitivity for insulin (increased insulin resistance, page 195),[3] and thus requiring large doses of bedtime insulin. Individuals without diabetes have increased levels of insulin in the blood to manage this.[226] If too little insulin is given during these "growth spurt" years, the young person's final height may be ½ - 1 inch less than predicted.[226] In earlier years, it was common for children with diabetes to be stunted in their growth, but today this is very rare (see also page 192).

If you are growing fast, you are likely to need to increase your bedtime insulin considerably. For example, teenagers often find they have to increase their NPH insulin (Novolin N, Humulin N) from 12 to 20 or 24 units within a short period. Then, this may need to be increased even further, up to 30 units, a couple of months later. A teenage girl using multiple injection treatment increased her bedtime dose of NPH insulin from 6 to 20 units within a year. A teenage boy increased his 24 hour dose from 1.2 units/kg to 1.7 units/kg (0.5 to 0.8 units/ during his growth spurt.

Increase your bedtime insulin by 2 units at a time until the blood glucose at 2-3 AM approaches 110 mg/dl (5-6 mmol/l, see page 149). Wait a few days before increasing the dose again to make certain that the effect is fully established. If your blood glucose level is still high in the morning, despite your 2-3 AM being 110 mg/dl (6 mmol/l), you may need to try another type of insulin for bedtime injections, for example Levemir. Long-acting type insulins, such as Lantus (see page 155), may also be a

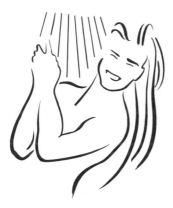

Try to make diabetes part of your daily routine. For example, you could test your blood glucose when you get up in the morning and then inject insulin before or after taking a shower, depending on your blood glucose level.

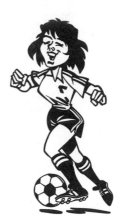

It can be tough if your parents seem to be nagging you about your diabetes during your teen years. But at the same time you need their support. Try to look upon them as "diabetes coaches" instead of "diabetes parents". A successful team player always has a good coach in the background.

better alternative. An insulin pump (see page 160) that will deliver sufficient amounts of insulin during the later part of the night could be even better.

No one can claim that remembering to take all your insulin injections is easy. But missed doses can contribute to a raised A1C, especially during puberty. One study in children and adolescents using insulin pumps showed that 2 missed premeal bolus doses/week raised A1C by as much as 0.5%.[121] A Scottish study compared the amount of insulin that young people (under the age of 30) with diabetes collected from the pharmacy, against the amount that was actually prescribed for them by their doctor.[557] As many as 28% obtained less insulin than their prescribed dose. On average, these individuals left themselves short of insulin adding up to 115 days in the year. People obtaining less insulin had higher A1C levels, and were more likely to be admitted to hospital with ketoacidosis.

Try to find a way of reminding yourself to take your insulin regularly without getting repetitive or boring yourself. One pen injector (Innovo®) has a memory so that you can see how long ago you took the last injection, and how many units it was. If you are using an insulin pump, it will have a memory that records the premeal doses,

along with the total amount of insulin given per day. It may be a good idea for parents and teenagers to read this memory together every now and again.

Insulin adjustments during the remission phase

A couple of weeks after the onset of your diabetes, your insulin doses will probably have been lowered considerably and they will go down even further in the weeks to come. There is no reason to worry if your blood glucose level is high on one occasion. Don't take extra insulin. Rather, you should wait and check the level again before your next meal. It is likely that it will have returned to normal by itself.

When the daily insulin dose is less than 0.5 units/kg (0.2 units/) of body weight the individual has entered the remission phase (honeymoon phase, see page 193). The duration of this phase varies widely among individuals but will often last 3-6 months, sometimes even longer.

Rapid-acting insulin (NovoLog/NovoRapid and Humalog) can be used for premeal doses during the remission phase since the body's own insulin

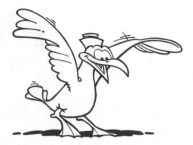

Come down to earth gently! Don't change too much at any one time when you are adjusting your insulin doses, or you will have difficulty establishing what caused what afterwards.

production will often be enough for the basal needs in between meals. The basal insulin injection in the morning can then be omitted for a longer or shorter period of time but you will usually need to take a small dose of Novo-Log/NovoRapid and Humalog before each main meal. In a study of adults with diabetes, the frequency of hypoglycemia after the meal decreased with this type of insulin treatment.[590]

Insulin requirements during the remission period may be very low, often only a few units to a meal. You may then need to temporarily withdraw the lunchtime and evening snack premeal insulin doses, if even half or a single unit results in low blood glucose readings. This would leave only three doses per day (premeal insulin for breakfast and dinner, and bedtime insulin). When the blood glucose level increases after lunch, or after the last meal of the day, this means it is time to reinstate these other doses. Another common policy is to give 2-dose treatment during the remission phase. Daily glucose monitoring is important during this phase, as it lets you know when to increase the insulin doses again.

During the remission phase it is important to increase the insulin doses if the blood glucose level is high on consecutive readings. This situation might occur if you have an infection, for example. Check your blood glucose levels before each meal and increase the dose by one

unit at a time (two if the dose is more than 10 units), if you find that the blood glucose is 145-180 mg/dl (8-10 mmol/l) or higher and your appetite is unaffected. You may have to get near to doubling the dose very quickly (more than 1 unit/kg, 0.4 units/lb) during an illness accompanied by fever (see chapter on illness, page 258). Always telephone your diabetes healthcare team if you have a child with diabetes who is ill for the first time since being diagnosed.

During the remission phase, you need to take smaller doses of additional insulin if you eat something extra (for example ice cream or pizza) compared with later in your diabetes life. This is because, during the remission phase, you will be producing some insulin of your own (see "How much extra insulin should you take?" on page 228).

There is some evidence that better blood glucose control and intensive insulin treatment early in diabetes makes the remission phase more likely to last longer.[592,696,199] High blood glucose levels seem to be harmful to the insulin producing beta cells. The capacity to produce insulin is decreased, even at a blood glucose level of around 200 mg/dl (11 mmol/l), and at 305 mg/dl (28 mmol/l) one can see alterations

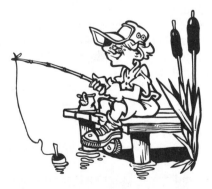

Not everyone likes physical exercise. Some people feel more like having a lazy time fishing or sunbathing. You must find the approach that suits you best, and and it is the job of your diabetes healthcare team to help you find a way of adjusting the insulin doses to your preferred lifestyle. However, you will undoubtedly be healthier in the long run if you can find some kind of exercise that you

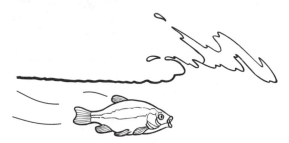

"You must swim upstream if you want to find the spring"

Saying from Middle east

When you feel that you understand the basics of your diabetes, it is important to have the courage to explore new pathways.

inside the cells.[242] See also page 193. From this it follows that if your "aim" is better when adjusting the insulin treatment during the remission phase, the chances of a prolonged remission increase. It is important that you check your blood glucose regularly, even when you are feeling perfectly well, in order to be able to see when the dose needs to be raised to deal with an increasing blood glucose level.

Hypoglycemia

Problems with hypoglycemia are less common during the remission phase. This is because the amount of insulin you produce yourself is regulated according to your blood glucose level. Therefore, it can be stopped completely if the blood glucose falls too low. For example, if you take three units of insulin for breakfast, your own pancreas can contribute by making another couple of units. These units will not be secreted at all if your blood glucose is decreasing to a low level, thereby preventing the hypoglycemia. The ability of your pancreas to secrete the hormone glucagon that increases the blood glucose level is better during the remission phase.[592]

If you have symptoms of hypoglycemia, with a blood glucose lower than 65 mg/dl (3.5

mmol/l), and you are not sure why (e.g. whether you are having too little to eat or more exercise than usual) you should lower the "responsible" dose of insulin (see page 137) by one unit (½ if the dose is < 3U, 2U if > 10U) the next day. See page 61.

Hypoglycemia before a meal

During the remission phase you can give rapid-acting insulin after the meal. This often works very well for children who are unpredictable in what they eat. When using regular short-acting insulin, you may need to shorten the recommended interval between the injection and eating to 15-20 minutes.[590]

Low blood glucose readings

Reduce the insulin in the same way as above if your blood glucose is 70 mg/dl (4.0 mmol/l) or lower at the same time of the day for 2 days in a row (even if you have no symptoms of hypoglycemia).

Experiment!

We encourage young people to experiment with their injections in different situations. It is important to try and avoid terms like "permitted" or "forbidden". The point is to find out what is suitable just for you. Do remember to measure your blood glucose level and record the results in your logbook so that you know what you are doing. The worst situation you are likely to encounter (and it is not particularly serious anyway) is that you can find yourself, after trying something new, hypoglycemic or with a temporary high blood glucose level. Gradually, you will get to know yourself better, finding out which insulin doses your pancreas would have supplied if it had worked as usual. There is a saying that goes: "You can only learn by your own mistakes". Remember that most lessons in life are learned by trial and error!

Insulin pumps

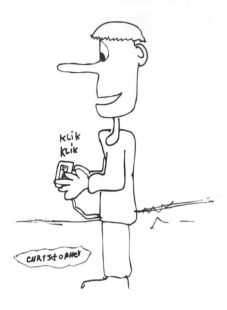

An insulin pump delivers insulin to your body in a way that much more closely mimics that of a normal pancreas. If treatment by injections does not give acceptable glucose control, many children and teenagers will feel much better after changing to pump therapy. More than 40% of those in the intensive treatment group in the DCCT study (see page 314) chose an insulin pump. In 2002 there were approximately 200,000 people with diabetes on insulin pumps in the US.

Insulin pump therapy (also called CSII, continuous subcutaneous insulin infusion) is more expensive than conventional syringe or pen therapy. In countries where insulin pumps are not reimbursed, they may be difficult to afford. If this applies to you, ask your diabetes team whether you might be eligible for any grants or other financial help from local organizations or national charities.

Only short-acting or rapid-acting insulin is used in the insulin pump. In the past, short-acting insulin with a special solvent was used to avoid

the catheter becoming blocked (Velosulin BR Human). The action time and effect of this insulin is similar to ordinary short-acting insulin (Novolin R, Humulin R). Today most pumps are started using rapid-acting insulin (NovoLog/Rapid [88] and Humalog,[827] see page 186). A study comparing NovoLog/NovoRapid and Humalog found no difference between the two insulins in the effect on blood glucose levels and A1C when used in pumps.[92] There was also no difference in the rate of hypoglycemia or the number of blockages in pumps and infusion sets.

The insulin pump will deliver a basal rate of insulin for 24 hours every day. Most modern pumps can be adjusted for different basal insulin rates during the day and night. Extra insulin is given with meals (a "bolus dose") by pushing a button on the pump. The insulin is pumped through a thin tubing (catheter) that is connected to a metal needle or indwelling cannula placed under the skin (subcutaneously).

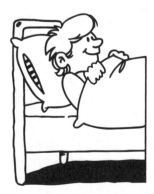

"How do I wear the pump at night?" is usually one of the first questions asked by someone interested in trying a pump. You will be surprised by how quickly you get used to this, and find a solution that fits in with your sleeping habits.

Advantages of using an insulin pump

➠ The basal rate will give you sufficient amounts of insulin in the early morning to avoid a high blood glucose level when you wake up (dawn phenomenon).

➠ Some people need more insulin than others between meals. An insulin pump can provide this.

➠ The continuous supply of basal insulin makes it less essential to eat at regular intervals.

➠ You will always have your insulin with you.

➠ It is easier to take a bolus dose with the pump than to take an injection with a pen or syringe, especially if you don't feel like injecting when you are out.

➠ Your premeal doses can be adjusted in 0.1 unit increments or even 0.05 units on some pumps.

➠ You will be able to adjust it to take account of the differing needs of basal insulin during the day and night.

➠ The pump uses only short-acting or rapid-acting insulin. These are likely to be more predictable in their effect than intermediate or long-acting insulins.

➠ The risk of severe hypoglycaemia is usually lessened by using an insulin pump.

➠ The fact that the body's insulin store is small will mean that additional insulin is less likely to be released in an unpredictable fashion during physical exercise.

➠ During and after exercise, a temporary basal rate can be used.

➠ Pumps are easy to adjust if you are travelling across time zones.

Disadvantages of using an insulin pump

➠ A small store of insulin in your body means you will be sensitive to any interruption in insulin supply, which puts you at risk of rapidly developing ketoacidosis.

➠ You need to do more regular monitoring tests if you are using an insulin pump.

➠ The pump will be attached to you 24 hours a day (except when disconnecting it). Some people feel this makes them more tied to their diabetes.

➠ The pump will be very obvious, for example if you go swimming in a public pool. So you will not be able to keep your diabetes secret. Other people may be curious about the pump, something people who are not yet entirely comfortable with their diabetes might find difficult to deal with.

➠ The pump's alarm is likely to go off every now and then, and you might need to stop your activities to change the infusion set at an inconvenient time.

and the absorption will be more even.[476] In a research study, insulin absorption after a premeal dose was constant for four days when the cannula was inserted in an area free of lipohypertrophy (fatty lumps).[583]

The total insulin requirement per 24 hours usually decreases by around 15-20% after starting with insulin pump treatment.[87,175,719] A US study of adults found an average decrease of 26%, with greater percentage reductions for patients on Humalog, and for those with higher daily dosages.[90] In a study of children with diabetes, those who had not reached puberty showed little change in insulin requirements, while those of the adolescents decreased by an average of 18%.[150] The basal dose with a pump was reduced by around 40% compared to the basal dose (intermediate or long-acting insulin) needed by young people on multiple injections.

A common problem with pen injectors and syringes is that the insulin will not always give quite the same effect even if the dose is exactly the same. With an insulin pump, the insulin will be deposited in the same site for several days

Reasons for starting with an insulin pump

▹ High A1C.

▹ Complications of diabetes.

▹ High blood glucose levels during the night or morning (dawn phenomenon).

▹ Wide fluctuations in blood glucose.

▹ A1C is OK with multiple injections but it takes too much work.

▹ Missed injections.

▹ Pain from insulin or injection needle.

▹ Recurrent severe hypoglycemia.

▹ Hypoglycemia unawareness.

▹ Possibility of sleeping in

▹ Need for flexible meal sizes and schedules.

▹ Need to manage diabetes while exercising.

▹ Shift work / variable working patterns.

▹ Quality of life issues.

▹ Use of a pump from the time diabetes is diagnosed in pre-school children?

At one time, we would only give people insulin pumps if there were definite medical reasons, but now more attention is being paid to quality of life issues and the use of pumps is becoming more widespread. We have recently started several pre-school children on pumps from the onset of diabetes with very good results. Pre-school children often have an irregular lifestyle and the use of pumps for this age group can be very positive.[495,763]

Insulin pump treatment will be easier if you: (adapted from [742])

▹ Are comfortable with the pump cannula being constantly attached to your body and understand how it works.

▹ Check your blood glucose regularly, at least 4 times a day (including morning and evening) and preferably before each meal.

▹ Regularly monitor ketones when you are ill or feeling nauseous, or when your blood glucose is repeatedly above 250 mg/dl (14 mmol/l) (preferably blood ketones).

▹ Recognize symptoms of low blood glucose. Always carry glucose tablets.

▹ Recognize early symptoms of ketoacidosis. Always carry extra insulin and a pen or syringe to be able to treat this condition.

▹ Make sure you keep in regular contact with your diabetes clinic.

▹ If you live alone, you should make sure you can always contact a close friend or relative.

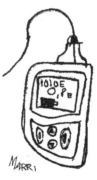

The glucose control often improves, resulting in a lower A1C.[87,175,337] Some patients (especially teenage girls) will gain weight when they start using an insulin pump if they don't decrease their food intake as their glucose control improves. The extra glucose that, beforehand, was lost in the urine now remains in the body and is transformed into fat instead.

The risk of severe hypoglycemia usually decreases with pump treatment,[87,175] even when used in children under the age of 6.[763] The risk of ketoacidosis (diabetic coma) may increase according to some studies [175] but appears to decrease in others.[87,763] Ketoacidotic episodes may occur soon after starting with a pump, before the person has got used to the new form of treatment.[539] Those teenagers who are prone to frequent episodes of ketoacidosis caused by interrupted insulin supply, may find the frequency and severity of these to be drastically reduced by using an insulin pump that makes a continuous insulin supply possible.[77,719]

Starting the pump

We start new pumps on an outpatient basis, except for the very youngest children (under 3 or 4 years old) who are admitted to hospital for a night or two. Patients attend a three-day pump school at the day care ward together with their parents (even older teenagers need to bring their parents to the sessions). No intermediate-acting insulin (Novolin N, Humulin N, Insuman NPH) is taken in the morning they start using the pump, and only half the dose the evening before for those using long-acting insulin (Lantus, Ultralente, Humulin U). Only the premeal bolus of short-acting or rapid-acting insulin is taken in the morning. The pump cannula is inserted after anesthetizing the skin (with EMLA®, ELA-Max® or similar) and using a skin disinfectant. The first pump bolus is given at lunchtime. Today, we start almost all new pumps on rapid-acting insulin. For a few patients, the slightly larger insulin depot when using short-acting insulin (Velosulin BR Human) can help to avoid recurrent episodes of ketones/ketoacidosis.

Even though the amount of insulin you are receiving goes down when you start using a pump, you will probably find your blood glucose levels will be in the lower range at first. If so, it is very important to lower your pump doses even further to avoid problems with hypoglycemia. The reason you will need even lower doses is that when your blood glucose readings decrease, your insulin resistance will decrease as well (increased insulin sensitivity, see page 195). This implies that a certain insulin dose will be more effective at lowering your blood glucose level than the same dose was just a few days before.

The basal rate

The small amounts of insulin that the pump automatically delivers every hour is called the basal rate. An appropriate basal rate lets you keep your blood glucose levels stable when you are not eating, for example during the night or

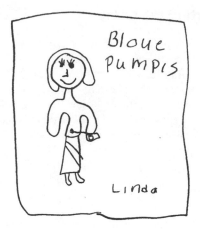

Many people come to look upon their pump as a reliable friend that they will use for many years. Little Linda has even given her pump a name "Bloue Pumpis".

between meals. When starting a pump we usually set five basal rates: after midnight (12-3AM), early morning (3-7AM), morning (7AM-12noon), afternoon (12-6PM) and evening (6-12PM). The charts on page 167 give more details. It is important to emphasize that starting doses are only estimates, also that it is essential to monitor your blood glucose very frequently (including at night) during the first few weeks in order to establish correct basal rates and bolus doses. If the basal rates are set correctly, the pump user will usually be able to delay or skip meals, and sleep longer in the morning when they want to.

Approximately 40-50% of the daily insulin requirement is given as the basal rate (often close to 1 U/hour for an adult person).[368] The remainder is given as premeal bolus injections. For older children and teenagers, a starting dose of up to 60% as basal rate has been recommended with rapid-acting insulin (50% if using short-acting insulin in the pump).[434] Younger children often need a lower percentage of their daily dose as basal insulin. In a US study, children before puberty had 41% of their daily dose as basal insulin and the pubertal group had 46%.[150]

Night time basal rate

Check your blood glucose levels during a night after an ordinary day when you have been feeling well and have not had extra exercise. Adjust the premeal bolus dose before the evening snack to reach a blood glucose level of about 125-145 mg/dl (7-8 mmol/l) at 10-11 PM.[103]

Blood test at 3 AM and in the morning	Measure
< 110 mg/dl < 6 mmol/l	Decrease the basal rate after midnight and/or early in the morning by 0.05U/h if the rate is <0.3U/h, 0.1 U/h if the rate is < 1U/h, 0.2 U/h if the rate is >1U/h.
>160-180 mg/dl >9-10 mmol/l	Increase the basal rate after midnight and/or early in the morning by 0.05U/h if the rate is <0.3U/h, 0.1 U/h if the rate is < 1U/h, 0.2 U/h if the rate is >1U/h.

If your pump cannot be adjusted for different basal rate profiles, you should adjust it to fit the night time need of basal insulin to reach a blood glucose level of 110-125 mg/dl (6-7 mmol/l) at 3 AM.[103]

Make the changes in basal rates in collaboration with your doctor and diabetes nurse.

After a change in the basal rate, it will take 2-3 hours before the blood glucose level is affected when using short-acting insulin,[361] and approximately 1-2 hours with rapid-acting insulin. The basal insulin may be absorbed twice as rapidly if the person has a thin layer of subcutaneous fat (less than 10 mm in a lifted skin fold) compared to a thicker subcutaneous fat layer (more than 20 mm).[363]

The body's insulin requirement in adults is often about 20% lower between 1-3 AM compared to 5-7 AM.[103] If you are using a pump with the possibility of different basal rates, you can administer a lower basal rate from 11-12 PM to 3 AM to avoid night time hypoglycemia.[103] If you have problems with high glucose readings in the morning, you can try a slight increase in the basal rate (0.1-0.2 U/hour) between 3 and 7 AM. Many children below the age of puberty need a higher basal rate late in the evening (9 PM to 12 AM) [100,150] and it is not uncommon for the basal rate to need to be higher in the middle of the night (midnight-3 AM) than later in the morning (3-7AM).[765] This may be caused by an early rise in the level of growth hormone shortly after the child falls asleep.[150]

Do not make too great a change in the basal rate at any one time. It is usually sufficient to change by 0.1 U/hour if the basal rate is < 1 U/hour and by 0.2 U/hour if the basal rate is > 1 U/hour. You should not change the basal rate more than twice in any week as, otherwise, it may be difficult to see which change leads to what. To avoid hypoglycemia you should be prepared to decrease the basal rate (especially at night) when blood tests start to show lower readings.

The advice on basal rates in this chapter are written for a pump that can be adjusted for different basal rate levels throughout the day and night. Some pumps can be adjusted for different basal rates every hour, and others can be set for different profiles for a longer or shorter period of time. However, if you have a pump that can be programmed for only one basal rate, you should adjust it according to your night time blood glucose values. You will then have to adjust the premeal bolus doses to fit the fixed basal rate.

Temporary change of the basal rate

Most pumps allow you to make temporary changes of the basal rate for one or several hours. This is practical if, for example, you have problems with low blood glucose and repeated hypoglycemia for sustained periods despite extra food intake. It will usually help to decrease the basal rate or stop the pump com-

Changes in the basal rate

Insulin absorption U/h. (y-axis: 2.2, 1.8, 1.4, 1.0, 0.6, 0.2)

x-axis: 0 1 2 3 4 1 2 3 4 1 2 3 h.

Basal dose   1,1   2,2   1,1 U/hour

When you change the basal rate using rapid-acting insulin analogs, it will take approximately 1-2 hours before the uptake of insulin into the bloodstream is increased. The reason for this is that when you increase the basal rate, part of the insulin will stay in the subcutaneous tissue as an insulin depot. When you decrease the basal rate, the insulin from the depot will continue to be released and absorbed into the bloodstream for another 1-2 hours until the depot has decreased in size. The graph is from a study where regular short-acting insulin was used, showing that the time before a change occurs is 2-3 hours with this type of insulin.[361]

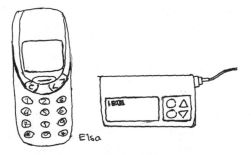

A modern insulin pump is small and easy to manage. You will soon master the different controls. Many teenagers with labile diabetes find life easier with an insulin pump. Even small children can benefit from using a pump. For example, one of our patients, a 3-year old boy, had better morning blood glucose levels in addition to less night time hypoglycemia after starting with an insulin pump.

When should basal rates be changed?

(adapted from [86])

You should not change the profiles of the basal rate too often. When you are used to the pump it may be practical to change the basal rates once or twice in a month according to what your 24 hour blood glucose profiles show. Change the premeal bolus doses to adjust for temporary changes in diet or blood glucose readings or use the temporary basal rate. In the following situations it may be necessary to make changes to the basal rates:

➠ Illness with fever and increased need of insulin.

➠ Change in school or work activities with a new schedule or different physical activity.

➠ Change in body weight of 5-10% or more.

➠ Pregnancy.

➠ Women may have different insulin needs during different phases of the menstrual cycle (see page 277).

➠ Initiation of treatment with drugs that increase the need of insulin (such as cortisol / prednisolone).

➠ Prolonged physical exercise (such as a hiking or cycling trip lasting 12-24 hours or more).

Changing the basal rate

Since it takes 2-3 hours with regular insulin and 1-2 hours with NovoLog/NovoRapid or Humalog before a change in the basal rate will take effect (see chart on page 165), you must plan ahead.

① Change the dose 2 hours before you want it to take effect, e.g. increase from 3 AM if you want an increased insulin effect from 5 AM on.

② If you want a rapid increase in the effect of the basal rate (e.g. if you are ill with fever) you should administer an extra dose of insulin (corresponding to 2 hours of the basal rate) before increasing the basal rate. This will result in a rapid increase of the insulin depot resulting in a quicker absorption of insulin into the blood.

③ If you want to decrease the effect of the basal rate fast (e.g. if you are going to exercise) you should stop the basal rate for 2 hours and then start it again at a lower level. The insulin depot will then rapidly decrease in size and the change in basal rate will take effect sooner.

pletely for an hour or two. If your blood glucose is high at bedtime you can temporarily increase the basal rate by 10-20% (~0.1-0.2 U/hour) for a couple of hours. If your blood glucose is low during the early part of the night, you can temporarily decrease the basal rate for a few hours by 10-20% (~0.1-0.2 U/hour). The temporary basal rate is very useful for prolonged exercise. For example, during a 5 hour bike ride, try decreasing the basal rate by 50%. If you have exercised in the afternoon or evening, you should decrease the basal rate by 10-20% (~0.1-0.2 U/hour) for the whole night.

If you work shifts, it may be a good idea to use the temporary basal rate during the nights you

are working or use a separate profile program if your pump has this feature. It is common to find you need to increase the basal dose during the latter part of the night to compensate for the stress effect of staying awake.

Premeal bolus doses

Take a bolus dose 30 minutes before the meal when you are using regular insulin in the pump, and just before the meal if you are using rapid-acting insulin (NovoLog/NovoRapid and Humalog). However, the timing will also depend on what your actual blood glucose level is (see page 135 and 139). Adjust the bolus doses up or down in the same way as you would if you were on multiple injections. See graph on page 143 for adjusting rapid-acting

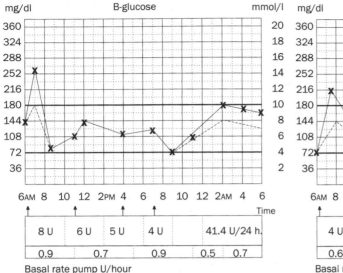

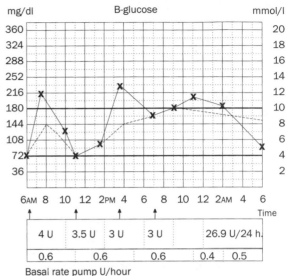

Basal rate pump U/hour

Interpreting the 24 hour profile
(boy 40 kg, 88 lb)

It is best to take tests for a couple of days in a row to be sure that the results of any one day were not unusual. Start by looking at the evening snack since that affects the level your blood glucose will be on going to bed. The dotted line shows what the blood glucose values might have been with the suggested changes.

Evening snack: The blood glucose after the meal is a bit low. Decrease the dose by 1 unit. Adjust the dose so that you will have a blood glucose of about 110-145 mg/dl (6-8 mmol/l) when you go to bed.

Night: Early in the night the basal rate needs to be increased slightly to 0.6 U/hour as the blood glucose is rising until 3 AM. The blood glucose level from 3 AM to 7 AM is stable so this rate does not need to be changed.

Breakfast: The blood glucose rises very quickly after breakfast. If you use NovoLog/NovoRapid or Humalog you can try increasing the pre-breakfast dose to 9 U and lowering the basal rate to 0.8 U/hour. With short-acting insulin, the breakfast dose could have been given even earlier before breakfast to prevent the peak at 8 AM.

Lunch and dinner: No changes.

Sit down when you have some time for yourself and consider all the doses for the next day. Don't change all doses at the same time as it can be difficult to see which change resulted in what. Let a few days go by between changes to make sure that the profiles look similar from day to day. Read the pump memory and write down in your logbook the total number of units your pump has delivered each day.

Interpreting the 24 hour profile
(girl 30 kg, 66 lb)

See the previous profile for general interpretation.

Evening snack: No changes in premeal bolus. Young children often need to have their highest basal rates before midnight. The rise in blood glucose before midnight indicates that an increase in basal rate of 0.1 U/hour from 9PM to midnight may be appropriate.

Night: The blood glucose does not change much between midnight and 3 AM. However, late at night it drops significantly, so reducing the basal rate from 3 AM to 0.4 U/hour is recommended. Young children often need less insulin during these hours and a further decrease to 0.3 U/hour may be appropriate.

Breakfast: The blood glucose rises quickly after breakfast and the dose should preferably be increased to 5 units. The basal rate is probably sufficient as the blood glucose is lowered at lunch again. However, when the breakfast bolus dose is increased to 5 units the basal rate might need to be decreased.

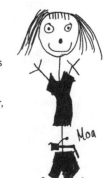

Lunch: The blood glucose two hours after the meal is only slightly increased indicating that the pre-meal bolus dose is correct. However, as the blood glucose rises prior to dinner, the basal rate could be increased to 0.7 U/hour.

Dinner: No changes.

insulin. The breakfast dose is usually slightly larger than the other premeal bolus doses. Since the basal need of insulin between meals is now supplied via the pump, your premeal bolus doses will be lower than when on multiple injections. You will probably need to decrease the size of extra insulin doses as well if you eat something extra. On many pumps the type of bolus dose can be varied from rapid delivery (standard bolus), administered over a period of time (square or extended bolus), or a combination of both (dual or combination bolus). See the figure on page 168.

You can calculate the amount of insulin needed for a given amount of carbohydrates by dividing the total amount of carbohydrates eaten during the day by the amount of insulin taken as premeal bolus doses.[185] One unit will usually cover 10-15 grams of extra carbohydrate. If, for example, you eat ice cream containing 26 g of carbohydrate, 2 units of extra insulin will probably be enough. See page 216 for advice on carbohydrate counting.

With an insulin pump, you will not be bound to maintain a regular interval between meals (and insulin doses) as when you were on multiple injection treatment with short-acting insulin. The basal rate will probably make it possible to

Square or dual bolus doses: when can they be useful?

⇒ When you are eating pasta, as this gives a slower blood glucose rise;

⇒ When you eat a meal rich in fat or protein that is digested more slowly, for example a pizza;

⇒ When your meal is larger than usual;

⇒ When you eat a meal that takes a longer time than usual, for example a three course dinner;

⇒ When several small meals are eaten within a short period of time, for example at a birthday party;

⇒ When you eat slowly, for example popcorn or chips while watching a movie;

⇒ If you have problems with delayed stomach emptying (see page 313).

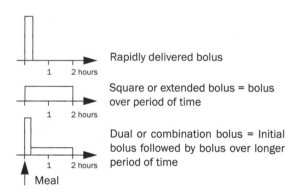

Rapidly delivered bolus

Square or extended bolus = bolus over period of time

Dual or combination bolus = Initial bolus followed by bolus over longer period of time

Meal

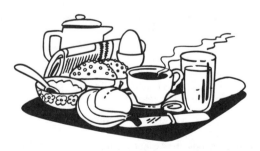

With a pump you can adjust the premeal bolus to match the carbohydrate content of your meal. Breakfast usually contains a high proportion of carbohydrates. You may find that 1 unit of insulin can take care of a slightly lower amount of carbohydrates for breakfast compared to other meals. See page 216 for further advice on counting carbohydrates.

The type of bolus dose can be varied on most pumps. A square or dual bolus may be preferred for a large meal that is rich in fat or proteins, a meal with low glycemic index (see page 208), or when you will be eating over a longer period, at a party for example. These bolus doses may also work well if you have problems with delayed emptying of the stomach (gastroparesis, see page 313). In a study of a meal high in carbohydrates, calories and fat, the square (whole dose over 2 hours) and dual (70% as an immediate bolus and 30% over 2 hours) bolus provided the lowest glucose levels over a 4-hour period.[138]

increase the time period between meals to 6-7 hours, which might be an advantage if you keep irregular hours.

You should, however, be aware of eating and taking premeal bolus doses with intervals of less than 2-3 hours as there will be a risk of overlapping insulin doses when using rapid-acting insulin in the pump. Try reducing the second premeal bolus by 1 or 2 units if the previous meal was only 2 hours earlier. Many modern pumps can subtract insulin "on board" before giving the second bolus dose to compensate for this effect.

Change of insertion site

The most common insertion site is the abdomen. Avoid your waistline, belt line and underwear line and a 5cm (2 inch) circle around your belly button (see illustration on page 123). With small children, it is preferable to use the buttocks as well to be able to spread the infusion sites, thereby decreasing the risk of fatty lumps (lipohypertrophies, see page 189). You can also use the thigh or the upper arm but both sites can result in an increased absorption of insulin when exercising. There is also a greater risk of the cannula catching on the clothing and being pulled out.

Individual advice is needed on how often the cannula should be replaced. We usually start by recommending the use of a soft teflon catheter,

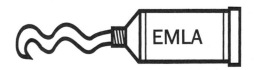

Always use a topical anesthetic cream such as (EMLA®, ELA-Max®) before replacing the infusion set when beginning with pump treatment in children. Apply the cream 1½-2 hours ahead of time to get full effect. An alternative way of lessening the pain is using an automatic inserter. Applying an ice cube is a quick way of decreasing the pain of insertion in less difficult cases.

When should you replace the accessories?	
Teflon cannula	Start by replacing it 2-3 times a week. If there are no problems try using it 4-5 days before replacement. Some people, especially small children, may need to replace every second day.
Metal needle	Replace every second day, more often if signs of irritation are noted.
Tubing	Replace the tubing at least every other time you replace the cannula/needle and when you replace the reservoir.
Insulin reservoir	Some pumps have prefilled reservoirs, others need to be filled. Do not reuse them as the silicon on the plunger wears off, resulting in an occlusion or blockage alarm.

but some people prefer a short steel needle. Start by replacing the catheter twice a week and then try to increase the number of days between replacements. You can usually let the catheter remain in place for 3-4 days if your blood glucose readings do not become raised. Some people, especially young children, will need to replace it every 2 days. The longer the catheter remains in one site, the greater the risk of developing fatty lumps (lipohypertrophies) and infections. A steel needle usually needs to be replaced every second day.

Disinfect the insertion site with Hibiclens™, IV Prep™ or similar product. Skin-Prep™, Mastisol™ and Tincture of Benzoin™ leave a sticky film after drying to help the adhesive get a firm grip. Don't use products containing skin moisturizers, as these may cause the adhesive to loosen more easily. If you are allergic to the adhesive, it can cause redness or itching. Try another type of adhesive or infusion set. Another solution is to apply a thin transparent adhesive (like Tegaderm™, IV 3000™ or Polyskin™) and then insert the cannula through it. In this way the cannula adhesive will not get into contact with the skin. A thicker stoma type

Replacement of infusion set

➠ If you replace the infusion set before taking a premeal bolus it will be flushed by the larger volume of fluid.

➠ Avoid replacing your infusion set before bedtime as you will need to be awake for a couple of hours to see that it functions properly.

➠ Start by washing your hands with soap and water.

➠ Choose an insertion site well away from your beltline.

➠ Disinfect a skin area that is a little larger than the adhesive you are going to apply. Use Hibiclens™, IV Prep™ or a similar product. Applying Skin-Prep™, Mastisol™ or Tincture of Benzoin™ will make the adhesive stick better. Use a disinfectant for hand-washing as well if you have problems with skin infections.

➠ Be careful not to touch the sterile needle. Do not breathe or blow directly onto the needle, as this may contaminate it.

➠ Pinch a two-finger skin fold and insert the needle at a 45° angle (see illustration on page 123) or according to the instructions for other types of needles.

➠ Remove the protective tape and apply the adhesive carefully. If it sticks unevenly don't try to move it. There is a considerable risk of removing the catheter at the same time if you try to move the adhesive.

➠ Fill the cannula with insulin after removing the insertion needle. Depending on the length of the cannula, it needs to be filled with 0.3-1 unit of insulin to fill up the dead space.

➠ Withdraw the old catheter after the insertion of the new one. Pull the adhesive from the side where the tip of the infusion set is located and it will come off more easily.

➠ If you have problems removing sticky traces of adhesive, try a remover such as Detachol™ or Uni-Solve™.

adhesive (like Duoderm™ or Compeed™) will often help in especially difficult cases. A small hole needs to be cut for the catheter in these thicker types of adhesives.

Avoid inserting the cannula in skin folds, close to the belly button or under the waistline. Straighten your back before you apply the adhesive to avoid tight skin. Always check your blood glucose level 2-3 hours after replacing the infusion set to make sure that it works properly.

Insert the new metal infusion set before you remove the old one. If you do it the other way around, you will be at greater risk of contaminating your hands on the old site and therefore of transferring bacteria to the new site. Insert the new infusion set at least 4-6 centimeters (2 inches) away from the old one to avoid developing fatty lumps. The adhesive should not cover a previous infusion site until it has healed completely. It is best to change sides on the abdomen (left/right) with each replacement.

Some sets of tubing and cannulas need to be filled with insulin before the needle is inserted. With others you need to give a small amount of extra insulin (around half to a full unit) after insertion to fill up the air inside it (called dead space). Even if you have filled the tubing by pressing the reservoir plunger you need to build up the pressure in the tubing by giving a priming dose with the pump to make sure insulin appears at the tip of the tubing.

The blood glucose level should always be checked 3 hours after changing the infusion set to ensure proper insulin delivery. It is not a good idea to change infusion sites just before going to bed. Since the basal rate runs very slowly during the night, it may take longer for the alarm to be triggered if something is wrong with the new insertion site. Many pump users find it more convenient to replace the infusion site straight after coming home from school or work. This leaves plenty of time to find out if something is wrong with the new infusion site. If you replace the cannula and tubing before

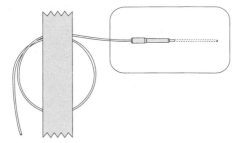

For young children it may be a good idea to put the tubing in a sling and fix it with some adhesive to minimize the risk of pulling the cannula loose if the tubing is pulled or jerked, for example if you drop the pump.

taking a meal bolus dose, this will clear away any tissue from the cannula or needle.

Problems with irritation or infection at the insertion site can be prevented by careful hand washing, disinfection and infusion set replacement every second or third day. Use chlorhexidine in alcohol (Hibiscrub™) or similar agent for hand-washing. If you have recurring problems with infected sites in spite of good hygiene routines, it might mean that the bacteria originate from your armpits or nostrils. If tests show you have bacteria (staphylococci) in your nasal cavity, you may need antibiotic treatment. Another approach is the application of local antibiotics to each nostril nightly, and chlorhexidine body washes on a daily basis.

If you have problems with fatty lumps or redness of the skin you should replace the infusion set more frequently. If the redness doesn't disappear soon after you have replaced the cannula, you can speed up the healing process by applying a dressing soaked in warm soapy water for 20 minutes four times daily. You can also try an antibiotic ointment or hydrogen peroxide cream. If the redness increases or starts hurting, you might need antibiotic treatment. Contact your diabetes healthcare team or doctor.

How many tests should you take when using an insulin pump?

➡ Blood glucose at least 4 times daily (including morning and before going to bed), preferably 4-5/day, especially if you are using NovoLog/NovoRapid or Humalog in the pump.

➡ One or two 24 hour profiles every or every other week with readings taken before and 1½-2 hours after each meal and at night.

➡ Before each meal if you are ill or feeling unwell for any reason at all.

➡ Check for ketones if you are nauseous, when you are ill, or when your blood glucose level is high (>250 mg/dl (14 mmol/l)).

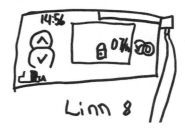

More frequent home monitoring

Since there is a greater risk of insulin deficiency with a pump, you must be willing to test your blood glucose level more often. At the very least, you will need to be doing 4 tests a day including morning and late evening. Preferably you should test before each meal. You must also be careful to check for ketones if your blood glucose is high, or if you are feeling unwell, as ketones are a sign of insulin deficiency. It is a good idea to keep reagent strips for blood ketone monitoring at home, so that you can monitor the effect of extra insulin doses given in this situation (see page 101). A 24 hour blood glucose profile with tests before and 1-1½ hours after each meal is needed every week or every second week to allow you to adjust your doses correctly. You should also take night time

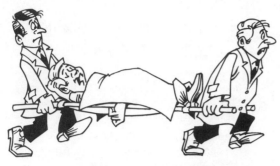

There is an increased risk of ketoacidosis in pump users if there is any interruption to insulin delivery as the insulin depot is so small. Ketoacidosis must be treated in the hospital with intravenous insulin and fluids. To avoid risking ketoacidosis, **always use a pen or syringe** when taking extra insulin if your blood glucose is high and you have ketones in your blood or urine.

tests when compiling a 24 hour profile (at 2-3 AM and if necessary at 5 AM as well).

Record your test results in a logbook where you can document clearly the pump's basal rate. We find it best to use a logbook where every entry is written on a blood glucose chart. Doing this will help you to see patterns in your blood glucose readings (see charts on page 167). Make it part of your routine to check the pump daily for the total number of units delivered every 24 hours and record this in your logbook.

Insulin depot with a pump

The disadvantage of using an insulin pump is that the insulin depot will be very small, since only rapid or short-acting insulin is used. This

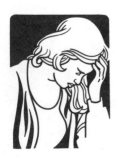

If you are not feeling well, remember to test your blood or urine for ketones as a matter of course!

KETONE ALERT!

If you are using an insulin pump, you are at greater risk of ketoacidosis because you have a very small insulin depot.

ALWAYS check your blood glucose and ketones when you are not feeling well. Check for ketones in the following situations too:

➡ If you wake up with a blood glucose of more than 250 mg/dl (14 mmol/l).

➡ If your blood glucose has been higher than 250 mg/dl (14 mmol/l) for more than a couple of hours.

➡ If you are ill and running a temperature (for example with a cold or flu).

➡ If you have any symptoms of insulin deficiency (nausea, vomiting, abdominal pain, rapid breathing, or your breath smells "fruity" or of "pear drops"').

If your ketone levels increase, this means that you are becoming more and more insulin-deficient. You will need to contact your doctor to discuss what to do next!

Be aware that insulin deficiency leading to increased ketone production shows in the urine within a couple of hours. With a blood ketone test, you will detect ketones even earlier. If you take extra insulin, the production of ketones will stop and the level of blood ketones will decrease within an hour or two (you may notice an increase in the first hour after extra insulin is given but the level should then drop). The excretion of ketones in the urine will continue for many hours but you should notice the concentration stabilizing, then decreasing, as the hours pass.

If you are the least bit concerned, or cannot get hold of someone who is familiar with insulin pumps over the phone, you should take an injection of insulin by pen or syringe and then go to your nearest hospital emergency room.

Always bring extra insulin to give with a pen or syringe wherever you go, even if you expect to be away from home for only a couple of hours or so.

High blood glucose and ketones?

If your blood glucose is higher than 250 mg/dl (14 mmol/l) and you have ketones in the blood (>0.5 mmol/l) or urine (moderate or large), this indicates a blocked insulin supply or increased need of insulin, for example, because of an infection.

① Take 0.1 U/kg (0.5 units/10 lb) body weight of short-acting insulin (or preferably rapid-acting NovoLog/NovoRapid or Humalog) **with a pen or a syringe.** Don't use the pump as you cannot be sure whether or not it works properly.

② Measure blood glucose every hour. If it doesn't decrease, the insulin dose of 0.1 U/kg (0.5 units/10 lb) body weight can be repeated (every 1-2 hours with rapid-acting insulin, every 2-3 hours with regular short-acting insulin). Measure blood ketones if you have such strips available (see page 101). Often there will be an increase in the first hour after insulin is given but after that you should find the level decreases.

③ Check the pump by disconnecting the tubing from the cannula/needle. Activate a prime dose. Insulin should immediately appear from the tubing. If not, replace the tubing.

④ Replace the cannula/needle if the tubing works well. Check for signs of redness in the skin and of moisture close to the infusion site as this would indicate insulin leakage.

⑤ Be sure to drink large amounts of sugar-free fluids. If your blood glucose is approximately 180-200 mg/dl (10-11 mmol/l) or below and you still have high ketone levels in the blood, you will need to drink fluids containing sugar and repeat the extra dose of rapid-acting insulin.

Causes of ketoacidosis

➡ Insulin delivery is interrupted, for example by a leak in the piece connecting the tubing to the reservoir or a cannula that has come out.

➡ Increased insulin requirements caused by illness (e.g. a cold with fever) without the insulin dose being increased.

➡ Inflammation or infection at the infusion site (indicated by redness or pus).

➡ Decreased insulin absorption, for example caused by inserting the infusion set into a fat pad (lipohypertrophy).

➡ Decreased insulin potency, for example after it has been frozen or exposed to heat or sunlight.

Thicker layers of subcutaneous fat will result in a larger insulin depot of the basal dose. In one study a basal rate of 1 U/h was used. The insulin depot for those people with a subcutaneous fat layer of 40 mm (1½ inch) was close to 6 U while those with less than 10 mm (1/3 inch) subcutaneous fat had only 1 U in their depot.[363] This suggests that thin people will be more sensitive to an interrupted basal rate since their insulin depot is smaller.

Ketoacidosis

A small insulin depot will result in early insulin deficiency symptoms if something goes wrong with the pump or the tubing. Your blood glucose will be high within 2-4 hours of interrupted insulin delivery (see chart on page 176). One night's interrupted insulin supply is enough to cause incipient ketoacidosis in the morning with symptoms of insulin deficiency such as nausea and vomiting. Be extra careful to check both blood glucose and ketones whenever you are feeling at all unwell.

It is very important to be able to recognize symptoms of insulin deficiency early on (nau-

will be important if the pump gets blocked, or if you intentionally turn it off when playing sport or swimming, for example. If the insulin supply is interrupted you will very soon develop symptoms of insulin deficiency such as high blood glucose, nausea and vomiting (see "Depot effect" on page 79).

Causes of a lack in insulin delivery

➭ The connector between the tubing and the insulin reservoir can be cracked. Feel it with your fingers. It may smell of insulin even if you do not see a leak.

➭ Hole in the tubing. (A cat bite in the tubing resulted in leakage which lead to ketoacidosis for a teenage girl.)

➭ Air in the tubing is not dangerous as such but will give you less insulin.

➭ If the tubing is squeezed or bent, e.g. by a belt or tight jeans, it will take several hours before the pump's blockage alarm is triggered.

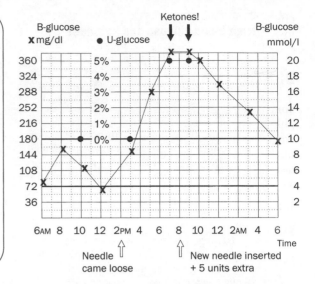

Needle came loose

New needle inserted + 5 units extra

sea, vomiting, abdominal pain, rapid breathing, fruity smell on the breath). To avoid episodes of ketoacidosis, we admit the person to the day care ward a few weeks after pump start and the pump is stopped for 6-8 hours (except in the younger children). See graph on page 176. Pump wearers (and family members) will learn to recognize the individual symptoms caused by lack of insulin, and can practice taking extra insulin with a pen or syringe under safe conditions. None of the patients who have undergone this form of test have had more than a mild degree of nausea with ketone levels of up to 2 mmol/l (with a normal pH). This reassures them that they can tolerate being without the pump for 6-8 hours ("a night's sleep") without risk of ketoacidosis. This procedure has also been recommended for adult pump users.[640]

If your blood glucose is above 270 mg/dl (15 mmol/l) and you have ketones in the urine or blood you should take an extra dose (0.1 U/kg or 0.5 U/10 lb. body weight) of insulin (preferably rapid-acting NovoLog/NovoRapid or Humalog if available). The dose can be repeated after 2-3 hours if necessary (1-2 hours with NovoLog/NovoRapid or Humalog). Contact the hospital if you vomit or feel nauseous and are unable to drink. If you often have episodes

A few hours of interrupted insulin supply is sufficient to make the blood glucose rise quickly. The blood glucose will rise even if you don't eat because the liver will produce glucose when there is a lack of insulin (see page 32). When the blood glucose level was raised in the evening, this teenager was feeling nauseous. He checked for ketones and discovered that something was wrong. When he examined the needle, he found that it had come out so the insulin could not get into his body. He gave himself 5 extra units (0.1 U/kg, 0.5 U/10 lb) with a pen injector, replaced the needle and started the pump. The blood glucose level returned to normal during the night.

If the blood glucose rises quickly you should remove the infusion set. Give a bolus dose and see if insulin comes out from the tip of the catheter. Bend the catheter and give another bolus dose. The pump should now give a blockage alarm. Check the tubing and connections for leaks. Replace the infusion set and check the blood glucose level frequently to make sure it goes down. Take an extra injection (with a pen or syringe) of 0.1 U/kg (0.5 units/10 lb) body weight if you have raised ketone levels, and check your blood glucose again after 1-2 hours. Repeat the dose if necessary.

of raised ketones or ketoacidosis, it may be a good idea to replace part of the night time basal rate with an injection of long-acting insulin in the evening. This will make insulin deficiency less likely to occur. We have found using a low dose of Lantus (0.1U/kg) to be particularly effective in this situation (you may need to lower the basal rate in the pump slightly).

Disconnecting the pump

Sometimes you will want to disconnect the pump for one reason or another, for example when playing sports, doing aerobics, or swimming. Most infusion sets allow you to disconnect the tubing by using a silicon membrane as a one way valve.

Taking a bath or shower

Most pumps can tolerate some water but we recommend disconnecting them when taking a bath or shower. You should also disconnect the pump if you have a sauna since insulin can't take the heat. The heat in a sauna will also cause previously injected insulin to be absorbed much more quickly (see page 80).

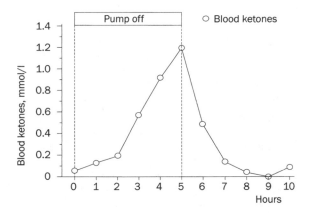

In this study of adults, the pump was stopped for 5 hours.[320] Blood ketone (beta-hydroxybutyric acid) levels increased rapidly to around 1.2 mmol/l. When the pump was started again, a bolus dose was given along with a meal and 1-4 U of extra insulin, resulting in a quick decline in ketone levels. Monitoring blood ketones is an effective method of monitoring the degree of insulin deficiency if you are having pump problems (see page 101). The ketone levels are comparable to those we have found in children and teenagers (see page 176).

Causes of high blood glucose

(adapted from [715])

① **The pump**
Basal rate too low
The pump has triggered an alarm and shut itself off
Other problems with the pump

② **Insulin reservoir**
Wrong position in the pump
Empty reservoir or plunger is stuck
Leakage in the connection with the tubing

③ **Infusion set**
Forgetting to fill the tubing when replacing
Leakage in connections or hole in tubing (feel the tubing and smell your fingers)
Adhesive and/or cannula has come loose
Air in the tubing
Blood in the tubing
Infusion set has been in place for too long
The tubing was replaced in the evening without checking blood glucose after 3 hours to ensure proper insulin delivery.
Bent or squeezed tubing
Blocked cannula/needle or tubing

④ **Infusion site**
Redness, irritation / infection
Fat pad at the infusion site
Placement close to belt or waistband

⑤ **Insulin**
Cloudy insulin
Expiry date passed
Exposed to heat / sunlight or extreme cold

Pump alarm

Insulin pumps seldom malfunction. If yours does, the pump will stop and give an alarm. There is no risk that the pump will pulse or surge, giving you too much insulin. The pump alarm will go off when something is wrong, for example if the tubing is blocked, the insulin container empty or the batteries dead. However, the pump cannot detect if the insulin is leaking somewhere, for example if the cannula has come out, the connections have come loose or

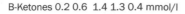

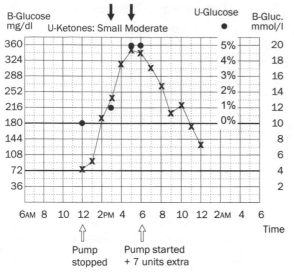

6AM 8 10 12 2PM 4   6   8   10 12 2AM 4   6

Time

⇧   ⇧
Pump   Pump started
stopped   + 7 units extra

It is important to familiarize yourself with the symptoms of insulin deficiency (nausea, vomiting, abdominal pain, rapid breathing, fruity smell on the breath) and we therefore plan a "pump-stop" some weeks after pump initiation. This graph was recorded at our day care ward when a planned pump stop was performed (see page 173). This 15-year old boy stopped his pump with Humalog at 5 AM. He was without insulin for 6 hours and felt slightly nauseous when his blood glucose increased and ketones were present. When he started the pump again at 1 PM he had his lunch and gave himself 7 units extra (0.1 units/kg) besides his normal premeal dose. Typically, blood ketones will rise to around 1.5 mmol/l when performing a pump stop like this. A few patients have been slightly nauseous, but the stop has not caused ketoacidosis in any of them (pH has not been affected).

If your blood glucose rises like this and you have raised ketone levels, you should take an extra dose of approximately 0.1 U/kg body weight (0.5 U/10 lb). **Always use a pen or syringe to be on the safe side!** Remove the cannula and take a bolus, watching whether insulin appears from the tip. Bend the cannula and take another bolus. The pump should now give an occlusion or blockage alarm. Check the tubing and connections for leakage (smell your fingers). Replace the cannula. Test your blood glucose again after 1-2 hours and repeat the bolus if necessary.

Disconnecting the pump

Time that the pump has been disconnected	Measure
< ½-1 hour	No extra insulin needed.
1-2 hours	Take an extra dose when you connect the pump corresponding to the basal rate you have missed.
2-4 hours	Take an extra dose before you disconnect the pump corresponding to the basal rate that you should have had during the missing 1-2 hours. Check your blood glucose when you connect the pump and take an extra bolus dose corresponding to 1-2 hours' basal rate if needed.
> 4 hours	Dose as above before disconnecting. Using a pen injector or syringe, take extra insulin every 3-4 hours corresponding to the missed basal rate. Take the pre-meal bolus dose with a pen or syringe.

If you remove the pump to exercise, you will probably need to lower the doses more than suggested above. Test this to find out what is right for you. Always leave the pump in "run" mode when disconnecting for a shorter time, as this prevents you from forgetting to turn it on again when you reconnect it.

Make sure there is no air in the tubing when reconnecting it. Prime it with some insulin if necessary. Do not put the pump lower than the insertion site when reconnecting (for example on the floor when in the gym). If you do, there is a risk that gravity will pull some air into the tubing.

see what the different alarms stand for and how to respond to them.

Most pumps have an alarm that is triggered if you have not pushed any of the buttons after a certain number of hours. It may wake you up

there is a hole in the tubing (pets can bite through it). Check the operating instructions to

Problems with the pump?

Problem	Measure
Infection/irritation at the infusion site	Wash hands and skin with chlorhexidine in alcohol. Replace infusion set more frequently.
Blocked infusion set	It can be bent or blocked by coagulation or insulin crystals. Replace it.
Blocked tubing	Can be caused by precipitation of insulin. Disconnect the cannula from the tubing and give a prime dose. Replace if the alarm is triggered.
Blood in the tubing	Replace the infusion set
Air in the tubing	No insulin delivered. See page 178.
White spots on the inner layer of the tubing	Most tubing is made from double plastic layers that can come apart, showing as white spots. This does not affect the function or the insulin.
Leakage of insulin at the insertion site	Has the needle/cannula come loose? Is there a bent cannula? Replace the infusion set.
Moisture under the adhesive	This indicates insulin leakage. Replace the infusion set.

Problems with the pump, cont.

Problem	Measure
Moisture under the adhesive	This indicates insulin leakage. Replace the cannula/needle.
Adhesive comes off	If EMLA®- cream has been used, wash it off carefully with water. Disinfect the skin with Skin-Prep® that leaves a sticky film when drying. Warm the adhesive with your hand after application. Apply extra tape if needed.
Itching, eczema from adhesive	Apply hydrocortisone cream. Use a stoma-type adhesive.
Sticky traces of adhesive	Wipe off with special remover or medical benzine.
Scars in the skin from old catheters	Often more visible with dark skin. Replace cannula/needle more frequently. Try using a metal needle.
Redness of the skin over the cannula tip	Can be caused by insulin allergy. See page 190
Nothing works	Try running the pump with both insulin and tubing removed.

early in the morning if you didn't take your evening snack insulin or forgot to push one of the buttons before going to bed. We usually recommend this alarm be set for 14-16 hours.

Occlusion or blockage alarm

The pump alarm will be triggered if there is an increased resistance when pumping insulin. But it cannot tell whereabouts in the system the problem may be. It may be that the insulin reservoir is empty, the plunger may be sluggish, or the tubing or cannula blocked. The tubing can be bent or squeezed, for example by a belt buckle. If the occlusion or blockage alarm is triggered, start by checking the tubing for bends or pinches. Then give the remainder of the pre-meal bolus. If no alarm is triggered, all is well now and you have received the intended amount of insulin. If the alarm goes off again, the next step is to stretch out and try careful massaging of the infusion port and catheter under the skin (only for infusion sets that do not have perpendicular cannula). If the tubing hasn't been disconnected, there is no need to take any more than the remaining premeal dose

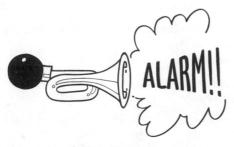

The pump alarm will tell you if there is a blockage in the tubing or cannula/needle. The alarm is triggered by the increased pressure in the tubing. However, if the pressure goes down, for example because of a leaking connection, a cannula that has come out, or a hole in the tubing, the alarm will not go off. This type of delivery failure can only be detected by repeated monitoring of glucose and ketones. If you suspect a leak, feel along the tubing and smell your fingers; insulin has a very distinctive smell. **If the pump alarm goes off, and your blood glucose is high, you should first give yourself an extra injection with a pen or syringe and then check all possible reasons for the alarm.**

of insulin if the pump now works without an alarm (unless the blood glucose level is still raised).

If the cannula or tubing is blocked it may take several hours before the pressure has increased enough to trigger the alarm. During this time you will not have received any insulin. Find out how much is needed to trigger the alarm in your pump. It may also depend on what kind of tubing you have, and how long it is. Test it by pushing the steel needle into a rubber cork or pinch the end of the cannula. If you then give a bolus dose you will see how many units are pushed into the tubing before the alarm is triggered. For example, if your pump has given 4.3 units of the meal bolus dose when the alarm goes off and 2.6 units are needed to build up pressure to trigger the alarm, you will have only received 4.3 less 2.6 units, or 1.7 units of the bolus dose.

For smaller children we often use insulin of 40 or 50 U/ml, for infants 10 U/ml. This means that fewer units are needed before the alarm goes off since the fluid volume is larger. If 2.5

units of 100 U/ml are needed to trigger the alarm, this will equal 1 unit of 40 U/ml.

Sometimes the pump will trigger the alarm for a block in the tubing even after you have replaced both the tubing and the cannula. If this happens, remove the insulin reservoir from the pump. Then start the pump again. If the alarm still goes off, the problem is an internal one, such as a motor problem. Don't reuse the pump reservoir. If doing so, the silicon on the plunger wears off, and this may result in a occlusion or blockage alarm.

Leakage of insulin

The pump can't trigger the alarm if there is an insulin leak. It will only trigger if the motor runs against an increased resistance. Insulin can be deposited outside the infusion site if the cannula has been retracted. Often this can only be detected when you take a bolus dose. When the basal dose is running, the amounts of insulin are so small that it can be difficult to pick up leaks.

The tubing connector on the pump end can crack, causing leakage, especially if you apply too much force when connecting it. Feel the connector with your fingers. If it is leaking, you can often detect the smell of insulin. Sometimes a cat or dog may be able to warn you that there is a leak as they often like the smell of insulin.

Air in the tubing

When you connect the tubing to the pump there is always a risk of air coming in, especially if you fill it with cold insulin. Air will come out of the solution when the temperature rises. Always make sure that the insulin is at room temperature before refilling the reservoir. Introducing air into the subcutaneous tissue is not dangerous in itself, but you will miss out on the corresponding amount of insulin. The alarm will not be triggered since the pump's micro-

Occlusion or blockage alarm

① Check the tubing for bends and pinching. Try a careful massage of the infusion port and the catheter under the skin. If the alarm was triggered when taking a premeal bolus, take the remaining portion.

No alarm → OK, no problems
Alarm ↓

② Disconnect cannula/needle from tubing. Start a prime dose with the pump.

No alarm → Replace cannula/needle
Alarm ↓

③ Disconnect tubing from insulin reservoir. Start a prime dose with the pump.

No alarm → Replace tubing
Alarm ↓

④ Remove the insulin reservoir from the pump and start a prime dose.

No alarm → Replace reservoir
Alarm ↓

⑤ Something is wrong with the pump. Contact the pump dealer and deliver insulin with a pen or syringe.

Insulin pump and illness

➠ Continue with your ordinary meal bolus doses even if you eat less, increasing them by 1 Unit if necessary (2 Units if your dose to start with is 10 Units or more, ½U if dose is < 3 U). Begin by increasing the basal dose if you have a raised temperature.

➠ Increase the basal rate by 10-20% (0.1-0.2 U/hour, 0.2-0.4 U/h. if the basal rate is > 1U/h.) if your blood glucose continues to be high.

➠ Check your blood glucose every 2 to 4 hours. Check for ketones frequently. Keep good records in your logbook.

➠ Take extra insulin (1 U/10 kg or 0.5 U/10 lb body weight), preferably NovoLog/NovoRapid or Humalog, if your blood glucose is high and you have ketones. Give another 1 U/10 kg (0.5 U/10 lb) every second hour until the blood glucose is below 180 mg/dl (10 mmol/l) and the level of ketones is decreasing.

➠ Give all extra doses of insulin with a pen or syringe if your blood glucose has risen suddenly. This is in case the high blood glucose has been caused by a problem with the pump.

➠ Try to drink large amounts of fluids as this will increase the excretion of ketones and lessen the risk of dehydration. As long as there is glucose in your urine, you will lose extra fluid. Drink glucose-free fluids when your blood glucose is above 180-215 mg/dl (10-12 mmol/l) and change to something containing glucose when the blood glucose is below this level. If you feel nauseous, try to drink small amounts (a couple of sips) at a time.

➠ Try to drink something sweet if hypoglycemia is a problem. You may need to lower the basal rate but never discontinue it completely.

computer cannot tell the difference between air and insulin in the tubing.

If you see air in the tubing when you are about to take a premeal bolus dose you can compensate with a little extra insulin. Five to seven cm (2-3 inches) of air in the tubing usually corresponds to 1 unit of insulin. To find out the exact dimension of your pump tubing, give a bolus dose of 1 unit when you are priming the tubing. Make a mark on the tubing with a felt tip pen corresponding to the length that the insulin travels for that unit.

If the air in the tubing corresponds to more than ½-1 unit when the basal rate is running (e.g. between meals) it is best to disconnect the tubing from the cannula in the skin. Prime the tubing to purge the air and fill it with insulin once again.

When to call the hospital or your diabetes team

➡ The first time you become ill after you have started with the pump.

➡ If you have been feeling too nauseous to eat for more than 6-8 hours.

➡ If you have vomited more than once during a 4-6 hour period.

➡ If your blood glucose level has not come down, or the ketone level is still running high after the second extra dose of insulin.

➡ If your general well-being is deteriorating.

➡ If you are at all uncertain as to how to handle the situation.

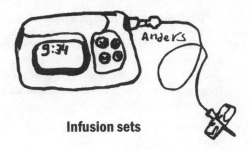

Infusion sets

Brand	Length cm	inches
Classic	60, 80, 110	24, 31, 43
Cleo 90 ®(6, 9 mm)	55, 80, 110	23, 31, 43
Comfort ®	30, 60, 80, 110	12, 24, 32, 43
Inset (6, 9 mm)	60, 110	43, 23
Silhouette ®	60, 110	43, 23
Simple Choice Easy	60, 110	43, 23
(12mm or 17 mm cannula length)		
Sof-set ®	61, 107	24, 42
Sof-set ® Micro (6mm)	61, 107	24, 42
Tender	60, 80, 110	24, 31, 43
Quick-Set ®(6, 9 mm)	60, 110	43, 23
Ultraflex (8, 10 mm)	60, 80, 110	24, 31, 43
Steel needles:		
Rapid (6, 8, 10, 12 mm)	60, 80, 110	24, 31, 43
Polyfin ®	61, 107	24, 42

For most tubings, 5-7 cm (2-3 inches) contain approximately 1 unit of insulin. Test your tubing by putting a felt pen mark on its end, then deliver one unit at a time as a bolus dose.

The Silhouette, Sof-set and Quick-Set infusion sets can be used with an automatic inserter that lessens the pain.

Sick days and fever

When you are ill, especially if you are running a temperature, your body will increase its insulin requirements, often by 25% for each degree Celsius (every 2 degrees Farenheight) of fever (see page 258). It is advisable to begin by increasing the basal rate. Start by a 10-20% increase when you notice that your blood glucose is rising. You will probably also need to increase the meal bolus doses in response to your blood glucose readings. It is important that you test your glucose level before each meal if you are ill, and preferably 1½ -2 hours after the meal as well. Usually, you will need to monitor your blood glucose levels during the night as well.

Pump removal doses

It is very important always to carry extra insulin wherever you go in case your pump fails to work properly. Check to see that the insulin has not expired. You should have your pump removal doses written down and with you in case you need to use a pen or syringe as a temporary measure. The total number of units over 24 hours will probably need to be increased by

10-20% if you stop using the pump for a whole day or more.

Use the old doses

It is easiest to start with the same doses that you had when you used a pen injector or syringes, provided that you have written down the doses and not too much time has elapsed since then so that you still have more or less the same insulin requirements.

Rapid-acting insulin (NovoLog/NovoRapid or Humalog) in the pump

You can continue taking the same premeal bolus doses with a pen or syringe. Replace the basal dose with intermediate-acting insulin. Divide the total basal dose during the day, taking one third in the morning as NPH insulin, and two thirds at bedtime. You will probably need to increase the total NPH dose by 10-20% compared to the total pump basal/24 hours.

Regular short-acting insulin in the pump

Look at the pump doses. The breakfast dose with a pen will be the sum of the pump pre-breakfast bolus dose and the number of basal units the pump would have delivered between breakfast and lunch. If you have a high basal rate (>1.5-2 U/hour), start by counting just 1-1.5 U/hour when calculating the dose when using a pen or syringe.

Calculating the bedtime dose

The bedtime dose of intermediate-acting insulin (Novolin N, Humulin N, Insuman NPH) is calculated by adding the basal rates between 10 PM and 8 AM (see example on page 181). You can also use short-acting insulin (*not* NovoLog/NovoRapid or Humalog) during the night, giving two doses, at 10 PM and 3 AM, corresponding to the sum of the basal rates during the night.

Long-acting basal insulin

Another alternative is to replace the basal dose in the pump with long-acting insulin (Lantus, Ultralente, Humulin U) and to use the same

Pump removal doses

NovoLog/NovoRapid or Humalog in the pump:

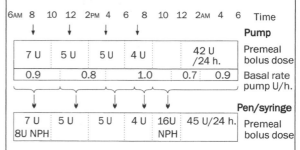

Sometimes you must use an insulin pen or a syringe for a while, for example if something is wrong with the pump. Continue with the same doses of NovoLog/NovoRapid or Humalog before meals as when on the pump. Replace the basal dose with an intermediate-acting insulin (NPH) given twice daily. Take the basal rate in pump, add 20% (20 U+20% = 24U) and divide it into 2 doses of intermediate-acting insulin. Give 1/3 in the morning and 2/3 in the evening and adjust according to blood glucose monitoring. If you will be without the pump for more than one day, you may try substituting the basal rate with the same number of units, taken as Lantus once daily.[93]

Short-acting insulin in the pump:

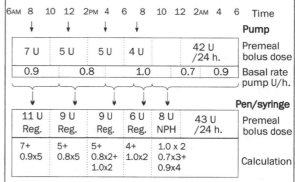

NPH = Intermediate-acting bedtime insulin

With short-acting insulin, you can calculate which dose to use if you add the meal bolus dose in the pump with the basal rate. You will probably need to increase the night dose since the pump is more effective, giving more insulin late at night and early in the morning than you would get from the intermediate acting bedtime insulin. Check with your diabetes nurse if you are unsure what doses you used when you were on multiple injections.

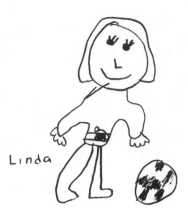

Linda

Many people with diabetes are successful in competitive sports. Others, like most children, just play for the fun of it. In either case, the pump helps keep the blood glucose at an appropriate level both during and after exercise.

bolus doses (and type of insulin) before meals as when using the pump. However, it will take several days for the doses of long-acting basal insulin to have a stable effect, so this may be a better alternative only if you know that you will be without the pump for more than a day or two. Take the total basal dose during 24 hours, and take the same dose of Lantus as one dose at dinner or the evening snack.[93] For Ultralente and Humulin U, add 10-20% and divide into two equal doses that you take with breakfast and dinner around 5-6 PM. Take the same amount of bolus insulin as when on the pump.

Admission to hospital

If you are admitted to hospital in an acute situation, you may well find that none of the staff members on duty are familiar with your pump. So, if you have any problems using it, it would be best to begin injecting insulin with a pen or syringe until the daytime staff arrive. If you are vomiting or have signs of ketoacidosis, the best treatment may be by intravenous insulin (see page 69).

Physical exercise

Try wearing the pump in a case on a strong elastic waistband during exercise. If you are involved in contact sports, you can disconnect the pump for 1-2 hours without taking any extra insulin. If you are exercising for longer than 2 hours, it will probably be better to keep the pump connected and temporarily decrease the basal rate. Try half the basal rate while exercising and for the following hour or two. You may need to lower the basal rate even more, but the only way to know for sure is to try it yourself. Another alternative is to connect the pump again for a short while when you are halfway through the exercise (for example at half-time in a game of sport), and take a small bolus dose. If you have problems with hypoglycaemia early in your exercise session, you will need to disconnect the pump at least 2 hours before the session starts.[286]

If you are using rapid-acting insulin, your blood glucose level may plummet if you exercise shortly after the premeal bolus dose (see graphs on page 249) without decreasing it. With short-acting insulin you can try taking half the meal bolus dose if you are exercising within 1-3 hours of a meal, or even skipping it if the exercise is particularly strenuous. However, you will probably then need to keep the pump connected to get the basal rate during the entire time of the exercise.[795]

Don't forget to refill your glucose stores after exercise (see page 245). After strenuous exercise (e.g. a ball game or skiing) you must decrease the basal rate by 10-20% (0.1-0.2 U/hour) or even more during the night to avoid hypoglycemia. Try this out yourself and note the blood glucose test results in the logbook for future reference should you be faced with the same situation again.

When you go to a diabetes or sports camp you will be very active for several days in a row. Try lowering the basal rate 10-20% (0.1-0.2 U/

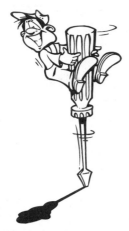

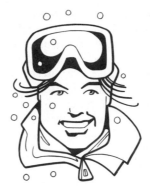

In the winter when it's cold, you must keep the pump close to your body. The tubing is very thin and no part of it must be outside the clothing, or it will easily freeze. It may be a bit awkward taking the bolus dose but since the insulin can't be allowed to freeze, you must protect it from low temperatures.

An insulin pump needs to be looked after, and tubing and batteries need to be replaced. When the alarm goes off, you must know how to respond. You will be the "first line pump mechanic" and will probably find that you soon learn how to take care of the practical details.

hour) when you arrive at the camp, and then adjust it according to your blood glucose levels.

Using the pump at night only

Some people feel that the pump has obvious advantages during the night but that multiple injections are better during the day. This may be the situation for a child who is not yet ready to manage the pump alone without adult supervision. A night time pump may be a good alternative for children who are using intermediate-acting insulin (Novolin N, Humulin N, Insuman NPH) at bedtime and experience problems with night time hypoglycemia or high blood glucose levels in the early morning.[435] It is perfectly acceptable to connect the pump in the evening, let it stay in place overnight, and disconnect it the next morning. During the day you can use a pen injector or syringe for premeal bolus doses. Talk to your diabetes doctor if this sounds like the right approach for you.

In a group of children aged 7-10 years, the pump was used for the dinner and evening snack bolus doses and for the basal rate during the night.[435] Intermediate-acting NPH was given in the morning and premeal boluses during the day were given as injections of rapid-acting insulin. The children's blood glucose readings were lower with the night time pump than when using bedtime NPH insulin. In one study of night time pumps in adults, the morning blood glucose levels were more even and the patients also experienced fewer episodes of hypoglycemia in the daytime.[425]

Nighttime pump may be a good alternative if you are on a beach vacation. Disconnect the pump in the morning and take your meal bolus doses with a pen or syringe, then connect the pump again when you come back to the hotel in the afternoon or evening. Since you will probably be exercising more than usual, you may not need to take any injection of basal insulin in the morning.

Is the pump a nuisance?

You must keep your insulin pump next to you 24 hours a day. Many people ask us, "How do you sleep with it?" But they are then surprised by how quickly they get used to wearing the pump at night. Some people who lie quite still put the pump beside or under the pillow and wake up in the morning with it still there. Others, who are more restless, find it better to have the pump on a waistband, leg band, or in a pajama pocket.

On rare occasions, some people have taken bolus doses while sleeping. It may well be that they have dreamt of eating and are so used to the pump that they have taken a bolus dose without waking up. If you have hypoglycemia unexpectedly in the morning, it is a good idea to check the pump memory to find out if you have taken a dose in your sleep. If this is the case, you should wear the pump in a case at night to prevent you from pressing the buttons. in error. Another solution is to lock the pump at night, or to use a remote control for bolusing and place this far away from your bed at night.

An 18 year old girl said that the first question friends asked her was, "What do you do with the pump when having sex?" Fortunately, it is easy to disconnect the pump for a short while to stop it getting in the way. Making love also involves physical exercise, so be aware that you might need a little less insulin for a while. Just don't forget to reconnect the pump afterwards.

Does using a pump cause weight gain?

If you have an increased A1C, there is a risk of gaining weight when your blood glucose improves since less glucose will be lost via the urine. If you have frequent hypoglycaemic episodes you will be likely to gain weight since you will find yourself needing frequent snacks. If you start treating yourself to candy and chips you are bound to put on weight. Talk to your dietitian about how to find a way around these problems. It might be easier to lose weight without an increase in A1C if you have an insulin pump because you can then decrease both your food intake and meal bolus doses but be able to ensure you meet your basal insulin requirements.

Sleeping in

With an insulin pump it is easier to sleep longer in the morning as your basal need for insulin is

When should I disconnect the pump?

⇒ In the bath tub

⇒ In a public bath or swimming pool

⇒ In a sauna or

⇒ During an X-ray, Cat scan or MRI scan

covered automatically. To find a suitable basal rate, skip breakfast (don't take the breakfast bolus dose either) and test your blood glucose several times until lunch. If the level hasn't changed you know it will work well when you sleep in late. Before you know how your body reacts, it is a good idea to have a parent or relative help check your blood glucose at 7-8 AM and adjust the basal rate accordingly. If it is below 65-70 mg/dl (3.5-4.0 mmol/l) it may be easier for them to shut off the pump for a while than to wake you up in order to eat something.

Travel tips

Always take extra insulin and an insulin pen or syringes wherever you go. Don't forget to adjust the pump's clock if you travel across time zones. Change the clock to the new time when you arrive at your destination. Since you will be sitting still on the plane, it may be a good idea to increase the basal rate slightly on a long trip. Measure your blood glucose before each meal and make necessary adjustments to the bolus dose. You may need a certificate for customs declaring that you need to wear an insulin pump. The pump does not usually trigger the metal detector at airports. If you travel in a very hot climate, the insulin may lose its potency. You may need to change insulin cartridges every 1-2 days. If you fill your reservoirs yourself, do not fill with more insulin than you will use in this time. Keep your insulin supply in a refrigerator, if possible. See page 294 for further travel tips.

Toddlers using pumps

No child is too young to use a pump. It has been used successfully even in babies only a few weeks old. In a US study of toddlers aged 2-5 years, A1C decreased from 9.5% to 7.9% and the numbers of severe hypoglycaemia decreased from approximately one episode every 2 months to approximately one episode every 10 months.[495] For young children with basal rates < 0.3 U per hour U-40 or U-50 can be used, for babies often U-10. Small children may need a lower percentage of the total daily dose as the basal rate (down to 40%). Young children often need the highest basal rate in the late evening from 9PM-12AM.[100]

Especially picky and unpredictable eaters will benefit from repeated small bolus doses in

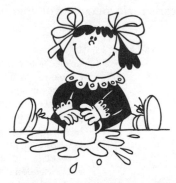

Using an insulin pump works well for all age groups; no child is too young to try one. Even babies only a few weeks old have used insulin pumps successfully. If your child has unpredictable eating habits, it is very practical to be able to give small bolus doses every time he or she eats something. The best insertion site for the infusion set in toddlers is the buttocks.

accordance with their eating habits. Dual/combined or square/extended bolus can be very effective if there is any doubt about just how much a child will eat. The pump can be kept out of reach of the toddler by being worn in a harness between the shoulders. Children from the age of 4-5 years can often wear the pump in the same way as older children. In our experience, they very quickly learn not to interfere with the pump. If in doubt, use a pump on which the buttons can be locked.

The buttocks are often used for infusion sites for the very youngest, since the cannula then is out of sight. If the child wears diapers, position the insertion site so that it won't be soiled by the diaper contents.

Pregnancy

Using an insulin pump is an excellent way to obtain blood glucose values close to those of a person without diabetes.[419] With a close to normal blood glucose, the risk of complications during pregnancy decreases to the same levels as for women without diabetes (see page 273). In pregnancy, basal needs are usually only 40% of the total daily dose.[224] The insulin requirements will gradually increase during pregnancy, but will often plummet after delivery (see page 275). During the later part of pregnancy it might be difficult to have the pump cannula on the distended abdomen. Instead, it would be a good idea to use the buttocks, the upper part of the thighs or the upper arm.

There is an increased risk of ketoacidosis during pregnancy. You should check your blood glucose more often and also change tubing and cannulas more often (every day with metal needles and every other day with teflon catheters). Contact the hospital immediately if your blood glucose level is high and you have raised levels of ketones in your blood or urine. Adding a bedtime dose of intermediate-acting insulin (0.2 U/kg) to cover part of the normal basal dose delivered by the pump has decreased the risk of ketoacidosis considerably.[526]

Rapid-acting insulin in the pump

As rapid-acting insulin (NovoLog/NovoRapid and Humalog) acts more quickly and more closely mimics the non-diabetic insulin response, it seems logical to try it when using an insulin pump.

One problem when using insulin with an even shorter duration is that your body's insulin depot will go down considerably as well (see page 172). This implies that symptoms of insulin deficiency will arise fast if the pump fails. The production of ketones will start after approximately 4 hours when a pump with Humalog is stopped.[759] One can compare a pump-free period of about 4 hours with rapid-acting insulin to about 6 hours with regular short-acting insulin. However, this can vary considerably from one individual to another.

NovoLog/NovoRapid and Humalog are now both approved for pump use in most countries and their use is increasing fast. The experiences to date are positive. In our department, we start all new pumps with rapid-acting insulin. However, if you develop symptoms very quickly after an interruption of the insulin supply, you may be better off using regular short-acting insulin.

When switching from short-acting to rapid-acting insulin in the pump, you may need to lower the bolus doses slightly (by approximately 1-2 units) since the bolus doses of regular short-acting insulin supplied part of the basal insulin, overlapping with the next meal as well. To compensate for this you may need instead to increase the basal rate slightly, when you are using either NovoLog/NovoRapid [91] or Humalog.[146]

The onset of action with a premeal bolus dose of NovoLog/NovoRapid or Humalog may be too rapid in certain situations, such as eating a meal that is digested slowly because it is rich in fat and carbohydrates (e.g. pasta or pizza), or a long drawn-out dinner with many courses. You can then try taking the bolus dose after the meal. If you have a pump that can deliver the dose more slowly (square or extended bolus, see illustration on page 168) this is an ideal solution in these situations. You can use this type of bolus dose even if you have problems with gastroparesis (slower emptying of the stomach due to diabetic neuropathy, see page 311). See the chapters on insulin adjustments on page 140 and diet on page 206 for further advice on the use of NovoLog/NovoRapid and Humalog.

If you use regular short-acting insulin in the pump and want to sleep half an hour longer in the morning, you can take the pre-breakfast dose with rapid-acting insulin in a pen or syringe immediately before eating instead of 30 minutes earlier. NovoLog/NovoRapid or Hum-

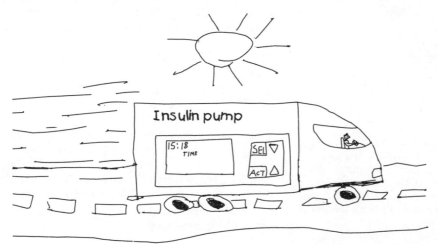

An insulin pump will enable you to "fine tune" your insulin doses and will give you more "horsepower under the hood" for taking care of your diabetes. However, greater knowledge and attention will be needed if it is to work well, just like a stronger and faster car. Used correctly, an insulin pump is a very good tool that can give you wonderful support on your long diabetes journey.

Research findings:
Rapid-acting insulin and pumps

♠ Long-term studies show that individuals can achieve a 0.5% lower A1C when using Humalog in the pump without increasing the risk of severe hypoglycemia or ketoacidosis.[683,540]

♠ In a Canadian study, regular short-acting insulin and rapid-acting insulin were used in insulin pumps during a 3 month double-blind cross-over study.[827] All bolus doses were given immediately before the meals. A1C was significantly lower (7.7% compared to 8.0%) when using rapid-acting insulin but there was no difference in the frequency of hypoglycemia.

♠ In a French pump study, blood glucose levels were more stable and the number of readings below 36 mg/dl (2.0 mmol/l) decreased when using Humalog.[540]

♠ In a German study of adults, the pump was stopped from 10 PM in the evening until 7 AM in the morning. With Humalog, the changes in blood glucose and ketones developed 1.5-2 hours earlier than with regular short-acting insulin.[640] Blood glucose increased with about 200 mg/dl (11 mmol/l) in 6 hours using Humalog compared to about 110 mg/dl (6 mmol/l) with short-acting insulin. One patient stopped the test after 7 hours due to headache and nausea but no one developed ketoacidosis.

♠ In an Italian study of adults, the pump was stopped for 5 hours in the morning without eating breakfast. During these hours, glucose levels increased by 100 mg/dl (5.6 mmol/l) on average when using short-acting insulin (Velosulin) compared to 165 mg/dl (9.2 mmol/l) with Humalog.[320] Blood ketone levels rose to about 1.2 mmol/l when using Humalog compared to 0.9 mmol/l with Velosulin (see figure on page 175).

♠ In an American study, the differences between regular short-acting insulin and Humalog were not as pronounced when the pumps were stopped for 6 hours.[41]

Remember to bring extra batteries and other accessories when you are away from home for more than a couple of hours. Also bring a pen or syringe and rapid-acting insulin so you can take extra insulin if your pump stops working properly.

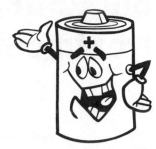

Which type of treatment do the health professionals prefer?

In an American study, professional members of AADE (American Academy of Diabetes Educators) and ADA (American Diabetes Association), mainly nurses, doctors and dietitians, were asked how they treated their own diabetes.[309] The results showed that as many as 60% of the AADE members with diabetes and 52% of the ADA members with diabetes used insulin pumps. Only 3-4% used 1-2 injections per day. The rest used multiple injections with 3-4 doses per day. The average A1C for pump users was 6.7%, for multiple injections 7.2%. One interesting observation was that diabetes (type 1) was 13 times more common among the AADE and ADA members than in the general population. The explanation may be that since diabetes generally develops at a younger age (average age at onset in the US is 16 years), the disease may influence a person towards choosing a career involving diabetes care.

For further reading on insulin pumps, try either of the following: *The Insulin Pump Therapy Book* by Linda Fredrickson (Ed.), Minimed Inc 1995, Sylmar, CA, USA; *Pumping Insulin* by John Walsh and Ruth Roberts, Torrey Pines Press 2000, San Diego, US; *Think like a pancreas* by Gary Scheiner, Marlowe 2004, New York, USA and *Insulin Pump Therapy Demystified* by Gabrielle Kaplan-Mayer, Marlowe 2002, New York, USA.

alog is also a good alternative if your blood glucose is high before you eat.

Side effects of insulin treatment

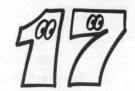

Pain

If an injection is particularly painful you have probably hit a nerve (see illustration on page 111). If you can stand the pain you can readily inject the insulin, otherwise you must pierce the skin once again. If your injections are often painful, see the chapter on injection equipment, page 122.

Insulin leakage

It is not uncommon for a drop of insulin to come out on the skin after the needle is withdrawn. Two to three drops from a pen needle contain approximately one unit of insulin (100 U/ml). In one study on children and adolescents with diabetes 68% encountered leakage of insulin after injections during one week.[721] And 23% of these injections were followed by leakage of up to 18% of the injected dose (2 units out of an intended dose of 11 units).

It may be difficult to avoid insulin leaking, but the risk will be reduced if you lift a skin fold and inject at a 45° angle (see illustration on page 113). Try to inject more slowly. You can also try to withdraw the needle halfway and then wait 20 seconds before withdrawing it completely. Some people find it helpful to press a finger on the injection site or to stretch the skin immediately after removing the needle. At one time, the standard advice was to stretch the skin sideways before injecting to avoid insulin leakage, but this is not a good idea because you risk giving yourself an intramuscular injection by mistake.

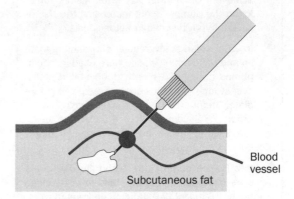

If you penetrate a superficial blood vessel with the needle it may bleed a little. Bleeding under the skin will feel like a small bubble, which is often bluish in color.

Blocked needles

Sometimes the needle will be blocked when you inject long or intermediate-acting insulin. This can be caused by the crystals in the insulin that build up. It seems to depend on how quickly you inject the insulin. The problem is more likely to occur if you perform the injection slowly (over a period of more than 5 seconds). Try to inject the insulin quickly (within 5 seconds) of penetrating the skin. The risk increases when you reuse needles as any remaining insulin may crystallize inside the needle barrel.

Bruises after injections

If you penetrate a superficial blood vessel in the subcutaneous fat layer, there may be a small amount of bleeding. However, the blood vessels in the subcutaneous fat are so small that there is no risk of insulin being injected directly into one of them. The bleed will feel like a small bubble under the skin and may be bluish in color. Bleeding like this is quite harmless and is absorbed completely after a while.

Fatty lumps

Fatty lumps (lipohypertrophies) are caused by insulin's effect of stimulating growth of fat tissue. This is a common problem when you don't rotate your injection sites often enough. Fatty lumps contain both fibrous and fat tissue.[757] Up to 30% of patients have problems with fatty lumps.[595,648]

A child usually wants to prick the skin where it hurts the least, resulting in injections too close together. It is important to explain carefully why this is not a good idea, and help to find a system for rotating the injections sites effectively. Younger children (aged under 10-12 years) should have a parent helping them with one or two of their injections each day. The parent can then inject into areas that the child might have difficulty in reaching, such as the buttocks (see "Where do I inject the insulin?" on page 111).

Re-using needles causes blunting which means that repeated injections are not only more painful, they also cause more damage to the skin and may even contribute to an increase in the formation of fatty lumps.[725]

Injections in fatty lumps will usually result in a slower (and probably more erratic) absorption of insulin.[468,824] An area with lipohypertrophy should be left alone for a couple of weeks. One way to accomplish this can be to use an

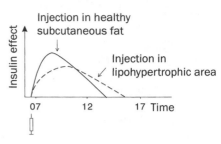

Insulin will usually be absorbed more slowly and probably more erratically if you inject in an area with fatty lumps (lipohypertrophy).

indwelling catheter (Insuflon, see page 122) with which the injection sites can be actively rotated. Another way is to use a guide with a rotation scheme, designed with holes or sections for different days of the week.[276]

In one report, the problems with lipohypertrophies decreased among individuals using Humalog.[648] The explanation may be that, as this type of insulin enters the bloodstream much faster, the time for which the fat cells are exposed to the insulin will decrease.

Remember that insulin will start to act sooner if you inject it in an area free from lipohypertrophy. You may have to lower the dose to avoid hypoglycemia when you switch your injections into a "fresh" site without lipohypertrophy.

Redness after injections

Redness, sometimes with itching, that occurs immediately or within hours of an insulin injection can be due to an allergy towards the insulin or a preservative. This type of reaction will usually subside after some years as you continue with insulin treatment.[600] Inform your doctor if you have problems with redness after injections. There is a special skin test available to find out whether you are allergic to the insulin or the preservative. There is often an increased level of insulin antibodies in the blood as well (see later). If problems with redness continue, so called antihistamine tablets can be helpful. Add-

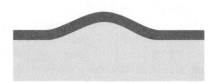

Insulin causes the subcutaneous tissue to grow if you inject frequently into the same spot. You will get a "fatty lump" (lipohypertrophy) in the skin that feels and looks like a bump.

ing a small amount of cortisone to the insulin may also help.[498] Switching to rapid-acting insulin (NovoLog/NovoRapid [12] or Humalog [466]) has decreased the problem with redness after injections in some cases. The slow infusion rate of an insulin pump was helpful for building up tolerance for insulin (so called "desensitization") in a girl who had problems with burning local reactions to insulin.[230] We have the impression that the problem of redness after injections has decreased considerably since we began giving all patients NovoLog/NovoRapid or Humalog right from the onset of diabetes.

It is important to make sure your insulin has not passed its use-by date and that it is stored correctly (see page 116). Inappropriate storage conditions can result in the insulin breaking down and give rise to harmful substances that can cause local allergic reactions.[315] A generalized allergic reaction after insulin injection is very rare.[143,466]

Allergy to the nickel in pen and syringe needles can cause redness after injections. The needles are covered with a layer of silicone lubricant. If you are allergic to nickel you should not use the needles more than once as the silicone layer wears off and the nickel will come in closer contact with the skin. Needles on syringes have a thicker silicone layer since they need to penetrate the membrane of the bottle when drawing up insulin. For this reason, they will be more appropriate if you are allergic to nickel. You can have a skin test to see whether this is the case. If you are allergic to nickel, you will usually react to it in other items as well, for example earrings, belt buckles or wrist watches.

EMLA®-cream (a topical anesthetic used for venepuncture or when replacing indwelling catheters) can cause an allergic redness that looks very much like an allergy to the adhesive.

Insulin antibodies

Your body will produce antibodies to "defend" itself against foreign substances. Insulin anti-

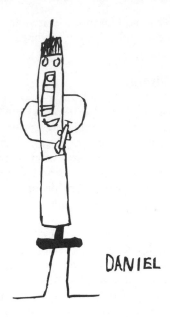

DANIEL

bodies with pork and beef insulin were common. With the use of human insulin it is not common to have high enough levels of antibodies to cause problems. Higher levels of insulin antibodies are more common when using multiple injections or insulin pumps compared to conventional treatment with two doses a day.[176]

Insulin antibodies work by binding insulin when there is a high level of free insulin, for example after a meal bolus injection.[30,176] When there is a low level of free insulin, for example during the night, they release insulin.[30,176] In this way the insulin concentration in your blood will be levelled off in a way that does you no good at all. When you want a high level of insulin after a meal, it will be lowered (resulting in high blood glucose); and when you want a low level in the blood during the night you will instead have too much insulin (resulting in hypoglycemia). It could be said that if you have high levels of insulin antibodies you will produce long-acting insulin on your own. In fact, one of the new long-acting insulin analogs (Levemir) is using the same principle: after entering the bloodstream, the insulin is bound to a protein (albumin) and then released very slowly.[350]

One possible method of reducing the impact of this reaction is to give yourself a fairly large dose of insulin in the morning to "saturate" the insulin antibodies. During the day, you can take smaller and smaller doses just before meals. At bedtime give only a very little dose of insulin to lessen the risk of night time hypoglycemia. As the injected insulin will have a prolonged action, it may help to keep in mind that rapid-acting insulin (NovoLog/NovoRapid or Humalog) will work like short-acting insulin (Novolin R, Humulin R) for a person with a high level of insulin antibodies; short-acting insulin will work like something in between short and intermediate-acting (Novolin N, Humulin N, Insuman NPH) while intermediate-acting insulin will work as long-acting (Lantus, Ultralente, Humulin U) normally does.

Switching to rapid-acting insulin (Humalog) substantially decreased the level of antibodies and problems with early morning hypoglycemia in one case report [472] and solved the problem of redness at the injection site and generalized insulin allergy in another.[466] Apparently, the structural differences between regular short-acting and rapid-acting insulin molecules prevented Humalog from binding to the human insulin antibodies. NovoLog/NovoRapid has also been used successfully in patients who are allergic to insulin.[12]

A blood test is available to measure how much of the total amount of insulin is bound to antibodies. Normally this level is approximately 6% but we have seen values above 90% in cases where the person has had particular diffi-culty both with redness after injections and with prolonged insulin activity. Insulin antibodies can be very troublesome but usually the negative effects will slowly subside after several years, even if you still have measurable levels of antibodies.

Lipoatrophy

Lipoatrophy appears as a cavity in the subcutaneous tissue. The reason for its development is not clear. It does not usually appear in areas that have been used too often as injection sites. Rather, it is believed to be an immunological reaction towards insulin which causes the breaking down of subcutaneous tissue.[600] Patients with lipoatrophy often have high levels of insulin antibodies. Lipoatrophy has also been described in a person using Humalog in an insulin pump.[317]

You can try treating the cavities by injecting insulin along the edges. This will cause the formation of new fatty lumps and eventually the cavities will disappear.

Insulin edema

Sometimes, local or generalized edema can follow a rapid improvement in blood glucose control (for example, shortly after diabetes has been diagnosed). This is caused by a temporary build-up of fluid in the body and usually subsides spontaneously over a period of days to weeks if the blood glucose control continues to be good.[701] In severe cases, ephedrine has been an effective treatment.[386]

Insulin requirements

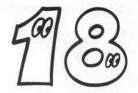

How much insulin does your body need?

An adult without diabetes produces approximately 0.5 units of insulin/kg (0.23 units/lb) body weight every day.[6] After the remission phase (usually within 1-3 years after the onset of diabetes) the insulin requirement for a growing child stabilizes, generally somewhere between 0.7 and 1.0 units/kg/day (0.3-0.45 units/lb/day),[505,701] and usually close to the 1 unit/kg/day (0.45 units /lb) mark. Sometimes only a few units less per day can result in quite a difference in A1C. If the young person becomes unwell, it will usually be necessary to increase insulin doses, especially if the illness is accompanied by fever (see page 258).

Puberty and growth

During puberty, the young person starts to grow rapidly, so larger doses of insulin are needed. Boys usually have their growth spurt at around the age of 14, and girls at around 12 years (a year before they start menstruating) but this does vary considerably. Boys usually require much higher doses during puberty, often as much as 1.4-1.6 units/kg/day (0.6-0.7 units/lb/day),[503] sometimes even more. Girls may also need to increase their doses to exceed 1 unit/kg/day during their growth spurt.[772] After they start menstruating, their growth slows down, and they have usually reached their full adult height within a further two years. At this time it is very important to lower the insulin dose, and regulate food intake, to avoid "gaining width" instead.

Within a few years after puberty, insulin requirements decrease to an adult level, usually 0.7-0.8 units/kg/day (0.3-0.35 units/lb/day). It

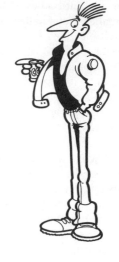

During the growth spurt of puberty, insulin doses often need to be increased considerably.

is a good idea to try and get used to counting insulin requirements in units/day in different situations as well as considering the number of units in each injection.

Height and weight should be monitored regularly. Children and adolescents with diabetes are often slightly taller than their healthy peers when they develop diabetes, but their final height falls within the normal range.[664,825] Poor diabetes control, especially during early puberty, can slow down growth.[226,811] Puberty may be delayed and girls' menstrual periods missed or their onset delayed.[226] Generally, the A1C will be high, but it may not be if a lack of insulin is combined with poor nutrition. Because of this, it is very important to consider both insulin and nutritional requirements in relation to growth patterns. Treatment with an insulin pump can considerably improve growth rate in poorly controlled diabetes by establishing a reliable supply of basal insulin.[719]

Remission ("honeymoon") phase

You are likely to need particularly large doses of insulin when your diabetes has just been diagnosed. This is because your body will not be as sensitive to insulin as it should be, on account of your high blood glucose levels during the weeks immediately before diagnosis (around the time you may have been feeling unbelievably thirsty). Once you start treatment, your body is likely to regain its sensitivity to insulin very fast so that, within a week or so, the amount of insulin you need is likely to have come right down.

When your blood glucose level has been normal for some time, the beta cells usually start to produce some insulin again, and this makes it possible to decrease your insulin doses further. Often this natural insulin production will continue to rise and, if the insulin doses can be lowered to 0.5 units/kg (0.23 units/lb) body weight or less, you can be described as having entered the remission phase (also called "honeymoon phase"). The advantage of insulin coming from your own pancreas is that it is secreted in relation to the blood glucose level, which makes it easier to manage your diabetes.

Even if the beta cells produce only a small amount of insulin, this can be enough to counteract the production of ketones. Insulin inhibits the breakdown of fat into fatty acids, which then can be transformed to ketones in the liver. Because of this, patients who produce their own insulin over a period of several years have a certain "protection" against ketoacidosis.[414] But if they are faced with a stressful situation or an infection, their need for insulin will increase considerably. This is because the increased levels of cortisol and adrenaline result in more fat being broken down into fatty acids and causing more ketones to be produced.

The remission phase usually lasts 3-6 months, sometimes a year or longer. Insulin requirements are usually at their lowest between 1 and

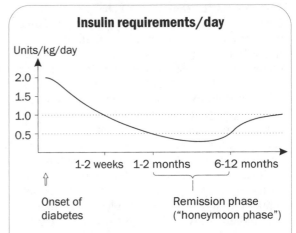

Insulin requirements/day

Large doses of insulin are usually needed during the first 1-2 weeks after diagnosis as blood glucose levels will have been high for a sustained period of time, resulting in considerable insulin resistance in your body. The amount of insulin needed usually goes right down during the first few weeks and months.

A growing child is likely to need an insulin dose of around 1 unit/kg body weight/day. When children need less than this, their pancreas is probably producing some insulin of its own. This is common during the first 6-12 months after the onset of diabetes. A child who needs less than 0.5 units/kg/day (0.23 units/lb/day) has entered the remission phase ("honeymoon phase").

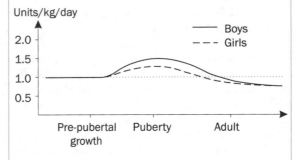

During puberty, teenagers grow fast, and larger doses of insulin will be necessary. It is important to be sure to take enough insulin at this time. Growth hormone is secreted mainly during the night and the bedtime insulin dose may need to be raised by a considerable amount. Young people who don't get enough insulin during puberty may lose ½-1 inch (a few centimeters) from their final height. Once the final height has been reached, insulin doses will need to come down again.

4 months after the onset of diabetes.[505] However, this varies from person to person. Some will not have a remission phase at all; for others it can last for more than a year. After 2-4 years of insulin treatment in young people, it is very unusual to be producing any insulin at all. If you had symptoms (thirst, needing to pass a lot of urine, weight loss) for only a week or two before starting insulin treatment, your chance of having a remission phase is higher. Younger children usually have a shorter remission phase. Children who were below the age of 5, or who had ketoacidosis at the onset of diabetes, are unlikely to have a remission phase according to one Italian study.[105] Intensive insulin treatment and better blood glucose control from the early start of diabetes is thought to give the beta cells an opportunity to rest, increasing the chances of enough insulin subsequently being produced to allow a longer remission phase.[182,199]

Insulin doses can sometimes be brought right down during the remission phase, to the extent that the person requires only a few units of insulin a day. It almost feels as if the diabetes will disappear, but unfortunately this doesn't happen. If you have it, you will need to take insulin for the rest of your life or until a cure for diabetes has been found. The remaining insulin produced by the beta cells reduces gradually, then usually disappears completely.

An infection will often trigger an increased need for insulin, and cause your blood glucose levels to rise. Insulin doses must be adjusted accordingly. If you are prompt in modifying your doses in response to your blood glucose readings, it is possible that your total insulin requirement per day will go down again once the illness is over.

The term "remission phase" might more accurately be described as "partial remission". Complete remission would mean needing no insulin at all for a shorter or longer period of time. All the insulin is usually not withdrawn, although the insulin requirement may be very low.[58] An exception to this rule is when a per-

---

Insulin requirements (after the remission phase)

☞ Pre-pubertal growth	0.7-1.0 U/kg/day, usually closer to 1 U/kg/day.
☞ Puberty	Boys 1.1-1.4 U/kg/day, sometimes even more.[503] Girls 1.0-1.2 U/kg.[772]
☞ After puberty	Girls: < 1 U/kg/day from a couple of years after the first menstrual period.
	Boys: ~ 1 U/kg/day at 18-19 years of age, less after a couple of years.
	(1 kg = 2.2 lb)

You can estimate your own insulin production during the remission phase by comparing the total insulin dose given per 24 hours with the numbers for different ages in the above table.

---

son with diabetes finds themselves experiencing hypoglycemia as a result of tiny doses such as 0.5-1 unit. The reason for not withdrawing insulin completely is that even small doses help to keep the beta cells working, which in turn makes a longer remission phase more likely.

How much insulin does the pancreas produce?

It is not possible to measure the insulin produced in the pancreas in a direct way as it is chemically identical to the insulin you inject. However, internal insulin production can be indirectly assessed by measuring C-peptide, a protein produced in equal measure to insulin in the healthy pancreas but not present in the insulin you inject (see page 320). A person with type 2 diabetes produces more insulin in his or her own pancreas, so measuring C-peptide can be used as a method of distinguishing between type 1 and type 2 diabetes.

Insulin sensitivity and resistance

The body's insulin sensitivity is essential for determining how much the blood glucose level will be lowered by a given dose of insulin. You might think that the same dose of insulin would have the same effect on the blood glucose in any single individual, but unfortunately this is not the case. Certain factors increase insulin sensitivity while others decrease it (see key fact box on page 196).

Insulin resistance implies that a higher insulin concentration in the blood is needed to obtain the same blood glucose lowering effect. You could also say that the insulin sensitivity is decreased. The decreased effect of insulin is caused by a restrained transport of glucose through the cellular wall when the blood glu-

Think of your blood glucose level as similar to your body temperature, the blood glucose meter as a thermometer and the regulation of the blood glucose as a thermostat (the same type that radiators have to maintain an even temperature). If you are faced with insulin resistance, i.e. decreased sensitivity for insulin, it is as if the "glucostat" has been turned up. Your blood glucose will be higher and more insulin than usual will be needed to lower it again. This is similar to having a fever which raises your body's thermostat and causes your temperature to increase.

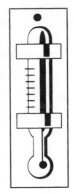

When you have recovered, your body will reset the thermostat so your body temperature returns to normal. In the same way the "glucostat" resets to a normal insulin sensitivity when the blood glucose level has been back to normal for a day or two.

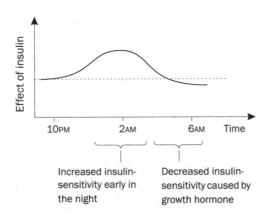

Increased insulin-sensitivity early in the night

Decreased insulin-sensitivity caused by growth hormone

Early in the night (midnight-2AM) when we don't eat, the body's sensitivity to insulin is increased. The secretion of growth hormone increases early in the night but the blood glucose raising effect does not appear for 3-5 hours.[103] Growing children have higher levels of growth hormone than adults do. Levels of growth hormone are even higher during puberty, which explains why the dawn phenomenon is more pronounced in adolescents. Young children who fall asleep early have their growth hormone peaks before midnight and it is common to see an increased need for insulin from 9PM-12AM.[100,150] Patients whose glucose control is poor have increased levels of growth hormone which make increased blood glucose levels in the morning more likely, as well as retarding growth (see page 38).[103]

cose level is high.[471,821] The decreased uptake of glucose into the cells can also be caused by a constriction of the blood vessels, resulting in a decreased blood flow.[292] Insulin resistance will, in this sense, be a defense for the insulin-sensitive cells that are prevented from taking up too much glucose.[822] These cells will not be exposed to glucose toxicity and will therefore not be affected by the long term complications of diabetes. The cells that are not dependent on insulin for their glucose uptake (e.g. the eyes, the kidneys and the nerves) will, on the other hand, have a high uptake of glucose. This will expose them to glucose toxicity leading to long term complications. See illustration on page 305.

If your blood glucose level has been high for a short period only (just one day, for example) such as during an infection, your body will require higher insulin doses to achieve the same blood glucose lowering effect. A meal of a given size and composition will accordingly need a higher dose of insulin than usual. This increased insulin need may continue for a week or so after the infection has subsided if your blood glucose level has been high for a longer period of time. Some people have noted higher blood glucose levels during periods when the pollen count is high if they have pollen allergy. This may be

Increased insulin resistance

Short-term factors

① High blood glucose level for 12-24 hours.[5,259,820]

② Rebound phenomenon (see page 49).

③ Later part of night (dawn phenomenon).

④ Infection with fever.

⑤ Stress.[550]

⑥ Surgery.

⑦ Inactivity, bed rest.[795]

⑧ Ketoacidosis.

Long-term factors

① Puberty.

② Pregnancy (the later part of).

③ Weight gain, being overweight.[36]

④ Smoking.[43,244,564]

⑤ High blood pressure.

⑥ Drugs, e.g. cortisol, contraceptive pills.

⑦ Other diseases like toxic goiter, chronic urinary tract infection, dental abscess.

Decreased insulin resistance

① Low blood glucose levels (improved glucose control).

② Weight loss.

③ After physical exercise.[801]

④ Early hours of the night (midnight - 2 AM).

Research findings: Insulin resistance

♠ In one study, the blood glucose level was held at 305 mg/dl (17 mmol/l) during part of the day and night, 15 hours in total.[259] The following day the patients had a decreased sensitivity for insulin.

♠ Another study showed that if the blood glucose level had been sustained between 220-360 mg/dl (13-20 mmol/l) during a 24 hour period, the effect of a given insulin dose was decreased by as much as 15-20%.[820] After 44 hours with a blood glucose level of 270 mg/dl (15 mmol/l) the insulin effect decreased by 32%.[273]

♠ In the same study it was found that admission to the hospital in itself resulted in a decreased insulin effect by 21%, probably caused by associated illness, bed rest and temporary changes in life style. The effect seems to be due to an increased blood glucose level as such, since the levels of the blood glucose increasing hormones (adrenaline, cortisol and growth hormone) were not increased.

♠ In a healthy beta cell, the production of insulin will be decreased if it is being exposed to high glucose levels even for as short a period as two days.[481]

because they are less active while suffering from pollen allergy.

After some time with high insulin doses (and normal blood glucose levels) you will start experiencing hypoglycemia, even though you have not changed either your insulin doses or the amount of food you eat. The body's sensitivity to insulin will change when the blood glucose level is low, and the same insulin concentration in the blood will now lower the blood glucose more effectively,[158] resulting in a lower dose of insulin for the same meal. As you experience this you will learn to decrease your insulin doses slightly as a preventive measure when your blood glucose levels have been normal for a day or two (or up to a week depending on individual differences), thus preventing hypoglycemia.

Compare your blood glucose level with a thermostat that regulates the central heating in a house. If the thermostat is adjusted to 20° C (68° F) more energy will be needed to maintain

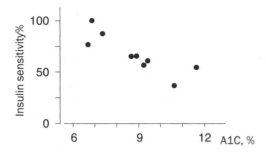

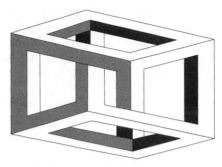

A vicious cycle can easily develop, in which a high blood glucose level can give an increased insulin resistance within 24 hours.[820] This will make your insulin less effective, you will find it more difficult to get your blood glucose levels down to normal, and your blood glucose levels will rise after some time as will your A1C. The graph above shows that a high A1C implies that twice the amount of insulin is needed to obtain the same blood glucose lowering effect.[821]

To start with, you must increase the insulin doses if you are to break this vicious cycle. However, in the long run the key issue is to become more "accurate in aiming" your insulin doses, not letting the blood glucose increase too much or too often again. After just 1-2 weeks with lower blood glucose levels, you will be able to decrease the insulin doses again. If you have been using pump treatment for 3-6 months, it may be possible to lower insulin doses by 10-30% as the insulin resistance decreases after a period with lower blood glucose levels.[821]

It is common to seek the "ideal insulin dosage". Just imagine, finding this would ensure "smooth sailing" for a long time to come. Unfortunately this is never as easy as it sounds. Sometimes you will find it very frustrating searching for the right insulin dose. It seems that no matter how you approach the problem you cannot make any sense of the relationship between your blood glucose measurements and the amount of insulin you take. This is made all the more frustrating by the fact that the speed at which injected insulin is absorbed varies enormously (see page 80). Often, your insulin doses are unlikely to be suitable for more than a couple of weeks at a time. After that, something in your daily life changes, the insulin sensitivity is affected and suddenly your doses are not appropriate any more. Of course, this can be very difficult to understand and to live with. But it is important not to have unrealistic expectations. Just as daily life differs slightly from week to week and month to month, so your insulin requirements will also change.

If you are unable to find a schedule that works, it can be helpful to keep to exactly the same doses for a week. You will then be better equipped to see a pattern in your glucose readings and insulin doses. Contact your diabetes healthcare team to discuss what to do next.

this temperature if the outside temperature is colder than usual. In the same way, more insulin will be needed to keep the blood glucose at the same level when insulin resistance is high. If the blood glucose level has been high for a while, the "glucostat" will adjust and you will start having hypoglycemia at a higher blood glucose level than before. If you have had very low blood glucose levels for some time, the glucostat will readjust in the opposite direction and you will not experience hypoglycemia until your blood glucose level is very low (see also page 43 and 57).

Weight gain increases insulin resistance while weight loss decreases it. This is one of the reasons why it is difficult to maintain a normal

blood glucose level if you are overweight. Male pattern obesity ("apple fatness") is particularly likely to increase insulin resistance.[500] Other factors can also contribute to the level of insulin resistance (see key fact box on page 196).

Increased levels of stress hormones (adrenaline, noradrenaline) will induce an insulin resistance that develops within 5-10 minutes.[500] Stress also causes release of cortisol, which increases insulin resistance within hours.

During puberty, an increase in the secretion of growth hormone raises the blood glucose level.

This causes a resistance to insulin that contributes to the need for increased insulin doses during puberty. Smoking leads to increased insulin resistance because nicotine decreases the uptake of glucose to the tissues of the body.[43]

Regular exercise (at least every other day) leads to a decrease in insulin resistance that lasts between exercise sessions, while inactivity (for instance caused by being bedridden) gives an increased resistance within days.[795] Active athletes, for example, need to lower all their insulin doses considerably. When the training season is over, doses are likely to need considerable adjustment upwards if higher blood glucose levels are to be avoided. Sometimes 30-50% more insulin will be needed during periods of reduced activity.

Ideal insulin doses?

Of course we all want to search for the ideal insulin doses, but unfortunately this is not a realistic goal since insulin requirements vary according to activity, other illnesses, insulin resistance (see page 195) and other factors. A good parallel can be seen with body temperature. Your body strives to maintain a temperature around 37° C (99° F) but this would be difficult if you always wore the same amount of clothing regardless of what the weather was like. Just as an outfit that is perfect one week can be much too warm the next, so a particular dose of insulin is likely to be ideal for a week or two only, before you need to readjust it. As with your clothing, you will need to make daily adjustments in your insulin doses if you are to remain comfortable.

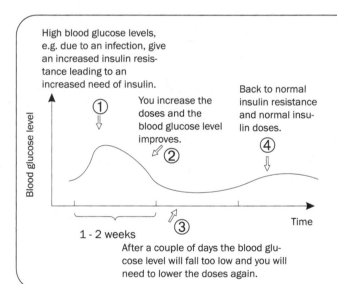

High blood glucose levels, e.g. due to an infection, give an increased insulin resistance leading to an increased need of insulin.

① You increase the doses and the blood glucose level improves. ②

Back to normal insulin resistance and normal insulin doses. ④

1 - 2 weeks

③ After a couple of days the blood glucose level will fall too low and you will need to lower the doses again.

When the blood glucose level is increased for some reason (for example an infection), more insulin is needed depending on the level of resistance. However, if you continue with the higher doses you will start having hypoglycemia before long. The best strategy is to lower the doses as a preventative measure when you start getting a lot of low blood glucose readings. These "waves" of insulin resistance usually appear with an interval of a few weeks.

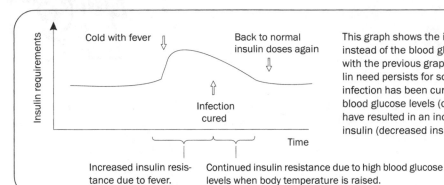

This graph shows the insulin requirements instead of the blood glucose level. Compare with the previous graph. The increased insulin need persists for some time after the infection has been cured since the high blood glucose levels (caused by the fever) have resulted in an increased resistance to insulin (decreased insulin sensitivity).

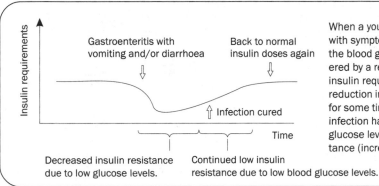

When a young person gets gastroenteritis with symptoms of vomiting and/or diarrhea, the blood glucose levels will usually be lowered by a reduction in food intake, causing insulin requirements to go right down. This reduction in need for insulin is likely to go on for some time (often 1-2 weeks) after the infection has been cured, as the low blood glucose levels cause a drop in insulin resistance (increased insulin sensitivity).

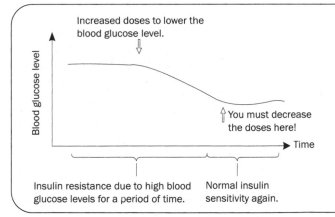

The same type of insulin resistance will arise if the blood glucose is high for a period of time due to other reasons, such as failing to follow your diet or eating too much candy Even if you stop eating much candy higher doses of insulin than usual are needed to bring the blood glucose back to normal levels. To avoid hypoglycemia, lower the doses once again when the blood glucose has been normal for 1-2 weeks. Otherwise there is a risk that you will go back to eating larger amounts to avoid hypoglycemia and thereby gain weight, ending up in a vicious circle.

Nutrition

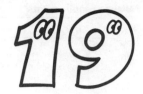

From a historical perspective, dietary advice for people with diabetes has been very restrictive when it comes to carbohydrate intake. Foods containing sugar were excluded from the diet. This created feelings of guilt in people with diabetes when the "rules were broken". To do as most other people do, i.e. to vary one's food intake and indulge in the occasional sweet "treat" was discouraged and by some looked upon almost as "sinning". But this is an outmoded and inappropriate approach. The inclusion of foods containing moderate amounts of sugar has not been found to worsen blood glucose control.

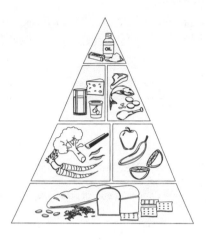

Sticking to a rigid pattern of meal times and selected food is unlikely to be necessary because of diabetes alone, especially if you are taking premeal insulin in a multiple injection or pump regimen, although regular eating habits and a knowledge of carbohydrate quantities is important. Many people with diabetes live full and varied lives, enjoy their food, and still manage to control their blood glucose levels effectively.

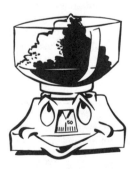

A kitchen scale can be useful for weighing food and extras to calculate the carbohydrate content when learning carbohydrate counting. After an initial learning period, this can often be estimated by eye. Carbohydrate gram counting will give you a more exact method of calculating premeal insulin doses when using multiple injections or a pump (see page 216).

The more knowledge you have about carbohydrate foods and their effects on your blood glucose, the more control you will have over your diabetes. This chapter will give you many details about blood glucose and different foods, but you will learn the general aspects of healthy eating from your dietitian.

It is important to be careful about what you eat, even if you don't have diabetes. But remember that food should not be looked upon as medicine. Food should look and taste good. Meals are meant to be pleasurable, we should enjoy food and feel satisfied afterwards. If you concentrate upon food being "good for you" to the exclusion of everything else, you will find no pleasure in it. It will be much more rewarding if you are able to discuss what you can eat with a dietitian who will help you draw up a meal plan based on the mealtimes, routines and preferences that are important to your family. "You should never eat what you don't like", is a wise comment from a dietitian.

"What can I eat?", "What should I avoid?" Such questions are commonly asked by people newly diagnosed with diabetes. Usually, the comment after the first consultation with a dietitian will be: "I am glad to discover I can eat most of the things as I used to before getting diabetes". Dietary advice should be directed towards the whole family from the very beginning. In a Finnish study of young children with type 1 diabetes, all family members increased their consumption of skimmed milk, low-fat cheese and low-fat cold meats. They also ate more fruit and vegetables.[789]

Nutritional recommendations will be based on requirements for all healthy children and adolescents.[274] Children need to double their energy intake between the ages of 6 and 12 years if they are to grow as much as they should.[792] At this time, they need to eat more food rich in energy and protein. However, if they do not reduce their energy intake once the growth spurt stops, they are at risk of becoming overweight.[792] At the present time, there is no good scientific evidence for recommending vitamin or mineral supplements.[792]

Absorption of carbohydrates

Glucose from food can only be absorbed into the bloodstream after it has passed into the intestines. It cannot be absorbed through the lining of the mouth, as used to be believed.[321,710] To reach the intestines, the food must first pass through the lower opening of the stomach (pylorus, see illustration on page 21) where a special muscle, the pyloric sphincter, acts as a "gateway" to the intestine below. The sphincter will only allow very small pieces to pass through.

Complex carbohydrates must first be broken down to simple sugars before they can be absorbed into the bloodstream. The length of the carbohydrate chain does not seem to affect

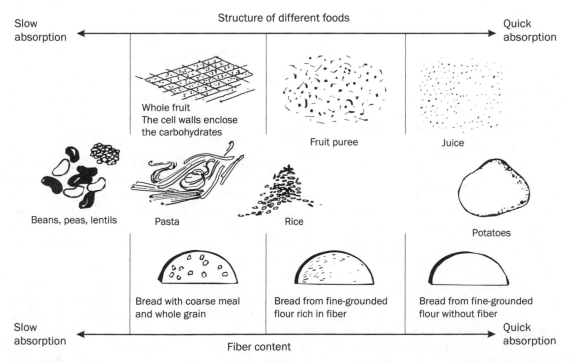

The structure and fiber content of different foodstuffs affect how quickly the carbohydrate content is absorbed. The illustration is from the book "Food and diabetes" by the Swedish Diabetes Association, printed with permission.

Factors that increase the blood glucose level more *quickly* (*increased glycemic index*)

① Cooking:

Boiling and other types of cooking will break down the starch in food.

② Preparing food:

Prepared food, e.g. polished rice will give a quicker rise in blood glucose than unpolished, mashed potatoes quicker than whole potatoes and grated carrots quicker than sliced.[753] Wheat-flour gives a higher blood glucose response when baked in bread than when used for pasta.[428]

③ Fluids with food:

Drinking fluids with a meal causes the stomach to empty more quickly.[760]

④ Glucose content:

Extra sugar as part of a meal can cause the blood glucose level to rise, but not by as much as was once believed. Particle size and cell structure in different food compounds give them different blood glucose responses in spite of their containing the same amount of carbohydrates.[36]

⑤ Salt content:

Salt in the food increases the absorption of glucose into the bloodstream.[754]

Factors that increase the blood glucose level more *slowly* (*decreased glycemic index*)

① Starch structure:

Boiled and mashed potatoes give a quicker blood glucose response (as fast as ordinary sugar) while rice and pasta give a slower blood glucose response.[784]

② Gel-forming dietary fiber

A high fiber content (as in rye bread) gives a slower rise in blood glucose by slowing down the emptying rate of the stomach and binding glucose in the intestine.

③ Fat content:

Fat in the food will delay the emptying of the stomach.[806]

④ Cell structure:

Beans, peas and lentils retain their cell structure even after cooking. Whole fruits affect the blood glucose level more slowly than peeled fruits and juice.[784]

⑤ Size of bites: [635]

Larger pieces of food take longer to digest in the stomach and intestine. Larger pieces also cause the stomach to empty more slowly.

absorption as much as was once believed since "cleavage" (breaking) is a fairly rapid process. Simple carbohydrates are cleaved by enzymes in the intestinal lining while more complex carbohydrates and starch are first prepared by amylase, an enzyme found in the saliva and pancreas. Starch fiber cannot be cleaved into carbohydrates in the intestine.

At one time, carbohydrates were divided into quick-acting and slow-acting, mainly depending on the size of the molecule. It is more accurate to speak of quick-acting and long-acting foods and to evaluate the composition, fiber content and preparation in order to determine the effect on the blood glucose level, rather than simply its content of pure sugar.[428,791] The term "glycemic index" (GI) is used to describe how the blood glucose level is affected by different food (see page 209).

Dietary fiber content and particle size seem to be particularly important according to recent studies.[36] The starch in vegetables is broken down more slowly than the starch in bread.[753] The starch in potatoes is quick to break down to glucose. The starch from pasta products is broken down much more slowly, even though it

Carbohydrates

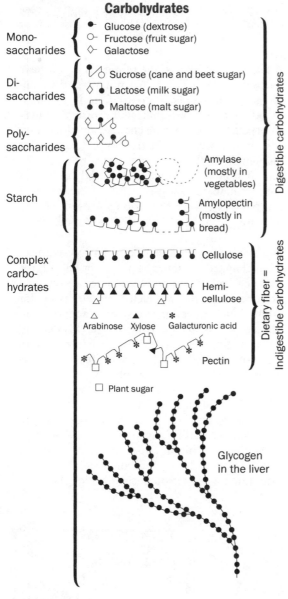

Carbohydrates are important for metabolism in the body. Only mono-saccharides can be absorbed from the intestine. Di-saccharides and starch must first be broken down by digestive enzymes. Dietary fiber cannot be broken down to saccharides in the intestines. The glycogen store in the liver is composed of very long chains of glucose. The illustration is modified from reference [36].

is made from white flour, which is low in fiber.[428]

How much you chew the food and the size of the food particles swallowed also influences the blood glucose response.[635] Industrially manufactured mashed potatoes contain a fine powder that is mixed with fluid. The glucose in mashed potatoes is absorbed just as quickly as a glucose solution.[784] Pasta and rice are swallowed in larger bites and must be digested before they can be absorbed. Likewise, a whole apple will give a slower rise in blood glucose than apple juice which contains smaller particles and is in a liquid form.

Heating decomposes starch, making sugar more accessible and faster to digest. Industrial food processing usually involves higher temperatures which gives food a quicker blood glucose raising effect compared to home-cooked meals.[753] Industrial baby food and semi-manufactured food (sometimes used in schools) can raise the blood glucose more than comparable home-cooked meals.

Indigestible carbohydrates (dietary fiber) cannot be broken down in the intestines and will therefore not give a blood glucose response. In the US, dietary fiber is listed on the food labels. Your dietitian can discuss this with you further.

Emptying the stomach

Everything that causes the stomach to release food more slowly into the intestines will also result in a slower increase of the blood glucose level [36] (see illustration on page 64). From this, it follows that the composition of the meal will be important, not only the amount of carbohydrates it contains. Fat [806] and fiber [579] cause the stomach to empty more slowly while a drink with the meal will make it empty more quickly.[778] A meal containing solid food (such as pancakes) is emptied more slowly than liquid food like soup.[778] Swallowing without chewing also causes a slower rise in blood glucose.[635] Extremely cold (4° C, 39° F) or hot (50° C, 122° F) food will also slow down stomach emptying.[728]

What is our food made of?[413]

The food that we eat is mainly made up of a mixture of:

Carbohydrates	Fat	Protein
Sugar	Butter	Meat
Bread/flour	Margarine	Fish
Cookies	Cookies	Egg
Potatoes	Oil	Cheese
Pasta	Cream	Milk
Rice	Milk	Yogurt
Fruit	Cheese	
Cereals		
Sweet corn, taro		
Milk, yogurt		

The emptying of the stomach is also affected by the blood glucose level. The stomach empties more quickly if the blood glucose is low and more slowly if it is high. Both solid and liquid food are emptied from the stomach twice as fast when the blood glucose drops from a normal level 72-126 mg/dl (4-7 mmol/l) to a hypoglycemic level (29-40 mg/dl, 1.6-2.2 mmol/l).[691] If your blood glucose level has been lowered by a large dose of insulin, you want your stomach to empty as quickly as possible so that the glucose can be absorbed into the blood. In this situation you should take something with a high glucose content, such as glucose tablets, glucose gel, or a sports drink.

A high insulin level in the blood (as if you have taken a too large dose) does not affect the emptying of the stomach in itself, it is the high blood glucose level that will cause a slower emptying.[458] Even small changes in blood glucose levels, well within the normal ranges for individuals without diabetes, seem to affect the rate of stomach emptying. One study of people without diabetes, showed a 20% decrease in the emptying rate when the blood glucose level was increased from 72 to 144 mg/dl (4-8 mmol/l).[692]

Non-strenuous exercise (like walking) will lead to unchanged or more rapid emptying of the stomach, while strenous exercise or physical exertion stops the stomach from emptying for 20-40 minutes after muscular activity finishes.[117] A possible explanation for this delayed stomach emptying after physical exertion is an increased secretion of adrenaline and morphine-like hormones (endorphins).

Stomach emptying can also be delayed if you have gastroenteritis.[52] This may contribute to the problem of prolonged low blood glucose levels that are often associated with vomiting and diarrhoea. There is a complication of diabetes known as gastroparesis in which the auto-

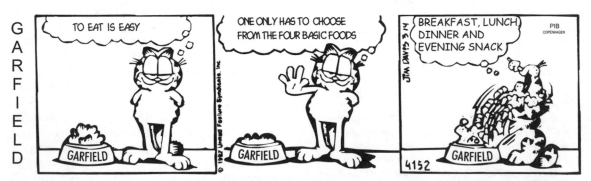

It isn't easy to balance food and insulin at all times. Many people seem to think that "It can't be that difficult, since a diabetes diet is what we all should eat". You may find well-meaning friends or relatives acting as "sugar-guards", telling you shouldn't be doing this every time you eat something sweet, even if you have hypoglycemia. Try to explain that at times it can be both healthy and necessary to eat sweet foods, and you may avoid some of the glances and remarks.

nomic nervous system is damaged. This damage involves the nerves that co-ordinate the movements of the stomach and intestine, resulting in the emptying of the stomach being mildly or even severely delayed. See also the section on complications on page 313.

Sugar content in our food

From a nutritional point of view, we do not actually need pure sugar at all. The liver is quite capable of producing the 250-300 grams of glucose that a healthy adult normally needs per day.

Small amounts of glucose along with a meal do not cause an increased rise in blood glucose according to several studies in which a small amount of starch has been exchanged for glucose at a meal.[36,274] This means that you can add 5 grams (1/5 ounce) of sugar to a meal without risk, for example in the form of ketchup.[732] Where sugar is an integral part of the meal, it should be balanced by a comparable reduction in carbohydrate, or an appropriate increase in insulin.[274] Dietary sugar does not increase blood glucose more than an equivalent amount of starch.[274] This is great news for people with diabetes as it makes following the food plans much easier. However, sugar eaten between meals affects the blood glucose level much more. Your blood glucose level will rise just as quickly if you eat candy or white bread (without butter or something on it) in between meals.[287] The important factor is whether the snack contains

Aims of nutritional management [792]

➡ To provide appropriate energy and nutrients for optimal growth, development and health.

➡ To maintain or achieve an ideal body weight.

➡ To achieve and maintain optimal glucose control for the individual by balancing food intake with insulin, energy requirements and physical activity.

➡ To prevent and treat acute complications of insulin therapy, for example hypoglycemia, crises with high blood glucose, illness and exercise-related problems.

➡ To reduce the risk of long-term complications through optimal glucose control.

➡ To reduce the risk of heart complications and blood vessel disease.

➡ To preserve social and psychological well being.

How can this be achieved?

➡ Healthy eating principles should be applicable to the whole family.

➡ Distribution of energy and carbohydrate intake to balance insulin action profiles and exercise (and adjustment of insulin doses to varying food patterns).

➡ Total energy needs should be sufficient for growth in children and adolescents, but should not cause overweight or obesity.

➡ Fruit and vegetables should be eaten regularly (five portions per day are recommended).

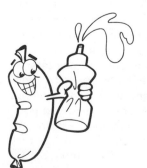

You can have a modest amount of ketchup with your food without any problems. However, if you use a large amount of ketchup, you will end up eating a lot of additional sugar.

fiber or fat (like chocolate-covered cookies) which delay stomach emptying. Far too many people in the US, Canada, UK, Australia and other countries are now becoming overweight, often seriously so. Therefore, you should be very careful to avoid high fat snacks if you have a weight problem.

The recommendation to decrease the sugar content in food is based on more general factors:

How is the emptying of the stomach affected?

More quickly	More slowly
Small bites	Large bites
Liquid food	Solid food
Drink with food	Drink after food
	Fatty food
	Food rich in fiber
	Extremely hot or cold food
Hypoglycemia	High blood glucose
	High levels of insulin
	Smoking
	Gastroenteritis
Light exercise	Heavy exercise

① Sugar gives "empty calories", i.e. sugar gives only energy and contains no other nutrients. This energy will cause you to gain weight, while reducing your appetite for more healthy foods.

② Sugar is bad for your teeth.

In an American study where children took insulin twice daily, there was no difference in their blood glucose levels when they had a diet with 2% of the carbohydrates as pure glucose (in fruit and bread) compared to 10% (in fruit and bread, cereal and toast with jelly for breakfast, chocolate chip cookies with lunch, chocolate for an afternoon snack and chilled milk with dinner).[499] This may be surprising, but can be explained by the fact that all the meals contained both fat and protein. The total carbohydrate content was the same for both types of meal.

It used to be common practice to decrease the carbohydrate content in a diabetes meal plan at all costs. The problem with this approach is that the fat content usually increases instead, and this results in the diet becoming inferior to the diet of many children without diabetes.[734,791] It is much more important to eat regularly and

to adjust the insulin dose according to appetite and the content of carbohydrates in the meal.

Taking fluids with food

You can affect your blood glucose level considerably, depending on what you have to drink with your meals. Sweet drinks like fruit juice can be used to raise your blood glucose if it is in the low range. But if your blood glucose level is high, it is better to have water. It is a good idea to drink plenty of calorie free drinks between meals if your blood glucose is high as this will help to bring it down (part of the excess glucose will be excreted into the urine). If you want ice cream for dessert, you can drink water instead of milk with your meal if you want to keep the amount of carbohydrate unchanged, or add 1-2 units to take care of the ice cream (see page 228).

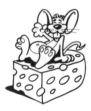

Dietary fats

The reason that individuals with diabetes should be careful with fat intake is that they have an increased risk of arteriosclerosis and heart disease (see page 305). A key goal for people with diabetes is to decrease the intake of total fat (including saturated fat and trans fatty acids) and cholesterol.[274] You need to be particularly careful with saturated fat and so called "trans fats".[274] Foods that contain large amounts of saturated fats include dairy products and red meats. They are also found in many snack foods such as chocolate, cakes and pastries and sometimes in chips. Trans fats are often listed as "partially hydrogenated vegetable oil" or "vegetable shortening" on the food label.[800] Try to use monounsaturated and polyunsaturated fats where possible instead. An increased intake of monounsaturated fats may even improve your A1C.[219] The softer the fat the better. Liquid margarine and oil do not contain any trans fats at all and also have a low content of saturated fatty acids. Be careful of palm, vegetable and coconut oil as all are high in saturated fat and used widely in different products.

Today, dietitians promote monounsaturated fats (MUFA) which have a protective effect against heart disease.[614] Choose a margarine that contains monounsaturated fat. Light margarine is not recommended for very young children, however, as they have an increased need for fat in their diet. Ordinary margarine and butter contain only 3% polyunsaturated fat. Olive oil and rapeseed oil contain large amounts of monounsaturated fat and are useful for frying. However, if the frying pan is very hot, the unsaturated fat can be broken down. Some types of light margarine cannot be used for frying. Sunflower oil is an example of oil which is good for frying as it is not broken down as readily as olive oil.

Up to the age of 5 years, it is expected that the proportion of energy derived from dietary fats will fall from about 50% (as it is in breast milk and infant formula) to levels recommended for adults, but this moderation should not occur

below the age of 2 years.[792] Below this age the energy density of foods is important and also low fat foods in toddlers may be associated with rapid gastric emptying and diarrhoea.[792]

Many people believe that fat increases the blood glucose level since people with diabetes are usually advised to cut down on fat in their diet. However, fatty food has no direct effect on the blood glucose level. Fat affects the blood glucose level indirectly by slowing the rate at which the stomach empties.[388,806] Studies on monkeys have found that their stomachs empty portions of food through the lower sphincter with the same amount of energy every minute.[537] As fat yields more energy than carbohydrate, the stomach is emptied more slowly when the fat content is high. A meal with a high fat content, therefore, will cause the blood glucose level to rise more slowly.

The fat in food must pass into the intestine before it can affect the emptying rate of the stomach.[806] This means that if you start a meal with something rich in fat, the signal that slows down the emptying rate will reach the stomach more quickly.

If you eat a meal very rich in fat, you may still have food remaining in your stomach when you are about to have your next meal. If you are using multiple injections, you will need to decrease the amount of food you plan to eat (without changing the insulin dose), if you are to avoid an increase in blood glucose. If you are using rapid-acting insulin (NovoLog/ NovoRapid or Humalog) you may be at risk of hypoglycemia shortly after a meal rich in fat. If so, try giving yourself the injection after the meal instead of before.

It is the total amount of fat over time that is important in the long run. You can cut down on fat during the week and then have a festive meal at the weekend, complete with a delicious cream sauce, or a takeaway meal. Most fat replacers, for example maltodextrin (modified

Food rules of thumb

⫸ Regular eating habits are encouraged in all children and adolescents, with or without diabetes.

⫸ Plan meal times and contents with other daily activities in mind, e.g. will you be taking physical exercise or sitting at a desk?

⫸ Take extra insulin when necessary, e.g. at parties, or when eating lots of candy.

⫸ Eat fresh fruit as a snack rather than drinking fruit juice.

⫸ Cut down on snacks and what you eat at every meal if you have weight problems.

⫸ Aim for a high fiber content in your food.

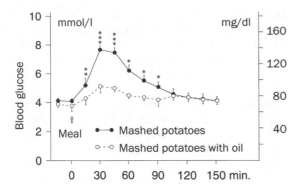

If the meal contains fat, the emptying of the stomach will be delayed, causing the blood glucose to rise more slowly. In this study, two helpings of mashed potatoes (50 grams of carbohydrate) were given with or without corn oil (approximately 30 ml, 2 tablespoonfuls). The study was done in adults without diabetes who can increase the amount of insulin in their blood very fast.[806] Notice that the blood glucose level increased quickly despite this, with a significant change appearing in 30 minutes, in the group of people whose mashed potatoes did not contain oil. If you have weight problems you need to be careful about adding fat to your food.

food starch), are made of carbohydrate which may affect your blood glucose.

Dietary fibers

The fiber content of food is healthy for many reasons. There are two kinds of fibers, soluble (gel-forming) and insoluble. Both help to prevent constipation but only the soluble fibers (found in fruit, vegetables, legumes, and oats) affect the glucose control. You will feel full for longer after eating coarse rye or wholemeal bread with a high soluble fiber content, than you would after eating the same amount of white bread without fiber. A high soluble fiber content will also decrease the cholesterol level in your blood.[579] Adding fiber (such as oats and barley) to a meal will increase the viscosity, causing the contents of the stomach and intestines to empty more slowly.[579,819] The fiber forms a thin film on the intestinal surface causing the glucose to be absorbed more slowly.[579]

When a glucose solution is mixed with large amounts of water-soluble, gel-forming fiber (i.e. guar, ß-glucan) the expected rise in glucose concentration will be reduced.[579] Soluble dietary fiber probably has the greatest impact on food intake with high glucose content (such as many snacks) since it has been difficult to show in long-term studies that the addition of dietary fiber has resulted in a better A1C.[579] These studies have mainly been done on individuals with type 2 diabetes. An Italian study of adults with type 1 diabetes compared a low-fibre diet with a high-fibre diet rich in fruit, legumes, and vegetables.[298] Both diets contained exclusively natural foodstuffs. The high-fibre diet resulted in lower blood glucose levels, 0.5% lower A1C, and decreased frequency of hypoglycemia. In a European study on 2065 adults with type 1 diabetes, a ~0.3% lower A1C was found in people whose fiber intake was high.[123]

Fruit and vegetables are good sources of fibre, but children eat on average less than half of the minimum of five portions recommended per day.[792] A piece of fresh fruit and multi-grain bread can be a good basis if the rest of the meal is made up mainly of "quick-acting" carbohydrates. Parents can make use of the "fiber effect" by offering a slice of coarse wholemeal bread with some fat (for example margarine or cheese) to their child before other concentrated sugary foods or snacks. The combination of fiber and fat in the meal will help to slow down any rise in the blood glucose level.

Glycemic index

The glycemic index (GI) is an attempt to describe the blood glucose raising effect of different foods. The glycemic index of a mixed meal can be predicted from the GI of single foods.[140] It may be difficult to estimate the GI for some combined meals from the GI of the single ingredients since the fat content also affects the speed with which carbohydrates are absorbed. A foodstuff with a low but easily accessible sugar content (for example carrots)

Glycemic index [272]

High glycemic index	GI	50g carb. in
Glucose	100	50g
Instant mashed potatoes	85	375g
Potato, baked	85	250g
Corn flakes	81	60g
Jelly candy	78	65g
White bread (gluten free)	76	100g
Waffles	76	135g
French fries	75	260g
Weetabix	75	70g
Oatmeal porridge	74	80g (dry)
Rice, puffed	74	180g
Potato, boiled	74	440g
Water melon	72	1000g
Popcorn	72	90g
White bread	70	110g
Sugar pop	68	370g
Sucrose (sugar)	68	50g
Rice, white	64	210g

Average glycemic index	GI	50g carb. in
Rye bread (wholemeal)	58	110g
Cola	58	480g
Rice, long grain	56	180g
Gluten free pasta	56 [589]	64g
Honey	55	70g
Banana, all yellow	51	230g
Pasta	46-52	200g
Lactose (milk sugar)	46	50g
Grapes	46	330g
Rye bread (whole-grain)	46	135g

Low glycemic index	GI	50g carb. in
Milk chocolate	43	90g
Banana, yellow and green	42	240g
All Bran	42	65g
Orange	42	550g
Apple	38	400g
Ice cream	37-61	190-280g
Yogurt	36	1100g
Lentils, green	30	440g
Kidney beans	28	300g
Milk, 3% fat	21	1000g
Fructose (fruit sugar)	19	50g
Soya beans (dried)	18	1250g
Peanuts	14	415g

See also reference [542] for an extensive list of foods.

Glycemic index

The glycemic index is an attempt to describe the blood glucose raising effect of different foods. A certain amount of carbohydrate is given (usually 50 g) and the area under the blood glucose curve is measured for 2 hours. Glucose is used to give a baseline glycemic index of 100. The glycemic index can be misleading if you want to know how the blood glucose level is affected during a shorter period of time (e.g. 30-60 minutes) or if the food has a low, but easily accessible, sugar content. The list to the right is based on reference [272].

has a high glycemic index but you must eat a great deal if your blood glucose is going to be increased. Although the use of low GI food may reduce blood glucose levels after meals, more research is required before GI can be used as a general tool in diabetes care. In Australia, the GI concept is much more accepted and widely used than, for example, in the US and UK. According to the ADA there is not yet sufficient evidence of long-term benefit to recommend the general use of a low GI diet.[274]

Potatoes (GI 74) give a faster blood glucose response than pasta (GI 46-52). Adding a small amount of oil or polyunsaturated or monounsaturated margarine to mashed potatoes (GI 85) will slow down the glucose peak. If you replace one item in a meal with another (for example potatoes with pasta) the GI of the individual foods will help you determine the likely effect on the blood glucose. For example, it may be a good idea to have something with a low GI for supper as this could lower the risk of night time hypoglycemia.

GI is very useful when you are looking at eating between meals (single items of food often such as yogurt, an apple, a bun, ice cream, chips etc.). Professionals and parents alike have the difficult task of explaining to children how they should handle items such as these.

If you know that an ice cream made from dairy products has a GI of 37-61, you can recommend this as a good diabetes snack to be eaten in moderate amounts together with siblings or friends. When treating hypoglycemia we want to use something with a high GI to obtain a quick glycemic response. Milk (GI 21) and chocolate bars (GI 43) are widely used for treating hypoglycemia but the rise in blood glucose is actually very slow.[116,132] However, white bread (without margarine, GI 70) with some sugar soda (GI 68) will cause the blood glucose to rise much faster. Glucose tablets have a GI of 100 and are appropriate when symptoms are more pronounced or the blood glucose level is lower (<65 mg/dl, 3.5 mmol/l).

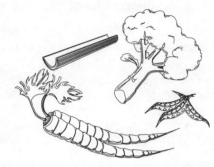

The starch in vegetables is broken down more slowly than other types of starch. Vegetables also contain soluble fiber which is good for the digestion and prevents constipation.

Milk

Many children drink milk with their meals. Different types of milk have different fat contents. However, all types have the same amount of milk sugar (lactose, 12 grams per 8 oz.) and usually the same amount of vitamins and minerals, including calcium. Small children (up to 2-3 years of age) need more fat in their diet and should drink whole milk. In practice, this means that the change from whole fat milks to semi-skimmed (partly skimmed) or even skim milk should only be instituted after the age of 2 years.[792] Which type of milk is most suitable also depends on how much the child drinks per day. Half a liter or 1 pint a day is recommended for its calcium content.

Vegetables

You can eat freely from this food group (except sweet corn) as the carbohydrate content is very low (see table on page 211). Vegetables are also high in dietary fiber. Put the vegetables on the table before the children come to eat and they will probably help themselves to them while waiting for the food to be served.

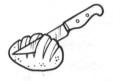

Potatoes

Potatoes, sweet potatoes, taro, and yam belong to this type of food stuff. The carbohydrate content of raw potatoes is absorbed slowly, but boiling causes the cell walls to burst. This allows the carbohydrates to be absorbed more quickly from the intestines. The carbohydrate content of mashed potatoes is absorbed as quickly as pure glucose [813] (see graph on page 208). This can give a quick rise in blood glucose after the meal but may also result in hypoglycemia 2-3 hours later, since all the carbohydrates in the mashed potatoes will have been absorbed during a fairly short time after the meal. If you change the surface of a potato (for example, by frying, deep frying, or storing it in the refrigerator) the glucose will be absorbed more slowly than if you eat it freshly boiled.[178] The manufacturing process and the high fat content in potato chips cause the glucose contained in these to be absorbed very slowly (see graph on page 234).[132]

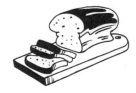

Vegetables

	Quantity	Carb.	% fiber
Bamboo shoots, canned	½ cup	4g	50%
Broccoli, frozen	½ cup	5g	60%
Carrots, raw	½ cup	5g	27%
Corn, canned	½ cup	20g	30%
Corn on cob, cooked 1 medium size	19g	10%
Cucumber	1 cup	3g	<1g
Lettuce	1 cup	1g	<1g
Onions, cooked	½ cup	11g	18%
Peas, green, cooked	½ cup	13g	31%
Peppers, green, raw	½ cup	3g	33%
Radishes	½ cup	2g	50%
Tomatoes, raw	½ cup	4g	25%

Data from reference [381].

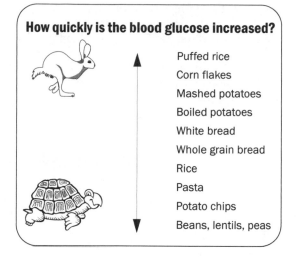

How quickly is the blood glucose increased?

Puffed rice
Corn flakes
Mashed potatoes
Boiled potatoes
White bread
Whole grain bread
Rice
Pasta
Potato chips
Beans, lentils, peas

In one study of adults, chocolate cake was substituted for a baked potato without an increase in blood glucose levels.[605] If the chocolate cake was added to the baked potato, the glucose level increased. However, remember that chocolate cake and baked potato are very different in nutritional and energy value!

Bread

At one time, people with diabetes were strongly advised to eat unsweetened bread. Today, we know that white bread raises the blood glucose level every bit as rapidly as ordinary sugar. However, margarine and something with a high fat content (e.g. cheese) on the bread will slow the rise in blood glucose by delaying emptying of the stomach. Bread (such as whole grain) that is high in fiber will also slow down any rise in blood glucose levels.

If you bake your own bread, it is perfectly acceptable to use an ordinary recipe. It should not be necessary to leave out sugar or experiment with alternative sweetening agents. Three to 6 tablespoons (45-90 ml) of sugar or syrup for a dough made from 2 cups (500 ml) of liquid can be used as only a small amount will remain in the bread after baking. It is more important to choose bread that is rich in fiber rather than omitting small amounts of sugar. Gluten free wheat bread gives a quicker rise in blood glucose compared to the same amount of bread containing gluten.[542]

Nutritious meals do not always need to be hot.[413] A sandwich or roll with tuna, egg, lean meat, chicken or cheese and salad, along with yogurt or fruit can be very enjoyable.

Unsweetened breakfast corn cereal (corn flakes) contains 90% starch, most of which rapidly becomes available as glucose. Sweetened (sugar-frosted) flaked corn cereal, on the other hand, contains around 50% starch and 50% sugar. Initially, both give the same blood glucose rise but sweetened corn flakes give slightly lower blood glucose levels after 3 hours.[807] This may surprise you, but corn starch raises the blood glucose faster than ordinary sugar. The volume of sweetened corn cereal is around 25%

less for the same carbohydrate content, so pre-sweetened corn cereals can be used in a meal plan without increasing the blood glucose if the total amount of carbohydrate is taken into consideration when estimating the insulin dose. However, increasing the number of calories you consume will cause you to put on weight in time.

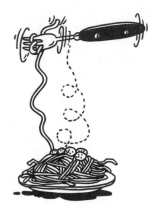

Pasta

Pasta gives a slow rise in blood glucose since it is prepared from crushed or cracked wheat, not wheat flour which causes the starch to be enclosed within a structure of protein (gluten).[379,543] This makes pasta a suitable food for people with diabetes. It has the additional advantage of being popular with children. If you are using rapid-acting insulin (Humalog), however, the rise may even be too slow, resulting in hypoglycemia within 30-60 minutes.[396] If this applies to you, you should take your Novo-Log/NovoRapid or Humalog after your meal, or use regular short-acting insulin when eating pasta (or beans as in chili con carne). If you have a pump, you can use a prolonged bolus dose (see page 166).

Thinner pasta, such as macaroni, gives a quicker blood glucose response than spaghetti.[379] Cooking time is not a factor in how quickly the blood glucose is raised by spaghetti except in extreme cases of overcooking. Canned spaghetti increases the blood glucose just as quickly as white bread.[379] As the gluten content of pasta contributes to the slow rise in blood

glucose,[819] gluten free pasta allows blood glucose levels to rise faster.[589]

Meat and fish

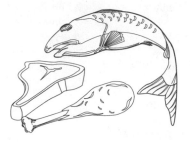

Meat and fish have a high protein content. Sometimes the fat content is high as well. They do not contain any carbohydrates that will increase your blood glucose levels directly. Dietary protein does not slow the absorption of carbohydrate, and the adding of protein to a carbohydrate snack does not prevent late-onset or night time hypoglycemia.[274]

Intake of protein does not increase blood glucose in people who do not have diabetes.[274] However, proteins stimulate the release of glucagon, and this in turn helps to convert protein into glucose (a process called gluconeogenesis, see page 32).[312] If there is not enough insulin, the blood glucose may be increased as a result. This increase comes rather late (after 3-5 hours)[606] so counteracting it with a premeal dose of rapid-acting insulin may not be the best approach. For a meal very high in protein (like a big steak) it may be better to use regular short-acting insulin or, if you use an insulin pump, to use a prolonged type of bolus (see page 166). If you have diabetic kidney disease, you may need to reduce the amount of protein in your diet. Consult your doctor and dietitian about this.

If you are preparing food with a very low fat content (e.g. white fish such as cod or haddock, or very lean meat) it is a good idea to add a little extra fat. This can be in the form of oil or margarine when frying or baking, or with a sauce containing butter or cream. If your meal is entirely fat-free, your stomach will empty very quickly, leaving you at risk of hypoglycemia after a couple of hours. As the energy content of boiled fish is fairly low, you may find having a larger helping is necessary to avoid getting hungry soon again. However, be careful about adding extra fat if you have weight problems, and check first with your dietitian.

Pizza

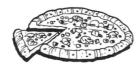

Pizza contains bread, cheese, meat or fish, and possibly vegetables. In other words, it is a balanced meal. One problem if you have diabetes is that a pizza meal will usually contain more bread than a traditional meal. The bread is baked hard which causes the carbohydrates to be absorbed more slowly. Cheese has a high fat content, which causes the stomach to empty more slowly. Try taking 1-2 extra units of insulin (or according to the actual carbohydrate content if you have calculated this) with the pizza or avoid eating the crust. If you use rapid-acting insulin (NovoLog, Humalog), it may be better to take this after the meal or substitute a dose of short-acting insulin (Novolin N, Humulin N, Insuman NPH) instead. If you have a pump you can use an extended bolus dose.

Salt

Salt intake is generally far too high. In Western countries, it is difficult to decrease this as salt is added to many processed foods (only 20% of total intake is added at the table and in cooking).[792] Extra salt in the form of sodium chloride (table-salt) will increase the blood pressure and can be a risk factor especially as diabetes itself increases the risk of heart and vascular diseases (see page 305). Eating salty food can

cause glucose to be absorbed more effectively from the intestine.[754] Salt is also available as potassium chloride but this is more expensive than common table-salt and tastes rather different. Sea-salt and herb-salt usually contain the same amount of sodium as table-salt. In many countries iodine is added to table salt. If this is available, it is a good choice since iodine is important for the function of your thyroid gland (see page 300).

Herbs and spices

Herbs will not affect your blood glucose at all. However, it is important to be aware that some herbal "seasoning" preparations also contain a lot of salt. If the flavouring is strong enough to make you drink more, your stomach may empty more rapidly, resulting in a quicker rise in your blood glucose level.

Fruit and berries

Fruits and berries have a high carbohydrate content (see table on page 221). The higher the fiber content, the less the effect they will have on the blood glucose level.

Meal times

Each family has its own routines for meal times, and they are likely to be the ones that particularly suit them. A dietitian should use the family's own eating habits and routines as a starting point when drawing up dietary advice for a person with diabetes. If you are using rapid-acting insulin (NovoLog/NovoRapid or Humalog) it is less important to have strict meal times since the basal insulin covers the time between meals. An insulin pump will also give you freer meal times. However, if you use multiple injection treatment with regular short-acting insulin, you should never leave more than 5 hours between the meals accompanied by insulin.

Snacks

People who don't have diabetes have low insulin levels in between meals. If you are using rapid-acting insulin (NovoLog/NovoRapid or Humalog) with multiple injections or an insulin pump, you will be less dependent on snacks in between meals. This is because its action is closer to the way blood glucose rises after a meal. This results in a lower insulin level between meals. Most children can have a fruit (10 g of carbohydrate) as a snack without extra insulin but if it is larger, you will probably need a small dose of insulin along with it.

Some younger children (up to 9-10 years of age) need a larger afternoon snack when they come home from school. When on multiple injections, many families find it easier to give insulin with this afternoon snack and have dinner a little later. The evening snack is then omitted. Try giving the same amount of insulin with the afternoon snack eaten earlier, as you would have done with the evening snack (or according to the carbohydrate gram count).

In diabetes, when regular short-acting insulin is injected, it lasts for 5 hours, and intermediate-acting insulin even longer if taken in twice daily injections. This results in having a higher insulin concentration between meals, than would be found in individuals without diabetes. This is why snacks are important with this type of insulin regimen. Since the morning injection is usually larger than the lunchtime one, it is even more essential to eat a snack in the morning. A child in school will usually require a sandwich (or something equally substantial) as the mid-morning snack. However, if the school lunch is served early, a piece of fruit might do. In the afternoon a piece of fruit will usually be an adequate snack.

If your blood glucose level is high, you won't need a snack. Try having half the snack if your blood glucose level is close to 180 mg/dl (10

mmol/l) and skip it completely if it is above 230-270 mg/dl (13-15 mmol/l). If this happens more than occasionally, you will need to adjust your insulin doses.

Common meal planning

Time	Meal	Example of doses for a child weighing 33 kg (73 lb)
7.30 AM	Breakfast	9 U Premeal dose
12 Noon	Lunch	6 U "
5.30 PM	Dinner	6 U "
8.30 PM	Evening snack	4 U "

Alternative meal planning

Time	Meal	Example of doses for a child weighing 33 kg (73 lb)
7.30 AM	Breakfast	9 U Premeal dose
11.30 AM	Lunch	6 U "
3.00 PM	Afternoon snack	4 U "
7.00 PM	Dinner	6 U "

With a multiple injection therapy or an insulin pump, you can be more flexible with your meal times and can switch mealtimes, for example between weekdays and weekends.

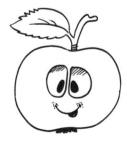

Some fruit is a good and healthy snack.

Can mealtimes be changed?

If you eat your meal up to one hour earlier or later than usual, you are unlikely to have problems as long as you don't change the time gap between taking your insulin and eating. Just remember not to exceed 5 hours between the doses of ordinary short-acting insulin. A child will usually be hungry and need something to eat every 3-4 hours anyway. If you use rapid-acting insulin (NovoLog/NovoRapid or Humalog) and twice daily basal insulin (or once daily Lantus), you will probably not have to be so strict about the hours between meals. If you check your blood glucose, you could try shifting meal-times by up to 2 hours.

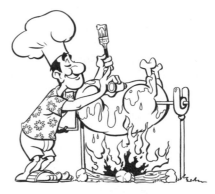

Counting the carbohydrates in your food will help you determine the size of your premeal bolus doses. Main sources of carbohydrates in your food are bread, pasta, rice, potatoes, chapatti, togas and tortillas. Meat and fat contain no carbohydrates at all.

Hungry or full?

A person whose diabetes is well controlled can often rely on feeling hungry or satisfied at the appropriate time. In one adult study, where fullness after a meal was measured, individuals with higher blood glucose levels experienced more fullness.[415] It is particularly important, if you are caring for a child with diabetes, to trust the child to respond sensibly to the promptings of appetite. Continuing to tell children that they must eat more or less regardless of how hungry they feel, will cause them to cease recognizing these feelings after a while. Children often experience lowered appetite if their blood glucose level is high. It is important, therefore, to give children time to reflect and build up their own opinion about what size meals should be. On the other hand, it is important for parents to be vigilant about how much children drink with any meal, especially if the drink contains carbohydrate (e.g. milk) or sugar.

Beware! If you are lacking insulin and your diabetes is badly regulated, you may feel hungry even when your blood glucose level is high (see page 45).

Infant feeding

The glucose content of infant formula is absorbed fairly quickly. With a multiple injection regimen, the child will need short or rapid-acting insulin for every bottle of formula milk (5-6 insulin doses/day). You may need to adjust in half units or even lower increments to find the right dose. If the child drinks formula milk at night, a small dose of short or rapid-acting insulin can be given with this. If the child has problems with night time hypoglycemia, a corn flour mix or commercial products made with uncooked cornstarch may help (see page 53).

If the child is breast-fed and takes full meals, you can give insulin in the same way as described above for formula. However, if the child feeds more frequently, taking a little at a time, a 2-dose treatment may work better. Lantus or a pump may also be a good alternative.

Toddlers' food (adapted from [413])

Food fads, picky eating, and food refusal are common in this age group. In fact, such behavior can be considered almost "normal" for toddlers, even though it is frequently worrying and frustrating for parents. Not surprisingly, such problems will cause even more anxiety to the parents of a child with diabetes. The following tips may be useful:

♠ Most children grow and thrive without being "told" how much to eat. Don't worry. Even if you feel your child is not eating enough, it is likely he or she is. Talk to your dietitian and diabetes team if you feel concerned and check your child's growth chart with your pediatrician.

♠ Rigid meals and snacks don't work well. Try to think what sort of food you would have provided, and when, if your child did not have diabetes and try to adjust the insulin accordingly.

♠ Plan meal times and menus taking into account the child's other activities, e.g. has the child been running around or sitting still?

♠ Children never respond to being force-fed. Even though it can be difficult, try to play down the emphasis on food. Usually a falling blood sugar will make the child hungry and more inclined to eat.

♠ Avoid using sweet foods or sugary drinks to "make up" for a low carbohydrate intake. Children soon learn to refuse food if the "reward" is a sweet drink or chocolate cookie.

♠ Fresh fruit, eaten as a snack, is better than fruit juice to drink.

♠ Give the child extra insulin when necessary, for example at birthday parties or when they are given candy.

♠ Breakfast time can be difficult, as it is quite common for children not to feel hungry early in the morning. Try a glass (or half a glass) of juice or milk to start with. After half an hour or so, when the blood glucose has risen a little, the appetite often improves.

♠ Glucose gel (or Cake Mate icing gel) and juice can be very useful in this age group as children need not chew the glucose tablets when they are hypoglycemic.

♠ Toddlers are growing and may often change their food habits. Talk to your dietitian for further advice.

Carbohydrate counting

Insulin is needed mainly to balance the carbohydrates eaten. The practice of carbohydrate counting differs between centers and countries. In many countries, carbohydrate counting is part of routine diabetes care (see page 216) and detailed tables are available for this.[381] Another method is to "judge by eye" for the size of the helpings (mainly the carbohydrate content, for example potatoes) and adjust the insulin dose accordingly.

Check with your dietitian what the local traditions are. Young children can be unpredictable eaters, so carbohydrate counting can be valuable for calculating the appropriate insulin dose for this age group.

The total carbohydrate content of meals and snacks is more important for the premeal insulin dosage than the type or where they come from.[274] However, some carbohydrates that are listed on food labels do not have any effect on the blood glucose level (dietary fiber, resistant starch).[814] If a food contains 5g dietary fiber or more, the fiber grams should be subtracted from the total carbohydrate grams for that food.[303,800] When counting carbohydrates, only half the amount of sugar alcohols (polyols) should be included.[800] Glycemic index and fiber content of foods do not affect the premeal insulin requirements.[274] In the DCCT study (see page 314), individuals who adjusted their premeal insulin dosages based on the carbohydrate content had 0.5% lower A1C than those who did not adjust their premeal insulin.[208]

Different methods of carbohydrate assessment

Many methods of counting or estimating carbohydrate intake are used in clinical practice. There is no consensus in favour of one particular method and some methods are better suited to particular individuals, children and families. What is becoming clearer is that if we are aim-

> ## Foods that contain carbohydrate
>
> ⇢ Bread, cereals, grains.
>
> ⇢ Pasta, rice, potatoes.
>
> ⇢ Starchy vegetables, such as corn and peas.
>
> ⇢ Fruit and fruit juices.
>
> ⇢ Dairy products, such as milk and yogurt (cheese usually contains no carbohydrate).
>
> ⇢ Chocolate, cookies, sugar, and candy

ing at really tight glucose control to improve diabetes outcomes, there seems to be a need for some form of carbohydrate estimation to counterbalance insulin doses.[792] Three levels of carbohydrate counting have been identified by the American Dietetic Association and can be considered as a step by step approach:[303,792]

Basic level

For counting carbohydrates, there are printed food tables in which you can find the carbohydrate content of different foods. Or you can use exchange lists where servings of (for example) starch, fruit and milk contain between 8 and 15 grams of carbohydrate each. Your dietitian can help you compile lists giving the carbohydrate contents of different products in special categories such as treats, ice cream or holiday fare.

In the simplest form of carbohydrate counting, your dietitian teaches you how to calculate the amount of carbohydrate you need for different meals and snacks during the day. You also learn to read food labels, and how to use food lists to count carbohydrates. With fixed insulin doses, it is important to eat about the same amount of carbohydrate for meals and snacks at the same time every day to keep your blood glucose levels within the target range.

Intermediate level

At this level you learn to recognize patterns of blood glucose response to carbohydrate intake and how it is modified by insulin and exercise. You make your own adjustments to insulin doses, or alter carbohydrate intake or timing of exercise to achieve blood glucose goals. Alterations of insulin should be made in response to a pattern of blood glucose results over a few days, not based on a single high or low blood glucose reading. A more flexible method is to correct the premeal dose for changes in size of the carbohydrate content of a meal (without counting the exact carbohydrate content). See page 136 for advice on how much to adjust the insulin dose. Simple insulin adjustments are used to manage intake of extra carbohydrate (see page 228).

In an Australian study, children tested both a flexible meal plan (servings based on appetite) and a fixed carbohydrate exchange model (servings based on carbohydrate content).[300] The exchange model included recommending artificially sweetened alternatives whenever available. In the flexible model, by contrast, sugar-sweetened products were preferred except for diet drinks. The children on the flexible meal plan appreciated their food much more than those on the exchange model. They also had, on average, a 0.3% lower A1C. In addition, children from this group experienced less family conflict. With multiple injection therapy or an insulin pump, you can enjoy flexible food habits together with the opportunity of adjusting your insulin doses in line with the carbohydrate contents of your meals.

Advanced level

Individuals taking short or rapid-acting insulin before meals (via either injections or a pump) can vary the amount of insulin depending on the carbohydrate content of the meal. Use food labels and/or a food table to calculate how

How many carbohydrates will one unit of insulin cover?[185]

Example:	Carb (g)	Units	Insulin:carb ratio
Breakfast	60	6	1:10
Lunch	50	4	1:12
Dinner	55	5	1:11
Evening snack	35	3	1:12
Whole day	200	18	1:11

The above example considers a 12 year old boy (weighing 38 kg, 84 lb). One unit of insulin will take care of 10 grams of carbohydrate for breakfast without changing the blood glucose level, and ~12 grams of carbohydrate for the other meals.

General advice on balancing carbohydrate intake against the insulin action profile [792]

➡ Regular and frequent carbohydrate intake including snacks is advisable to prevent hypoglycemia during inevitable periods of high insulin levels when the insulin regimen is twice daily mixtures of quick and slower acting insulins.

➡ A flexible carbohydrate intake is possible when mealtime doses of insulin are given with multiple injection regimens or during insulin pump treatment.

➡ Carbohydrate intake is required before bedtime to prevent night time hypoglycemia with a 2-dose treatment.

➡ Extra carbohydrate is required before, during and after increased exercise and sport to balance increased energy needs and prevent hypoglycemia.

➡ A "grazing" or "little and often" style of eating, often seen in younger children, may be suited to an insulin regimen consisting mainly of longer acting insulins or an insulin pump.

many grams of carbohydrate there are in the meal. In the advanced form of carbohydrate counting, you need to determine the amount of insulin to take for the amount of carbohydrate you wish to eat. This is called an insulin-to- carbohydrate (insulin:carb) ratio (the number of grams of carbohydrate covered by one unit of insulin). This method gives a more flexible meal schedule and, once you have learned it, you can apply it both at home and when eating out. Basically, you count the grams of carbohydrates in a meal and divide by the number of units of insulin required to keep the blood glucose at a similar level 2-3 hours later. Test your insulin:carb ratio only when you have not had hypoglycaemia in the last 4 hours before the meal. Another method of calculating the insulin:carb ratio is to divide the total number of grams of carbohydrate consumed for all meals in a day by the total bolus (mealtime) insulin taken during the day (see key fact box on page 218).[185] Do not include intermediate or long-acting insulin (or pump basal rate) doses in this calculation.

A third method of calculating the insulin:carb ratio is the "500 Rule".[797,800] Divide the number 500 by your total daily dose of insulin (adding all types of insulin, both premeal doses and basal insulin). The answer is the number of grams of carbohydrate covered by 1 unit of rapid-acting insulin (NovoLog, Humalog). The number 450 can be used for short-acting insulin (Novolin R, Humulin R).[800]

Check the appropriate ratio by calculating the insulin dose from the carbohydrate content of the meal. When you take this dose, the blood glucose should be within approximately 36 mg/dl (2.0 mmol/l) of the initial blood glucose after 2-3 hours if you use rapid-acting insulin, after 4-5 hours if you use regular short-acting insulin. Checking your blood glucose after the meal is the only way to find out how well your bolus dose has worked.

One unit of insulin will usually cover 10-15 grams of carbohydrate in a meal for an adult.

For a school child who is more insulin-sensitive, one unit may cover up to 20g of carbohydrate, perhaps even 30g if they are in the remission ("honeymoon") phase. An overweight person who is extremely insulin resistant may require one unit of insulin for every 5 gram of carbohydrate.[185] You may find that one unit of insulin covers a slightly lower amount of carbohydrate in the morning. This may be explained by temporary insulin resistance due to the dawn phenomenon (see page 54) and less physical activity at this time of the day.[185] In a Canadian study of adults, an average of 1.5 U was needed for every 10 g of carbohydrate for breakfast, 1.0 for lunch and 1.1-1.2 for dinner (insulin:carb ratio ~1:7 for breakfast, 1:10 for lunch and 1:8-1:9 for dinner).[627] In this study, the glycemic index, fiber, fat, and caloric content of the meals did not affect the premeal insulin requirements. People who are physically active need to lower their insulin doses, changing the insulin:carb ratio. So, if you take part in seasonal sports you will probably need to adjust your insulin:carb ratio. If, for example, it is 1:15 (i.e. 1 unit per 15 grams of carbohydrate) in the active season, you may need to change to 1:10 when the season is over.

When focusing on the carbohydrate content of a meal, food and insulin can be matched more precisely as you will eat different amounts of carbohydrates depending on your appetite or regime. However, if you concentrate only on the carbohydrate content, you may forget that some foods contain a lot of fat as well, and this is not healthy in the long run.

School

These days, it is unlikely that there will be any problem over a child with diabetes receiving appropriate types of food and snacks at school. However, older children don't always want to have special diabetes food at school. It may not be as appetizing, and they may be unwilling to be seen as "different" from their peers. It is difficult to give general advice for this situation.

Nutrition behaviors associated with lower A1C

➧ Adherence to the prescribed meal plan.

➧ Adjusting food and/or insulin in response to high blood glucose levels.

➧ Adjusting the insulin dose for carbohydrate content.

➧ Consistent consumption of agreed snacks within the meal plan.

➧ Appropriate treatment of hypoglycaemia (not over-treating).

The average A1C among intensively managed patients in the DCCT study who reported that they followed specific diet-related behaviors was 0.25 to 1.0% lower than among subjects who did not follow these behaviors.[208]

These behaviors were associated with a higher A1C:

➧ Over-treating hypoglycemia.

➧ Consuming extra snacks outside the meal plan.

Some children and teenagers cope well, adjusting their insulin dose to ordinary school meals, while others find this more difficult.

It may be difficult to get school staff to understand that a child with diabetes will not always eat the same amounts of food. When using multiple injection therapy or an insulin pump, the insulin dose can be adjusted according to the appetite and size of portion. Sometimes children may need additional snacks to avoid hypoglycemia if there is a long interval between breaks. The dietitian can speak to the staff if necessary.

With a fixed meal plan, school lunches are best eaten at the same time every day, not too early since the time until the next insulin dose may be a long way off for a young person on multiple injection treatment. See the suggestions for meal schedules on page 214. Schools should be given

School meal

It may be a good idea to note the child's insulin dose right on the packaged food items or on the container holding entrees.

Units	Food
5U	Spaghetti and meat sauce
4U	Fish with rice
6U	Mashed potatoes and sausage
4U	Lasagna
2U	Banana

Check with your dietitian if you are not sure about the food contents.

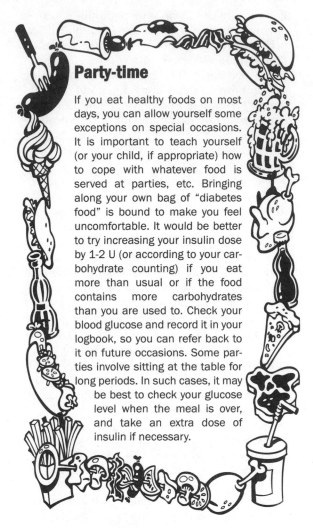

Party-time

If you eat healthy foods on most days, you can allow yourself some exceptions on special occasions. It is important to teach yourself (or your child, if appropriate) how to cope with whatever food is served at parties, etc. Bringing along your own bag of "diabetes food" is bound to make you feel uncomfortable. It would be better to try increasing your insulin dose by 1-2 U (or according to your carbohydrate counting) if you eat more than usual or if the food contains more carbohydrates than you are used to. Check your blood glucose and record it in your logbook, so you can refer back to it on future occasions. Some parties involve sitting at the table for long periods. In such cases, it may be best to check your glucose level when the meal is over, and take an extra dose of insulin if necessary.

the necessary information about appropriate meal times in order to be able to make the appropriate timetabling adjustments.

When school friends buy candy, children with diabetes may find it difficult to resist joining in. There is always a risk that, instead of being sensible, they will "show off" by eating even more candy than the others. A compromise could be to buy a small number of candy to have after lunch, when the stomach already contains some food. At that time and under those conditions, the blood glucose level will not be affected to such an extent, especially if the lunch dose is adjusted to cover the candy. Skipping lunch and buying candy instead, as some teenagers do, can be harmful for those with diabetes. Children who do buy candy would be better advised to buy chocolates than candy made from pure sugar (see page 231) unless they have a weight problem.

Special "diabetic" food?

So called "diabetic" food (often found in health food stores) is not recommended for children with diabetes [701,791] and is not suitable for adults either.[232] It is often both more expensive and higher in energy content than similar "normal" food. Besides, many find the taste unappetizing. Children may feel singled out as "different" if they are not allowed to eat the same food their friends eat. Diabetes food often contains sorbitol as a sweetener, which may produce side effects such as abdominal pain and diarrhea. It is much better to learn how to handle ordinary food if you have diabetes.

Fruits

	Quantity	Carb.	Fiber	% fiber
Grapes	4 oz.	17g	1.6g	9%
Blackcurrant	4 oz.	16g	4.9g	32%
Blackberries	4 oz.	16g	7.2g	46%
Pineapple, canned	4 oz.	16g	1.0g	6%
Redcurrant	4 oz.	13g	3.4g	27%
Pineapple, fresh	4 oz.	12g	1.2g	9%
Cherries, sweet	4 oz.	12g	1.7g	13%
Strawberries	4 oz.	10g	2.4g	24%
Watermelon	4 oz.	9g	0.6g	7%
Raspberries	4 oz.	8g	3.7g	46%
Honeydew melon	4 oz.	8g	0.9g	11%
Banana	1 fruit	21g	1.5g	7%
Pear	1 fruit	16g	3.0g	19%
Apple	1 fruit	14g	1.9g	13%
Kiwi fruits	2 fruits	14g	3.8g	27%
Orange	1 fruit	13g	2.0g	16%
Plums	2 fruits	9g	1.2g	13%
Grapefruit	1 fruit	9g	2.0g	22%
Raisins	1 tbs	8g	1.0g	12%

A higher percentage of fiber will cause the glucose to be absorbed more slowly. Bananas contain very little dietary fiber and will raise the blood glucose level more quickly than other fruits. It is therefore a suitable fruit to take if your blood glucose is low, or during exercise. When counting grams of carbohydrate, the fiber content should be subtracted if it is 5g or more.[303,800]

Carb. = carbohydrates

"Fast food"

Many children, teenagers and adults like fast food, and it has become a fixture of modern life. As fast food often contains a lot of fat, it is not a good idea to make a habit of eating it. However, occasional eating of fast food shouldn't cause problems, and after a couple of times you will have found out what insulin doses are appropriate for your favorite items.

Food at diabetes camps

Children who attend diabetes camps are likely to be very active physically while they are there, and usually very hungry at meal times. It may be difficult for the staff to judge how much individual children are used to eating. The basic rule must be that they are allowed to eat enough to feel satisfied to compensate for the increased energy expenditure. Sometimes you see a child eating very large helpings, and it may then be a good idea to cautiously limit their food intake and then check with the parents how they handle such situations at home. This may present a good occasion for a discussion on how the carbohydrate amounts eaten, and what drinks are consumed with a meal, will affect the blood glucose levels. The increased activity will often require lowered insulin doses, especially at bedtime. A later evening snack (8.30-9 PM) will help young people withstand the night better. The total daily insulin dose was lowered by around one third, on average, in children aged 7-12 years, attending a physically active (mainly water sports) camp in New Zealand.[112]

Vegetarian and vegan diets

A pure vegetarian or vegan diet may result in a disturbed balance between the amount of protein and carbohydrate in the diet. This is because vegetarian nutrients contain much less protein than animal nutrients. A lactovegetarian diet includes milk and milk products resulting in a higher protein content. A vegan diet including a high proportion of fruits and berries may even have a higher content of sugar than a mixed diet.[40]

However, if reasonable attention is paid to achieving a balanced diet, many vegetarians do very well and avoid vitamin and mineral deficiencies despite having diabetes. As many of these young people are in their mid teens or older, problems with growth are likely to be avoided too.

A strict vegetarian or vegan diet is not recommended for children, as it will put them at risk of a deficiency of protein, vitamins and minerals. Not eating meat, fish or eggs is not necessarily synonymous with being a vegetarian. In vegan or lactovegetarian diets, the animal products are mostly replaced by products from leguminous plants. The intake of vitamin B_{12} will be cut in half when the vitamins in animal products are not replaced. This will lead to a considerable risk of anemia which can show as tiredness. You should always talk to your dietitian or doctor before changing your diet.

Different cultures

Families from different cultures and different religions often have quite different eating habits. The number of meals can be fewer and sometimes certain foods are excluded due to religious reasons (Muslims and Jews are not supposed to eat pork, Hindus should not eat beef). The way of cooking is usually different. Lactose intolerance is more common among children from some countries.

In every case, it is of course important to take the family's customary food habits into consideration when discussing nutrition with a person who has diabetes. With a multiple injection treatment and premeal injections there are usually no difficulties in adjusting the diabetes diet to fit family routines.

Religious fasting days

Special religious fasting days, such as Yom Kippur for Jews, can easily be accommodated by appropriate attention to monitoring and adjustment (downwards) of insulin doses. Consult your diabetes healthcare team for advice if you are at all unsure about how to handle the situation, and keep records in your logbook for the next time!

Ramadan: the fasting month

During Ramadan, the ninth month of the Islamic year, Muslims fast from dawn until sunset. Sick people, and women who are pregnant, breast feeding or menstruating are exempted, as are young children. Fasting is not recommended for individuals with type 1 diabetes according to some health professionals [11] but even so, many devout Muslims with diabetes prefer to fast during Ramadan. If this applies to you, it is important that you find a way of accommodating both your body's need of a low basal insulin level during fasting hours, and the need for an increased insulin level for the meals you take just before sunrise and at sunset. This means frequent monitoring of your blood glucose and adjusting your insulin doses, so that you can avoid low levels during the day as well as high levels after ceasing your fast in the evening.

Fasting accelerates the breakdown of fat and ketone production, by increasing glucagon levels. So, if you cut down your insulin doses too much during the period of fasting, you will put yourself at risk of ketoacidosis. One patient, a 15 year-old boy, was admitted to hospital in ketoacidosis after fasting and omitting his lunchtime dose of insulin in combination with dehydration during Ramadan.[284]

In addition to the problem of fasting, there is risk of over-eating high-calorie candy in the evenings during Ramadan.[11] Two doses per day of rapid-acting (Humalog) and NPH insulin gave better blood glucose levels and less hypoglycemia than regular short-acting insulin and NPH in one study.[424] The two doses were taken before the morning and evening meals. Lantus should be a good alternative as basal insulin in this situation. Ask your diabetes team for practical advice if you plan to fast during Ramadan.

Sweeteners

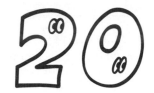

Sugar free?

When manufacturers state that a product has "no sugar added", this does not always mean it is completely devoid of sugar. It usually implies that no sugar is added, whereas the natural sugar from berries or fruits are still present. No added sugar chocolate or ice cream can contain more calories than ordinary alternatives. Sweet foods like this often contain sorbitol, which eventually will be transformed into glucose in the liver. Check the food label carefully.

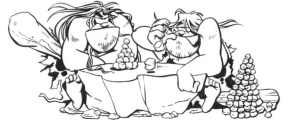

Since prehistoric times, humans have craved sugar. This is believed to be because sweet natural products are seldom poisonous while many bitter ones can be so.

Non-nutritive sweeteners

Aspartame

Aspartame is 200 times sweeter than sugar and is used in such small amounts that the energy

---

Free from sugar?

Unsweetened	No compound with sweet taste has been added to the product. However, it can contain natural sugar (fruit sugar, milk sugar).
Without added sugar No added sugar No sugar added	Contains no type of sugar, either natural or substitute. Other sweeteners without energy may be added (but these should be on the food label).
Sugar free	Less than 0.5 g sugars per serving.
Reduced sugar	At least 25% reduction on the original product.

---

content is negligible. It can lose its sweetness through cooking and baking.

Aspartame is made up of two amino acids called aspartic acid and the methyl ester of phenylalanine. Amino acids and methyl esters are found naturally in foods like milk, meats, fruits and vegetables. When digested, the body handles the amino acids in aspartame in the same way as those in foods we eat daily.[421] Although aspartame can be used by the whole family, individuals with a rare genetic disease called phenylketonuria (PKU) need to be aware that aspartame is a source of the protein component, phenylalanine. Those who have PKU cannot properly metabolize phenylalanine and must monitor their intake of phenylalanine from all foods, including foods containing aspartame. In many countries, including the US and Canada, every infant is screened for PKU at birth.

Unfortunately, many myths about aspartame are circulating, scaring people with diabetes and others who use drinks. The fact is that aspartame has been studied extensively in humans. The safety of aspartame has been well established and it has been shown that eating or drinking products sweetened with aspartame is not associated with adverse health effects.[421] A

240 ml (8-oz.) glass of milk has six times more phenylalanine and thirteen times more aspartic acid than an equivalent amount of soda sweetened with NutraSweet. An 8-oz. glass of fruit juice or tomato juice contains three to five times more methanol than an equivalent amount of soda sweetened with NutraSweet.[421]

The FDA (Food and Drug Administration) in the US has set the Acceptable Daily Intake (ADI) for aspartame at 50 mg/kg of body weight/day. An adult would have to consume 20 cans of a sugar-free drink every day before reaching the ADI, assuming the sweetener was used in the drink at the maximum permitted level. In practice, most drinks use aspartame in combination with other sweeteners so that the level is considerably lower. Aspartame intakes have been shown to be considerably below the recommended maximum level, even among children and people with diabetes who consume large quantities of sugar-free drinks.

Saccharin

Saccharin is a synthetic product. It is 300-500 times sweeter than sugar and contains no energy. It gives a slight metallic taste when heated above 70° C (158° F) and should therefore be added only after cooking.

Acesulphame K

This sweetener is 130-200 times sweeter than sugar. It withstands heating well and can be used for baking. It is mixed with milk-sugar (lactose) but in amounts too small to give any significant amount of energy.

Sucralose

Sucralose is 600 times sweeter than ordinary sugar. It is made from sugar but does not affect blood glucose. Sucralose tastes like sugar and is heat stable. It can be used both for baking and for cooking.

Cyclamate

Cyclamate is 30-50 times sweeter than sugar and contains no energy. It is stable in high temperatures and therefore suitable for cooking and baking. It is often used in soft drinks, dairy products and chocolate.

Cyclamate was removed from the US market in 1970, but FDA approval is now being sought. It is approved by the Canadian FDA and most other countries' food regulatory agencies.

Nutritive sweeteners

These all contain energy which should be considered if weight is a problem.

Hot and cold drinks

	Quantity	Carb.	Fat	Kcal
Low-fat milk	1 cup	10 g	1 g	75
1.5%-fat milk	1 cup	10 g	3 g	96
3%-fat milk	1 cup	10 g	6 g	120
Chocolate milk	1 cup	~20 g	*add milk	
Orange juice	1 cup	~25 g	-	100
Fruit drink	1 cup	~15 g		60
Soft drinks	1 cup	~20 g		100
Sugar soda	8 fl. oz.	~30 g	-	120
Diet soda	8 fl. oz.	0 g	-	1
Diet Cola	8 fl. oz.	0 g	-	1
Coffee	1 cup	0.3 g		2
Tea	1 cup	0 g		2
Herb tea	Can have a high sugar-content!			

Carb. = carbohydrates, kcal = kilocalories

* The fat and energy content of chocolate milk depends on how much fat there is in the milk used.

Fructose

Fructose is almost twice as sweet as sugar. Even if fructose does not affect your blood glucose level directly, it is transformed into glucose in the liver, and the calorie content can cause weight gain. Because of this, fructose is not considered as a suitable sweetener for people with diabetes in some countries. In other countries (such as Finland and Germany) many "diabetes products" containing fructose are sold (see also page 65).

Sugar alcohols

Sugar alcohols (also called polyols) are used by food manufacturers to lower carbohydrate and/ or fat content and are often used in chewing gum, "sugar-free" candy, ice cream, and pastry. Sugar alcohols provide approximately half the energy (2.5 kcal/g) compared to other carbohydrates (4 kcal/g). Chemically, they are neither sugars nor alcohols but eventually they will be converted into fructose and glucose by the liver. The names of sugar alcohols usually end in "-ol", for example Sorbitol, Xylitol, Mannitol, Maltitol, and Lactitol. Hydrogenated starch hydrolysates and Isomalt are also sugar alcohols. The sweetness of sorbitol is about half that of sugar. When counting carbohydrates, it is currently suggested that only half the amount of sugar alcohols should be included.[800]

Sorbitol is a natural component of plums, cherries and other fruits and berries. Sorbitol and other sugar alcohols absorb water from the intestines and provide nourishment for intestinal bacteria. Large amounts of sorbitol can cause abdominal pains and diarrhea, which may put an automatic limit on the amounts eaten.

Sweeteners without energy

Substance	Trade name	Common in
Acesulphame K	Sunett Hermesetas Gold (aspartame + acesulphame K) KetoSweet	Beverages, jams, baked goods, candy
Aspartame	NutraSweet Equal	Chewing gum Candy Soft drinks Table top sweetener
Cyclamate	Sucaryl, Sugar Twin Weight Watchers,	Tabletop sweetener
Saccharin	Sweet'n Low Hermesetas Original	Tabletop sweetener
Sucralose	Splenda	Tabletop sweetener, drinks, baked goods, frozen and canned fruit

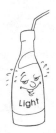

Diet drinks and "light" foods

Diet drinks are usually sweetened with aspartame and do not contain any sugar. Most of these drinks are "unrestricted" for people with diabetes in the sense that they do not raise the blood glucose. However, cola drinks often contain caffeine so it is not healthy to drink large amounts of them.

When a foodstuff is labeled "light", the situation is more complex. Such products are not necessarily sugar-free. In some countries a foodstuff may be described as "light" if the sugar content is decreased. Products containing fat can be labeled "light" if the fat content has been decreased. Most countries have regulations to ensure that terms such as "light" or "low fat" are explained on food labelling. As the rules for labelling may vary from country to country, you should check with your dietitian about what is applicable where you live.

In the US, "light" or "lite" refers to fewer calories or less fat compared to the regular food. However, this does not say anything about the initial and total sugar content. "Fat free" on the food labels means less than 0.5 g per serving. "Reduced fat" means at least 25 % less fat than comparison food. Light (low-fat) ice cream contains around one third of the fat content found in regular ice cream. "Fat free" means the product contains no fat, while "no sugar added" may mean sugar alcohols are added instead.

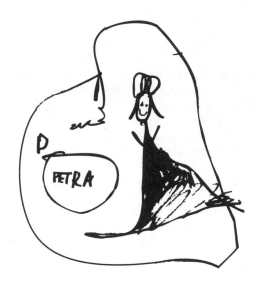

Candy, treats and ice cream

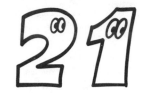

Sooner or later all young people with diabetes will be tempted by their friends and peer group to indulge in treats like ice cream or candy. At home, families often try to regulate this by allowing ice cream on special occasions and candy only on certain days. This is something all parents may find difficult to enforce, regardless of whether or not a child has diabetes. The obvious problem for a young person with diabetes is that all these delicious things will also increase the blood glucose (if they don't take extra insulin or exchange for other sources of carbohydrates). This is often the reason parents feel they have to say, "No, you can't have that. It is bad for your diabetes".

In saying this, it is easy to forget that the answer is likely to have been "No" even if the child did not have diabetes: "No, you will damage your teeth", "No, we can't afford it", or "No, in our family we have candy only on Saturdays". The practical effect will be the same (no candy) but, for the child, the difference is important. If you always refer to the child having diabetes when saying "No!", the child will soon start hating the illness which appears to lie behind the limitations. He or she will start to believe that it is the diabetes alone that makes this and everything else impossible.

We don't want to ban candy from children (or adults) with diabetes, but we do not in any way want to say that they are unrestricted either.

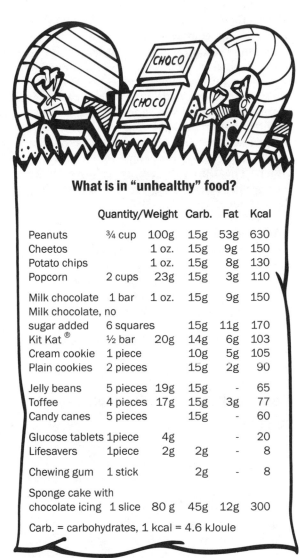

What is in "unhealthy" food?

	Quantity/Weight	Carb.	Fat	Kcal
Peanuts	¾ cup 100g	15g	53g	630
Cheetos	1 oz.	15g	9g	150
Potato chips	1 oz.	15g	8g	130
Popcorn	2 cups 23g	15g	3g	110
Milk chocolate	1 bar 1 oz.	15g	9g	150
Milk chocolate, no sugar added	6 squares	15g	11g	170
Kit Kat ®	½ bar 20g	14g	6g	103
Cream cookie	1 piece	10g	5g	105
Plain cookies	2 pieces	15g	2g	90
Jelly beans	5 pieces 19g	15g	-	65
Toffee	4 pieces 17g	15g	3g	77
Candy canes	5 pieces	15g	-	60
Glucose tablets	1piece 4g		-	20
Lifesavers	1piece 2g	2g	-	8
Chewing gum	1 stick	2g	-	8
Sponge cake with chocolate icing	1 slice 80 g	45g	12g	300

Carb. = carbohydrates, 1 kcal = 4.6 kJoule

Read the list carefully! Fifteen grams of carbohydrate corresponds to one slice of bread. Which would you prefer? Four pieces of candy or 3 cups of popcorn (25 g of unpopped popcorn)?

The message is that **of course you can have some** candy **or ice cream — but you need to think about how and when to eat them so your blood glucose will not be affected too much.** Most adults allow themselves a treat every now and again. So children, too, should be given opportunities to manage their insulin and food in a way that enables them to enjoy something sweet on occasion, without their blood glucose rising too high. Going to parties is far more fun if you can eat the same food as everyone else. However, just as adults won't feel well if they go out partying all the time, we emphasize to children that this is something they can do only on special occasions, not every day. Too many sweets are not good for people without diabetes either. They provide empty calories which increase the risk of weight gain and cause damage to your teeth.

It is all about freedom with responsibility and to master this you need to practice and experiment. It is important to monitor your blood glucose before and after you have tried something new. It will often not be perfect at your first attempt but after a few times you will learn better how your body works. The logbook is important so that, later, you will remember what you did and how it turned out.

How much extra insulin should you take?

One additional unit of insulin for every 10-15 g of extra carbohydrate (i.e. sugar) is usually enough.[185] Use your insulin:carb ratio if you have calculated this (see page 217). With fixed insulin doses, only the carbohydrate content which is in excess of that of your ordinary snack should be counted if candy or ice cream are eaten instead of the usual snack. Of course, the effect on your blood glucose level will not be ideal, so this is not something we recommend you do on a regular basis. But it can be a good method for special occasions. Remember that exceptions must be exceptions — if you do it every day it will become a habit and such a

habit is not compatible with your diabetes. How and when to eat candy and ice cream is something that you and your family will need to discuss together. Your diabetes team can only tell you how the sugar in these treats works in your body and how to adjust your insulin.

The amount of extra insulin needed will depend on your total insulin requirement. If you are in puberty and your total insulin dose is high (more than 1 U/kg/24 hours, 0.5 U/lb/24 hours), you may need more than 1 U of insulin for every 10 g of carbohydrate. If you are in the honeymoon phase (low insulin requirements during the first 6-12 months after the onset of diabetes, see page 193) you should only take a quarter to half a unit extra per 10 g of extra carbohydrate. Your own insulin production will supply the rest. Measure your blood glucose level ½-1 hour after you have eaten your candy and experiment to find out what works well for you. See "Carbohydrate counting" on page 216 for a more exact method of finding your individual need of insulin for a given amount of carbohydrates.

Rapid-acting insulins (NovoLog/NovoRapid or Humalog) are effective if you are eating candy containing pure sugar, but may be too quick for treats containing fat, such as ice cream and chocolate bars. If you find this to be the case, it may be better to take the dose after you have had the treat. If you use a pump, you can set it to deliver a prolonged bolus dose if needed (see illustration on page 168). If you use short-acting insulin, you can take extra insulin at the same time as you have chocolate or a regular ice cream. But you should take it 30 minutes before having candy containing only sugar as this will

When should you test your blood glucose level?	
Candy	After ½ hour
Ice cream, chocolate bar	After 1-1½ hour
Potato chips	After 2-3 hours

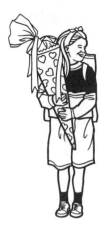

It is easy to develop a "candy-mania" if you have diabetes. Some children with diabetes eat more candy than their friends although they know this is not healthy for them. Try not to make sweets too big a thing in your life. Aim at managing to eat only small amounts on appropriate occasions. Even if you can't manage this just at the moment, you can make a decision to do it when you are a little older. The question will then not be **if** you will succeed, it will be **when** you will succeed...

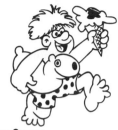

Contents of some common ice creams

Ice Cream	Weight	Carb.	Fat	Kcal
Klondike Bar,	148g, 1 bar	35g	35g	488
(vanilla ice cream with chocolate coating)				
Eskimo Pie Bar	50g, 1 bar	12g	12g	165
(vanilla ice cream with dark chocolate coating)				
Ice Cream Sundae	100g	29g	6g	185
(prepackaged)				
Skinny Cow Sandwich	78g	29g	2g	145
	1 bar			
Vanilla Light Ice Cream	72g	20g	3g	120
	½ cup			
Vanilla Regular Ice Cream	72g	17 g	8g	145
	½ cup			
Vanilla Rich Ice Cream	107g	24g	17g	266
	½ cup			
Vanilla Soft Serve	88g	19g	2g	110
	½ cup			
Ben & Jerry's				
Cherry Garcia	(½ cup)	26g	16g	260
Chocolate Chip Cookie		34g	16g	300
Chubby Hubby	(½ cup)	33g	21g	350
Orange and Cream		23g	14g	230
Popsicle				
Fruit 'N Juice Bar		16g	0g	70
Juice Bar, no sugar added		6g	0g	25
For comparison				
glass of whole milk	6oz	10g	6g	120
Cheese sandwich		15g	8g	150
(½ or open-faced)				

Carb. = carbohydrates, 1 kcal = 4.6 kJoule

The content of the ice creams can change from time to time as recipes are adapted. The more fat that is added, the slower the blood glucose rise will be but the more calories it will contain.

affect your blood glucose more quickly. Popsicles (those that are not special "no added sugar" ones) contain a lot of sugar that can affect your blood sugar considerably. They may come in handy, however, if your blood sugar dips while you are on the beach, for example.

It is good idea to have your candy or ice cream as dessert after a regular meal. The sugar content will then be mixed in your stomach with the rest of the food, so it will not affect your blood sugar too quickly. You can take your ordinary insulin dose if, for example, you replace a glass of milk (8 oz., ~200 ml) with 10 g of carbohydrates in candy or ice cream. Substituting sweets for other carbohydrates in your meal plan is probably the best way to deal with this if you have a "sweet tooth". You can, for example, have smaller servings of bread, potatoes or fruit. If you add a dessert you will have eaten more carbohydrates than usual, in which case you will need to increase your insulin dose as described above. Like everyone else, doing this often will put you at risk of gaining weight.

Ice cream

A summer without ice cream is no summer at all in the eyes of many children. Of course you can eat ice cream even if you have diabetes. The usual advice applies: think ahead and experi-

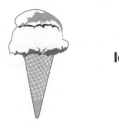

Ice cream cones

Ice cream cones usually contain:

Soft-serve ice milk	20-30 g of carbohydrate
Ice cream (3 scoops)	20-25 g "

ment to find out what is best for you. There are mainly two types of frozen treats: popsicle and ice cream made from dairy products. Popsicles are like frozen fruit juice (often with added sugar or sweetener) and affect the blood glucose level in the same way as juice except that it takes longer to lick a popsicle than to drink a glass of fruit juice. Popsicles can be perfectly suitable if you have hypoglycemia, for example while you are at the beach. You will need to be sure, however, that what you are eating is an ordinary popsicle, and not a "light" or low sugar variety, as the latter would have little or no effect on your blood glucose level.

Ice cream made from dairy products contains fat that causes your stomach to empty more slowly. Thus the increase in blood glucose level will not be seen until 45-90 minutes after eating ice cream.[568] From this it follows that dairy-based ice cream is not suitable for reversing hypoglycemia. However, it can be a good alternative if you are playing soccer, for example, as an activity such as this requires extra sugar over a longer period of time. Dairy-based ice cream goes well with regular short-acting insulin in the sense that the insulin will start working at about the same time as the ice cream starts raising the blood glucose level. However, rapid-acting insulin (NovoLog/NovoRapid or Humalog) may have too quick an action for dairy-based ice creams. If this is the type of insulin you use, it may be better to take it after

finishing the ice cream or use a prolonged bolus if you have a pump.

During our diabetes camps, we do some experimenting with ice cream and caramels. The dietitian tells the children about the contents of different ice creams. We then have an "ice cream test" at snack-time. The children measure their blood glucose levels beforehand and then discuss with their leaders what they should do next in order to have their favorite ice cream. If it is necessary, they will take an extra dose of insulin along with the ice cream. It may not be the most sensible thing to have a large ice cream if your blood glucose level is 270 mg/dl (15 mmol/l) — but life is full of such situations and it is a good idea to know how to handle them. The children can have their choice of ice cream, but only if they take extra insulin. When

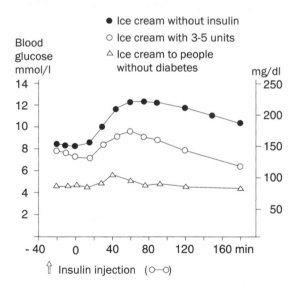

Ice cream gives a slower blood glucose rise than you might expect. The reason for this is that the high fat content causes the stomach to empty more slowly. The graph is from an American study of adults with diabetes who ate 100 g (3/4 cup) of vanilla ice cream (24% carbohydrate and 11% fat content). When they injected regular short-acting insulin (3-5 units) 30 minutes before the ice cream, the rise in blood glucose was reduced considerably.[568]

"Ice cream test"

① Measure your blood glucose level at snack-time.

② Calculate the carbohydrate content of your snack in grams (one open sandwich = 15 g, one glass of milk = 10 g, for fruit see table on page 221).
Decide which ice cream you want (not popsicles — they only contain frozen sugar-water).

③ Calculate the carbohydrate content of the ice cream.

④ Take one unit of extra insulin for every 10 g of excess carbohydrate in the ice cream (or according to your insulin:carb ratio).

⑤ Decrease the dose by 1-2 U if your blood glucose level before the ice cream is less than 70-90 mg/dl (4-5 mmol/l) or if you are about to exercise. Increase by 1-2 U if the blood glucose level is above 180 mg/dl (10 mmol/l). You can also use the correction factors on page 131 if you are used to this system.

⑥ If you are in the remission phase (honeymoon phase, see page 193) you should only take a quarter or half the above mentioned extra doses of insulin.

⑦ Measure your blood glucose level 1-1½ hour after you have finished the ice cream to see if things worked out the way you expected.

⑧ Record what you did in your logbook and you will be better placed to know what to do the next time you want to eat ice cream.

Remember that, whether or not they have diabetes, children do not eat ice cream every day. It is their parents who decide when they eat it, and the same rules should apply to children both with and without diabetes.

the children measure their blood glucose level 1-1½ hours after the ice cream, the average level is lower than it was before eating the ice cream.

Chocolate

Chocolate contains fat which will slow down the absorption of glucose by emptying the stomach more slowly. For example, you may eat a small chocolate bar (24 g, 1 oz. = 14 g carbohydrate) for a snack instead of an open sandwich. This may be fine occasionally, but (in common with anyone who does not have diabetes) you should not snack like this every day. However, when you are physically active you will probably be able to take a small chocolate bar in addition to your usual snack without problems.

Candy

During our diabetes camps, we exchange the apple of the afternoon snack (on the "treasure hunt") for a box of candy that contain jelly making them tougher to chew, and causing the sugar to be absorbed more slowly. Other candy which taste sweet and easily break into small pieces during chewing, contain mostly pure sugar. Sugar-free candy usually contain sorbitol which is better for your teeth and raises the blood glucose level more slowly. We tell children these facts at the same time as they taste candy of various types, in order to help them recognize the difference.

One box of jelly-type candy sweetened with sorbitol (about 15 g) has the same blood glucose raising effect as an apple or a pear. However, the contents of a box of sugar-type fruit pastilles gives the same effect as 6 lumps of dextrose (18 g). If a child chooses to eat one small piece of candy of this type at some stage in the course of an afternoon, it will not affect the blood glucose level at all. By saying this we don't mean that children should have candy every day. Keeping candy intake low is a good rule for all children whether or not they have diabetes. This situation should be the same for families without diabetes, in that it is the parents who decide which rules apply. The important thing is that children with diabetes feel

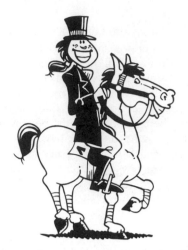

Use the opportunity to eat your regular portion of candy while you are doing some physical exercise. One girl had her "Friday candy" every week while horse-riding and they did not affect her blood glucose level at all.

that, as far as possible, they receive equal treatment as their friends without diabetes and siblings when it comes to candy.

These principles for managing eating both ice cream and candy combine freedom and responsibility. In order to learn how to manage different situations well, you will need to practice and experiment. It is important to measure your blood glucose level both before and after trying something new. It is likely that your blood glucose level will not be quite as it should be the first time around, but after a couple of times you will get to know your body better. The logbook is important — afterwards you can go back and determine what worked well and what did not.

Weekend candy

In some places it is common to restrict candy for children to the weekends. The best approach then is probably to give the candy as part of a regular snack or meal, substituting the carbohydrates. If you want to have sweets for a snack, start by having a sandwich (preferably bread with a high fiber). The combination of fat and dietary fiber contained in this snack will slow down the emptying of the stomach, thereby lessening any effect on the blood glucose level. Rapid-acting insulin (NovoLog/NovoRapid or Humalog) is effective much more quickly, so you may not need the slow absorption effect of the sandwich. Check your blood glucose before and after you eat candy to find out what works best for you.

How much in the way of treats and candy can a young person have? You must try this out individually. Eating too many sweets will cause you to gain weight, in exactly the same way as it would if you didn't have diabetes. A rule of the thumb is that half to three quarters of the weight of any candy is pure sugar. The carbohydrate content of an open sandwich corresponds to approximately 20-30 g (1 ounce) of candy. Candy containing fat give a slower blood glucose rise but contain more energy. This applies to treats such as milk chocolate or chocolate type candy. toffees and others candies containing almost pure sugar will increase your blood glucose level much more quickly. The sugar content of licorice candy is about the same as of other types of candy.

A good way to enjoy candy is to eat them while you are engaged in some sort of active outdoor pursuit — for example, during an afternoon walk, playing soccer, or when you are out riding

Weekend candy

A child's typical afternoon snack:

1 sandwich (2 slices of bread)	= 30 g carbohydrate

Saturday snack:

½ sandwich	= 15 g carb.
20 g candy	≈ 15 g carb.
	30 g carb.

15 g candy extra	≈ 10 g carb.	➡	1 U extra
30 g candy extra	≈ 20 g carb.	➡	2 U extra

If the candy contains fat (e.g. chocolate, which contains ~50-60% carbohydrate), this produces a slower emptying of the stomach and thereby a slower rise in the blood-glucose level. If you have access to both regular short-acting insulin (Novolin R, Humulin R) and rapid-acting insulin (NovoLog, Humalog) you may find that short-acting insulin works better with sweets like these.

What does the labeling on candy packets mean?

Types of sugar	Fructose
	Lactose
	Xylose
	Dextrose
Sugar alcohols	Xylitol
	Mannitol
	Sorbitol
	Isomalt
	Maltitol
	Lactitol
Other carbohydrate terms	Hydrogenated starch hydrolysate (HSH)
	Maltodextrins
	Corn Syrup
	High-maltose syrup
	High fructose corn syrup (HFCS)
	Corn starch
	Unmodified starches

Tip: Ask your dietitian to learn more about food ingredients, sweeteners and types of carbohydrates and their impact on blood glucose.

or running around on the beach. The additional activity will use up the extra calories gained from the candy.

Taking a break from eating candy

It is not easy to manage diabetes if you are eating large amounts of candy as everyone who has tried can testify. Even so, many individuals with diabetes do this. This is a bit like smoking for some people — just cutting down doesn't work. Try then to avoid eating candy completely, at least for a while. If it is difficult to say "no" to yourself, do not keep them in the house. Unfortunately, excessive candy eating must remain exceptional behavior for any person with diabetes. And if you do something every day, it ceases to be exceptional.

Many families practice a system of taking a break from eating candies, whether or not they have diabetes in the family. Children may then receive money instead or some other kind of

bonus if they can manage without candy for six months or a whole year. This system works well for children who benefit from not having candy for other reasons as well, such as those who are overweight. Adults can try giving themselves some kind of bonus, such as a new dress or a vacation, if they manage without candy for a longer period of time.

If you have weight problems you will find it difficult balancing eating candy with diabetes. If you eat candy containing fat, this will have less of an effect on your blood glucose, but it will cause you to put on weight. If you eat candy containing less fat, they will have a greater effect on your blood glucose level. A total break from eating candy may be your only chance in

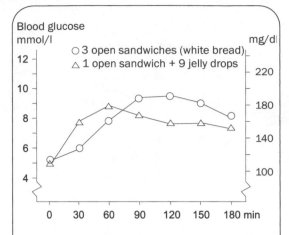

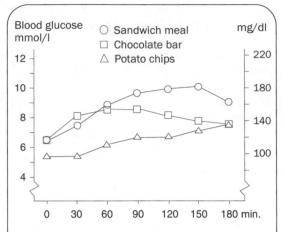

In a Swedish study, teenagers replaced 2 out of 3 open cheese sandwiches with jelly drops at snack time.[131] The blood glucose rise is slightly more rapid with jelly drops and the sandwich, but considerably less rapid than if they had eaten jelly drops alone. White bread contains almost no fiber but gives a larger volume compared to jelly alone, causing the stomach to empty more slowly. The fat in margarine and cheese also leads to a slower emptying of the stomach.

A sandwich made of bread rich in fiber, along with the jelly drops, would probably have made the blood glucose response even less pronounced. From this it follows that a good way to eat your candy is to eat them after a meal and your blood glucose level will be less affected.

In another study, different types of snacks with the same calorie-content were compared: 2½ slices of dark rye bread with cheese and an apple, a bar of milk chocolate (67 g, 2.3 ounces) and potato chips (70 g, 2.5 ounces).[132] The ordinary snack containing slightly more carbohydrates gave the highest blood glucose rise while potato chips gave the slowest rise. The bar of milk chocolate gave a slow rise making it unsuitable for anyone with hypoglycemia.

The fat in chocolate and potato chips causes the stomach to empty more slowly and the increase in blood glucose level will therefore be slower. The food processing used in the manufacturing of chips causes the sugar to be less accessible to digesting enzymes, thereby being absorbed more slowly.

The message from the dietitian, Gunilla Cedermark, who carried out these studies is not that we should have chocolate and chips for snacks every day. Most children don't, even if they would very much like to... The difference is that saying "No!" to chips and bars of chocolate should be done on the same terms as it is for children without diabetes. It is very important to avoid referring to diabetes more often than necessary when saying "No!".

A bar of chocolate is a good snack for children with diabetes who are going on a hiking or skiing trip, in the same way as it is for friends and siblings without diabetes. One day a week you can replace a snack or parts of the evening snack with potato chips. The whole family can enjoy these together with an easy conscience.

this situation if you want to manage both your weight and your A1C.

Potato chips

Potato chips are not a healthy snack option since they contain a lot of fat and calories which easily can create a weight problem. Potato chips will raise the blood glucose very slowly over a period of at least 3-4 hours (see graph on page 234).[132] Twenty-five grams of potato chips (the amount that can be held in the palm of an adult hand) have approximately the

Different types of candy

	Quantity	Carb.	Fat	Kcal
Gelatinous candy	100 g	79 g	0 g	355
Caramels/ pastilles	100 g	97 g	0 g	400
Wine gums	100 g	75 g	0 g	300
Jelly Beans	100 g	100 g	0 g	400
Marshmallows	100 g	80 g	0 g	360
Milk chocolate	100 g	54 g	33 g	570
Dark chocolate	100 g	60 g	32 g	560
Toffee	100 g	69 g	18 g	470

Carb. = carbohydrates

The contents are approximate as they vary from brand to brand. Chocolate with a high fat content increases your blood glucose level more slowly. Gelatinous candy raise the blood glucose level slightly slower than candy that are easy to chew. If you have access to both rapid-acting insulin (Novo-Log, Humalog) and short-acting insulin (Novolin R, Humulin R) you may find that short-acting insulin works better with chocolate candy.

The best time to eat candy is when you are physically active, when you have a low blood glucose level or immediately after a meal.

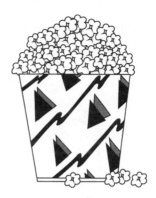

Popcorn makes a good "diabetes treat". Two cups of popcorn contains about the same amount of carbohydrate as one open sandwich (1 slice of bread). Micro-wave popcorn contains the same amount of carbohydrate as ordinary popcorn.

same content of both fat (8 g) and carbohydrate (15 g) as an open cheese sandwich. It may be a good idea to eat chips as an extra bedtime snack after a game of soccer to avoid night time hypoglycemia. But remember that moderation is all and make sure you get chips with unsaturated fat (vegetable oil). If you eat a whole 200 g () bag, your blood glucose will certainly rise.

Chewing gum

Chewing gum contains such small amounts of sugar (about 2 g/stick) that chewing one piece at a time over a couple of hours will not cause you a problem. If you chew in this way, you will find little disadvantage, from the point of view of your diabetes, in using ordinary chewing gum, as opposed to the "sugar-free" variety. Your dentist will almost certainly recommend the latter of course. If you prefer chewing half a packet at a time, it is better to choose a brand with an artificial sweetener, like NutraSweet®.

Weight control

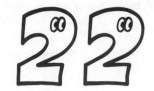

Many young people, particularly teenage girls, find they have problems with keeping their weight at a desirable level, whether or not they have diabetes. There are plenty of girls without diabetes who put on quite a lot of weight during the years following their first menstrual period (menarche), especially if they decrease the amount of regular exercise they do. This is caused by continuing to eat the same amount of food even though they have stopped growing in height. Most girls only grow another 6-8 cm (2-3 inches), after the menarche. The problem is made more complicated for girls with diabetes, as they find it particularly difficult to lose weight. It is very important, therefore, that teenage girls with diabetes reduce both their food intake and the insulin doses when their growth rate is slowing down and especially when they have reached their final height.

Body Mass Index (BMI) is an index for assessing body weight in relation to height. BMI can be calculated by dividing a person's weight by their height in meters square (kg/m^2). Overweight is defined as a BMI above 25.0, obese is above 30.0 and severely obese is above 35.0 kg/m^2. Overweight is a result of consuming more energy than is expended. Even moderate activity of just 30 minutes per day has been shown to improve insulin sensitivity, and this is what really helps weight loss.

A British study found females with diabetes to be overweight as adolescents, and both sexes to be overweight as young adults. Approximately 30% of the young women (but none of the young men) had given themselves less insulin than prescribed, in the hope this would help them control their weight.[120] A Swedish study found girls with diabetes to be on average 6.5 kg (14.3 lb) heavier than their peers without diabetes. Between the age of 18 and 22 their weight was unchanged but A1C improved and

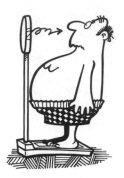

the daily insulin dose was significantly reduced.[217]

Satisfied or "feeling full"?

We believe children should always eat enough to satisfy them, but we should differentiate between being comfortably satisfied and "feeling full". Eating until you feel satisfied is not the same as eating as much as you want. Even children in their very early years at school should understand this distinction, and can be aware that over-eating will lead to weight gain.

Many children prefer to eat large helpings at every meal and this can easily become a habit. So, stop eating just as soon as you begin to feel satisfied and wait for 10-15 minutes. By this time, your feelings of hunger are likely to have disappeared without your having eaten any more. Vegetables will satisfy your hunger without providing significant amounts of carbohydrates or calories, and are a good alternative if you still want more to eat.

When a child or teenager has weight problems, some parents make a deliberate decision to avoid cooking more food than is needed for a normal helping for every family member. Once all the food prepared has been eaten, there will be less room for discussion about second helpings and how much more it is appropriate to eat. Parents can also make sure there are no candies, cookies or cakes available at home to tempt children to eat food when it is better they don't.

Many parents are quite strict about their children finishing what is on their plate. But if you are trying to lose weight, you might find it difficult to judge by eye how much you are going to eat. If you have weight problems, therefore, you should ask permission to leave food on the plate if you find that you have taken too much and feel satisfied before you have finished. If your blood glucose level is high, you won't need to eat as much as usual, and you are likely to find you feel unusually full.[415]

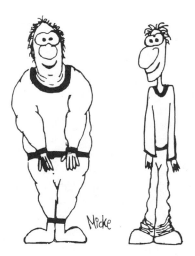

It seems unfair that some individuals can eat as much as they want, while others gain weight by just "looking at" food. The reason for this is that our bodies work differently when it comes to using energy and storing it. During the Stone Age it was useful for survival to be able to store energy as fat when food was not available on a daily basis. But in today's world, for those with an unlimited supply of food, this ability has become a disadvantage.

Reducing weight

Talk to your dietitian about adjusting food intake and insulin doses. Losing weight can easily lead to a vicious circle if you have diabetes. Taking insulin forces you to eat even if you are not hungry at the time. Try to decrease your food intake and, at the same time, decrease the amount of insulin you give yourself. It can be difficult to find the appropriate balance between insulin and food.

You may find it hard to know what foods you can cut down on. Write down everything you eat in the course of a three-day period, recording the exact quantities. Include everything, food, drink, candy, ice cream and so on. Ask your dietitian to calculate the energy amounts and advise you on reducing the amount of fat and calories you consume.

If you decrease the amount of food you eat, you run the risk of becoming hypoglycemic — and if this happens you will need to eat to reverse the situation. But the next day you can think about reducing both food and insulin to lose weight sensibly. Remember to check that you really have low blood glucose (less than 65-70 mg/dl (3.5-4.0 mmol/l) before eating something extra. Be careful not to eat too much if your blood glucose level is too low. Ten to fifteen grams of glucose is usually enough (see page 62). Then wait 10-15 minutes before eating anything else, even if you are still hungry, as this will give your blood glucose level time to rise.

You should avoid losing weight too quickly. A slow and steady loss resulting from a change in habits is better than a quick loss caused by reducing your food intake to a minimum. A sufficient rate is usually 1-3 kg/month (2-6 lb). It may not sound like much, but will result in many kilograms in one year. Complete fasting can be dangerous for a person with diabetes and it is something that is positively discouraged (see also page 240).

How do you count calories?

All food is made up of from different ingredients. Check the table of contents to calculate how many calories you will get.

Fat	9 kcal/g
Sugar	4 kcal/g
Protein	4 kcal/g
Alcohol	7 kcal/g
Sugar alcohol (e.g. sorbitol in candy	~2.5 kcal/g

Calorie table

The following will give you 100 kcal		Activities which will spend 100 kcal	
Whipped cream	1 cup	Walking	
Sugar	2 tbs	slow	40 min.
Oil	2 teasp.	quick	15 min.
Mayonnaise	1 tbs	Bicycling	
Waffle	1	normal	35 min.
Danish pastry	½	quick	10 min.
Chips	20 chips		
Peanuts	½ oz.	Running	10 min.
Candy	8-10 pieces		
Chocolate	2/3 oz.	Skating	25 min.
Doughnut	½	Dancing	25 min.
Light beer	12 fl. oz.	Chopping logs	15 min.
Beer	8 fl. oz.		
White wine, dry	5 fl. oz.	Swimming	10 min.
Spirits	1.5 fl. oz.		
Liqueur	1 fl. oz.		

1 US fluid oz. = 30ml, 1 ounce ≈ 28 grams

The little extras

A little extra food, such as candy, chips, or cookies every day, will amount to quite a lot before the year is over. About 7000 Kcal are needed to build up 1 kg (2.2 lb) of fat in the body. An extra bun a small sandwich each day (100 kcal) will cause you to put on 5 kg (11 lb) of weight in one year! A small bag of peanuts (175 g, 6 ounces) *every week* will result in almost 8 kg (17 lb) weight increase in one year!

Never skip a meal. If you eat regularly, your blood glucose levels will be more steady and prevent you from getting too hungry. A missed meal is often followed by binge eating on something less healthy, such as chips, which contain a lot of empty calories.

High A1C and weight loss

Having a high blood glucose level will result in the loss of large amounts of glucose in the urine. You might say that you "eat for two" since you not only eat to cover your daily energy requirements but also for the glucose lost in the urine. When your A1C is between 9 and 10%, it is not unusual to lose glucose in the urine in amounts of up to 100-200g of glucose in a day.

Having a high A1C can be an effective but dangerous way to lose weight.[180] Many teenagers will deliberately skip insulin injections to avoid gaining weight. In an American study, 15% of teenage girls with diabetes (but no boys) had used this method to diet.[609] You may get rid of a few pounds or kilograms temporarily, but the high blood glucose level that follows will increase your risk of long term complications. If you feel tempted to use this method, try speaking instead to your diabetes team. They will make every effort to help you find a safe means of controlling your weight. The parents of young people with diabetes should be alerted if their teenager loses weight, or fails to show a normal weight increase at the appropriate time.

Increasing insulin doses will cause your body to take up the glucose that was being lost in the urine, and this will cause you to put on weight. Unfortunately, you have to increase the insulin doses initially because the high blood glucose level itself has induced increased insulin resistance (see page 196). What you must do is to increase the insulin doses for a short while (one or two weeks) to overcome the insulin resistance, and then lower them again as quickly as possible. This is because your blood glucose level goes down when the insulin resistance is back to normal. If you also reduce your food intake you will have a good chance of success.

Remember that if your blood glucose level has been high for some time you will have early symptoms of hypoglycemia even at a low normal blood glucose level of 70-90 mg/dl (4-5 mmol/l).[110,369,417] Because of this, you should always take a blood glucose test when you feel hypoglycemic. Eat only if your glucose level is less than 55-65 mg/dl (3.0-3.5 mmol/l). If your blood glucose level is higher, try to avoid eating despite symptoms. Your body may be giving you warning symptoms, but remember that it believes you want a higher blood glucose level as this has been the case for some time. (See "Blood glucose levels and symptoms of hypoglycemia" on page 43.) You must be prepared for a difficult time during the first 1-2 weeks, but after this you should start to experience warning symptoms at a lower blood glucose level. It is a good idea to have a friend or

Exchange list

It is more important than one might imagine to choose an alternative with fewer calories. The table shows the difference (Diff.) between foodstuffs in calories and weight gain.

If you replace	with	Diff. in kcal	Diff. in Weight
2 cups of standard milk	2 cups of low fat milk	120 kcal/day	12 lb/year
3 open sandwiches with margarine and full fat cheese	3 open sandwiches with low-fat cheese but without margarine	205 kcal/day	20 lb /year
1 fried egg	1 boiled egg	40 kcal /day	4 lb/year
2 tbs mayonnaise	3 tbs sour cream	155 kcal	2 lb/ 45 times
1 bar of chocolate	1 apple	235 kcal	2 lb/ 30 times
1 helping of french fries	1 helping of boiled potatoes	145 kcal	2 lb/ 50 times
1 bottle of beer	1 bottle of light beer	45 kcal	2 lb/155 bottles
1 bag of peanuts (175g)	2 cups of popcorn	1000 kcal	3 lb/ 10 bags

1 kg = 2.2 lb

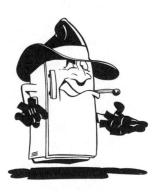

You might sometimes find it necessary to put a guard on the refrigerator in case you find yourself craving something tasty... One extra sandwich per day turns into 16 kg of extra fat in one year!

parent present while you are getting accustomed to this. You will need support and understanding from someone close to you, if you are to make it work.

Eating disorders

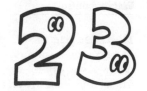

Both anorexia and bulimia (binge eating) are symptoms of weight phobia, in that the person concerned finds it impossible to eat without worrying about gaining weight. A person with an eating disorder always has a distorted picture of their own body, but it is the emotional disturbance which is the most important. Eating disorders are much more common among girls, but can occur in boys as well. Anorexia usually starts between the ages of 13 and 16 years, bulimia somewhat later.[252] A person with an eating disorder is unlikely to appreciate the seriousness of the problem and may not feel it at all necessary to seek medical help.

Anorexia

In anorexia there is a weight loss of at least 15% of the estimated normal weight for age or not being able to reach this weight at all. There is also an extreme fear of gaining weight and a very distorted idea of what the body looks like. Typically, someone with anorexia will see themselves as fat when looking into the mirror — even though, to others, they appear very slim. Food fixation is common, i.e. being interested in cooking for others while avoiding eating anything themselves. A person with anorexia is usually quite active physically, often running many miles a day in an attempt to keep their weight down.

The starvation that a person with anorexia is going through can result in physical symptoms such as headaches, lowered body temperature, increased body hair and irregular or disrupted menstrual periods. Psychological symptoms may include depression, feelings of inadequacy, sleeping difficulties and obsessions.

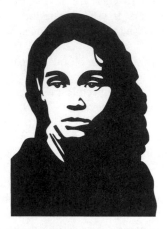

Having an eating disorder is difficult. It is common for young people with anorexia or bulimia to try and manipulate their insulin doses and individuals often have problems with low or high blood glucose levels. Anyone with anorexia or bulimia will definitely need help. If this applies to you, tell your diabetes nurse or doctor, or another adult whom you trust. You will probably need to be referred to a specialist in these problems. It is also very difficult to calculate the insulin doses to match your irregular food intake if you have an eating disorder, so you will need help from your diabetes team with this.

Bulimia

People with bulimia engage in binging large amounts of food, much more than a person without the disorder would eat at one sitting. There is sense of loss of control and an inability to stop eating unless, for example, another person comes into the room. Self-inflicted vomiting or laxatives, excessive exercise or fasting may be used to control the weight. These individuals are often very impulsive and, if they also have diabetes, may find the regular routines necessary to manage it effectively, really very difficult.[644]

Diabetes and eating disorders

A UK study found that 9% of 11-18 year olds met the criteria for eating disorders, and that the proportion was the same among girls with or without diabetes.[609] However, a Swedish study found that teenage girls with diabetes were at greater risk of eating disorders (binge eating and self-induced vomiting) than their peers without diabetes.[252] The combination of diabetes and eating disorders has been called "diabulemia".[115] Physical or sexual abuse or any form of trauma can be the root cause of eating disorders such as anorexia and bulimia.[796]

Having diabetes and an eating disorder usually implies problems with blood glucose control and a tendency to manipulate insulin doses to control weight.[609,644,645] Not eating enough causes low blood glucose levels, and reducing insulin doses results in high blood glucose peaks.

Individuals with diabetes cannot starve themselves the same way as people without diabetes are able to, because insulin levels will not adapt to the situation of hunger as it does in people without diabetes. If you have diabetes, it is much more dangerous for you to make yourself vomit or take laxatives than it would be if you did not have diabetes. Your body will be easily thrown off balance, especially if you change insulin doses up and down as well. Your condition can deteriorate to a dangerous level and hospitalization may be necessary. A BMI below 14-15 usually indicates that you need medical attention. The risk of dying a diabetes-related death is considerably higher if you have anorexia too.[574] A high A1C will increase your risk of developing late complications of diabetes in the future.

Anorexia and bulimia in someone with diabetes demand expert psychological and psychiatric care in addition to diabetes care. Anyone suffering from such a combination may also require a long hospital stay because of the risks of death and diabetic ketoacidosis if insulin is omitted. Family involvement should be an integral part of the treatment of eating disorders in young people.[180] Most people with these disorders can recover if they receive proper treatment.

Physical exercise

Everyone should do some form of physical exercise if they are to keep healthy. A body in good general condition can withstand hardships better. However, exercise must be enjoyable and should not be something one is forced into. Younger children usually run around a lot while they are playing, but older children are very different. Some like sports while others prefer to sit quietly with books, the television or a computer. We must adjust the insulin treatment to the individual, not the other way around.

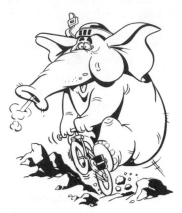

Walking to and from school or riding your bicycle will give you some exercise every day. It is easier to find an appropriate dose of insulin when you are exercising daily than if you sit still one day and do a lot of exercise the next.

The effect of exercise on the blood glucose level

➠ Exercise increases absorption of insulin from the injection site that you move during exercise, for example the thigh when running or playing soccer.

➠ It also increases the consumption of glucose without increasing the need for insulin.

➠ BUT — insulin must be available or the muscle cells will not be able to take up glucose!

➠ **Beware!** Be careful with exercise when there is not enough insulin available in your body (blood glucose above 270-290 mg/dl, 15-16 mmol/l and elevated levels of ketones). You might need an extra insulin injection (0.05-1 units/kg, 0.25-0.5 units/10 lb) and abstain from exercise for 2-3 hours until the blood glucose level has gone down.

➠ You will be at risk of hypoglycemia many hours afterwards (in the evening or night) because you have used the liver's store of glycogen after a lot of exercise.

➠ If you exercise regularly you will know how much the blood glucose is affected but if you exercise occasionally only, your blood glucose may drop much more than you expect during and after exercise.

Controlled studies have not been able to show that physical exercise improves the management of diabetes.[732,801] Because of this, exercise is not considered as a treatment for diabetes.[349] However, everyone should be encouraged to take part in some form of regular physical activity, even if it is only riding a bicycle to and from work or school, and people with diabetes are no exception to this. Regular physical exercise also lowers the risk of cardiovascular diseases in people with diabetes.[483] In contrast, the pronounced lack of exercise and muscular activity in some teenagers seems to contribute to an increased insulin resistance, a tendency to be overweight and a deterioration in blood glucose control.[505]

When your muscles are working, the store of glucose in the muscles (muscle glycogen, approximately 400 g in an adult person) is used first. After this, glucose from the liver and fatty acids (breakdown products from fat) are used as fuel. Exercise lowers the blood glucose level by increasing glucose uptake into the muscle cells without increasing the amount of insulin needed. This is because more glucose is consumed by your muscles during exercise. After exercise, the muscles will have increased insulin

How do insulin and exercise work together?

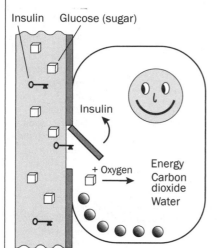

Insulin   Glucose (sugar)

Insulin

+ Oxygen

Energy
Carbon
dioxide
Water

Blood vessel   Muscle cell

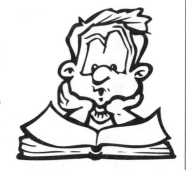

Sitting still

Insulin "opens the door" to the cell for glucose to enter. The size of your insulin dose decides how quickly your blood glucose level will fall. Your regular insulin doses during school or work days are adjusted in line with your usual level of physical activity.

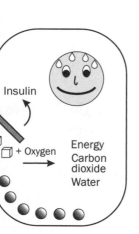

Insulin

+ Oxygen

Energy
Carbon
dioxide
Water

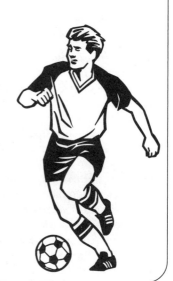

Physical exercise

If you play soccer or take part in some other type of intensive physical activity you will need to lower your insulin dose. Exercise will cause the same amount of insulin to keep the door open for a little longer, i.e. more glucose will be transported into the cell, and the blood glucose level can easily fall too low. Decrease the insulin dose slightly.

The effect of strenuous exercise may last for at least 8-10 hours which means that you should decrease your bedtime insulin as well (by 1-2, up to 4 units) and have a substantial bedtime snack to avoid night time hypoglycemia.

sensitivity for 1-2 days [795] (see also "Insulin sensitivity and resistance" on page 195). This means that exercise 3-4 times/week will result in increased insulin sensitivity even between the training sessions and the total insulin dose can probably be lowered. Sometimes the increased insulin sensitivity does not begin until 4-6 hours after the exercise [795] which may occur during the night if you exercise in the evening.

If you have been exercising your leg muscles, insulin injected into the thigh will be absorbed rather more quickly from the subcutaneous tissue (more so with short-acting than with rapid-acting insulin).[280] If you inject insulin deep enough to enter the muscle it will be absorbed much more quickly and you will risk having hypoglycemia (see page 81). *It is important to remember that exercise alone will not*

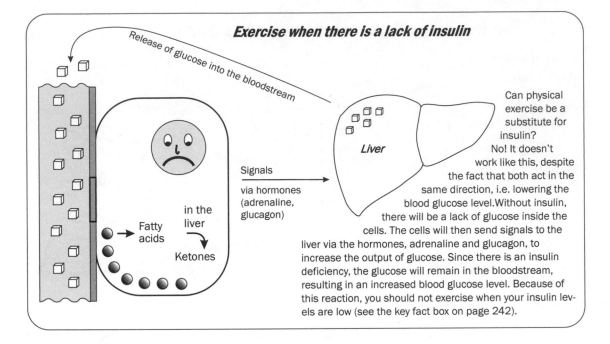

Exercise when there is a lack of insulin

Release of glucose into the bloodstream

Signals via hormones (adrenaline, glucagon)

Fatty acids → in the liver → Ketones

Liver

Can physical exercise be a substitute for insulin? No! It doesn't work like this, despite the fact that both act in the same direction, i.e. lowering the blood glucose level. Without insulin, there will be a lack of glucose inside the cells. The cells will then send signals to the liver via the hormones, adrenaline and glucagon, to increase the output of glucose. Since there is an insulin deficiency, the glucose will remain in the bloodstream, resulting in an increased blood glucose level. Because of this reaction, you should not exercise when your insulin levels are low (see the key fact box on page 242).

lower the blood glucose level at all. Insulin has to be present to enable this to happen. Glucose from the bloodstream needs insulin in order to enter the muscle cells.

The rate of glucose uptake into the muscles of an adult is approximately 8-12 g/hour when exercising at an ordinary rate, and is more than doubled with heavy exercise.[801] The levels of the hormones, adrenaline, glucagon and cortisol in the bloodstream increase during physical exercise. Glucose is released from the liver depot (liver glycogen, see page 32) and new glucose is produced in the liver from proteins. If the liver was unable to increase its glucose production, the blood glucose level would drop by about 2 mg/dl (0.1 mmol/l) per minute during exercise, soon resulting in hypoglycemia.[801] A high level of insulin in the blood counteracts the pro-

duction of glucose in the liver which, in turn, increases the risk of hypoglycemia. In people without diabetes, the level of insulin in the blood drops during exercise.[801]

Can the blood glucose level increase through exercise?

The blood glucose level will increase on account of exercise if there is not enough insulin. The cells don't "understand" that there is plenty of glucose in the bloodstream. On the contrary, they act as if the body was starving (see figures on page 24). This is caused by the muscle cells having a lack of glucose following a period of exercise in the presence of insulin deficiency. The muscle glycogen is used up, and insulin deficiency prevents new glucose from entering the cells. Hormonal signals will then tell the liver to release more glucose from its glycogen depot.

The signals to the liver are communicated by the hormones glucagon and adrenaline. The

You can never replace insulin with exercise!
When exercising, you will need less insulin. But if you exercise without enough insulin in your body, your blood glucose level will rise.

increased amount of glucose in the blood comes from both a breakdown of the liver's glycogen and a production of glucose in the liver. At the same time, when there is a lack of insulin, there will be a breakdown of fat to fatty acids which are transformed into ketones in the liver. This puts you at risk of developing ketoacidosis.[801]

When your blood glucose level is above 250 mg/dl (14 mmol/l), and there are raised ketone levels indicating insulin deficiency, exercise should be postponed while extra insulin is taken. Running to lower a high blood glucose in this situation is not a good idea. It might even be dangerous.

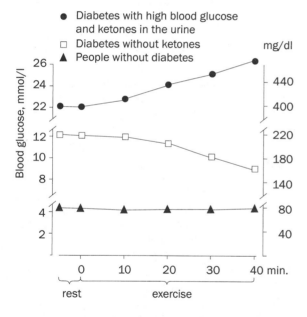

Your blood glucose level will rise if you exercise when the insulin level in your body is low. This is due to the lack of sugar inside your muscle cells causing different hormones to increase your blood glucose level. Your body still "thinks" as if it did not have diabetes, so it cannot adapt to the fact that you already have too much sugar in your blood. If your blood glucose level is high (above 250 mg/dl, 14 mmol/l) and you also have elevated ketone levels, you should take some extra insulin and wait a while for it to start working before exercising. The graph is from reference.[790]

Some friends of mine met a 45-year old man when starting out on a mountain hike. He asked them if he could accompany them as he was alone, and they agreed. During the second day the man felt nauseous, began vomiting and appeared very tired. Then he told my friends he had diabetes. He was under the impression that exercise lowers the blood glucose level and had thought that exercise might cure his diabetes. He had left all his insulin at home. One of my friends ran 20 km (13 miles) to the nearest telephone, and called for a helicopter. But by the time it reached the camping site, the man was already dead. He died from a diabetes coma caused by a total lack of insulin, made more severe by the hard physical exercise.

This happened many years ago. Knowledge has improved since then and people with diabetes know it is dangerous to not take insulin. In spite of this, episodes of serious ketoacidosis, caused by missed insulin injections, and requiring hospital treatment, are not uncommon. Many of these cases involve teenagers who do not realize how dangerous it can be to leave out insulin injections.

Hypoglycemia after exercise

As the glycogen stores in the liver are depleted during heavy exercise, there is a greatly increased risk of hypoglycemia several hours after the exercise. The muscles will have increased insulin sensitivity for at least another 8-10 hours, sometimes up to 18 hours after the exercise is finished. This means that you are likely to be at risk of night time hypoglycemia after strenuous physical activity. If you find yourself in this situation, you should begin by trying to refill the glycogen stores in your liver and muscles, by eating during and after the exercise. Count on needing an additional 10-15 grams (1/3-1/2 ounce) of carbohydrate (15-30 grams, 1/2-1 ounce, for an adult) for every 30 minutes of exercise after the initial 30 minutes.[795]

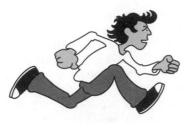

To be able to run quickly your muscles need glucose. If your exercise session lasts longer than 30 minutes, you will need extra food, approximately 10-20 grams of carbohydrate for every 30 minutes of exercise.

You might find it valuable to experiment with different amounts of carbohydrate during a game of soccer for example, and when you find a suitable amount, follow this up by eating the same amount of extra carbohydrate every time you play. If you start playing within one hour of your injection, the insulin uptake will be increased and you will probably need to increase your carbohydrate intake again or decrease the insulin dose.[745]

Remember that it takes more than one meal to refill the glycogen stores in your liver and muscles after heavy physical exertion. This means that even if you have eaten a substantial meal after the game you may become hypoglycemic later in the day or evening, since the glycogen stores have not had time to be refilled completely. If you play sport in both the morning and the afternoon, you will be more likely to have problems with hypoglycemia during the afternoon game for the same reason.

What this means, in practice, is that you are likely to need an extra helping at your evening snack if you have been playing sport all afternoon. Your appetite may well remind you of this! However, even though you are eating more, you may still find your need for insulin has gone down, and you need to decrease the dose at the evening snack by 1-2 units. More often than not, the bedtime insulin dose should be decreased as well to avoid night time hypoglycemia (by 1-2 units for a younger child, 2-4 units for a teenager or adult).

Tips for heavy exercise

4-5 PM	**Dinner** (pasta is fine) Decrease 1-2 U if you are using Novo-Log/NovoRapid or Humalog, preferably taking the dose at least 1 hour before the game. Take your ordinary insulin doses if you are using short-acting insulin.
	Take a blood test before the game:
<125 mg/dl <7 mmol/l	Eat extra carbohydrates.
125-180 mg/dl 7-10 mmol/l	OK to get started
200-250 mg/dl 11-14 mmol/l	Go ahead but take a blood glucose test again after 30 minutes -1 hour. If the level is decreasing, there is insulin available and it is OK to continue. If the level is increasing, there is a lack of insulin and you should stop exercising and take extra insulin.
>250mg/dl >14 mmol/l	Check for ketones in blood or urine. If positive take 0.05 units/kg (0.025 units/lb) body weight of short-acting (or preferably rapid-acting) insulin and wait 1-2 hours for it to have an effect.
5-6 PM	**Game:** Eat half (or a small whole) banana at half-time.
8 PM	**Evening snack** (rich in carbohydrates): Eat more than usual. Take your ordinary dose but usually one will need to decrease it by 1-2 units.
10 PM	**Bedtime insulin:** Try lowering the dose by 1-2, up to 4 units, sometimes more, and take a bedtime snack. Lower the basal rate by 10-20% (0.1-0.2 U/hour) if you have a pump (use the temporary basal rate).

It should be borne in mind that exercise can take many forms. It could include, for example, spending a full day swimming at the beach, a long bicycle ride, a day of skiing or ice skating,

Tips for heavy exercise, cont.

Rule of thumb: For every 30 minutes of heavy exercise you will need about 10-15 g (1/3-1/2 ounce) of extra carbohydrate (15-30 g, 1/2-1 ounce, for an adult). Take half as "quick-acting" carbohydrates (like juice, sports drink) and half as slower carbohydrates (like a chocolate bar) or eat half to a whole banana (about 10-20 g of carbohydrate).

Hypoglycemia: Make sure that your coach and team-mates know how to help you should you need it.
Always carry glucose in a pocket!

the first (or possibly the second) class after lunch is likely to be best when using regular short-acting insulin. The second class after lunch is less suitable for younger children as they are more likely to be active during the lunch break as well.

Talk to the P.E. teacher about the schedule well in advance to find out if it is possible to adjust the schedule. Indeed, it is important to be sure that the P.E. teacher, and any other members of staff who have regular contact with young people, are aware if any pupil has diabetes, what their particular needs are, as well as how to recognize hypoglycemia, what to do when it occurs and how to call others for help. The P.E. teacher and the school nurse should both have access to glucose tablets and know when and how they should be used. This should be a key part of the education plan for children with diabetes in all grades of the education system.

It would be helpful for children to have an extra snack before the P.E. lesson if their blood glucose is low. Many children need an extra snack after this sort of activity, in order to prevent delayed hypoglycemia. Because of the risk of hypoglycemia, a schoolchild who has diabetes should always be accompanied by a friend or teacher (who knows how to help) when climbing or balancing or on outings such as nature walks, cross country running, swimming or school trips.

as well as many hours dancing in the evening. The after effects of such aerobic exercise are all similar and often include delayed, activity-induced hypoglycemia in the middle of the night or the next morning. Sleeping late the next morning can be especially dangerous under such circumstances. Mixing this increased activity with alcohol can cause particular problems since alcohol blocks the body's ability to respond to hypoglycemia. Unconscious hypoglycemic reactions or hypoglycemic seizures may result if you forget to decrease your bedtime insulin or to have an extra snack before going to bed.

Physical education

Children and teenagers with diabetes can and should take part in physical education (P.E.) to the same extent as youngsters without diabetes. The risk of hypoglycemia will be lower if P.E. activities can be timetabled for the second or third class following a meal if a child is using rapid-acting insulin (NovoLog/NovoRapid or Humalog), as the insulin level increases rapidly during the first hour after an injection (see graph on page 249). The first (or possibly the second) class in the morning, or alternatively

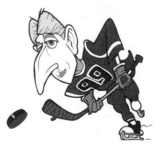

Top level competitive sports

You can certainly take part in competitive sports even if you have diabetes. There are many successful sportsmen and women with diabetes playing in international teams or at a professional level. A normal blood glucose level

Physical exercise — some rules

① Plan ahead so that you have eaten and taken your premeal insulin 1-2 hours before you start exercising, otherwise you risk having the greatest blood glucose lowering effect right at the beginning. If you are using NovoLog/NovoRapid or Humalog it may be better to reduce the dose by 1-2 units if you are going to exercise within 1-2 hours of the injection.[767]

② Test your blood glucose before starting the exercise. If it is below 250 mg/dl (14 mmol/l) you should eat something before starting.[801] If you have ketones in your blood or urine too, this is a sign that your cells are starving. You should wait until your blood glucose level has increased before you start your exercise.

③ If your blood glucose is above 270-290 mg/dl (15-16 mmol/l) you should check for ketones before starting the exercise. If your ketone levels are raised, you should not exercise until 1-2 hours after you have taken extra insulin (0.05-1 units/kg, 0.25-0.5 units/10 lb).

④ Eat something extra during exercise if the session lasts more than 30 minutes. Depending on your body size, half to a whole banana (or other source of 10-20 g of glucose) is usually about right. Find out what suits you best. Take blood tests while you are exercising and note them in your logbook for future reference.

⑤ Eat a large meal after the exercise, preferably something with a high carbohydrate content, like sandwiches.

⑥ Decrease the insulin doses following exercise (evening premeal by 1-2 units and bedtime dose by 1-2, up to 4 units or 10-20% decrease using temporary basal rate with a pump). If you exercise more than 3-4 times a week, the increased insulin sensitivity that your exercise causes will probably be effective "round the clock". You will therefore be unlikely to need to lower your insulin doses as much in this situation since they will already be adjusted for it. For seasonal sports you may need to lower your insulin 24 hour dose considerably during active season, e.g. up to 40% when playing ice hockey.

⑦ If you exercise to lose weight, it is important to lower the premeal dose instead of eating more after exercising.

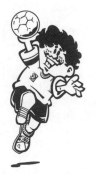

The blood glucose lowering effect of exercise will last for at least 8-10 hours.
Always lower the bedtime dose by 2-4 units after heavy exertion, such as a game of handball or soccer.

is essential if you are to achieve maximum performance. You may need to decrease the amount of insulin you take just before the physical exercise, for example a match of soccer or basketball. Remember that, if you have a difficult bout of hypoglycemia, it will take you several hours to return to a level of maximum performance. Check your blood glucose level frequently to find out how your body reacts in different situations during training and competition. This will make it easier to plan food intake and insulin doses for the training sessions if they take place at regular times. For example, Sir Steve Redgrave who has won 5 Olympic gold medals in rowing, a tough endurance sport, needs to consume 6,000 calories a day, which he does in six meals, each accompanied by an insulin injection. And he measures his blood glucose before each meal to know how much insulin to take.

The best time to begin exercising varies slightly, depending on whether you are using regular short-acting insulin (Novolin R, Humulin R, Insuman Rapid) or rapid-acting insulin before meals (when on multiple daily injections or a pump). During the first hour after an insulin injection, the level of insulin in the blood increases quickly — particularly with NovoLog/NovoRapid or Humalog. If you were to exercise during this time, insulin would be absorbed even faster (especially if you have injected yourself in the thigh) making hypoglycemia more likely. You should therefore avoid injecting premeal doses in the thigh before exercising.

Testing the effect of exercise on blood glucose levels

♠ In an American study, teenage boys consumed a sports drink (Gatorade®, 6.5% sucrose/glucose) corresponding to 2 ml/kg (1.3 grams of carbohydrate/10 kg body weight) and exercised for 10 minutes followed by 5 minutes rest.[745]

♠ In spite of this the blood glucose level fell by in average 70 mg/dl (4.0 mmol/l) after 90 minutes (6 bouts of exercise).

♠ The boys performed the same test for 2 days and there was a clear similarity between the glucose lowering effect of exercise for each person during the testing.

♠ Experiment yourself to find out how much extra carbohydrates are needed for your type of activity.

① Short-acting insulin

Exercise within one hour of the injection is usually OK.[767] If you start your exercise 3 hours after the meal and the injection, you will need an extra snack before starting.

② Rapid-acting insulin

If you are using NovoLog/NovoRapid or Humalog, it may be better to decrease the dose by 1-2 units if you are going to exercise within 1-2 hours after the injection [767] (see page 144).

If you have problems with night time hypoglycemia following evening training sessions, it may be better to reschedule them to the afternoon.[801] Avoid being alone for strenuous training sessions as you may need the help of a friend if you have difficult or severe hypoglycemia. Don't forget to decrease your bedtime insulin by 2-4 units after strenuous exercise, such as a soccer or football match. If you are using Lantus you may need to reduce the dose by 2-4 units the evening before a daytime exercise session that will last more than 2-3 hours.

If you use an insulin pump, try taking the premeal dose as usual (or perhaps 1-2 units less) and disconnect the pump during the period you are exercising (provided it is not for more than 1-2 hours). Another alternative is to try skipping the premeal injection before you start exer-

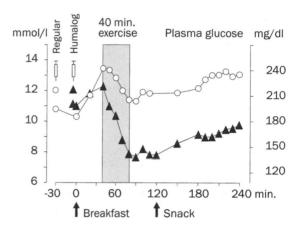

A Finnish study compared the use of Humalog and regular short-acting insulin prior to moderate exercise on a cycle exerciser (comparable to jogging).[767] This tells us that, even with relatively moderate exercise, the blood glucose level can decrease considerably if you time the exercise closely after a premeal dose of Humalog. With regular short-acting insulin you will have fewer problems with this intensity of exercise but as you see from the graph, there is still a drop in blood glucose levels which may get worse if you increase the load.

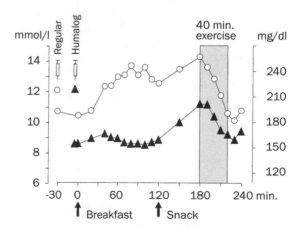

With the exercise timed late after the meal (3 hours in this study) there is a greater drop in blood glucose level with regular short-acting insulin than with Humalog.

cising, keeping the pump connected with the basal rate running during the exercise.

In competitive situations, your body may react a bit differently, even though you are doing the same physical work as you do during training. The stress will increase your blood glucose level with the help of adrenaline (by increasing the liver output of glucose). This usually reduces the risk of hypoglycemia and the need for extra carbohydrates during a competition as compared to a training session. On the other hand, it will be even more important to eat extra food afterwards, so that you refill the glycogen stores in the liver and muscles.

If you find your blood glucose levels go up when you compete, you can try taking the insulin dose less than an hour before you start. In some team sports (such as ice hockey) you will probably be sitting on the bench for a large part of the game so there will be less physical exercise in total compared to a training session.

The effect of stress will often reveal itself early on in a competition. It is usually short-lived, often lasting only 10 or 20 minutes.[707] Different individuals react differently and you should find out how you react, for example by testing your blood glucose level during the first break of the game (like the professional football, player Jay Leeuwenburg, see page 351). Very heavy exertion can cause excessive amounts of adrenaline to be secreted. This can make the blood glucose level rise even though insulin levels are adequate.[701] After a heavy bout of exercise, such as a game of soccer, the blood glucose will often be raised because of stress hormones in people who do not have diabetes. They can compensate for this with doubled levels of insulin in their blood. People with diabetes have the same reaction, but as their insulin levels are not increased, the blood glucose level will rise sharply instead.[546] It is difficult to match this situation with extra insulin. Wait an hour or two and your blood glucose will usually start coming down by itself. If you have this reaction

---

Should you lower your premeal insulin doses before exercising?

A study of adults using Ultralente and Humalog, found that blood glucose was lowered approximately 55 mg/dl (3.0 mmol/l) after 60 minutes of light exercise or 30 min. of heavy exercise.[628,] This should be taken into consideration when you take your premeal insulin dose of rapid-acting insulin. If your blood glucose level is a bit high, such a drop in the level may be a good thing, but if it is lower (< 110-145 mg/dl, 6-8 mmol/l) the premeal dose can be lowered according to the table below in order to reduce the risk of hypoglycemia. This is very individual, of course, but after some attempts you will know which levels and doses suit your body best.

Reduction of premeal insulin dose

Intensity of exercise	30 min.	60 min.
Walking, swimming (¼ of VO$_2$max)*	25%	50%
Jogging (½ of VO$_2$max)	50%	75%
Soccer, handball (¾ of VO$_2$max)	75%	100% (no dose)

*Maximum oxygen uptake

How much energy is spent per hour? (adults)

Slow walking	100-200	kcal
Bicycling (leisure)	250-300	kcal
Table tennis, golf tennis (doubles)	300-350	kcal
Dancing	300-400	kcal
Gymnastics	300-400	kcal
Tennis (singles)	400-500	kcal
Gym work-out	~ 500	kcal
Jogging, downhill skiing, soccer	500-600	kcal
Swimming	~ 600	kcal
Cross-country skiing	800-1000	kcal

often, you could try taking some insulin at half-time.

Keeping fit with diabetes

One study of teenagers with diabetes showed that those with higher A1C had poorer capacity for physical work.[53] This means that if you want to achieve top performance you must also have an optimal A1C. Competitive athletes risk decreasing their insulin too much in an attempt to avoid hypoglycemia, thus resulting in higher A1C levels compared to those doing moderate physical exercise.[234] Although physical training enhances insulin sensitivity, it improves A1C levels only if blood glucose is carefully monitored.

Regular exercise (at least every other day) leads to a decreased insulin resistance (see page 195) that lasts between the sessions. Correspondingly, inactivity (for instance caused by being confined to bed) gives an increased resistance within days.[795] Active athletes in training will therefore need to lower all their insulin doses considerably. When the training season is over, the doses are likely to need a considerable increase if higher blood glucose levels are to be avoided. Sometimes 30-50% more insulin is needed during the inactive season. A major benefit for all young people with diabetes is that regular daily exercise of one sort or another helps to keep the weight down and also in the long term improves heart and blood vessel fitness.

However, a person with diabetes-related eye damage, kidney damage or nerve damage should consult their doctor about what type of exercise is most appropriate. It is important to be careful with strenuous physical exercise if you have pronounced complications in your eyes, kidneys or nervous system. This is because vigorous exercise will increase the risk of high blood pressure or skin wounds.[801] People with complicated eye damage (so called proliferative retinopathy) should avoid strenuous exercise and anyone who has loss of sensation in their feet should limit weight-bearing exercise (e.g. running or playing soccer).[26] People with kidney damage often have a reduced capacity for exercise, which places an automatic limit on their activity level.[26]

Camps and skiing trips

If you are physically active for a prolonged period, on a skiing trip or an outward bound camp for example, you will have an increased insulin sensitivity after 1-2 days which will probably call for substantially lower insulin doses (decreased by 20% or sometimes even 50% especially if you are not used to hard physical exercise). You must increase your food intake to compensate for the increased energy output and it is usual to be hungry after a day of vigorous activity. The increased insulin sensitivity will continue for at least a couple of days after you return home. Check your blood glucose levels and you will see when it is time to increase the insulin doses again. It is important when skiing to eat extra sweet snacks before going on a long ski-lift ride to make these carbohydrates last through the next ski slope.

Marathon efforts!

If you are engaged in heavy physical activity for an entire day, you may need to lower your insulin doses considerably (often by 20% and sometimes even by 50%). You will need extra energy, glucose and fluid at regular intervals (approximately 40 g carbohydrate/hour [234]). When you are involved in prolonged physical work (many hours) it is best to try gradually to increase the time of activity by 1-2 hours each day. You will probably need to lower your basal insulin considerably. You may need short-acting or rapid-acting insulin more frequently (every second to fourth hour) together with extra energy in the form of quick carbohydrates.

Extreme physical performance can be achieved by very careful planning, although there may still be risks. The participants with diabetes in a

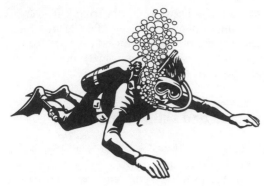

It is possible to dive if you have diabetes. You must be extra careful to avoid hypoglycemia as this can be very dangerous when you are under water. However, it is not justifiable from a medical standpoint to have a standard diving certificate. The diver who has diabetes should should have as their diving buddy, a person who is familiar with the problems of diabetes (but this person should not have diabetes). This can be either a regular diving partner or a trained medic/paramedic.

mountaineering expedition on Kilimanjaro decreased their insulin doses by half.[555] They had more symptoms of acute mountain sickness than the other participants. More worryingly, some experienced severe hypoglycemia and there were two episodes of ketoacidosis. So there would appear to be clear hazards associated with extreme altitude climbing for people with type 1 diabetes.

Meticulous planning can minimize problems, however. One father took a long distance canoeing trip with his two sons, covering the entire coastline of Sweden (more than 2000 km, 1250 miles). One of the boys was 15 years old, and had diabetes. He managed the whole trip without severe hypoglycemia. Talk to your doctor about how to plan insulin doses, food intake and glucose testing before you attempt any such extreme situations.

Anabolic steroids

Anabolic steroids are unfortunately used by many sportsmen and women in spite of all the warnings from the medical profession, not to mention the risk of being discovered in a doping control. How might anabolic steroids affect diabetes? They are known to disturb the glucose metabolism in people without diabetes, because they increase the body's resistance to insulin. So they are also likely to increase insulin resistance in people who have diabetes, but this has not yet been studied. There also appears to be a risk of hormonal changes, and some reports indicate problems with impotence. The long-term effects of anabolic steroids are still not very well understood, but it is likely they will prove to be very dangerous, especially for people who also have diabetes.

Diving

Diving is a fascinating sport, which places great demands on the individuals performing it. Tasks that are easy to accomplish on shore (like opening a package of dextrose) may be very difficult to do in the water even without any hypoglycemic symptoms. Hypoglycemia may proceed into sudden unconsciousness with the risk of drowning. It therefore implies additional risks also for the diving partner who does not have diabetes. Diving with diabetes has been much discussed and opinions on the subject differ. However, on the basis that the degree of caution called for is over and above that required of their counterparts without diabetes, most diving organizations now allow people with diabetes to dive under certain conditions (see key fact box).

Olle Sandelin, Swedish diving physician: [668]
— A declaration of health for a normal diving certificate is not possible when it comes to individuals having diabetes who are treated with insulin. Individuals with diabetes should dive with an instructor or with a so called handicap certificate which is only valid when they are accompanied by two people instead of one, which is the usual requirement.

Consulting physician Bengt Pergel from the Swedish Marine gives the following advice: [487]
— An ordinary diving certificate should not be

Limitations for the diver with diabetes [239]

➠ All members of the diving team must be informed that you have diabetes.

➠ It is advisable to dive only a maximum of 2 dives per day (and on not more than 3 consecutive days) to avoid the build-up of an excessive tissue nitrogen load.

➠ Do not dive deeper than 30 meters.

➠ Remain well within the diving tables or have no more than 2 minutes no-stop time left on a dive computer.

➠ Be aware that diving sickness ("the bends") has similar symptoms to hypoglycemia (e.g. confusion, unconsciousness, seizures). In this situation, treat as if the person has both conditions, giving both oxygen and glucose or a glucagon injection.

See reference [238] and [464] for further advice.

verify that the person doesn't have an increased risk of hypoglycemia when doing the heavy physical work associated with diving. This may be a difficult decision even for a qualified diabetologist. It is virtually impossible to adjust blood glucose levels while diving and it is very difficult even when swimming at the surface. Divers who count on having glucose available in their life jacket pockets have probably never been diving in rapid water or a rough sea.

Christopher Edge, UK diving physician (who is referenced in the key fact boxes):
— Don't forget that we don't allow the vast majority of adolescents to dive with diabetes, as their control is very rarely good enough, and a lot of the time there is parental pressure on them to "dive with dad". We've only allowed one 16 year old to dive. Certainly no-one under 16 has been considered.

While you are diving you must be able to recognize clearly symptoms of blood glucose levels below 70 mg/dl (4.0 mmol/l). If you have so-called "hypoglycemic unawareness" (see page 48) with blood glucose levels less than 55 mg/dl (3 mmol/l) without symptoms, *your life will be in danger if you dive*!

You should eat extra carbohydrates before diving, just as you would before any strenuous physical exercise, to keep your blood glucose

issued to a person with diabetes out of consideration for both the diver and the person she/he is diving with. If a person diving has diabetes it is essential that everyone in the diving team knows about it.

— When it comes to the physical examination, the doctor issuing the certificate must be able to

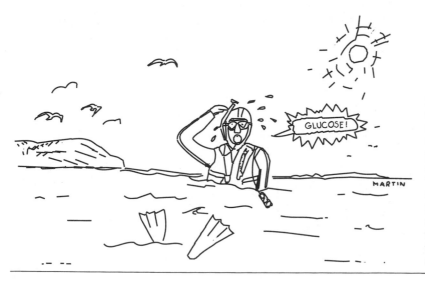

Hypoglycemia in or under water is the greatest problem when diving with diabetes. Getting dextrose out of a pocket can be difficult enough even at the surface. To do it under water while experiencing hypoglycemia may be close to impossible, as your symptoms make the task even more difficult. Practice finding dextrose both in and under water.

Diving and diabetes

The diving clubs in the UK (BSAC, SAA and SSAC) allow a person with diabetes to dive if certain conditions are fulfilled.[239] These rules are also referred to by the US diving organizations DAN and UHMS.

➡ The medication regime of the diver with diabetes should not have changed considerably during the course of the last year.

➡ No severe hypoglycemia (requiring help from another person, glucagon treatment or hospital admission) should have occurred during the last 12 months.

➡ No hospitalization during the last 12 months for diabetes-related conditions.

➡ Satisfactory glucose control throughout the last 12 months (A1C < 9%).

➡ There should be no evidence of long-term complications from diabetes (retinopathy, nephropathy including microalbuminuria, neuropathy and heart and blood vessel disease).

➡ The physician in charge of the diver's diabetes should confirm that he/she considers the diver both mentally and physically capable of undertaking the demands of sport diving.

➡ The diver with diabetes should be prepared to give an annual lecture to his/her club on the problems associated with diabetes and diving.

➡ An SOS (Medic Alert) bracelet stating that the diver has diabetes should be worn at all times.

Tips when diving (modified from [239])

➡ To be able to experience obvious symptoms of hypoglycemia below 70 mg/dl (4.0 mmol/l) on the day of diving, you must take care to avoid having any readings below 70-90 mg/dl (4-5 mmol/l)) 1-2 weeks prior to the dive.

➡ *Never* dive if you have hypoglycemia unawareness or if you have had any readings below 65 mg/dl (3.5 mmol/l) within 24 hours of the dive (otherwise your hypoglycemic warning symptoms will be inadequate, see page 48).

➡ Don't drink alcohol within 24 hours of the dive.

➡ Eat more carbohydrate than usual on the day of the dive and drink enough not to be dehydrated.

➡ Dive after a meal. Leave at least 1-2 hours between your premeal insulin dose and diving if you are using rapid-acting insulin. Try decreasing the premeal dose by 1-2 units. The blood glucose level should be at least 145, preferably 180 mg/dl (8-10 mmol/l) when you start diving. Eat extra carbohydrate just before diving.

➡ Have 2 packets of glucose tablets or gel/liquid in the pockets of your wet suit and practice taking them out in water and under water. The nozzle of a tube of glucose gel/liquid can be placed between the mouthpiece of the demand valve and the corner of the mouth, thus avoiding the need to remove the mouthpiece from the mouth. Glucagon for injection should be readily available in the boat and on the shore and someone should be available who can give an emergency injection.

➡ Always dive with a friend or trained medic/paramedic who is capable of giving you adequate help (such as glucose under water) if you develop hypoglycemia. Your diving partner should *not* have diabetes.

➡ Decide on a signal in advance to indicate when you begin to feel hypoglycemic.

➡ Measure your blood glucose after the dive and take extra food or insulin. If you deliberately keep your blood glucose level slightly high when diving, you can take extra insulin if it is still high after the dive. This will prevent your A1C from being negatively affected by frequent diving. Be aware that you are at greater risk of hypoglycemia after heavy exertion and use only small doses of extra insulin.

level reasonably high (around 180-215 mg/dl, 10-12 mmol/l). This will help, as far as possible, to prevent hypoglycemia under water. Cold water increases the body's energy consumption. If your blood glucose level is high due to an insulin deficit, you will not feel well and diving will be dangerous, even life-threatening. You should also check for ketones in your blood or urine before you dive (see page 100). The message here is that it is much better to have a higher glucose level because of eating too much, rather than because your body has too little insulin.

Stress

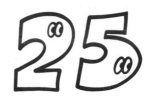

Stress and psychological strain affect your body and will at times increase the blood glucose level on account of the way different hormones behave. Different individuals are more or less sensitive to these reactions in their bodies.

When the body is exposed to stress, the adrenal glands secrete the hormone adrenaline which in turn increases the output of glucose from the liver. To explain this you must understand our Stone Age legacy. During this far off period, stress was usually associated with danger, for example an attacking bear. The alternatives were to stay and fight or to run away as quickly as possible. Extra fuel in the form of increased glucose in the blood is needed for both these responses.

Today, the same stress reaction can occur in front of the TV if you are watching something exciting, but you will not benefit from the increased blood glucose level. A person without diabetes will automatically release insulin from their pancreas to restore the glucose balance. In theory it is possible for a person with diabetes to take extra insulin in this situation. In practice this is often hard to accomplish since it is diffi-

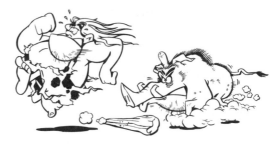

Your body is built to withstand the strenuous life of a Stone Age man or woman. In a stress situation, large amounts of adrenaline are secreted to help prepare the body for fight against, or flight away from, the danger.

cult to evaluate one's stress level, and the stress will be different from day to day. It is advisable to be careful when using extra insulin to treat high blood glucose levels caused by stress.

In one study, adults with diabetes performed a mental stress test for 20 minutes causing the blood glucose level to rise after one hour. It continued to be raised by about 35 mg/dl (2 mmol/l) for another 5 hours.[550] The blood pressure was increased as well and the stress induced a resistance to insulin (see page 195) via increased levels of the hormones adrenaline, cortisol and growth hormone. Patients who were able to produce some of their own insulin found the stress had less influence on their blood glucose level. After the earthquake in Kobe, A1C levels rose in people living in the affected area. The highest increase was found in those who had experienced the death or injury of a close relative, and those whose homes had been severely damaged.[401]

Studies of heart attack victims have shown that so-called positive stress is not as dangerous as other forms of stress. Positive stress is defined as the kind of tension that is produced when

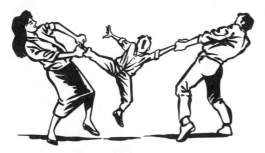

A divorce is always stressful for a child. If, instead of co-operating, the parents engage in a "tug of war" with the child, his or her situation will become very difficult. The child will feel bad in every sense and the blood glucose levels and A1C are likely to increase as a result.

Stress

⟹ Stress that cannot be influenced (such as problems in the family or at work) will have the greatest effect on your health.

⟹ Stress can also affect your blood glucose for the simple reason that you will not have as much time to care for your diabetes when life becomes busy and stressful.

⟹ Adrenaline (stress hormone) gives

① Increased blood glucose level by:
   A) Release of glucose from the liver.
   B) Decreased uptake of glucose into the cells.

② Ketones by:
   Breakdown of fat into fatty acids that are transformed into ketones in the liver.[463]

you have a lot to do, but you choose to do it yourself and you are in control of the situation. The type of negative stress that increases the risk for heart attack is when the person cannot influence the situation, for example, if they are having problems at work or at home within the family, such as relationship break-up or divorce. Similar situations may contribute to an increased blood glucose level as well. One of our patients was a little boy whose blood glucose level went up whenever an intravenous needle was inserted. The level remained elevated for several days in spite of increased insulin doses. It was the needle that bothered him. As soon as it was removed his blood glucose returned to normal and the insulin doses could be decreased again. In one study of adolescents, higher blood glucose levels were found after negative stress.[343]

Blood glucose readings taken at the hospital are often higher than those taken at home. Raised blood glucose levels have been observed in people with diabetes, in both outpatient [125] and inpatient [330] settings. This is also the case for blood pressure measurements, so called "white coat hypertension".

Stress in daily life

Everyday stress factors can cause a higher A1C.[153] For example, during school exams many people find that the stress causes higher blood glucose levels. The exams also involve a change to routines and you may forget to take your insulin, or forget to bring dextrose into the exams with you. It is not a good idea to take extra insulin before the exam, but when it is over, a small amount extra might well be justified.

Parents' stress reactions can be very important for children's psychological adjustment to diabetes. Metabolic control is better in families where the mother and, in particular, the child show initial injection anxiety and protest, but less generalized distress.[752] This implies that distress in itself makes adaptation more difficult and that families who focused their emotional upset on the practical aspects of the disease used problem-solving coping strategies. Since the daily management of diabetes involves such a great deal of practical application, it is probably necessary to control one's feelings in order to be more problem-focused.[752]

Learned helplessness is a phenomenon that can occur when you feel unable to control a situation and the reason for this is unrealistic expectations rather than insufficient ability on the part of the individual.[228] One example is when you follow every piece of advice given by the diabetes team and your blood glucose is still much too unstable. This "teaches" you that it is not possible to control your blood glucose and, after a while, you will stop trying. The reason for this is the unrealistic expectation that you can achieve a stable blood glucose level simply by "trying hard". This has also been called "diabetes burnout".[619] An example of a realistic expectation is that your blood glucose will swing between high and low values and that you will have at least one reading above 180 mg/dl (10 mmol/l) every day. It can be realistic to try to achieve a lower average blood glucose

Research findings:
Stress and A1C levels

♠ One study found that individuals with higher A1C levels reported poorer quality of life, and more anxiety and depression.[532]

♠ When the A1C value was increased or decreased during the scope of the study, the scores for quality of life, anxiety and depression changed accordingly.

♠ These results suggest that you will feel better with a lower A1C. However, another interpretation is that it is easier to obtain a good A1C when you feel well.

♠ Individuals who had experienced many severe stress factors (unpleasant life events, ongoing long-term problems, conflicts with other people) within the previous three months had higher A1C in one study.[497]

♠ Another study showed that stress causes a higher A1C but only in individuals who handle the stress in an ineffective way.[610] Anger, impatience and anxiety were examples of ineffective coping mechanisms. Stoicism (not reacting emotionally in stressful situations), pragmatism (handling stress in a problem-oriented way) and denial (disregarding the stress and thereby not letting it affect you) were effective coping mechanisms.

♠ However, in earlier studies, denial has been shown to have a correlation with impaired blood glucose control.[610] This might be explained by the fact that a problem must first be recognized before being solved. Appearing to accept a chronic disease initially, but then refusing to let it affect your daily life negatively, may be an effective form of denial.

♠ In an analysis of 24 studies (so called meta-analysis), depression in persons with diabetes was associated with a higher A1C.[514] However, it is difficult to conclude whether the elevated A1C is the result of depression or the other way around.

♠ Some data indicate that anti-depressive medication can improve A1C in people with depression.[514]

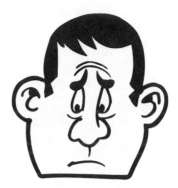

"Negative stress" is experienced when a person cannot change a stressful situation. Insurmountable problems at work, or at home within the family, may contribute to a raised blood glucose level.

(A1C) without laying yourself open to an increase in hypoglycemia-related problems. Realistic expectations for the long term might include being able to manage school or work, for example, without being inconvenienced to any great extent by your diabetes.

Fever and sick days

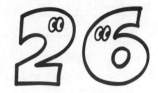

If you have an infection, especially with fever, the secretion of blood glucose-raising hormones (particularly cortisol and glucagon [793]) is increased. This effectively also increases your insulin requirements. However, it is common to eat less and rest more when you are ill, so these factors usually balance each other out. The basic rule, therefore, is to resist decreasing your insulin doses despite a drop in food intake.

Start by taking your usual dose. Measure your blood glucose level before each meal and adjust the dose before eating. If your blood glucose level is above 180 mg/dl (10 mmol/l) you can increase by one unit at a time (half a unit if your premeal dose is less than 3 U, two units if it is greater than 10 U) until your readings are better.

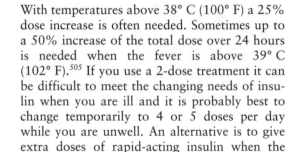

With temperatures above 38° C (100° F) a 25% dose increase is often needed. Sometimes up to a 50% increase of the total dose over 24 hours is needed when the fever is above 39° C (102° F).[505] If you use a 2-dose treatment it can be difficult to meet the changing needs of insulin when you are ill and it is probably best to change temporarily to 4 or 5 doses per day while you are unwell. An alternative is to give extra doses of rapid-acting insulin when the blood glucose is high (see algorithm on page 133).

Feeling ill or well?

① **Feeling well**

⟹ Start out with your need for food and your appetite.

⟹ Adjust your insulin dose in relation to the size of the meal.

⟹ Aim not to let the blood glucose level rise too much.

② **Feeling ill**

⟹ Start out with your need for insulin.

⟹ Take your usual insulin dose to begin with (unless your blood glucose is low, or you have diarrhoea) and make sure that you can eat enough to supply the insulin with carbohydrates "to work with".

⟹ Aim at preventing your blood glucose level from falling too low by drinking something sugary when necessary.

Illness and need for insulin

⟹ Fever increases the need for insulin.

⟹ **But** — decreased appetite and food intake decrease the need for insulin.

⟹ **Thus** — you will probably have at least the same need for insulin/24 hours as usual.

⟹ **You are likely to** need up to 25-50% more insulin when you are feverish.

⟹ You could also be at risk from **ketoacidosis** caused by insulin deficiency. Check for ketones in your blood or urine!

⟹ **But** — you may need less insulin if you have gastroenteritis with vomiting *and* diarrhea.

> ## IMPORTANT!!
> *Do not adjust insulin doses "by eye" or by carbohydrate counting when you are ill!*

During the remission phase (honeymoon phase, see pages 193 and 157), the insulin doses often need to be increased considerably if you are unwell. A child will usually need up to 1 U/kg/24 hours (1 U/2.2 lb), sometimes more, an adult slightly less. The rapid increase in need for insulin is due to the fact that your own pancreas no longer contributes substantial amounts of insulin.

Good glucose control increases the body's defense against infections. Document your blood glucose and ketone readings (as well as insulin doses) in your logbook and contact your diabetes healthcare team or the hospital if you are in the least unsure about your condition or how to handle the situation. This is equally, if not more, important advice for the parents of children with diabetes.

The increased insulin requirements during illness (e.g. a cold with fever) usually last for a few days, but sometimes they can last up to a week after recovery. This is due to the increased blood glucose level which, in turn, gives rise to increased insulin resistance (see page 195 and graphs on page 198). Sometimes there are increased insulin requirements during the incubation period for a few days before the onset of the illness.[700]

> ### Diabetes and illness in children
> (adapted from [701])
>
> ① **Treat the current illness**
> The reason for the child's illness must be diagnosed and treated in the same way as for children without diabetes.
>
> ② **Symptomatic treatment**
> If the child has a fever or headache, paracetamol/acetaminophen (Tylenol®, Tempra®, Panadol®) or ibuprofen (Advil®, Motrin®) can be given to relieve symptoms.The child will feel better and often have a better appetite.
>
> ③ **Staying home from school**
> It is advisable to let a sick child with diabetes stay at home as blood glucose levels are affected by infection and fever.
>
> ④ **Fluid balance**
> It is important to give plenty of liquids to a child who is running a temperature, especially if they also have a high blood glucose level (>215-270 mg/dl, 12-15 mmol/l) as this will cause them to produce larger volumes of urine than usual. The risk of dehydration may increase rapidly if the child vomits or has diarrhea.
>
> ⑤ **Nutrition**
> It is important that the child gets insulin, sugar and nourishment. Serve something the child enjoys and is likely to eat.

If the child does not feel like eating regular meals you should still try to convince him or her to eat regular amounts of carbohydrates. Offer food the child likes, such as ice cream, fruit or soup.

Nausea and vomiting

Nausea and vomiting are common symptoms of many "bugs" and illnesses, particularly in children. At the same time, nausea and vomiting in a child with diabetes can often be the first signs of insulin deficiency. This is why it is always important to check both blood glucose and

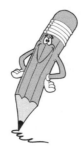

Write down all insulin doses and test results in your logbook. You will find it easier to adjust insulin doses and food intake next time you are faced with the same situation. Make a note of how many units you have taken over 24 hours. This is the best way of measuring how the illness has affected your diabetes.

Insulin treatment during sick days (except gastroenteritis)

➥ Always start out by taking your usual dose (except when you have gastroenteritis).

➥ Monitor your blood glucose before each meal and in between when needed. **Check for ketones regularly.**

➥ Adjust insulin doses according to the results of the blood tests. Increase the premeal doses by 1-2 units when needed (see text for guidelines).

➥ Give extra insulin (preferably rapid-acting NovoLog/NovoRapid or Humalog) 0.1 unit/kg (0.5 units/10 lb) body weight if the blood glucose is more than 250 mg/dl (14 mmol/l) and you have elevated levels of ketones in the blood or urine. Repeat the dose if the blood glucose level has not decreased after 2-3 hours.

➥ An alternative rule is to give an additional dose of 10-20% of your total daily insulin dose every 3-4 hours.

➥ Contact your diabetes healthcare team or the hospital if you start vomiting or if your general condition is affected.

How do different illnesses affect blood glucose? (adapted from [701])

① **Not much influence at all**
Illnesses that have no significant effect on your general condition do not usually affect your insulin requirements either. Examples are common colds without fever and chickenpox with few symptoms (in children).

② **Low blood glucose levels**
These illnesses are characterized by difficulties in retaining nutrients due to nausea, vomiting and/or diarrhea. Examples are gastroenteritis or a viral infection with abdominal pain.

③ **High blood glucose levels**
Most illnesses that give obvious distress and fever will increase the blood glucose levels, thereby increasing the need for insulin. If insulin doses are not increased when the blood glucose level rises, there may be a risk of developing ketoacidosis. Examples are colds with fever, otitis (inflammation of the ear), urinary infection with fever or pneumonia. A genital herpes infection may also result in a substantial increase in insulin requirements.[749]

ketone levels when these symptoms appear. If the blood glucose level is high and ketones are present, the child is probably feeling nauseous on account of insulin deficiency. The insulin level may not be high enough, despite the usual doses being taken, because an intercurrent illness can increase the body's need for insulin.

If, on the other hand, the blood glucose level is low, the illness itself is probably contributing to the nausea. Ketones may still be present in the blood or urine as a sign of a lack of food (carbohydrates) when the child has no appetite and can then contribute to the nausea.

The same principal also applies with adults. If you feel nauseous while you are ill, and if you eat less, it is important that the food you do eat

contains sugar and carbohydrates, both to give your body nourishment and to lessen the risk of hypoglycemia. The nausea will usually get worse if you drink large amounts of liquid at one sitting. It is better to drink small amounts frequently, for example a couple of sips every 10 minutes. Oral rehydration solution (ORS), available at the pharmacy, is very useful in this situation, particularly if you are caring for a

Remember to check both blood glucose and ketones in your blood or urine frequently when you are ill! Always carry on taking your insulin, and make sure you eat or drink something containing carbohydrates.

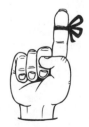

The signs that tell you when to go to hospital (adapted from [701])

The signs that tell you when to go to hospital (adapted from [701])

⟹ Voluminous or repeated vomiting.

⟹ Increasing levels of ketones in the blood or urine, or laboured breathing.

⟹ Blood glucose levels remaining high despite extra insulin.

⟹ It is unclear what the underlying problem might be.

⟹ Severe or unusual abdominal pain.

⟹ Confusion, or a deterioration of general well-being.

⟹ The sick person is a young child (2-3 years old or under) or has another disease besides diabetes.

⟹ Exhaustion on the part of the person or their carer, for example due to repeated night time waking.

⟹ Always call if you are in the least unsure about how to manage the situation.

sick child with diabetes. However, older children may not accept the taste (since it is quite salty). Try adding some juice to improve its taste. Sports drinks such as Gatorade can be helpful in this situation as they already contain both glucose and salts, thus helping to prevent dehydration and salt imbalance. A small dose of metoclopramide (Reglan®, Maxolon®, Clopra®, Octamide®) can be helpful in preventing vomiting.

If a child with diabetes vomits and cannot keep liquids down, you should contact your diabetes healthcare team or emergency ward!

It is very important to give insulin, even if the child cannot eat regular meals. Give something sweet to drink, so that the blood glucose level will not fall. *Make sure that the drink contains real sugar.* Children usually like juice, fruit smoothies or ice cream and will take at least small helpings of these foods without problems. Sugar-free drinks should not be used at all in this situation but extra water can be given, especially with fever, once enough sugary drink has been taken to keep the blood glucose level up.

Gastroenteritis

Gastroenteritis is an infection of the intestinal tract, which usually causes both vomiting and diarrhea. Very little nourishment will stay in the body and there are generally problems with low blood glucose levels, and you will need to lower the insulin doses considerably. Gastroenteritis and food poisoning are therefore exceptions to the rule that the need for insulin will increase during illness. This reduction in need for insulin is likely to go on for some time (often 1-2 weeks) after the gastroenteritis has been cured, as the low blood glucose levels cause a drop in insulin resistance (increased insulin sensitivity, see graph on page 199).

A slower emptying of the stomach [52] contributes to a low blood glucose level when a person has gastroenteritis. You may need to lower the insulin doses by 20-50% in order to avoid hypoglycemia. For prolonged problems with low blood glucose, repeated mini-doses of glucagon can be helpful (see page 36).

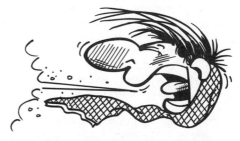

A cold with fever increases your insulin requirements, often up to 25%, sometimes even up to 50%. Begin by increasing all your doses by 1-2 units if your blood glucose levels are high. Increase further if needed, depending on results from blood glucose and ketone tests.

Insulin and gastroenteritis in children

Make sure that it really is gastroenteritis:

➠ Vomiting *and* diarrhea.

➠ Low blood glucose levels.

➠ Slight or moderate elevation of levels of ketones in blood (see page 101) or urine. The blood level of starvation ketones seldom exceeds 3 mmol/l. In adults, eating 150-200 g carbohydrate daily (45-50 g every 3-4 hours) will reduce or prevent starvation ketones.[274]

① Always call the hospital if it is the first time your child has gastroenteritis after developing diabetes or if you are in the least unsure about what to do. If your child is vomiting repeatedly, you should go to the hospital. He or she might require treatment with intravenous fluids and insulin in this situation.

② Give a drink containing real sugar *(not "light" or "diet" drinks!)* in small and frequent portions (several sips every 10-15 minutes) when the child feels nauseous or is vomiting. Suitable drinks include fruit juice, tea with sugar and oral rehydration solution and sports drinks, such as Gatorade. Write down how much fluid the child has taken.

③ Measure blood glucose every other hour (every hour if at risk for hypoglycemia) and check the blood or urine for ketones every 1-2 hours.

④ If prolonged low blood glucose is a problem, the best approach may be to inject a small dose of glucagon, (see page 36). The dose can be repeated with good effect.

⑤ The insulin doses usually need to be lowered. There will be a balance between how much the child can eat and how much the insulin should be lowered. Low blood glucose levels will increase the insulin sensitivity (decreased insulin resistance, see page 195) and the doses usually need to be lowered by 20-50%. If the child uses a 2 dose treatment, start by decreasing the short-acting insulin which at times may even be omitted. The intermediate-acting insulin may need to be decreased as well.

⑥ Begin with solid food as soon as the vomiting decreases or stops.

Vomiting but no diarrhea?

Beware! Remember that nausea and vomiting are often symptoms of insulin deficiency.

Vomiting without diarrhea should always prompt you to suspect insulin deficiency. This also causes high blood glucose levels and elevated levels of ketones in the blood or urine. See also "Not enough insulin?" on page 27 and "Ketones" on page 99.

Remember to drink plenty of fluids containing sugar, but take small sips at a time as long as you are feeling nauseous or vomiting. When you have stopped vomiting, you can start taking ordinary food. However, we no longer recommend the diet that used to be prescribed after gastroenteritis (boiled fish, rice, toast etc.). This diet meant it was often difficult to obtain enough glucose and calories, so is rarely (if ever) used now. It is better to eat what you like. The only exception is milk for small children. If diarrhea continues to be a problem, milk and milk products should be excluded from the child's diet for a week or two.

Be aware that vomiting can often be a symptom of insulin deficiency which should be treated with increased insulin doses.

You should check both the blood glucose and the ketone levels (in blood or urine) if you, or a child with diabetes, feels nauseous or vomits. If you are short of insulin, your blood glucose level will be high and the ketone test will show high readings. Extra doses of rapid-acting insulin are urgently required to prevent ketoacidosis. Talk to your diabetes doctor or nurse about the results before changing any doses if you are not sure about how to interpret them.

Wound healing

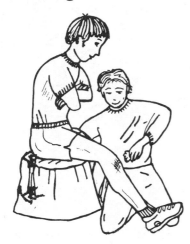

It is commonly believed that when people with diabetes injure their feet, they will heal more slowly and because of this regular podiatric care is needed. This is certainly true for individuals who have had diabetes for many years, and who are beginning to suffer from complications in the form of reduced circulation and loss of feeling in the feet and toes (see also page 311). However, if a child or young person with diabetes is injured, and the blood glucose control is good, the wound will heal just as well as it would in anyone else of the same age, provided good care is taken to prevent the wound from becoming infected.

On the other hand, the body's defense system will not work as well as it should if the diabetes is uncontrolled and the blood glucose level high. This will increase even young people's susceptibility to infection.[474]

Surgery

People with diabetes should be taken care of in hospital if they need surgery, even if the operation is only a minor one. The operation should be scheduled for as early in the day as possible. During operations of more than 20-30 minutes with general anesthesia, it is advisable to give insulin intravenously (see page 69).[431,611] This system is very easy to adjust and will ensure appropriate blood glucose and insulin levels throughout the operation and during the recovery phase. During shorter operations, it is better to continue with the ordinary basal insulin, which can be supplemented with intravenous insulin, if necessary. When the person can eat and drink again, they can return to their usual method of insulin administration. It is important to adjust the insulin doses carefully during and after surgery, since high blood glucose levels (over 200-230 mg/dl, 11-13 mmol/l) have been found to increase the risk of infections after surgery.[307]

If your child is admitted to a pediatric surgical ward, you should be put in touch with a pediatric diabetes team to discuss appropriate insulin treatment. As parents of a child with diabetes, you have every right to express your own views on the treatment. Remember that your knowledge about your child's diabetes is likely to be much more extensive than that of the staff on a surgical ward.

It would also be appropriate to ensure that you, along with the anesthesiologist and all members

---

Take care of small wounds and poor friends... (Swedish saying)

☞ Wash the wound with soap and water.

☞ Apply a clean, dry dressing.

☞ Signs of infection? See a doctor!

① Pain / throbbing from the wound after the first 1-2 days.

② Increasing redness of the skin.

③ Red streak in the skin going from the wound towards the body (infection of the lymph vessel).

④ Painful nodule in the groin or armpit (infected or inflamed lymph node).

⑤ Fever

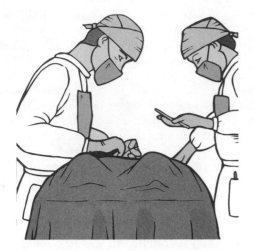

During surgery it is advisable to administer insulin intravenously. This is a convenient and safe way to obtain a stable blood glucose level without risking hypoglycemia.

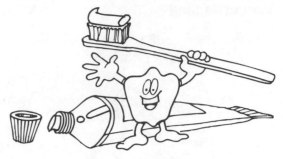

Even if you eat less candy than your friends, you are at risk of tooth decay. This is caused by glucose in the saliva when your blood glucose level is high. Don't forget to brush your teeth at least twice a day.

of the operating team, can contact your diabetes team in the case of any elective surgery. This will help to ensure that diabetes care and appropriate monitoring, as well as insulin adjustment, can be carried out effectively. For emergencies, it would be appropriate to insist that the diabetes team physician on emergency call be contacted, if at all possible, or the local diabetologists or endocrinologists contacted, as a minimum. It is important for teenagers to be accompanied by a parent to help them keep track of their blood glucose levels.

Drugs that affect blood glucose

Drugs that contain sugar can affect blood glucose. However, the sugar content is often low enough not to raise the blood glucose appreciably. If a medication is given with a meal, 5 g (1/6 ounce) of extra sugar is unlikely to make a noticeable difference to the blood glucose level. If it does rise, however, you can give a small extra dose of insulin (½-1 unit/10 g of sugar).

Other drugs may affect the glucose level without containing sugar. Treatment with cortisol or other steroids (e.g. prednisolone, dexamethasone) causes a marked increase in the blood glucose level, often to above 360 mg/dl (20 mmol/l). This can happen even when the steroid is given as a single dose, for example to treat asthma or croup. When taking cortisol medication for several days or longer, the insulin doses need to be increased considerably. The total dose for a 24 hour period often needs to be doubled, increasing both the premeal doses and the intermediate or long-acting insulin. Steroids for inhalation affect glucose levels far less. At times, a slight increase in glucose levels is seen as a small amount of the given drug is absorbed into the bloodstream. You should try to find the lowest possible dose that is effective for the asthmatic disease. It may be advantageous to take the maintenance dose at bedtime. This will make it easier for you to increase your bedtime insulin if necessary to counteract the effect of the steroids. In acute severe asthma, the combination of beta-sympathomimetics, such as salbutamol, with prednisolone often raises the blood glucose level considerably.

Teeth

It is a good idea to see your dentist regularly, and ask for advice about your dental hygiene so that you can minimize any risk for damage. Be sure to tell your dentist that you have diabetes!

It is unusual for children with diabetes to have more tooth decay (dental caries) than other children. On the contrary, they often have fewer such problems than many children of the same age.[447] It might be seen as surprising that they have any decay at all, as they often eat less candy than their friends. The explanation may be that children with diabetes eat snacks regularly. In addition, they might often need to take dextrose or something else with sugar if they become hypoglycemic, and this contributes to an increased number of bacteria in the oral cavity. One study on adults, found that the subjects who had diabetes had the same amount of caries as those in the control group who did not have diabetes.[746]

Another contributing explanation is that glucose is excreted into the saliva when the blood glucose level is high, and this may contribute further to cavities.[746] The saliva would not normally contain glucose but, if the blood glucose level is above a certain threshold, increased amounts of glucose will be found in the saliva. In this sense a person with very high or variable blood glucose level has a higher risk of tooth decay. Unfortunately the agreement between the glucose level in blood and saliva is not very good, so it not possible to use tests on saliva to estimate the blood glucose level.[746]

Gingivitis is an inflammation of the gums caused by bacteria accumulating in the tooth sockets. The bacterial deposits on the teeth harden into tartar. The gums go red and bleed when you brush your teeth. Gingivitis and periodontal disease are slightly more common in people who have diabetes than in people who don't, even in young people.[615] They are also more common when the blood glucose level is high. People with diabetes may also find their gingivitis progresses more rapidly, and causes more damage than it does in people who don't have diabetes. Periodontal disease is also more common in smokers.

Removal of the wisdom teeth is a common procedure usually carried out on older teenagers or

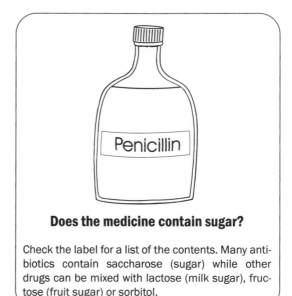

Does the medicine contain sugar?

Check the label for a list of the contents. Many antibiotics contain saccharose (sugar) while other drugs can be mixed with lactose (milk sugar), fructose (fruit sugar) or sorbitol.

young adults. If the person concerned has diabetes, however, the dentist will need to take special precautions. The procedure is often carried out on a "walk in" outpatient basis, or "in the dentist's chair". The dentist or oral surgeon should have a formal protocol to follow when treating a person with diabetes as you will need intravenous glucose treatment during the procedure, and possibly insulin as well. Your insulin dose is likely to be adjusted in advance, but make sure you know what is happening and who is responsible for monitoring your blood glucose levels and making any necessary changes to your insulin dose. For a procedure such as this, it is essential that you ensure everyone involved in treating you knows well in advance that you have diabetes.

Vaccinations

Children with diabetes should have the same vaccinations as other children. See page 295 for more information about vaccinations when travelling abroad.

Smoking

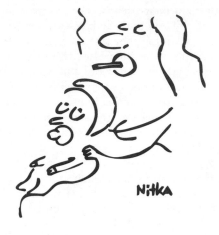

Everyone knows that smoking is unhealthy. Despite this, a large number of people smoke while nobody seems to care. While we don't seem to be very concerned about this aspect of smoking from a moral point of view, many people with diabetes feel that society at large employs double standards by disapproving of them for eating "the wrong sort of food" but completely ignoring people with all sorts of health problems who smoke. For example, if a person with diabetes stands in a line to buy candy, others seem to feel it is perfectly acceptable to act as "candy police", and stare at them as if they are thinking "you are not allowed to do that". Many will even make hurtful comments. On the other hand, if a smoker is standing in the same line to buy cigarettes, nobody will say anything despite the fact that smoking can cause even more health problems than excessive candy-eating in a person with diabetes.

About the same number of people with diabetes smoke as do other people. And smoking results in a substantially increased risk for lung cancer, chronic bronchitis and diseases of the heart and blood vessels. Having diabetes, in itself, puts you at increased risk of heart and blood vessel diseases such as arteriosclerosis, heart attacks and stroke. In diabetes the risks are cumulative. If you imagine diabetes as a balancing act on a slack rope, smoking may be the extra factor that tips you over. Many studies in adults confirm that the risk of premature death for a person with diabetes who smokes is 1.5-2 times that of a person with diabetes who does not smoke. But research also indicates that giving up smoking reduces this risk.[139,564]

At the 1994 World Congress on Tobacco it was established that every second smoker will die from a disease that is connected with smoking. Smoking was called the greatest epidemic of the 20th century causing more deaths than both the plague and AIDS. A 14-year old who has begun smoking should be treated like a contagious tuberculosis patient, considering the risk that such a person can influence other teenagers to start smoking too!

Nicotine from smoking affects the blood glucose level by contracting the blood vessels, resulting in a slower absorption of insulin from

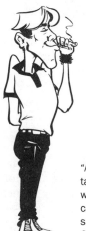

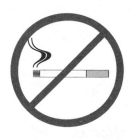

"A 14-year old smoker is about as contagious as a patient with tuberculosis, when you consider the risk that he/she can entice other adolescents to start smoking" (message at the 1994 World Congress on Tobacco).

the injection site.[451,454] Nicotine will also cause increased insulin resistance [43,244] (a poorer blood glucose lowering effect of a given dose of insulin), which makes diabetes more difficult to manage (see page 195). The risk of acquiring type 2 diabetes is twice as high for a person who smokes, especially if that person is a woman.[564]

Smoking causes the inhalation of carbon monoxide, which binds strongly to hemoglobin in the red blood cells and prevents oxygen from binding to them. The number of red blood cells increases to compensate for this. Scientific studies show that in a person with diabetes, smoking increases the risk of renal failure, visual impairment, foot ulcers, leg amputations and heart attacks.[561,564,675]

Passive smoking

Even passive smoking will damage your health. It has been shown that children absorb nicotine into their bloodstream at twice the rate of adults through smoking passively. Smaller children are even more sensitive. Children of smoking parents also have increased levels of lead and cadmium in their blood. Smoking near an extractor fan (e.g. in the kitchen) will not prevent smoke from spreading into the house. It has been claimed this is "about as effective as urinating in a corner of a swimming pool."

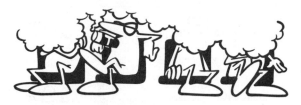

Passive smoking is dangerous to your health. Small children are often exposed to passive smoking by their parents. One woman who never had smoked developed a fatal type of lung cancer normally seen only in smokers. It was established that she had developed her cancer because people were smoking in the room where she worked.

Giving up smoking

The easiest way to give up is never to start. Most smokers have started in their teens. It is difficult to withstand the "peer pressure" but it can save many years of your life. Besides, giving up smoking will save you a lot of money.

It may be difficult to quit smoking on your own. Your diabetes healthcare team can help you with advice and nicotine chewing gum or patches that may be effective. However, unless you are motivated yourself, you will never succeed in giving up! In one study the A1C levels decreased from 7.7% to 7.0% in a group of people with diabetes who ceased smoking.[322] There is a risk that you will put on weight when

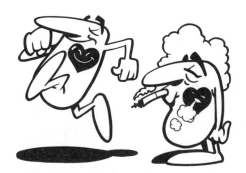

You will stay much more healthy if you give up smoking!

Can you die from smoking?

Statistics presented at the 1994 World Congress on Tobacco [608] estimated that out of 1.000 20-year old habitual smokers:

➠ 1 will be murdered.

➠ 6 will die in traffic accidents.

➠ 250 will die in middle age from smoking-related diseases.

➠ 250 will die in older age from smoking-related diseases.

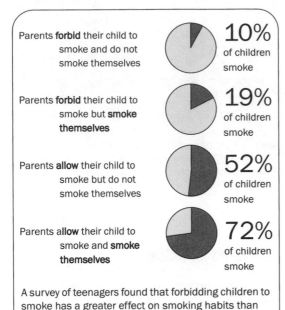

Parents **forbid** their child to smoke and do not smoke themselves

10% of children smoke

Parents **forbid** their child to smoke but **smoke themselves**

19% of children smoke

Parents **allow** their child to smoke but do not smoke themselves

52% of children smoke

Parents **allow** their child to smoke and **smoke themselves**

72% of children smoke

A survey of teenagers found that forbidding children to smoke has a greater effect on smoking habits than whether or not parents smoke themselves.[1]

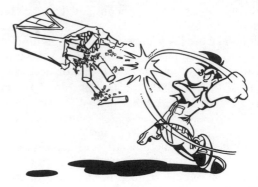

It is never too late to give up smoking. For every day without a cigarette, the damaging effects of tobacco in your body are reduced.

you stop smoking, but this will not necessarily happen. So it may depend on how you go about trying to quit. You should talk to your diabetes health care team for specific advice to maximize your chances of success while minimizing your chances of any adverse effects during the actual process of giving up.

Snuff

In Sweden 30% of all men under the age of 30 use snuff and it is common in other countries as well. Nicotine from snuff is absorbed through the oral lining as quickly as from an intravenous injection. Whether you smoke it or sniff it, nicotine has strong effects on your heart, blood vessels and blood pressure. It may increase the risk for kidney damage when having diabetes.[251] The addiction to nicotine is just as strong as that for cocaine or heroin. Because of nicotine addiction, it is just as difficult, if not more so, to give up snuff as it is to give up smoking.

Alcohol

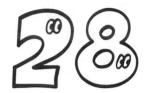

We do not recommend a total ban on drinking alcohol if you have diabetes. However, it is important to know how alcohol works and that you take it easy, making sure you stop drinking before you get drunk. If you are not old enough to be able to drink legally, your parents should have the final say about whether or not you can drink. The age when you are allowed to buy alcohol differs from state to state. Your diabetes team can neither allow you to do something, nor forbid it. They can only tell you how things work and where and why you should be particularly careful.

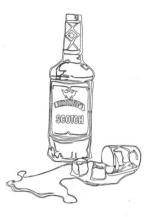

Alcohol and the liver

Alcohol counteracts the ability of the liver to produce new glucose (a process called gluconeogenesis) by keeping the enzymes occupied with the breakdown of alcohol.[45] The liver can still release glucose from the glycogen store (see page 32) but when this is depleted you will experience hypoglycemia.[45] The concentration of cortisol and growth hormone in the blood will decrease after alcohol intake.[45] Both hormones have an enhancing effect on the blood glucose level, and this appears 3-4 hours after they are released into the bloodstream (see page 31). This will contribute to an increased risk of hypoglycemia many hours after alcohol intake. The liver's ability to produce free fatty acids will also be impaired.[45] These biological factors come together, making the risk of hypoglycemia much greater after drinking alcohol. This effect of alcohol will last the entire time it takes the liver to break down the alcohol in your body. The liver will break down 0.1 g (1.5 grains) of pure alcohol/kg body weight per hour. For example, if you weigh 70 kg (155 lb) it will take one hour to break down the alcohol in a bottle of light beer, two hours for 40 ml of liquor and 10 hours to break down the alcohol in a bottle

of wine. Therefore, if you drink during the evening you will be at risk of hypoglycemia all night as well as part of the next day.

Why is it dangerous to be drunk with diabetes?

When you have diabetes you must be able to think clearly in many situations, so you can take the correct amount of insulin at the right time and be aware of feeling unwell if your insulin levels are low or you are becoming hypoglycemic. You cannot do this if you have had too much to drink, in exactly the same way as you cannot drive a car safely after taking more than a small amount of alcohol. Severe hypoglycemia after drinking alcohol has caused the death of young people with diabetes on rare occasions. Scientific studies show the role of alcohol in causing hypoglycemia has more to do with losing the ability to recognize the signs of impending hypoglycemia than with reducing the liver's ability to produce glucose.[285,440,455]

In one study, people with diabetes drank either white wine (approximately 600 ml, 3 average-sized glasses) or water 2-3 hours after the

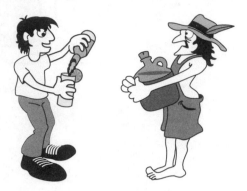

It is not dangerous for an adult person with diabetes to drink a glass or two, but if you drink too much you will find it difficult to think clearly...

evening snack.[770] The morning blood glucose was 55-70 mg/dl (3-4 mmol/l) lower after drinking wine and five of the six individuals experienced symptomatic hypoglycemia 2-4 hours after breakfast. This suggests it is advisable to be prepared for late-morning hypoglycemia after an evening spent drinking, and it is advisable to lower the insulin dose both at bedtime and before breakfast.

Basic rules

For a person with diabetes, the intake should be limited to one drink (defined as a 12-oz. beer, 5-oz. glass of wine, or 1.5 oz. glass of distilled spirits) for women and two drinks for men in one day.[274] Make sure that your friends know you have diabetes and wear some type of diabetes ID (necklace or Medic-Alert bracelet) when you are socializing. Always eat something at the same time as you are drinking alcohol. Remember that what you eat should be "long-acting" carbohydrates as the risk of hypoglycemia extends into the next day. Alcohol containing sugar (liqueur, for example) will cause your blood glucose level to rise for a short time, but then it will drop and you will be at risk of hypoglycemia. A glass of beer contains about the same amount of carbohydrate as a glass of milk. Adults with diabetes can drink moderate amounts of alcohol if they eat food at the same time. If an adult drinks one or two glasses of wine or 2-3 fluid oz. (60-80 ml) of liquor along with food for dinner, it will not increase the risk of hypoglycemia during the night.[113]

It takes a long time for your liver to break down alcohol, which increases the risk of severe hypoglycemia. Because of this, sleeping late is particularly dangerous the morning after you have been drinking. If you have also been espe-

Alcohol and calories

Drink	Alcohol content	Kcal	Carb. g
1 bottle, (12 fluid ounces)			
Non-alcoholic beer	<0.5%	~60	~16
Low alcohol beer	0.5-1.2%	~40	~7
Light Beer	~3-5%	~90	~5
Beer	>4%	~160	~13
1 glass, (5 fluid ounces)			
Red wine	9.9%	114	3.5
White wine, dry	9.5%	99	0.7
White wine, sweet	10.7%	147	8.9
(2 fluid ounces)			
Sherry	16%	91	6
(1.5 fluid ounce)			
Vodka	32%	100	0
Whisky	32%	100	0
Punch	20%	132	14
Liqueur	19%	150	24

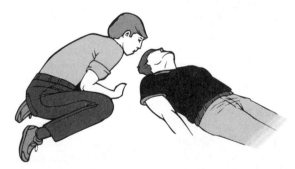

If you develop severe hypoglycemia after drinking alcohol, the person finding you is likely to assume that you are simply drunk. Especially if you don't wear a pump, it is essential that you wear a Medic-Alert necklace/bracelet. (You can also carry an ID card, but it will likely not be discovered as promptly.)

cially active, playing team games or dancing at a club for example, the combined risks of extra activity with alcohol intake put you at much greater risk than usual of severe hypoglycemia. Under such circumstances, preventing hypoglycemia becomes imperative.

What if you've had too much to drink?

Eat extra food immediately before going to bed. You can eat potato chips in this situation as they give a slow increase in blood glucose over several hours (see page 53). The blood glucose level should not be less than 180 mg/dl (10 mmol/l) when you go to bed. Decrease the dose of bedtime insulin by 2-4 units to avoid hypoglycemia. Don't go to bed alone; if you have severe hypoglycemia during the night you will need someone to help you. If you come home very late, make sure to wake a parent or partner, and let them know about your condition. Your life may actually depend upon it, even if you find the situation embarrassing. Set your alarm clock. Don't sleep in late! Be sure to eat a proper breakfast as soon as you wake up the next morning If you feel nauseous, check your blood glucose level. It may be caused by high glucose levels rather than a hangover.

You also need to understand that even giving a glucagon injection may be less effective in correcting severe hypoglycemia in this situation because the liver will be "busy" breaking down the alcohol and therefore unable to respond and raise the blood glucose levels.[274] This is because alcohol counteracts glucagon's ability to

If you are under the age when it is legal for you to drink alcohol, remember that the staff at your diabetes team can neither give you permission nor prohibit you to drink alcohol. This is something to be discussed with your parents. What they can do is to tell you how alcohol affects your body if you have diabetes and what the risks might be.

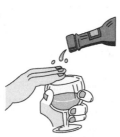

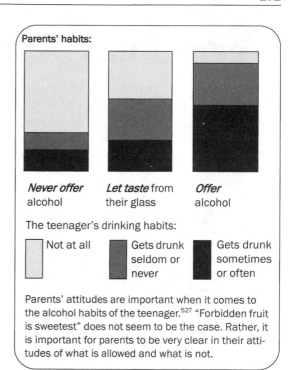

Parents' habits:

| *Never offer* alcohol | *Let taste* from their glass | *Offer* alcohol |

The teenager's drinking habits:

☐ Not at all   ▨ Gets drunk seldom or never   ■ Gets drunk sometimes or often

Parents' attitudes are important when it comes to the alcohol habits of the teenager.[527] "Forbidden fruit is sweetest" does not seem to be the case. Rather, it is important for parents to be very clear in their attitudes of what is allowed and what is not.

increase the production of glucose in the liver. If a person becomes unconscious or has seizures due to hypoglycemia following alcohol intake, they may need to be put on a glucose drip in hospital.

Can you drink at home?

Many assume that "stolen pleasures are sweetest", i.e. that it is better for teenagers to try alcohol at home under parental supervision than to sneak a drink on the quiet. However, studies have shown that more children start drinking alcohol if you have a permissive attitude towards trying alcohol in the home. A total prohibition of alcohol for teenagers seems to have a better preventative effect than the idea that it is advisable to test at home.[527] The same is true for smoking.[1] Whether or not parents allowed experimenting in the home had a greater impact in these studies than if the parents drank alcohol or smoked.

Illegal drugs

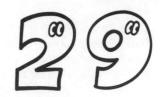

Drugs affect the brain and nervous systems and will make it much more difficult to manage something like diabetes. Many drugs make you forgetful and the risk of ketoacidosis (diabetic coma) will increase if you have not taken enough insulin or missed your injections. A person taking drugs is at high risk of developing hypoglycemia since drugs make you think less clearly. If friends know about your diabetes and how to treat hypoglycemia, they may be able to help (unless they also are too heavily affected by drugs or alcohol). Unless the drug user wears a diabetes ID, it may take some time to get appropriate help, even if the police or ambulance staff intervene.

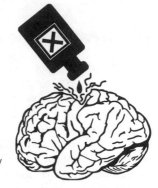

Illegal drugs act as poisons on your brain, and are likely to be extremely addictive.

Narcotics and other illegal drugs are likely to be very addictive, so if you start using them you will have great difficulty giving up without help. If you have diabetes, you must understand that it is completely inappropriate from a medical point of view, as well as extremely risky to use, or even try, any type of illegal drug.

Certain drugs may have specific extra risks associated with the blood vessels. Amphetamine is known to damage the linings of blood vessels [519] thereby increasing the short-term and long-term risks of diabetes complications. Many people who are drug users would find it extremely difficult to take good care of themselves and their diabetes while continuing their drug use, because of the behavioral aspects of drug use. Casual drug users would have the same problems as those of other medications that interfere with rational self-care at the time.

Marijuana

Use of marijuana (cannabis, hash, blow, weed) is often viewed as less harmful than the use of "hard drugs" such as heroin, cocaine or amphetamines. In terms of making rational decisions about complex activities such as driving or diabetes self-management, marijuana is likely to be at least as risky as alcohol. Combining marijuana with alcohol (as often happens) adds special risks for making diabetes-related decisions about, for example, when to wake up the next day. Many people who take marijuana find themselves becoming especially hungry and want to eat everything in sight, especially junk food (the "munchies") which will raise the blood glucose level considerably.

"Uppers"

Uppers like amphetamine (speed, whizz, sulph), ecstasy (E, eckies, doves), and cocaine (coke, charlie, snow) are used to give more energy and confidence and have been popular at rave parties. There is a risk of dehydration when the body loses fluid through continuous dancing or other strenuous activity. Uppers can suppress appetite, and combined with dancing there is a risk of experiencing severe hypoglycemia. In this sense these drugs can be extremely dangerous for a person with diabetes, especially if not enough extra fluid is taken or the extra bedtime snack is forgotten.

Pregnancy and sexual issues

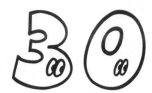

One of the first things a girl with diabetes and her family will ask is whether she will be able to have babies. Being pregnant exerts a certain strain on every woman, but there is no reason to discourage women with diabetes from having children. The mother's risk of developing diabetes complications later in life is not affected by pregnancy.[68]

Of the children born in UK and US, approximately 0.3% have a mother with diabetes.[108,347] About 90% of these mothers have type 1 diabetes.[69] Gestational diabetes (a temporary form of diabetes occurring during pregnancy) affects 3-5% of pregnancies.[712] The symptoms of diabetes usually disappear after the birth but these women have an increased risk (40-60%) of acquiring type 2 diabetes later in life.[155,587]

If the woman has good glucose control with an A1C similar to that of a person without diabetes at the time the baby is conceived and during early pregnancy, the risk of birth defects or miscarriage is no greater than average.[196,449,727] This is the case even if the mother has diabetes complications.[340] The risk increases with increasing A1C and is very great (close to 25%!) when A1C is above 11%.[602,727] It is therefore very important to plan your pregnancy, if at all possible, and to ensure that your A1C is below 7% before you get pregnant.[19] However, it is important to point out that even if your A1C is high during pregnancy, this does not necessarily mean your baby will have something wrong with it. A high A1C value is not, in itself, a reason for recommending abortion, for example.[602] Fifty percent of all women with a high A1C (above 10%) have quite normal pregnancies.[69]

If the mother's blood glucose level is high, there is a risk that the unborn baby will be affected. A high blood glucose level early in pregnancy (during the first 8 weeks) seems to give an

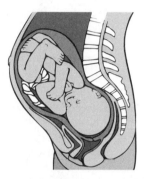

If you make up your mind to achieve a good A1C before getting pregnant, you will give your growing and developing baby a better start in life.

increased risk of birth defects, about 2-3 times the 1.6% risk that is present in all pregnancies.[69] In about half of these cases, the baby is so badly affected that it will not survive. Most major malformations can be identified by ultrasound or a blood test.[727] These studies were done on women with type 1 diabetes. There is a increased risk of birth defects [461] and difficulties at delivery [604] even with diabetes that is identified during pregnancy (gestational diabetes). However, these risks are associated with diabetes in the mother and do not apply if only the father has diabetes.

Insulin requirements may decrease early in pregnancy, especially if the woman has problems with nausea. Thereafter, the amount of insulin needed rises steadily, until close to full-term (36-38 weeks), when it is often as much as twice the level it was before the pregnancy.[224,602] This increased need for insulin is partly caused by weight gain during pregnancy but also by hormones excreted from the placenta, which counteract the blood glucose lowering effect of insulin. The average weight gain during pregnancy is around 11-12 kg (24-26 lb) but individuals vary greatly.

Although eye and kidney damage may be accelerated by pregnancy,[443] these changes have been found by the DCCT study to be reversible once the pregnancy is over.[201] However, if the mother's kidneys have been damaged by her diabetes, the risk of fetal growth retardation and premature birth will increase considerably.[69,443]

Short periods of hypoglycemia are not dangerous to the unborn baby.[598] However, severe hypoglycemia with seizures or unconsciousness can be dangerous.[602] Low blood glucose levels can increase nausea and vomiting during pregnancy.[224] Feeling very nauseous may make it difficult to eat regular meals, resulting in hypoglycemia. A vicious cycle may easily develop. The use of an insulin pump can be an effective way of minimizing these problems.

Glucose in the mother's blood will pass easily through the placenta into the blood of the unborn baby.[419] In this way, the baby is continuously consuming a large proportion of the mother's glucose, leading to a risk of hypoglycemia when she does not eat regularly. This may result in her needing more snacks during the day and increase the risk of night time hypoglycemia.[224]

If the mother's blood glucose level is increased, some of the glucose will be delivered via the placenta to the baby — whose own pancreas can produce enough insulin to take care of the extra sugar. However, insulin cannot pass back to the mother through the placenta. If the blood glucose level is high during a large part of the pregnancy, the baby will grow faster than it should, and will have gained excess weight by the time it is born. This may cause problems at delivery.

Even if the A1C during pregnancy is kept well controlled, the child may have gained excess weight by the time it is born. The blood glucose level after meals seems to be most significant according to one study.[148] The recommendation in this study was to aim for a blood glucose level of approximately 130 mg/dl (7.7 mmol/l)

Diabetes and pregnancy: risks for the unborn baby

① Early in pregnancy:

⟹ Increased risk of congenital malformations if the A1C is increased, especially if it is higher than 9-11%.

② Complications at delivery:

⟹ The baby will have the same blood glucose levels as the mother since glucose can pass freely through the placenta.
An increased amount of glucose to the infant will increase its growth, as it can produce insulin of its own.

⟹ The infant will be large in size which will increase the risk of a difficult delivery.

⟹ The infant will be at risk of developing hypoglycemia during the first few days of life as he or she will continue to produce considerable amounts of insulin.

---

one hour after the meal. With lower levels there was some risk that the baby will show a slight retardation in growth, instead of weight gain, by the time it is born.

Blood glucose levels should be as normal as possible during labor and childbirth, as high blood glucose levels cause increased insulin production in the unborn baby. This means that the baby will be less able to cope with the partial lack of oxygen that even a normal delivery entails.[68] When the umbilical cord is cut, the high insulin production by the baby's body will continue, causing the blood glucose level to drop. The child of a mother with diabetes, therefore, will be monitored carefully with extra blood glucose tests. If the baby becomes hypoglycemic, glucose will be given intravenously. The child will also receive extra food early on, before the mother has begun to produce breast milk.

The woman's daily insulin requirement decreases quickly after childbirth, returning to the pre-pregnant level after as little as one week.[567] Breast-feeding mothers usually need to decrease their insulin doses to levels lower than they were before pregnancy to avoid hypoglycemia. If doses are not lowered considerably, there is a clear risk of experiencing severe hypoglycemia.[798] After a few weeks or months, the insulin doses will usually be back to the levels they were at before the pregnancy. Breast-feeding lowers blood glucose, and a high-carbohydrate snack is often needed before or during breast-feeding. Evening or late night snacks may also be necessary.[567]

Pre-pregnancy care

If you are thinking about becoming pregnant, let your diabetes team know and they will help you to get your diabetes under best control before conception. Advice and counselling will be available.

It is better for a girl to wait at least until she is in her twenties before becoming pregnant as a teenage pregnancy brings about increased medical risks both for the baby (premature birth, complications in the new-born) and the mother (anemia, toxemia).

Caring for the mother

Pregnant women with diabetes are usually very highly motivated and will also receive closer attention from the maternity care services. Tell your diabetes healthcare team as soon as possible if you suspect you may be pregnant, or if you are hoping to become pregnant. They can help you get a pregnancy test (so called chorionic gonadotropin test) which will give a reliable result within a couple of days after you have missed a period.

A general consensus is that it is a full time job to be pregnant if you have diabetes. This means that it is quite hard work to maintain blood glucose levels at as normal a level as possible during pregnancy. The goal is for A1C during

Insulin requirements during pregnancy[224]		
	U/kg	U/lb
Before pregnancy	0.6	0.27
Week 6-18	0.7	0.32
Week 18-26	0.8	0.36
Week 26-36	0.9	0.41
Week 36-delivery	1.0	0.45
During delivery	Very low	
After delivery	Below 0.6	Below 0.27
Breast-feeding	Further decrease in insulin need	

pregnancy to be within the normal range for individuals without diabetes. Treatment with an insulin pump may be an effective way of achieving this.

During the latter part of pregnancy, it often becomes more difficult to recognize symptoms of hypoglycemia as the threshold for developing symptoms will be lowered because of frequent low blood glucose levels [652] (see "Hypoglycemia unawareness" on page 48). The A1C value for women without diabetes is approximately 0.5-1% lower at the end of pregnancy, which is

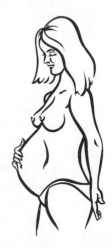

Nearly every woman has thoughts during pregnancy about something being wrong with her child. However, most women with diabetes have a quite normal pregnancy, leading to the birth of a healthy child. If you have a low A1C before and during pregnancy, the risks for your child are approximately the same as if you didn't have diabetes.

the reason for aiming for a A1C close to 6% (upper limit for individuals without diabetes) during the later part of pregnancy.[306,341] In a Scottish study, half of the women attained an A1C in the non-diabetic range at some point during their pregnancy.[306] Within one year, however, most of them increased in A1C to levels observed before pregnancy. This may be attributed to not having the time to take care of their diabetes in the most effective way at the same time as caring for an infant at home. Women giving birth to their second or third child had higher A1C during pregnancy, suggesting that the amount of work to be done at home affects how easy it to care for your diabetes during pregnancy.

During pregnancy, the ketone production during periods of insulin deficiency is increased, making ketoacidosis more likely.[68] Ketoacidosis during pregnancy is very dangerous, especially for the unborn child.[224,554] You should therefore check for ketones in blood or urine regularly, especially if you are feeling nauseous or vomiting, or have an infection with fever. A bedtime snack is usually necessary for pregnant women as it decreases the risk of night time hypoglycemia and fasting ketones. Ketones will show in the urine after only 12-14 hours of fasting.[274] Urine testing every morning will show whether or not you have "starvation ketones" from inadequate carbohydrate intake in the evening. Morning ketones are present in 30% of pregnant women who do not have diabetes.[25] A slight delay in development was found in children aged 2-9 years whose mothers had raised ketone levels during pregnancy.[642]

If you use an insulin pump, your risk of ketoacidosis will increase due to the smaller insulin depot (see page 172). If the pump infusion set fails during the night you will have high blood glucose levels and elevated levels of ketones in the morning. One method of avoiding this is to give a bedtime injection of intermediate-acting insulin (0.2 U/kg) in addition to the normal basal dose delivered by the pump.[526]

The renal threshold is usually lowered in pregnant women, causing an increased excretion of glucose via the urine. Urine tests for glucose cannot be relied upon therefore.

How will the child develop?

In a Swedish study, children of women with diabetes were seen to be developing normally at the age of 5.[68] The height and weight were also found to be normal in another study.[68] An Australian study followed children up to the age of 3 years.[694] Children of mothers having low A1C readings were found to be developing normally, while children of mothers with high A1C values during pregnancy had delayed language development and a smaller head circumference.

Will the child have diabetes?

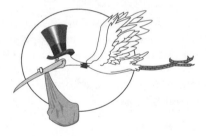

If you have diabetes you may ask yourself: "Should I have a baby when there is an increased risk of the child getting diabetes?" In one study 3% of the children of mothers with diabetes went on to develop diabetes themselves by the age of 10-13 years [603] (which is about 10 times the risk for the child of a mother without diabetes). Although it is believed that half the factors contributing to diabetes are inherited, only about one in every 10 children with newly diagnosed diabetes has a parent or sibling with diabetes.[164] The hereditary disposition for developing type 1 diabetes is very common, at least 40% according to certain studies.[166] From this it follows that a person with diabetes should not in any way be discouraged from having children. See also "Heredity" on page 323.

A few people may choose adoption instead. They do this because of increased risks, both for the child acquiring diabetes and, for the mother, of going through a pregnancy with diabetes, especially if she also has diabetes complications (see page 284).

It appears that the risk for a child of acquiring diabetes decreases as the mother's age increases. If a mother has diabetes and is older than 25 when she gives birth, the risk to the child of developing diabetes later in life is not significantly increased compared to mothers without diabetes.[799] Another study showed that 8.9% of children born to fathers with diabetes, but only 3.4% of children born to mothers with diabetes developed the disease before the age of 20.[78] If the mother was 8 years old or younger when she developed diabetes, the risk for the child was considerably higher, 13.9%, in this study.

Infertility

Women with average diabetes control have the same chances of getting pregnant as women without diabetes.[68] If you suspect problems with your fertility, contact your diabetes healthcare team who will refer you to a gynecologist.

Does the need for insulin change during menstrual periods?

Many women have noticed that their blood glucose level increases the days before they have their period.[6,513] In a Hungarian study, the premenstrual insulin doses were approximately 3 units higher than they were mid-cycle.[741] However, during the first couple of days of menstruation, the insulin requirements may fall, predisposing for hypoglycemia. If you notice that you have this type of problem, check your blood glucose level especially carefully the days close to menstruation. This will enable you to

adjust your insulin doses upwards just before your period, and lower them again afterwards.

It is quite normal for teenage girls' menstrual periods to be irregular and unpredictable during the first 6-12 months. A high A1C increases the risk of having irregular or missed periods.[688] The risk of menstrual disturbances in adolescents in this study was increased seven times if A1C was above 10% and 18 times if A1C was above 12%.

Sexuality

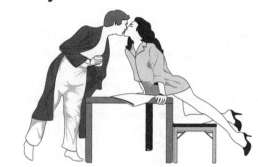

In terms of sexual relationships, teenage boys and girls with diabetes will function in exactly the same way as their friends of the same age. The only difference is that it is particularly important to use contraceptives to avoid an unwanted pregnancy. Remember that you may encounter hypoglycemia after having intercourse — making love can be energetic exercise! Some people find they don't function well sexually if their blood glucose level is high, but this can improve if the level is corrected.[49] According to some studies, sexual desire is negatively affected by long-standing diabetes, in both women and men.[250] Other studies, however, have not found this to be true.[250]

Impotence may be a complication of diabetes, which men who have had diabetes for many years will encounter. This can be caused by a combination of premature arteriosclerosis and a reduction in the intensity of physical response caused by disturbances in the autonomic nervous system (see page 311). In a population based study of men who were 21 years or older, and were less than 30 years of age at diagnosis of diabetes, 20% reported erectile problems.[409] These problems increased with age, from 1.1% in those 21-30 years of age to 47.1% in those 43 years of age or older. Another study found that the risk for developing erectile problems in men with diabetes in the age group 40-69 years was 1.8 times more common compared to the general population.[450]

Impotence commonly has a psychological (rather than a physical) cause in individuals both with and without diabetes. If you have erections in the morning, it is likely that the reasons for your impotence are psychological.[49] Temporary disturbances of erection are something that all men encounter once in a while. The difficulty for a young man with diabetes is that any temporary erection problem is likely to be attributed immediately to the diabetes, when the cause may be something as simple as tiredness or feeling nervous in a new relationship. A vicious cycle may arise with negative expectations and the fear of continued failure. Do not hesitate to talk to your diabetes doctor or nurse about the problems.

If the impotence is a complication of diabetes, there is a good chance of getting effective treatment. In the past, injection treatment was used but the impotence drugs Viagra® and Levitna® function well even for men with diabetes.[641] If you have heart disease you should consult your doctor before using this type of drug. Part of the treatment involves lessening other risk factors such as alcohol, tobacco and drugs (for example, certain drugs for blood pressure).

Poor diabetes control with a high A1C will increase the risk of impotence.[680] In the same way as with other complications (see page 303) the problems may be halted or even reversed if they are discovered early, and the diabetes treatment is changed, leading to a lowered A1C.

Female sexuality is less affected by diabetes.[49] Problems with vaginal discharge and fungal infections are more common in women with

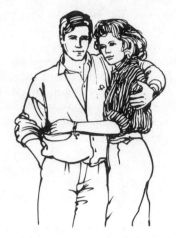

If you have diabetes, it is particularly important that your pregnancy be planned. Tell your diabetes team or doctor if you need contraceptives and they will refer you to the appropriate professional.

diabetes and may have a negative effect on sexual desire. The vaginal mucous membranes can become temporarily dry when the blood glucose is high, and this can be troublesome during intercourse. It is not yet established whether late complications to diabetes (nerve damage) can result in the same problem.[250] A pharmacist can advise you about suitable lubricants if you have this type of problem. The ability to reach orgasm does not appear to be affected by diabetes.[250]

Contraceptives

In the past, the "minipill" (containing only progesterone) was usually recommended to women with diabetes. However, this increases the risk of "spotting" between periods, and has a narrower time margin for taking the pills (not more than 30 hours between pills). Combined contraceptives ("ordinary" pills) are more effective in preventing pregnancy. They contain two types of female sex hormone. Estrogen prevents the egg from developing and being released from the ovary. Progesterone prevents the sperm from passing through the mucus of the

Contraceptive methods

Condom	The only contraceptive that protects against sexually transmitted disease.
Ordinary pills	Sometimes result in a slight increase in blood glucose levels.
Minipills	Risk of spotting. Less margin for error when forgetting to take tablets.
Depot injection	Can affect metabolic control. Sometimes troublesome side-effects.
Implant	Same as depot injection but easy to remove if side-effects are not acceptable.
Diaphragm and spermicidal jelly	Not so easy to use. Risk of itching as side-effect.
Intrauterine device (IUDs, coil)	Risk of pelvic infection is low but an IUD is not recommended before the first pregnancy.
"Morning-after" pills	For "emergency" situations. Needs to be taken within 72 hours.

Which contraceptive should you choose if you have diabetes? [68]

① Pills (not minipills) for teenagers.

② Coil (IUD) for women who have been pregnant.

③ Using a condom is always a good alternative and, besides, it is the only way of protecting yourself from sexually transmitted diseases. Always use a condom in a temporary relationship.

neck of womb (cervix). The use of oral contraceptives does not appear to increase the risk of later complications with the eyes or kidneys.[294]

At one time, combined contraceptive pills were thought to raise the blood glucose level slightly, but recent studies show no adverse affects on glucose control.[607] If the glucose control is different during the week without pills and it is difficult to adjust the insulin doses, it might be appropriate to wait longer before interrupting, that is, take pills for three months without interruption.[8] Today, combined pills are recommend to begin with. Combined pills are not advisable if you smoke (due to an increased risk

of thrombosis and heart attack), if you have high blood pressure, severe migraine attacks, or complications with your eyes or kidneys.[8]

An intrauterine device (IUD, coil) is a safe contraceptive for women with diabetes according to recent studies.[442] Problems with infections or spotting are no more common than for women without diabetes.[444] However, they are not recommended if you have irregular or heavy menstrual periods. As there is a small risk of infection of the womb or ovary (and thus a risk of becoming infertile), intrauterine devices are not recommended for women who have never been pregnant. However, for a woman who has diabetes complications affecting the eyes or kidneys, intrauterine devices may be a good alternative to contraceptive pills. [442]

Depot injections or implants contain the same hormone (progesterone) as minipills. However, they will give a higher hormone concentration and affect the blood glucose level more than minipills. Common side-effects are nausea, increased appetite or irritability, all of which make it more difficult to control the blood glucose levels. The contraceptive depot injection is not considered suitable for women with diabetes as the effects of one injection last for many months.

A contraceptive implant contains the same hormone as a depot injection. It is implanted under the skin using local anesthesia. The advantage is that it can be removed if the woman experiences serious side-effects. This makes it more suitable for a woman with diabetes than the depot injection.

Remember that most contraceptive methods only prevent unwanted pregnancy. It is as important to protect yourself against sexually transmitted diseases. Some of these diseases can be life-threatening, others can have a serious effect on women's fertility. A condom is the only contraceptive that offers full protection from sexually transmitted diseases. Talk to your doctor about which type of contraceptive can be suitable for you. Depending on local policies and practices, your doctor can give you a prescription or refer you to a gynecologist for further advice. Young women using oral contraceptives should have regular blood pressure monitoring and gynecological check ups.

Forgotten to take a pill?

If you discover that you have forgotten to take your contraceptive pill within 48 hours, you should take an extra pill when you realize this.[8] If more than 48 hours have passed (more than 30 hours with minipills) you will have no protection and you must use another method, such as condoms, during the following week.[8] If you forget this, you will need to take a pregnancy test.

Emergency contraception

Emergency contraception ("morning-after pills") is available in most countries for emergency situations, that is if you have had unprotected intercourse between day 8 and 18 (counting with 28 days between menstrual periods, and day 1 being the first day of bleeding).[305] The risk of getting pregnant after unprotected intercourse is 6-7% overall, and at the time of ovulation as high as 20-30%.[38] With "morning-after pills", this risk goes down to 1-3%.

**Morning-after methods
Only for "emergency" use!**

① Pills:

⟶ Two pills taken within 72 hours after unprotected intercourse and 2 pills after another 12 hours. Only special pills with high hormonal content can be used.

⟶ Contact a doctor or pregnancy advisory service as soon as possible. You will need to see your GP within 3-4 weeks to discuss which contraceptive to continue with.

⟶ A new type of pills (Norlevo®, Postinor®, Levonelle®, Plan B®) gives higher security and fewer side effects.

② Inserting a coil:

⟶ A **coil** should be inserted within 72 hours, at the very latest within 5 days.

⟶ Coils are recommended only for women who have been pregnant.

This type of medication prevents the fertilized egg from implanting in the membranes of the uterus. Unfortunately, nauseous or even vomiting is a relatively common side effect. A new type of tablet containing only one type of hormone (progesterone, Norlevo®, Postinor®, Levonelle®, Plan B®) decreases both the risk of unwanted pregnancy and the risk of nausea. "Morning-after pills" must be taken at the very latest 72 hours after intercourse,[305] which is why you should get in touch with your pregnancy advisory service, general practitioner, or local pharmacy as soon as possible. Emergency contraception requires a prescription but are easily available from emergency rooms, walk-in clinics, hospitals or private physician offices. The contraceptive effect is higher, the earlier the tablets are taken. Contact an emergency pharmacy, or the hospital if the need for these arises over the weekend or after office hours.

Social issues

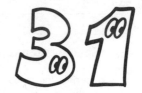

School

When you go back to school or work again after your diagnosis, it is important to tell your friends about your diabetes. It is very understandable not to want to talk about your diabetes at this stage and many people find this is how they feel. It takes real courage to tell your classmates and friends at home or at work. However, it really will make your life much easier if you can tell them right away and have done with it, rather than find yourself worrying about who knows and who doesn't. If it can be arranged, it is a good idea for a diabetes nurse educator to come to your class and talk about diabetes, inviting all teachers who come into contact with you, including the physical educa-

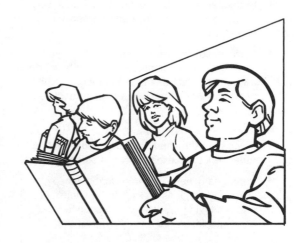

tion teacher. Invite the diabetes nurse to come to school again when you move to a new class or change to a new school.

It is very helpful when a teacher really understands a child or teenager with diabetes. Sometimes it may be difficult for them to know if something the child does or a particular behavior (such as tiredness or irritability) is due to a low blood glucose level or something else. It is important for the child to be able to measure blood glucose values at school when necessary. Some parents have the impression that the school and teachers take diabetes more seriously only after the child has had a difficult hypoglycemic reaction at school, but this is of course an unfortunate way to demonstrate how serious diabetes can be.

In the United States, Federal laws that protect children with diabetes include the Rehabilitation Act of 1973, Section 504, the Individuals with Disabilities Education Act of 1991 (originally the Education for All Handicapped Children Act of 1975), and the Americans with Disabilities Act of 1992. Under these laws, dia-

---

Hypoglycemia in school

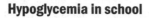

☞ An emergency plan should be set up to determine who does what if a child with diabetes is unwell or develops hypoglycemia.

☞ Your teacher or the school nurse (if there is one) should preferably be able to help you measure your blood glucose level if necessary.

☞ Make sure that your teachers and friends know where you keep your emergency glucose and when you need to take it.

☞ Snacks should be available so that you have something to eat if hypoglycemia occurs. Eating in the classroom must be permitted.

☞ The other children must be helped to understand why you may have to eat glucose tablets, a piece of fruit or a sandwich during class to prevent or treat hypoglycemia.

School routines (adapted from [64] and [23])

It is desirable for school routines to be adjusted in line with the needs of a child with diabetes:

➥ Understanding that the diabetes expert closest at hand is the young person and his or her parents.

➥ Staff need to have sufficient background knowledge about diabetes, and must be made aware of the fact that type 1 diabetes in childhood is not at all the same disease as type 2 diabetes.

➥ Reach an agreement with staff about how much help the young person needs, such as reminders to take insulin or test blood.

➥ Appropriate help with monitoring blood glucose and ketones, taking insulin injections, and managing hypoglycemic reactions should be available, according to the age of the child, both in school and on field trips.

➥ Understand the need for frequent trips to the bathroom when the blood glucose level is high.

➥ Young people with diabetes should be able to test their blood and urine in an undisturbed environment when necessary. They should also be allowed to test their blood glucose during lessons.

➥ Young people should be allowed to take their lunchtime dose of insulin undisturbed.

➥ Don't send a child who is in hypoglycemia on their own to the school nurse. Give dextrose first and then, if necessary, send the child accompanied by a friend or adult.

➥ Don't send a child with diabetes home on their own from school earlier than expected (especially not after a hypoglycemic episode) without first checking that someone is at home who can take care of him or her.

➥ Understand that the young person's school tests and exam results can be less reliable than they should be because of hypoglycemia. The young person should be allowed to retake the test as it is difficult to obtain full concentration for several hours after hypoglycemia.

School routines, continued

➥ Regular mealtimes should be established, with lunch as close to noon as possible.

➥ If the school serves food, it must be appropriate for a child with diabetes. However, it needs to be eaten if it is to do any good at all for the blood glucose level. It is important to be aware that young people with diabetes do not have the same choice as their peers to go hungry if they don't find the food appetizing. An alternative outside the regular menu must be available at all times. It may be helpful if parents check the school menu in advance, together with the young person.

➥ Physical education should preferably be scheduled the second or third lesson after a meal when using rapid-acting insulin (NovoLog/NovoRapid or Humalog), since there will be a quick increase in insulin level in your blood during the first hour (see graph on page 249). However, when using short-acting insulin physical education should preferably be scheduled as the first or second lesson in the morning or the first or second lesson after lunch. See also page 247.

➥ Report timetable changes to parents well ahead, such as visiting a public swimming pool or a games day.

➥ Organize a parent-teacher conference when needed, inviting the diabetes nurse or doctor to attend.

➥ School staff can visit the diabetes healthcare team along with the child, to increase their knowledge of diabetes.

➥ Give realistic vocational guidance.

betes has been determined to be a disability, and it is illegal for schools and/or day care centers to discriminate against children with diabetes. In addition, any school that receives federal funding or any facility considered open to the public must reasonably accommodate the special needs of children with diabetes. Indeed, federal law requires an individualized assessment of any child with diabetes. The required accommodations should be provided within the child's usual school setting with as little disruption to the school's and the child's routine as possible and allowing the child full participation in all school activities.

In Canada, The Canadian Diabetes Association (CDA) also supports the belief that children with diabetes have the rights to be full participants in all aspects of school life. Where requested, the CDA will work with school boards, administrators, teachers and parents to ensure delivery of accurate and current information about diabetes, and assist the development of policies and programs addressing diabetes management. The CDA can provide a practical guide to anyone needing to learn how to care for children with diabetes.

When a schoolchild has diabetes, it is a good idea to draw up an individualized Diabetes Health Care Plan as a collaborative effort between the child's parent or guardian, members of the diabetes care team, and the school or day care provider — as well as with the child him or herself. This plan sets out the basic medical needs the child has while at school, and how these needs will be met. Inherent in this process are responsibilities assumed by all parties, including the parent or guardian, the school personnel, and the child. For children with diabetes, this means that the school administration must provide appropriately trained adults (nurses or other school personnel) who can supervise or do blood glucose testing as well as insulin injections. Sometimes this causes major problems or battles between parents and school staff. More frequently, the school staff understand this is their legal obligation and make appropriate accommodation in accordance with the recommendations of the health care team and the parents. In addition to the medical issues covered in such a health care plan, children with diabetes must be permitted to eat wherever and whenever they need to, even if other children are not allowed to eat (for example, in class, on the school bus, during P.E. lessons).[424]

JDRF (the Juvenile Diabetes Research Foundation, see page 290) has a special pack for schools containing brochures, a Warning Signs card, a Low Blood Sugar Emergencies card, a book list and more. This is available on request.

Hypoglycemia

It is important and very helpful for the child to talk to friends about diabetes and the signs of hypoglycemia. Friends should know where to find dextrose tablets. Hypoglycemia will affect a child's performance at school, not only when the blood glucose level is low, but also up to 3-4 hours after it has been normalized. In a study of children and adolescents between the ages of 11-18 years, a significant decline in mental efficiency was found at blood glucose levels of 60-65 mg/dl (3.3-3.6 mmol/l). This was most evident in measures of mental flexibility, planning, decision making, attention to detail, and rapid responding.[658]

Exams

Always make sure that you have something extra to eat during an examination. Many students prefer to have a slightly higher blood glu-

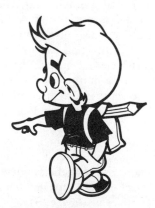

Don't send a child with diabetes home from school alone earlier than expected without checking that someone is at home. If the child experiences hypoglycemia on his or her way home and nobody is there to help, this may easily develop into severe hypoglycemia.

cose level during examinations to avoid hypoglycemia. Stress before an exam may make the blood glucose levels higher (see page 256).

You should feel free to measure your blood glucose if you experience difficulties in concentrating during an examination. You will then know if you need to eat something extra. It may also be important to be able to show a low blood glucose reading to your teacher, if you feel that your results from an examination are not as good as they should be, and you want to resit. In some cases, you might need a doctor's certificate to support this. See also page 67, 219 and 247 concerning low blood glucose levels, food and physical education in school.

Day-care centers and child care

A child with diabetes attending a day center will need more time and attention than children without diabetes of the same age. In some communities, children with diabetes can be counted as two in the accounting, giving the staff more time for the child. The rules and regulations differ from country to country.

In most countries, babysitters or day center staff have no formal obligation to help with blood glucose testing. However, you will usually find someone interested enough who will help, at least if the child is not feeling well. In some places the staff will also give insulin. This may be easier to do if the child has an injection aid, such as Inject-Ease®, PenMate™, or Insuflon (see page 122) or a pump. Sometimes it may be appropriate to have glucagon available if staff members know how and when to give it.

Regular babysitters will benefit from accompanying the family on a visit to the diabetes healthcare team, or the diabetes nurse may visit the day nursery to talk to staff and children about diabetes (see also page 87).

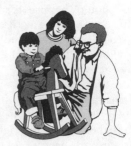

Child care allowance

There are no special bonuses or supplements available in the US because a child has diabetes and no special work allowances provided. However, certain family sick day benefits can be applied when caring for a child with a chronic illness.

Adoption

Some countries have restrictions on adoption by a parent with diabetes. Such restrictions are usually due to outdated information about life with diabetes but you may be required to get medical clearance indicating your ability to provide appropriate self-care.

Choice of job or employment

Almost all types of employment are open to people with diabetes. It is important that you, like everyone else, think first and foremost about what you would like to do. Jobs which include some type of physical work or at least not sitting still all day have the advantage of giving you regular exercise. However, considering the risk of hypoglycemia, you should avoid jobs where your own or other peoples' safety depend on you *always* functioning perfectly in all situations. Particularly dangerous situations can occur for police and fire personnel while most other situations (for example a physician or other health care professional) would include the possibility of stopping to check blood glucose levels and making appropriate adjustments with food and/or insulin accordingly. The risk of developing hypoglycemia may hinder some-

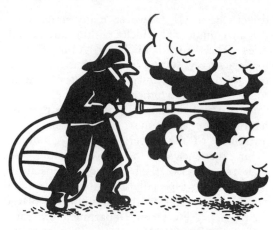

Police officers, fire fighters and pilots are examples of professionals who might be putting their own or other peoples' lives at risk if they develop severe hypoglycemia. In most countries, you are not allowed to work as a pilot or police officer if you have diabetes, but being a fire fighter or driving an ambulance may work well if you do not have problems with hypoglycemia.

one with diabetes from becoming a police officer, pilot, or flight attendant, joining the armed forces, and perhaps also driving a bus, taxi or train. Professional diving or working at high altitudes is usually discouraged since these are difficult situations in which to deal with hypoglycemic emergencies. The rules will vary in different states in the US (and provinces in Canada) since each state (province) is responsible for such governance.

Usually, you can adjust insulin doses to fit with most working schedules, even when irregular hours are included. When working shift patterns, or if there are frequent changes in work schedules and meal timetables, this may be more difficult to accomplish. A flexible insulin regimen or a pump with different basal rate profiles for work days and days off may help.

Examine the possibility of trying out different occupations to find out how well you can cope with your diabetes under the work situations; talking to people in different jobs may be helpful in terms of flexibility for food and snacks as well as insulin administration and blood glu-

cose testing. People with diabetes should be individually considered for employment, based on the requirements of the specific job but this is not always the case. There are many myths about people with diabetes and what they can and cannot do, so that you may have to educate folk about diabetes in such circumstances. Ask The American Diabetes Association (ADA) or Canadian Diabetes Association (CDA) for advice if you feel that your diabetes stops you from getting a particular job. The ADA and CDA believe that a person with diabetes should be eligible for employment in any occupation for which he or she is individually qualified. They feel that a person with diabetes has the right to be assessed for specific job duties on his or her own merits based on reasonable standards applied consistently. They also believe that employers have the duty to accommodate employees with diabetes unless the employer can show it to cause undue hardship to the organization. Both the ADA and CDA have a strong advocacy groups to help in situations where discriminations on the basis of diabetes has occurred.

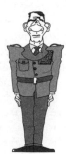

Military service

So far, although the ADA has agreed with such a position, the US government and the military authorities have not agreed to such a possibility. Young people with diabetes in the US are exempt from military service. If one develops diabetes while in the service, they are given an immediate medical/honorable discharge from the service including the service academies like West Point, Annapolis etc. Since there is no current automatic draft, they need to register like everyone else but receive a medical waiver and cannot even volunteer for any of the military academies or any of the armed services. Your diabetes healthcare team and the military authorities can give you further information if this will change.

Drivers license

While European governments have further restricted driver's licenses for insulin-treated drivers with diabetes, the restrictions on drivers in the US have been relaxed. In the US and Canada, driver's licenses are regulated by individual states and provinces. All states and provinces require people with diabetes to indicate this on their applications and to obtain medical clearance to drive. Commercial driving licenses have more specific rules to be followed.

However, each state's applications are not very clear about whether diabetes should be automatically listed. Some merely question if a person has a "condition which would influence their ability to drive" while others list diabetes specifically. Since there is no standard questionnaire or application, people with diabetes should honestly list their condition and then act responsibly to get a letter of medical clearance from their health care team indicating that they test appropriately, take their medications appropriately and are not a public health menace. There should be no reason to withhold such medical certification with reasonable self-care and responsible behavior unless severe and recurrent hypoglycemia occurs. Obtaining a driver's learning permit falls under the same rules and regulations of each state. Your diabetes team can tell you exactly what is applicable in each area of the US and Canada. All questions about driving applications, permits and rules should be discussed with local automobile registry officials.

In the US, people with type 1 diabetes are usually disqualified for interstate commercial driver's license.[531] However, many states allow driving commercial vehicles within state boundaries. The Federal Highway Administration made a survey, stating in 1996 that the driving of waived drivers with type 1 diabetes continues to be better than other drivers. The accident rate for the diabetes group was lower than the national rate and none of the accidents were attributed to the drivers' diabetic condition. "Our experience with these drivers is that, with high awareness of their unique circumstances, they are both especially careful as drivers and notably responsive to the requirements placed on them." (New Jersey Department of Transportation). From 1996, licenses for recreational pilots in the US are issued on a case-by-case basis. In 2001 the US Department of Transportation has concluded that some people with insulin-treated diabetes should be allowed to drive commercial vehicles.

In Canada, people with insulin treated diabetes can qualify for a commercial drivers's licence as long as certain criteria are met. The applicant must not have had an episode off severe hypoglycemia within the past 6 months; hypoglycemia unawareness; uncontrolled diabetes; or a recent significant change in their insulin regimen.

Driving and diabetes

Key safety issues with regard to driving for people with diabetes involve frequent blood glucose testing and hypoglycemia prevention, especially unawareness of hypoglycemia, to maximize the individual's safety while driving and to ensure public safety as well.

The risks associated with driving while suffering from hypoglycemia are obvious. Drivers with diabetes are generally not more prone to accidents than other drivers according to most studies.[160] However, there are case reports of serious accidents due to hypoglycemia.[215] In the DCCT study (see page 314) hypoglycemia was the main contributing factor in 36% of the traf-

Research findings: Driving with diabetes

♠ In an American study, subjects with diabetes were tested in a driving simulator.[152] They were not told their blood glucose readings (a blind study).

♠ At a blood glucose level of 65 mg/dl (3.6 mmol/l) only 8% showed impaired driving while at 45 mg/dl (2.6 mmol/l) 35% were driving more slowly, and had steering difficulties (more swerving, spinning, time over mid-line, and time off road). Only half of them were aware of their impaired ability.

♠ When the same investigations were re-done three months later, the results were similar in that the same individuals had impaired ability to drive at lower blood glucose levels.[626]

♠ In another study, the blood glucose level was reduced from 120 mg/dl (6.7 mmol/l) to 40 mg/dl (2.2 mmol/l) without the patients being aware of their actual blood glucose level.[804]

♠ At 120 mg/dl (6.7 mmol/l) 70% of the subjects judged they could drive safely. At 40 mg/dl (2.2 mmol/l), 22% still thought it safe to drive.

These studies illustrate the importance of checking your blood glucose before driving.

Commercial Driver's Licence

No restrictions	Certain restrictions	Not allowed
Argentina	Australia	Belgium
Brazil	Austria	Greece
Finland	Canada	Italy
Japan	Chile	Mexico
Libya	Israel	Poland
Puerto Rico	New Zealand	Romania
Tanzania	Great Britain	
Thailand	Sweden	
	US	

The rules for people with diabetes regarding driving trucks heavier than 3500 kg vary considerably between countries.[215] US and Canada are heading for fewer restrictions while the European Community is doing the opposite. If a person who already has a truck licence develops diabetes, the licence will be suspended in 8 countries, restricted in 7, and in 6 will continue to be free of restrictions.

fic accidents that the participants encountered during the nine years of the study.[194] In a Scottish study, 25% of the participants attributed their road accidents to hypoglycemia.[520] Of cases reported to British authorities, 16-17% of cases of collapse at the wheel were caused by hypoglycemia in a person with diabetes.[267] Although these studies exemplify an increased risk for traffic accidents in a small number of cases, the conclusion of a review is that, for the general population with diabetes, accident rates do not exceed the rates for drivers without diabetes.[521] As a comparison, a ban on all young male drivers would be more effective in terms of improving road safety, but would represent a totally unacceptable restriction in the freedom of individuals.[521]

You should check your blood glucose before driving and if it is below 70-90 mg/dl (4-5 mmol/l) you should eat something before beginning your trip. If you don't experience hypoglycemic symptoms at low blood glucose levels (hypoglycemia unawareness) you are not fit to drive. Even if you feel quite capable of driving when your blood glucose level is 45 mg/dl (2.5 mmol/l), your reaction time will be too slow for safety. This has been shown to occur below the level of approximately 50 mg/dl (2.8 mmol/l). See page 48 for further information on how to treat this phenomenon, which is caused by your body becoming accustomed to low blood glucose levels. It will take a while after a hypoglycemic episode before your reaction time is back to normal. In one study where the blood glucose was lowered to 48 mg/dl (2.7 mmol/l) the reaction time was still prolonged 20 minutes after the blood glucose level had returned to normal.[255]

To consider while driving:

① Check your blood glucose level before you take your place behind the wheel. It should not be below 70-90 mg/dl (4-5 mmol/l) when you set out. **Even if you feel quite well, your blood glucose level must never fall below 70 mg/dl (4.0 mmol/l), or your driving performance will be impaired.**[152]

② Don't start out on a drive or a bicycle trip if you have not eaten recently.

③ Always bring along extra food and carry dextrose tablets in your pocket or the glove compartment of the car.

④ Always pull over and stop the car if you have hypoglycemia and wait until you feel better before continuing. Remember that your thinking and judgement will not be back to normal until several hours later.

⑤ Be extra careful when the risk of hypoglycemia is increased, for example, after playing sport or when you have recently adjusted your insulin doses.

⑥ Alcohol increases the risk of hypoglycemia as well as making you unfit to drive. Make it a habit never to drive a car or motorcycle when you have been drinking.

⑦ Changes in your blood glucose level can result in transient blurred vision.

⑧ Refrain from driving for a week or so if you make major changes in your insulin regimen (such as changing from 2 to 4 or 5 doses/day or starting to use an insulin pump) until you find out how the new treatment affects you.

⑨ No matter how good a driver you are with a normal blood glucose level, you are never a safe driver if you have hypoglycemic unawareness (no warning symptoms until the blood glucose level is very low). See page 48 for advice on how to treat this problem.

Insurance policies

In the US, with usual health insurance coverage, the vast majority of diabetes clinical care as well as diabetes supplies are covered. Sometimes there is a small co-payment required for ongoing care and supplies. With usual health insurance coverage expensive supplies like insulin pumps are also usually covered but with a requirement for prior authorization because they are so expensive. Your diabetes health care team will know about the details of your insurance coverage and you should feel free to discuss any problems that you may have since members of the team will be aware of local circumstances and coverage options. It can be difficult for a person with diabetes to get health or life insurance although some companies may have special arrangements, which allow enrolment for a higher premium (impaired risk insurance). Shop around different insurance companies to get the best deal or ask ADA or CDA for specific advice.

In Canada, government drug plan coverage to help with the financial costs of caring for diabetes varies greatly across the country. Some provincial plans cover almost all of the medication, supples and devices, while other jurisdictions provide little or no coverage. Coverage levels are often subject to very high deductibles or

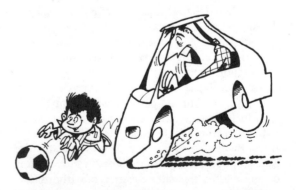

There are many situations in which one must be 100% alert when driving a car. Never drive with a blood glucose level below 70-90 mg/dl (4-5 mmol/l) even if you feel perfectly well!

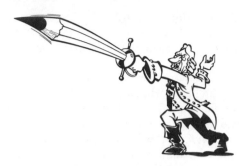

You may need to appeal if your health insurance conditions change after you are diagnosed as having diabetes.

co-payment formulas, meaning that even those who qualify for government programs may still be unable to benefit from them. In addition, the level of assistance based on income or age also varies widely across the country. For instance, although the cost of insulin for people on social assistance is covered in almost all provinces, in some areas the cost of syringes needed to administer the insulin is not.

You may need to appeal if your health insurance conditions change after you are diagnosed as having diabetes. Unfortunately, people with diabetes don't always take as much care of themselves as they should, and the insurance companies use this information to assign higher risk to all people with diabetes. People with diabetes use hospital and emergency room resources more than those without diabetes; people with diabetes require ongoing medications (syringes, pens, insulin, glucose and ketone testing equipment) and need more hospital or clinic visits to help manage their illness than those without chronic illnesses. Individual insurance companies which are not organized by governments but rather organize to be profit-driven, feel that such risks produce excessive costs; however, with new employment, most family members with diabetes are allowed to automatically enroll in employer-based health insurance indemnity programs as well as health maintenance organizations (HMOs) without prejudice. Because all such circumstances are so individualized, it is important for parents to be knowledgeable and to questions

exact policy details whenever jobs (and therefore insurance coverage) are changed.

Disability insurance policies and life insurance policies are often not allowed for people with diabetes since statistically they are at higher risk for being disabled at earlier ages compared to their peers, as well as of dying prematurely. While this is clearly improved with better self-care, more self blood glucose monitoring and better insulins, this is not always apparent to individual insurance providers or even to employers. Policies may be available but with much higher premiums so that one must weigh the benefits of such policies against their costs. Travel insurance may also be available at higher premiums because of a pre-existing condition.

The present practice of increased accident insurance premiums and limited coverage is not supported by scientific evidence. A Danish study of 7,599 adult individuals with diabetes found that the risk of accidents and permanent disability was no different from that in a control group without diabetes.[529] Furthermore, the authors found an increase in average life expectancy of 15 years or more over a 40-year period (mainly because of a decreased risk of kidney damage), which should motivate and encourage insurance companies to re-evaluate their policies.[106]

Diabetes ID

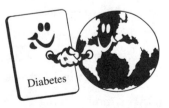

It is a good idea to always carry something on your person showing that you have diabetes, such as a special necklace or bracelet (Medic-Alert® or something similar). It is not uncommon for a person with diabetes to be mistaken for being drunk when in fact he or she is hypoglycemic. Even if you have only had a small amount to drink, people noticing the smell of alcohol are likely to pass by without helping you.

If you are travelling abroad, it is a good idea to have some kind of identification showing that you have diabetes and that you need to carry insulin and accessories. Insulin companies and Diabetes Associations often have special cards with text in different languages explaining what help you need if you become hypoglycemic.

Juvenile Diabetes Research Foundation International

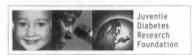

dedicated to finding a cure

The Juvenile Diabetes Research Foundation International (JDRF) was founded in 1970 by parents of children with juvenile diabetes. JDRF volunteers have a personal connection with diabetes in the young and this translates into an unrelenting focus on the needs of all people with diabetes and the commitment to finding a cure as soon as possible.

The mission of JDRF is to find to find a cure for diabetes and its complications through the support of research. Embedded in JDRF's mission are its three core goals:

➡ Restoring normal blood sugar levels.

➡ Preventing and reversing complications.

➡ Preventing type 1 diabetes.

JDRF is now leading the worldwide effort to replicate and expand upon the success of the Edmonton Protocol (see page 273), while continuing progress towards the goal of inducing tolerance to transplanted islets without the need for long-term immunosupression. To date, JDRF has established eight centers specifically for islet transplantation, co-funded the

NIH/JDRF Immune Tolerance Network, and has invested or committed more than $150 million for islet transplantation worldwide.

JDRF has more than 120 Chapters, Branches and Affiliates worldwide. There are Affiliates in Australia, Canada, Chile, Greece, India, Israel, Italy, Puerto Rico and the UK. In their magazine *Countdown,* you will find in-depth analysis of cutting edge diabetes research along with information on treatments, profiles and more. *Countdown for Kids* is especially for children with diabetes and includes information and opportunities for fun, as well as access to role models and pen pals.

Children with Diabetes

children with **DIABETES**

The mission of Children with Diabetes is to promote understanding of the care and treatment of diabetes, especially in children; to increase awareness of the need for unrestricted diabetes care for children at school and day care; to support families living with diabetes; and to promote understanding of research into a cure. www.childrenwithdiabetes.com is one of the largest web sites in the world for children and adolescents with diabetes, with over 25,000 pages of content. CWD organizes conferences for children with diabetes and their parents, including the annual Friends for Life Conference held in Orlando, Florida.

Diabetes Associations

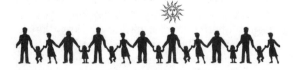

In nearly every country, there is a Diabetes Association protecting the interests of people with diabetes. Local branches can be found in most towns. Find out if there is a special section for children and adolescents in your area. We strongly recommend joining your local diabetes association. You will receive valuable information including a magazine.

American Diabetes Association (ADA)

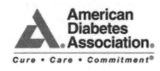

The American Diabetes Association is a non-profit health organization providing diabetes research, information and advocacy. The mission of the organization is to prevent and cure diabetes and to improve the lives of all people affected by diabetes. To fulfill this mission, the American Diabetes Association funds research, publishes scientific findings, provides information and other services to people with diabetes, their families, health care professionals and the public. ADA publishes journals for persons with diabetes (*Diabetes Forecast*) and for health care professionals (*Diabetes Care, Diabetes, Diabetes Spectrum,* and *Clinical Diabetes*). The Association is also actively involved in advocating for scientific research and for the rights of people with diabetes.

The International Diabetes Federation (IDF)

The International Diabetes Federation (IDF) is open to members of all countries. It promotes diabetes interests in many different areas. An international conference is organized every 3rd year. The 1994 conference was in Kobe, Japan, 1997 in Helsinki, Finland, 2000 in Mexico City and the year 2003 conference in Paris. The 2006 conference will be held in South Africa. You can obtain further information about IDF from your local diabetes association or over the Internet.

International Society for Pediatric and Adolescent Diabetes (ISPAD)

ISPAD is the only global (professional) advocate for children and adolescents with diabetes. It is an association for diabetes teams (doctors, nurses, dietitians, educators, psychologists, and all others involved in the care of children with diabetes. The society is committed to promoting the best possible health, social welfare and quality of life for *all* children and adolescents with diabetes, anywhere in the world. The aims of the society are outlined in the Declaration of Kos from 1993:

➡ To make insulin available for *all* children and adolescents with diabetes.

➡ To reduce the morbidity and mortality rates associated with acute metabolic complications or missed diagnosis relating to diabetes mellitus.

➡ To increase the availability of appropriate urine and blood self-monitoring equipment for *all* children and adolescents with diabetes.

➡ To develop and encourage research on diabetes in children and adolescents around the world.

➡ To prepare and disseminate written guidelines and standards for practical and realistic care and education of young patients with diabetes, and their families, emphasizing the crucial role of health care professionals (not just physicians) in these tasks around the world.

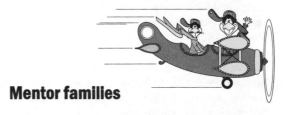

Mentor families

Many things about diabetes are difficult to learn from a book or from the staff at the diabetes clinic. For example, few of the health professionals you come into contact with will either have diabetes themselves, or have children with diabetes. Because of this, some clinics have a system for finding a mentor family with a child of a similar age, preferably living close by. Such a family will be able to give you valuable tips and information about practical ways of handling different situations such as school, birthday parties, travel and so forth. The mentor system may be equally valuable for an adult with diabetes.

Diabetes camps

Participating in a diabetes camp gives young people the opportunity to increase their self-confidence by establishing friendships with other children with diabetes who have to abide by the same rules about insulin, diet and testing. The program varies from camp to camp but most of these camps emphasize improving young people's ability to manage diabetes on their own. In small groups, they can learn about correct injection technique, testing and monitoring, diet, physiology and other issues relating to diabetes.

It is more fun to take insulin and see what your blood glucose level is when your friends are doing the same thing. Children who have difficulties taking insulin or testing blood glucose levels will soon learn all about this from peers at a diabetes educational camp. The children are often relieved to find that their friends at the camp already know what diabetes is. They do not need to explain what hypoglycemia is or why they take injections and so on, as is often the situation in daily life at home.

Many will meet new friends with whom they will keep in touch for years to come. At our camp for children below the age of puberty, we emphasize the importance of managing the basics of their diabetes independently. If they can handle major parts of diabetes on their own during their teenage years, they will be helped in their struggle for independence and hopefully diabetes will not play too large a role in the family conflicts associated with puberty (see also page 343). At the diabetes camp we aim primarily for the children to be able to participate fully in all activities. From this, it follows

---

Diabetes and the Internet

There is a vast amount of diabetes information available on the Internet. However, you must be aware that the information on the Internet often is not reviewed by health care professionals and may only be the opinion of the person writing it. Bring questions and thoughts about what you read to your diabetes team for continued discussions.

Associations:

American Diabetes Association (ADA)	www.diabetes.org
Canadian Diabetes Association (CDA)	www.diabetes.ca
Diabetes UK	www.diabetes.org.uk
Diabetes Australia	www.diabetesaustralia.com.au
International Diabetes Federation (IDF)	www.idf.org
International Society for Pediatric and Adolescent Diabetes (ISPAD)	www.ispad.org
Juvenile Diabetes Research Foundation International	www.jdrf.org
Diabetes Camping Association	www.diabetescamps.org

Links to patient information:

Children with Diabetes	www.childrenwithdiabetes.com
Betamed - home page of this book	www.betamed.se/eng

At www.betamed.se you will find many other links of diabetes interest. Since Internet pages are constantly updated and many sites change their addresses from time to time, we have chosen not to include more links in this book.

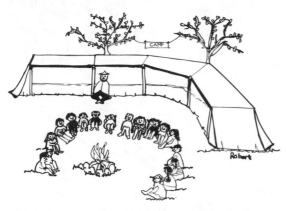

At diabetes camps, the children will meet friends who are "in the same boat" and understand what living with diabetes is like. The aim is to have fun together but also to prepare the children for a life with diabetes by increasing their knowledge and ability to manage on their own.

Most diabetes associations have journals where you can read news on diabetes research and many other helpful articles. It is a good idea to become a member of ADA or your local diabetes association.

that we will not achieve perfect control of diabetes. Some children may even have higher blood glucose levels than they managed at home. Most children will be more active than usual during the camp and, therefore, we often lower the insulin doses, especially at bedtime, to prevent night time hypoglycemia. Participating in a camp can also increase children's confidence in their own ability to manage without their mother or father. This will be especially true for children who are perhaps away from home for more than a night or two for the first time ever. Many parents find it a relief to be on their own, knowing that their child is being taken care of by professional staff.

Diabetes and the Internet

An increasing amount of information on diabetes is available on the Internet. Both medical companies and institutions have homepages displaying information and news. Use one of the search services to find the type of information you are looking for.

One thing is particularly important to remember when you are reading information on the Internet. Most of what you find will not have

been reviewed by health care professionals, and may often be only the opinion of the person writing it. However, if you judge the information somewhat critically, you may find out a lot of interesting information about diabetes and you can discuss it with your team at clinic.

When does a young person become an adult?

The precise age at which we enter adulthood may be difficult to determine, as most of us carry part of our childhood and adolescence with us throughout our lives. Practice and regulations about when diabetes care is transferred from pediatric to adult units differ between countries. It may also differ between cents depending on local policies. In the US, the American Academy of Pediatrics has indicated pediatricians should stay involved through age 21. Usually there is a discussion at the end of high school or college whether or not to stay or transfer to adult care. Systems of transition vary. One example is for the pediatrician to join the teenager for his or her first visit to the adult clinic. Another is for the diabetes nurse from the adult team to join the last pediatric visit before transfer. Some centers have joint adolescent or young adult clinics with both pediatric and adult physicians attending. Discuss with your care providers what is best for your individual circumstances.

Travel tips

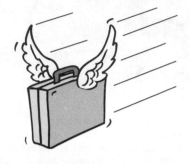

Travelling is an important part of life for many people, and you should not avoid this activity just because of your diabetes. If you think things over and plan the trip ahead, no destination or means of travel is impossible. However, you must be able to measure your blood glucose during the trip, and adjust your insulin doses in line with differing conditions, if you are to manage well.

It will be necessary to test your blood glucose levels more frequently. They could be raised if you have been sitting still in the car or on a plane or eating food with more carbohydrates than usual. The excitement involved in visiting a new city or country may also increase your blood glucose level.

Remember always to take spare insulin, at least 2-3 times the amount you expect to use. Keep insulin and pens/syringes in your hand-luggage but make sure that you have an extra set in another bag in case you lose one bag. Don't put insulin in the check in-luggage as there is a risk of it freezing in the airplane luggage hold at high altitudes. Besides, there is always the risk of your luggage being lost or arriving late. The X-ray in security controls will not affect your insulin. It is important to have some kind of ID showing that you have diabetes, as you may have to show it to the customs officer.

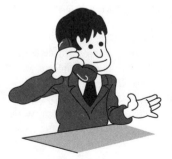

Remember that you are never more than a phone call away from your diabetes healthcare team when on vacation or a business trip.

Usually, you will have no problem obtaining insulin from a pharmacy abroad if you can prove that you have diabetes. Take a card on which your doses, concentration and brand of insulin are documented, or bring the original pharmaceutically labelled box. It may be difficult to store your insulin in a refrigerator all the time, but usually it will not be wasted during a short trip, as long as you avoid temperatures above 25-30° C (77-86° F). Remember that it can be extremely hot (up to 50° C, 120° F) in a closed car on a sunny day. Bring a thermos flask or similar with you, containing cold water (cool it with ice before putting insulin into it) during hot days. Remember that insulin is absorbed more quickly from the injection site if you are very warm and that this can result in unexpected hypoglycemia (see also page 82).

Insulin that has been frozen loses its effect. Don't leave it in the car on a skiing trip, for example. Keep your insulin bottles or pen injector in an inner pocket if it is below freezing outside. Damaged insulin will often turn cloudy or clumpy, sometimes with a brownish color. Some blood glucose strips can give too high a reading when it is very hot outside and too low a reading when it is very cold. Many glucose meters will give you a warning if the temperature is too high or too low.

Remember that some countries use other concentrations of insulin, mostly 40 U/ml. If you use insulin of 100 U/ml in syringes designed for 40 U/ml or vice versa, you will be in trouble. The insulin concentration appropriate for each syringe is clearly printed on the side of the syringe. If you run out of insulin it is probably better to buy both insulin and syringes for 40 U/ml if 100 U/ml is not available. You can continue taking your usual doses when counting in units. The units are the same and will give just about the same insulin effect with both 40 U/ml and 100 U/ml. The only difference is that insulin of 40 U/ml may give a slightly quicker onset of action. (See also "Units and insulin concentrations" on page 72.)

Blood glucose is measured in mmol/l in some countries and mg/dl in others (see page 90 for conversion table).

1 mmol/l = 18 mg/dl   100 mg/dl = 5.6 mmol/l

Make sure that you have dextrose and glucagon when travelling, sailing or hiking. With glucagon you can treat a serious hypoglycemia even if you are a long way from emergency care. Make sure that your friends know how and when dextrose and glucagon should be used.

Vaccinations

There are no special restrictions for vaccinations or gamma globulin injections due to diabetes. However, it is particularly important that individuals with diabetes make sure they get the recommended vaccinations, since illness often leads to difficult consequences with problems of diabetes control. Vaccination for hepatitis A, typhoid and other diarrheal diseases is a sensible precaution if you travel to areas where these may be a problem. It is a good idea to have the vaccinations well ahead of the trip, as some cause an episode of fever that can affect the blood glucose for a few days after the shot.

Names of insulin abroad		
Type	**UK**	**US**
Analog	NovoRapid Humalog	NovoLog Humalog
Regular insulin	Actrapid Humulin S Insuman Rapid	Novolin R Humulin R
NPH insulin	Insulatard Humulin I	Novolin Humulin N
Lente insulin	Monotard Humulin L	Novolin L Humulin L
Ultralente	Ultratard Humulin Zn	Ultratard Humulin U
Mixed insulin (70% NPH)	Mixtard 30 Humulin M3	Novolin 70/30 Humulin 70/30
Mixed analog (70-75% basal)	NovoMix 30 Humalog Mix 25	NovoLog Mix 70/30 Humalog Mix 75/25

Most insulins can be found under different names in different parts of the world. If you plan a longer trip, have the insulin vial and box available, or ask your doctor to write down what type of insulins you use so that you can get them from the local pharmacy if you lose your supplies. Be aware that the premixed insulins have their proportions stated in opposite ways in the US from in the UK!

Problems with travel sickness?

➡ Take medication: depot adhesives (e.g. scopolamine) or travel pills.

➡ You will be less likely to feel nauseous if you eat "little and often" rather than large helpings several hours apart.

➡ Avoid carbonated drinks.

➡ Sit in the front if you are in a car or bus, so you can see the road.

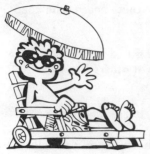

Remember that insulin cannot withstand heat and sunshine as well as you can. The trunk of a car or bus will be too hot for insulin in the summer and too cold in the winter.

Ill while abroad?

Remember to take documents relevant to your health insurance so that you receive compensation if you fall ill abroad. Check the small print on your insurance policy to find out whether your health insurance covers acute illness only, or whether it will also cover any deterioration of your diabetes.

Always say that you have diabetes if you need to see a doctor abroad. If you become ill while in countries other than Western Europe and the US you should, if possible, try to avoid surgical intervention, blood transfusions and injections. If you need medication, ask for tablets instead of injections. If possible, also avoid dental treatment as there may be a risk of acquiring a blood infection.

Diarrhea problems

Prophylactic antibiotic treatment aimed at avoiding diarrheal diseases while on vacation is a controversial issue. Since a person with diabetes will have problems with blood glucose levels and insulin adjustments when they ill, some doctors are more liberal about prescribing treatment for diarrheal diseases in advance.[129] It can be given during a short trip (3-4 weeks or less) to high risk areas (Africa, Asia or Latin America) with a 70-90% protective effect.[731] Without this, the risk of catching a diarrheal infection is 25-35%. On a longer trip, antibiotics should be given only if you actually have diarrhea. It is best to take the antibiotics with you. Avoid buying them locally as you may not know exactly what you are getting, thereby increasing the risk of side-effects.

Considering the risks of gastroenteritis, you should avoid drinking water in some countries if you cannot be sure it is entirely clean. Avoid all tap water (even frozen, i.e. ice cubes!) Bottled water and fizzy drinks (Cola, Fanta or similar) are usually safe. Oral rehydration solution

---

Oral rehydration solution

Oral rehydration solution can be found at many pharmacies, both at home and abroad. You can also mix your own rehydration solution. Remember though that the water you use must be pure! Buy bottled water if you are in any doubt.

☞ 1 lit pure water
½ teaspoon of salt
8 dextrose tablets (3 g each)
or 2 tablespoonfuls of ordinary sugar

Avoid the following in hot climates and places with poor standards of hygiene

Tap water (even when brushing your teeth)
Ice
Milk, cream, mayonnaise
Unsealed ice cream
Diluted juice
Cold buffets
Food kept warm for a long time
Shellfish
Salad, vegetables and fruit rinsed in water
Raw food
Poorly cooked chicken

Other advice:[812]
Wash your hands often.
Food should be freshly prepared and piping hot.
Don't eat food prepared in the street.
Drink only bottled, carbonated fluids.
Beer, wine, coffee and tea are also safe.

(Pedialyte®, Infalyte®) is a good alternative if you feel nauseous or are vomiting (see "Nausea and vomiting" on page 259).

If you travel in primitive conditions, water should be disinfected by boiling it briefly or by using water purifying tablets (Chlorine®, Puritabs®, Aqua Care® or similar).[812]

If you do not drink enough when outdoors in the heat, you will risk dehydration. This causes the insulin to be absorbed more slowly.[344] Later, when, you drink properly, more insulin will be absorbed and you will risk becoming seriously hypoglycemic. A high blood glucose level above the renal threshold (see page 92) will also cause you to lose extra fluid as you will be passing more urine.

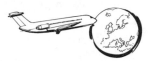

Passing through time zones

When you travel to other continents there will be a time difference. If you go westwards, the day will be longer, and if you go eastwards, it will be shorter. Calculate your total insulin dose for the travelling day by increasing or decreasing it by 2-4% for every hour of time shift.[430,669] If you are flying, don't order special diabetes food as this is often not very appetizing and the amount of carbohydrates served is often too small. It is better to adjust your insulin doses to the food being served on board.

Due to the pressure differences in the cabin, air bubbles easily accumulate in the pen cartridges. To avoid this, remove the needle immediately after each injection. If air bubbles are present, be sure to get rid of them before taking injections after you have landed (see page 121). It is common to feel a bit weary before adjusting to the new time zone (called jet-lag) and it will usually take a couple of days before your energy

levels are where they should be and your sleeping pattern returns to normal.

Multiple injection treatment

Use short-acting insulin and eat every 4 to 5 hours during the trip. If you fly westwards, take one or two extra doses. If you fly eastwards, you will need fewer doses. Take your usual bed-

---

Passing through time zones
(adapted from [430])

☞ **Multiple daily injections**

✦ Going west (longer day):
➡ Extra doses of mealtime insulin with 1-2 meals.
➡ Usual dose of bedtime insulin adjusted to the "new" night.

✦ Going east (shorter day):
➡ Decreased number of meals.
➡ Usual dose of bedtime insulin adjusted to the "new" night.

☞ **2-dose treatment**

✦ Going west (longer day):
➡ Extra doses of mealtime insulin with 1-2 meals.
➡ Usual dose of intermediate-acting insulin adjusted to the "new" night.

✦ Going east (shorter day):
Night time flight:
➡ Take the ordinary mealtime insulin with dinner.
➡ Reduce the intermediate-acting insulin by 3-5% per time shift hour.[669] If the night on the plane is shorter than 4-5 hours, you can try skipping the intermediate-acting bedtime insulin. Instead take an extra dose of rapid or short-acting insulin if necessary.
Daytime flight:
➡ Usual insulin dose with breakfast.
➡ Reduce the intermediate-acting insulin at dinner time on the plane by 3-5% per time shift hour.[669]

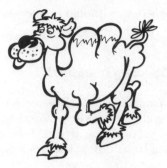

A camel can survive many days in the desert without drinking, on account of its humps. Diabetes makes you more sensitive to dehydration. Be sure always to drink plenty of fluid when you are in a hot country, especially if you have problems with diarrhea or vomiting. If you find yourself feeling nauseous or vomiting, you should drink often but only a few sips at a time. (See the chapter on illness page 258.)

time insulin in the evening when you arrive at your destination (at the "new" bedtime). It is important to check your blood glucose before every meal when improvising like this. If you sleep for many hours on the plane you can try taking a small dose of bedtime insulin. However, if you sleep less than 4-5 hours, it will probably be easier to adjust to the new time zone if you stick to rapid or short-acting insulin during the night (see also "Staying awake all night" on page 85).

2-dose treatment

If you use a 2-dose treatment it may be difficult to adjust to a shorter or longer day. You will probably be better off if you change temporarily to premeal injections 3-4 times daily while travelling. You should have tested this regime well in advance to know what doses are needed with different types of meals.

If you use a 2-dose treatment and travel westwards (longer day) take extra premeal insulin doses on the plane and take your usual afternoon dose when you arrive, adjusting it to the night time at the destination. If you travel eastwards (shorter day) take a dose of premeal insu-

Travel pharmacy

✈ Glucagon.

✈ Fever suppressing drugs. Acetaminophen/paracetamol and/or aspirin /salicylic acid (adults only).

✈ Nose drops (flying while you have a cold can be painful).

✈ Imodium®(loperamide) for diarrhea
(above 12 years of age).
Give if:≥ 4 loose stools a day or
≥ 2 loose stools a day and fever.
Dose: 2 tablets initially, thereafter 1 tablet after each bout of diarrhea.
(Maximum 8 tablets per day for 3 days.)
See a doctor if your general condition is affected, your symptoms worsen or if you do not improve within 3 days.[731]

✈ Oral rehydration solution, powder or tablets (Dioralyte® or similar).

✈ Antibiotics for diarrhea when travelling to Southern Europe, Asia, Africa or Latin/South America:

Lexinor®, Utinor®, Norfloxacin
Not for children younger than 12 years old or pregnant women.
Dose: 200 mg twice daily for prophylactic use or 400 mg twice daily for 3 days if you are having acute diarrhea.[731]

Co-trimoxazole, Colizole®(trimethoprim + sulphamethoxazole) or similar for children younger than 12 years old.

✈ Travel sickness pills or scopolamine adhesives.

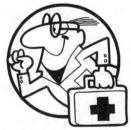

Always take glucagon wherever you go and you will have your own emergency treatment handy.

Safety rules for flying within the US

✈ Syringes or insulin delivery systems should be accompanied by the insulin in its original pharmaceutically labelled box.

✈ Capped lancets should be accompanied by a glucose meter that has the manufacturer's name embossed on the meter.

✈ An intact glucagon kit should be kept in its original preprinted, pharmaceutically labelled container.

✈ No exceptions will be made. Prescriptions and letters of medical necessity will not be accepted.

✈ A passenger encountering any diabetes-related difficulty because of security measures should ask to speak with a Complaints Resolution Officer (CRO) for the airline.

Diabetes equipment you may need on the trip

✈ ID and necklace or bracelet indicating that you have diabetes.

✈ Extra insulin pen and/or syringes (pre-filled pens are handy for this).

✈ Keep all your insulin divided into separate items of hand-luggage.

✈ Thermometer to check the temperature of the refrigerator (for insulin).

✈ Finger-pricking device, and lancets.

✈ Test strips for blood glucose, and meter.

✈ Test strips for ketones (blood and/or urine).

✈ Dextrose/glucose tablets and gel.

✈ thermometer.

✈ Telephone and fax numbers for your diabetes healthcare team at home.

✈ Insurance documents.

lin for the late evening snack on the plane. If the night on the plane is shorter than 4-5 hours, you can try skipping the intermediate-acting bedtime insulin. Instead take an extra dose of rapid or short-acting insulin if necessary. Take your usual dose of rapid or short-acting insulin with breakfast but decrease the intermediate portion by 20-40%.[430]

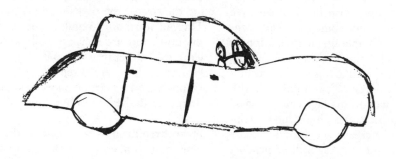

Tobias 9 years

Associated diseases

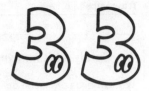

Some diseases are more common if you have diabetes. Celiac disease and hypothyroidism are examples of so called autoimmune diseases (see page 322) where the immune system is involved. Because diabetes is, in part, a hereditary disease, it is also more common for other family members, as well as the person with diabetes, to have other autoimmune diseases. Both hypothyroidism and celiac disease can be difficult to detect. Regular measurements with blood tests are therefore a part of annual checkups.

Celiac disease

Celiac disease (intolerance to gluten in wheat, oats, rye and barley) is ten times more common in children and adults with diabetes. Studies have shown that 3-6% of all children with diabetes have this disease as well.[398] If you have untreated celiac disease, you will have damaged bowel lining. Your body will have difficulty absorbing food and, as a result, your blood glucose levels are unlikely to be high even after meals. Your insulin requirement will tend to be low and hypoglycemia may be more common.[398,552] Often people with this disease have no further symptoms, but some may have generalized abdominal complaints, constipation or diarrhea and are sometimes anemic. Screening by a blood test for celiac disease is recommended for both children [673] and adults [380] with diabetes. The best way to manage celiac disease is to avoid all food containing gluten. Gluten-free food may increase the blood glucose level quicker than the corresponding product containing gluten.

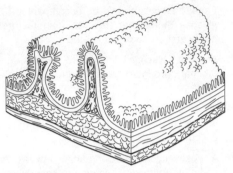

The bowel lining is arranged in narrow pleats with small projections that look like fingers (called villi). In this way the absorbent surface of the intestine increases to as much as 200 square meters (250 square yards). In celiac disease, these villi are destroyed and the surface that can absorb nourishment decreases considerably, down to as little as 2 square meters (2.5 square yards).

Thyroid diseases

The thyroid gland in your neck, just below the Adam's apple, can be damaged by auto antibodies which lead to a decreased production of thyroid hormones (called hypothyroidism). Your body will try to compensate for this by increasing the size of the thyroid gland (called goiter). Thyroid hormones regulate the metabolism in the body and a deficiency will cause tiredness, lethargy, intolerance to cold and constipation. However, there are often no symptoms at all. Hypoglycemia may be more common in children with diabetes and hypothyroidism.[553]

Hypothyroidism is a hormone deficiency disease (as is diabetes) but the treatment is much simpler. It involves taking 1-2 tablets per day containing thyroid hormone. Your body will use the hormone from the tablets when it is needed.

Toxic goiter (hyperthyroidism, increased production of thyroid hormone) is also more common amongst people with diabetes. Frequent symptoms are weight loss, feelings of warmth, and diarrhea.

Skin diseases

When the blood glucose level is high, fluid loss via the urine may cause the skin to become dry and itchy due to a degree of dehydration.

Irregular reddish-brown skin lesions, 2-10 mm (1/10-1/2 inch) in size, may appear on the lower part of the leg and are called shin spots. Sometimes they even appear on the forearm or thighs. The cause is unclear but they can develop after an accidental trauma such as bumping the leg on the edge of a table. This type of skin lesion is fairly common, especially in men, and usually arises after the age of 30.

Another skin condition found in around 1% of people with diabetes is necrobiosis lipoidica diabeticorum.[600,823] This shows as round or irregular red-brownish lesions with very thin skin, and sometimes ulcers. These skin changes are usually seen on the front of the lower part of the leg but can also be found on the feet, arms, hands, face or scalp.[407] The lesions usually appear in people who are in their 30s or 40s, but can occasionally arise in people who are still only in their teens.[600] They grow slowly over many years and are not affected by blood glucose control. The cause is unknown but some data indicate an autoimmune origin.[600] There is no known effective treatment but you can try applying a stoma-type bandage (such as Duoderm®). Skin transplants have been used successfully in more difficult cases.

Adults with diabetes can develop blisters on their fingers or toes. These look similar to burns, but the underlying skin is not irritated.[407] Usually they will dry within a week or so, but can lead to ulcers that heal slowly. The treatment of choice is to prick the blisters with a sterile needle and then apply a dry bandage.

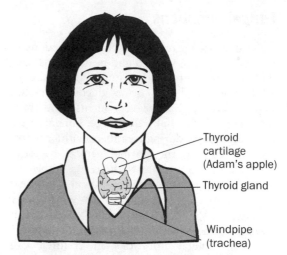

Thyroid cartilage (Adam's apple)

Thyroid gland

Windpipe (trachea)

The thyroid gland is located in front of the windpipe and is normally not visible. When the gland cannot produce enough hormone, it will increase in size, making it clearly visible (called goiter). Goiter can also be caused by an overproduction of hormones but is then referred to as toxic goiter.

Acanthosis nigricans is a skin disorder characterized by a dark pigmentation and insulin resistance which is sometimes found in people with type 2 diabetes (see page 13). As far as it is known, none of these skin conditions have any relationship to glucose control or A1C levels.

Infections

The white blood cells that help defend the body against infections work less efficiently if the blood glucose level is above 250 mg/dl (14 mmol/l). So this makes infection more likely.[48] This is particularly true for urinary tract infections and skin infections.[474,600] It follows, therefore, that your blood glucose level should be as close to normal as possible if you are fighting off an infection. One study found bacteria in the urine without symptoms in 26% of women with type 1 diabetes.[295] With a blood glucose below 200 mg/dl (11 mmol/l), the risk of infection after surgery decreased considerably in another study.[307]

Fungal infections

Genital itching caused by fungal infections is more common in women and teenage girls with diabetes after puberty. The fungus thrives better when the blood and urine glucose level are high.[194] Itching may be very intense and there may be a whitish flaky discharge. Fungal infections often arise during treatment with antibiotics that disturb the normal genital bacterial flora. The treatment of choice is improved blood glucose control and a topical antifungal cream until symptoms resolve, which may require 6-14 days of treatment.[96,600] Men can have the same type of fungal infection under the foreskin. Fungal infections in children can appear as cracks in the corner of the mouth, or sores in the cuticle or between the fingers.[600]

Diseases that can cause you to need less insulin

Cortisol deficiency:

A low cortisol production in the adrenal glands decreases the blood glucose level. This can be caused by a disease in the glands (adrenal insufficiency, Addison's disease) or disturbed function of the pituitary gland.

Growth hormone deficiency:

Low production of growth hormone (pituitary insufficiency) decreases the blood glucose level.

Gluten intolerance:

Intolerance of gluten (celiac disease) causes reduced food absorption from the intestine.

Deficiency of thyroid hormone:

Low production of thyroid hormone (hypothyroidism) causes a slower metabolism in the body.

Renal insufficiency:

Renal insufficiency causes a decreased degradation and excretion of insulin.

Complications in blood vessels

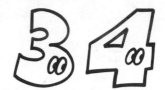

It may be distressing to think ahead about how things will turn out in the future. Many people have relatives or friends who have had diabetes for quite a number of years. Someone might tell you about a person with diabetes who has had all kinds of complications. It is important to remember that the diabetes complications we see today are caused by 30-40 years of diabetes with the type of diabetes treatment available during that time. The result may be discouraging with serious complications in the eyes, kidneys, feet and nerves. Individuals in this age group may have had a shorter life span due to kidney damage or heart disease.

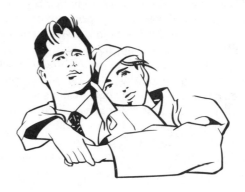

What causes complications?

We don't know for certain the reasons behind side effects and complications that develop after many years of diabetes. However, it is known that they are caused by high blood glucose levels, and that high A1C values and a long duration of diabetes will increase the risk of complications. Different people are more or less susceptible to developing these complications, but the reason for this difference is not yet known. The important message is that the better the blood glucose measurements and the lower the A1C is, the less likely the person is to develop diabetes complications in later years.

The risk of blindness and partial sight in people with diabetes is three times higher than the general population.[346] Approximately 2.3% of all individuals with type 1 diabetes in a European study were blind.[708] It is however very important to know that the outlook for someone developing diabetes today is not at all the same as for a person who has had the disease for 30-40 years. Insulin treatment is much better and the possibilities of both preventing and

treating eye complications have improved considerably in most countries.

It may be very difficult to know how much one should tell children about complications. Teenagers understand more and want to know about their situation. We feel it is important that "all the cards are on the table", so you know what type of complications can occur in the long run and what the risks are. It is important to know the facts, but it is not something you need to talk about on a daily basis.

A 13-year old girl believed that candy as such caused the risk for complications and blindness (and not the high blood glucose levels that can follow from excessive candy eating). No wonder she was in agony whenever she ate something sweet and still she just could not resist doing it.

During family teaching sessions on complications in diabetes I always encourage the young person to sit in although I do not force anyone to listen. Younger children need to know as much as they can understand, but perhaps not too many details. But I will ask a question every now and then to see how interested the child is in what we are talking about. If he or she wants to go off and play after a while, probably the topic has stopped being interesting.

In the home environment, it is a good idea to bring up the subject of complications in a careful way every once in a while, preferably when the young (or not so young) person with diabetes is in the mood for talking. Many children and teenagers store up their questions. They sometimes don't want to raise difficult issues with their mom or dad for fear of worrying them. Diabetes educational camps provide excellent opportunities for group discussions on the dangers associated with diabetes. In the course of these, many children reveal they have thought about such issues at one time or another.

Heart and large blood vessel diseases: Diagnosis

① Blood pressure measurements.

② Examination of pulses in feet and lower legs, with a doppler device if necessary.

③ Analysis of cholesterol and triglycerides in the blood.

Treatment

The same advice is given to all people with an increased risk of heart and blood vessel diseases, regardless of whether or not they have diabetes:

① Stop smoking.

② Increase the amount of physical exercise or physiotherapy.

③ Avoid putting on too much weight.

④ Avoid negative or undue stress (see page 255).

⑤ Don't drink too much alcohol.

⑥ Treat high blood pressure.

⑦ Eat foods that are rich in fiber and low in fat. Increase fruit and vegetable intake.

Complications

① Large blood vessels: Arteriosclerosis Heart disease.

② Small blood vessels: Eyes, kidneys, nerves.

If your child has diabetes, don't threaten them with kidney damage or blindness, no matter how worried you are. Frightening your child won't do any good. On the contrary, such threats will generate feelings of hopelessness, like "drawing a blank in the lottery of life". I have all too often met children who have told me that their parents have said "Don't eat candy because it will make you blind!" Such statements will only cause anguish since children cannot understand the time frame involved. Try instead to explain and motivate the child to think carefully about what, and how much, they should eat.

Diabetes is such a common disease that if we do not tell the children about complications when they are old enough to understand, then someone else will. Sooner or later, someone (with the best of intentions) will say: "Poor child, your diabetes will someday make you blind..." It is important that young people know the real facts and are able to answer: "That is how things used to be, but nowadays there are much better ways to treat diabetes!"

It used to be believed that the years before puberty were not significant when it came to the risk of developing complications. However, it has been shown that the A1C levels during the years before puberty contribute significantly to the risk of long-term complications.[141,218,538]

In some patients, early signs of complications can be found on close examination after 10-20 years of diabetes, depending upon how their blood glucose levels have been over these years. In any case, signs of complications usually do not cause practical problems before 20-30 years of the disease. Some people who have had their diabetes for 60 years have still not developed signs of complications.

Large blood vessels

Diseases of the heart and blood vessels are more common among people with diabetes, and the large blood vessels in your body are at greater risk of developing arteriosclerosis (hardening, narrowing and eventually blocking of the blood vessels). The increased risk for arteriosclerosis

and heart problems is thought to be caused in part by the high blood glucose level. Other contributing factors are cholesterol problems and high blood pressure.

If you keep your blood glucose levels under control, there is every chance that you will be able to put off the time when diseases like arteriosclerosis become a problem for you.[408,570] There is also research evidence to show that effective treatment reduces your chances of developing early heart disease.[480,570]

Why are only certain cells damaged by a high blood glucose?

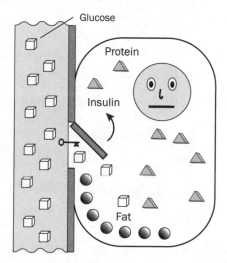

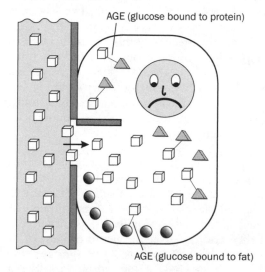

Even if the blood glucose is high, only a certain amount of glucose in the bloodstream will pass into the cell as it is dependent on insulin to "open the door". Most of the cells in your body work this way.

Many important cells in your body can take in glucose without the help of insulin. In these cells glucose will enter in direct proportion to the level in the blood. Example of such cells are found in the brain, nerves, retina, kidneys, adrenal glands, red blood cells and in the walls of the blood vessels. It may not seem logical that some cells can take in glucose without insulin but in a situation where there is a lack of glucose in a healthy body (for example, when starving) the production of insulin is stopped. This will lead to saving the available glucose for the organs in your body that are most vital. However, when a person has diabetes, this phenomenon will cause these cells to take in large amounts of glucose whenever your blood glucose is high. Glucose will bind within the cells to form so called AGE (advanced glycation end products) that has the potential of damaging the cells (see page 325).

The increased risk of diseases of the heart and blood vessels is the main reason that persons with diabetes are recommend not to smoke and to keep fat levels in their diet low. Fat has no direct effect on the blood glucose level other than causing the stomach to empty more slowly (see page 206). Increasing the number of fruit and vegetables eaten, and taking regular physical exercise, is also important in protecting against heart and blood vessel diseases.

Small blood vessels

If your blood glucose levels are high for long periods, this will lead to glucose building up in the cells in the walls of the blood vessels, causing these vessels to become more brittle.[670] The cells mainly affected by this glucose toxicity are those which don't need insulin in order to transport glucose, i.e. the eyes, kidneys, nerves and blood vessels. As glucose can pass freely into these cells, they will always be exposed to high glucose concentrations when the blood glucose level is high.

If a person has diabetes, glucose binds to a protein in the wall of the red blood cells. This makes the red blood cells stiff. These stiffened cells will have difficulties passing through the finest blood vessels (capillaries) as they need to if they are to deliver oxygen to the rest of the body's tissues.[556] So it is very important from the point of view of the red blood cells that blood glucose levels can be kept under control. Normal blood glucose levels for 24 hours restore the normal texture of the blood cell walls, remedying the problem.[556]

Complications affecting the eyes (retinopathy)

Risks

The risk of eye damage has decreased considerably with modern diabetes and eye care. As of today, a majority of people with 15-20 years of diabetes will have some kind of retinal changes, half of which need laser treatment.[18,732] Of 1000

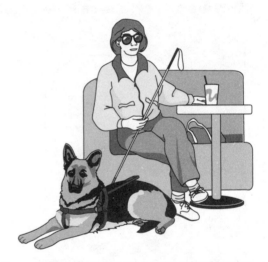

Many people feel that blindness is the worst thing that can happen if they have diabetes. You may worry about this, for example if you have been eating too much candy. However, it may be difficult to talk about this with your parents (or your partner) since they will be worried too.

If you develop diabetes today and have a good A1C during the years to come, there is a very little risk that you will lose your sight. This is because much better methods of treatment have been developed during recent years, both for diabetes and for eye damage.

Try to talk about this at home even if it is difficult. It is important that you know all the facts and that you realize you can influence the course of events yourself. Many adults have seen what has happened to people with diabetes in the past, especially if they have older friends or relatives who have been diabetic for a long time. They may find it difficult to believe that the same will not apply to someone developing diabetes today.

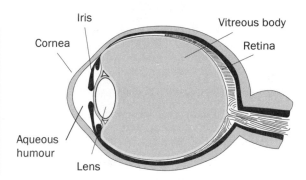

The eye seen in cross-section. Eye damage is first noted in the retina. At check-ups, the retina is examined after dilation of the pupil. Most often it is photographed (called fundal photography) and an eye specialist will have a close look at the pictures.

individuals with diabetes, one will sustain serious visual impairment (visual acuity 0.1 or less) each year but blindness due to diabetes is today very rare in countries where modern treatment methods are available.[679]

Brittle capillaries can give rise to small swellings called microaneurysms (see illustration on page 308). These are thought of as "background" problems that do not affect the sight. It is important to realize that this type of early lesion can get better if blood glucose control is improved. On the other hand, if you continue to have a high blood glucose and high A1C the process of change in your eyes will continue, and the lesions on the retina may worsen and new blood vessels form. These new blood vessels are brittle and can easily rupture resulting in bleeding and damage to your vision. Usually, the blood will be absorbed and the sight restored. Large or repeated instances of bleeding that are left untreated can result in permanent damage to your vision and, in the worst case, blindness. Impaired color or night vision can be a result of damage to the nervous system caused by diabetes.[577] Smoking also increases the risk of damage to your vision.[561]

Treatment

The most important treatment is good blood glucose control. This can reverse early changes to the retina. We inform newly diagnosed chil-

dren and teenagers that they should not need to risk becoming blind as, today, we have better methods both for treating diabetes and for avoiding possible eye damage. But you need to look after your diabetes, as having high A1C levels over a period of 20-30 years still puts you at quite high risk of becoming blind.

You may experience some worsening of eye damage if you improve your metabolic control considerably (as when starting with an insulin pump).[342,200] It is important to know that studies have shown that this situation is temporary only, even if some people need laser photocoagulation treatment. If you continue with the good glucose control, the changes to your eyes will reverse. It has been suggested that people with established eye damage should try to improve their blood glucose control slowly if they are to avoid damage to their sight.[342] However, in the DCCT study the risk was still there, even if the A1C was gradually improved.[200] A temporary deterioration was seen in women who became pregnant during the DCCT study, and this can be attributed to the rapidly improved blood glucose levels. At the end of the study, the level of eye damage had decreased and was back to average level again.[201]

Laser is an effective form of treatment which can spare the sight and sometimes even improve

Eye damage: Diagnosis

Eye examination
(preferably fundal photography [394]):

① Initially at diagnosis of diabetes.[184,701]

② Annually after 2 years of diabetes
(5 years in children before puberty), or from
the age of 10-11 years.[18,439,701,735]

③ To obtain a driving licence in many countries.

Treatment

① Good glucose control.

② Stop smoking. [561]

③ Laser treatment.

④ Surgery.

it. In a large study of individuals with high-risk eye damage, the progression to severe visual loss decreased from 26% in untreated eyes to 11% after laser photocoagulation.[22] Some eye lesions can be operated on.

To be able to discover changes as early as possible, all individuals with diabetes should be given an eye examination annually as soon as their diabetes has 2 years duration (5 years for those who have not yet reached puberty).[701] In

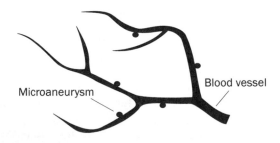

After many years of high blood glucose levels, the blood vessels of the retina will become brittle and small "bubbles" (called microaneurysms) can form. They do not affect your vision but can be seen on a photograph of the retina.

addition, you may need to have your eyes examined when you apply for a driver's licene. The most sensitive type of examination is a photography of the retina (fundus photography). Before taking the photograph, eye drops will be applied in order to dilate the pupils, so that a larger part of the retina can be seen on the photograph. The retina can also be examined with a special instrument (an ophthalmoscope) but this method is not as good as fundal photography in detecting changes.[560]

Disturbed vision at unstable blood glucose levels

Blurred vision for a couple of hours is a common symptom of unstable blood glucose levels. It is not in any way dangerous for your vision or associated with future visual impairment. This most often happens in the first week of diabetes when insulin is first started and the blood glucose levels fall considerably (see page 30). Unstable blood glucose can also cause disturbances in color vision.

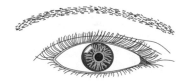

Temporarily blurred vision when blood glucose levels are high does not result in any permanent eye damage.

Sometimes the disturbed vision can continue for several weeks. This is caused by glucose being stored as sorbitol in the lens, disturbing the fluid distribution. This will have a temporary effect on the way the lens works, and make you nearsighted. However, if your blood glucose levels are high for long periods, there is some risk that permanent clouding will occur (cataract). For example, this may happen if an adolescent has had symptoms for a long time (many months) before diagnosis.[184] Cataract surgery can be performed and is usually successful.

Glasses

Your blood glucose levels should be stable when you try out new glasses. Otherwise, your vision will be affected by temporary changes in blood glucose. After the onset of diabetes, it may take 2-3 months of normal blood glucose levels before the lens has returned to its usual shape.[203] This means it is not a good idea to get glasses or replace them during this time.

Contact lenses

People with diabetes can wear contact lenses. However, you should avoid long-term lenses (that are replaced every second or third week) as the protecting cell layer of the cornea tends to be more brittle if you have diabetes.[144]

Complications affecting the kidneys (nephropathy)

Risks

The blood vessels of the kidneys are formed into small clusters where waste products in the blood are filtered into the urine. Damage to the walls of these blood vessels causes an increased leakage of protein into the urine. Tiny amounts of protein (known as microalbuminuria) can then be detected in the urine. If the leakage continues, the person is at risk of developing high blood pressure and continuous leakage of protein into the urine (proteinuria). This may occur after 10-30 years of diabetes and leads to uremia (urine poisoning because the body is unable to rid itself of its waste products). If the condition is left untreated, dialysis will be necessary in a further 7-10 years.[62] Only about 30-40% of all those with diabetes will develop microalbuminuria and its associated risk of permanent kidney damage.[62,732] Good diabetes control decreases the risk of kidney damage. It is still not known why more than half of all individuals with diabetes are not at all susceptible to kidney damage, but hereditary factors appear to play a significant part.[198]

Microalbuminuria is defined as more than 20 µg/min in a timed urine sample or more than 30 mg per 24 hours in two out of three consecutive tests [62,151] taken within a 2-3 month period. Proteinuria (manifest kidney damage) is defined as more than 200 µg/min in a timed urine sample or more than 300 mg in a 24 hour

---

Kidney damage: Diagnosis

① Measure blood pressure regularly.

② Check for microalbuminuria (small amounts of protein in the urine) annually:
In children after 5 years of diabetes or at age 11, or at puberty (whichever is earlier).[735]
In adolescents after 2 years of diabetes.[735]
In adults after 5 years of diabetes.[25]

Check at every visit if microalbuminuria has been detected.

③ Measure kidney function when necessary.

Treatment

① Good glucose control (A1C).

② Stop smoking.

③ Microalbuminuria is treated with ACE-inhibitors.

④ Treatment of blood pressure above 130/80 [28,62,565] or 95th percentile for age.[701]

⑤ Treatment of urinary tract infections.

⑥ Reduction of protein and salt in your diet if you have persistent excretion of protein in the urine.[274]

⑦ Dialysis.

⑧ Transplantation.

period. Overnight microalbuminuria can be measured as a concentration test on early morning urine (such as Micral-test®, with a cut-off 30 mg/l).[735] A newer method (now recommended by ADA and CDA) of measuring microalbuminuria in a morning spot sample is the ratio between albumin and creatinine (A/C ratio or ACR). With this method, microalbuminuria is defined as more than 2.5 mg/mmol (>30 mg/g) [25] in men and > 3.5 mg/mmol in women [735] because of lower muscle mass according to ADA and 2.0 mg/mmol and 2.8 mg/mmol respectively according to CDA.[127] Because exercise within 24 hours, infection, fever, smoking, menstruation, a very high blood glucose level and blood in the urine may increase the level of microalbuminuria, an abnormal value should be repeated.[27,703] The level is lower in a morning sample as you have been lying down all night.

The ACR microalbuminuria cut-off for a random daytime urine sample (spot urine) has been defined as more than 4.5 mg/mmol for boys and more than 5.2 mg/mmol for girls.[771] Some adolescents have been found to have microalbuminuria although they have had diabetes for only a short time.[771] This may be caused by puberty as such but these individuals may also have an increased vulnerability in their kidneys leading to a greater risk of kidney damage later on if they have high A1C values. Proteinuria can have other causes apart from diabetes.

In one study of adults, the risk of progression to established kidney damage was increased in people whose diastolic blood pressure was higher than 80 mm.[565] In another study, 53% of those smoking, 33% of those who had smoked previously, but only 11% of those who had never smoked, experienced an increase in the damage to their kidneys in the course of one year.[675]

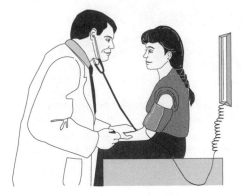

Control of blood pressure is very important to prevent and reduce kidney damage. Your blood pressure should be checked routinely at clinic visits.

Treatment

Just as for eye lesions, the most important treatment for nephropathy is tight insulin and blood glucose control. This is because, if microalbuminuria is discovered early, it can be reversed by lowering the blood glucose level and A1C.[98] It is equally important to treat raised blood pressure early on. Weight control helps to keep blood pressure within target range. The average blood pressure reduction per kilogram of weight loss is 1-2 mm Hg.[274]

Treatment of albuminuria with a special type of anti-hypertensive drugs (ACE inhibitors) has shown good results even if the blood pressure is normal. This is recommended as routine treatment as soon as permanent microalbuminuria is discovered.[62,785] However, ACE-inhibitors should not be used during pregnancy since they can cause damage to the unborn child. One study showed that the risk of microalbuminuria progressing into manifested kidney damage decreased from 21.9 to 7.2% when it was treated with ACE inhibitors.[545]

The progression of renal disease can be successfully slowed by a reduction in dietary protein.[599] Renal failure can be treated with dialysis or kidney transplantation.

Complications affecting the nerves (neuropathy)

Risks

Your body's nerve fibers, which are made of very long and thin cells, can be affected after many years of diabetes. The blood vessels supplying the nerve fibers can be damaged resulting in a decreased supply of oxygen.[750] This causes damage to the nerves' insulating covering (myelin sheath) and ultimately results in poorer nerve impulses. Sensation decreases and there can be accompanying numbing or tingling. The longest nerves are the most vulnerable, thus problems arise primarily in the feet, fingers or lower parts of the legs. Later on, a more general sensation loss can occur, starting from the toes and spreading upwards. Pain caused by nerve damage can even be felt in the hands and shoulders.

If the blood flow in your small skin capillaries is decreased, along with sensation, you will not feel the pain from small wounds and healing will be slow. Decreased perspiration in your feet can make the skin dry and cause it to crack. With inadequate foot care, small wounds get worse. If untreated, this may lead to ulcers, gangrene, and in the worst case, amputation. If you have problems with decreased sensation you should avoid sports that involve the risk of foot damage (blisters, cuts) such as running or soccer.

If you step on a nail or splinter there is always a risk of wound infection. If you have nerve damage with diminished sensation, the risk of infection increases as you may be unaware of the wound. Impaired sensitivity to pain often means that a person with diabetes will seek medical care for such a wound later than they

otherwise would (9 days after the trauma compared to 5 days for a person without diabetes in one study [478]). The infection will then have had time to spread and the risk for a complication, i.e. tissue or bone infection, becomes much greater. In the above mentioned study, 35% of the individuals with diabetes had an infection compared to 13% of individuals without diabetes. It is also worth mentioning that 42% of those with diabetes had injured themselves

The autonomic nervous system

Different organs can be affected by damage to the autonomic nervous system after many years of diabetes (modified from reference [729]). The risk for these complications is decreased with modern diabetes care.

Organ	Problem
Heart	Dizziness when standing up.
Blood vessels	Reduced capacity for physical work.
Esophagus	Difficulty in swallowing.
Stomach	Vomiting. Slow emptying of the stomach.
Intestines	Constipation, night time diarrhea.
Rectum	Incontinence.
Urine bladder	Difficulties emptying the bladder. Frequent voiding.
Penis	Erection problems/ impotence (see page 277). Ejaculation backwards into the bladder (can result in infertility).
Vagina	Dry mucous membranes.
Sweat glands	Profuse sweating in the face and neck after eating hot food, spices or cheddar cheese. Decreased sweating in feet, legs and trunk.
Skin	Increased skin temperature.
Pupils	Small pupils.

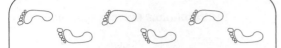

Children with diabetes have healthy feet and don't need special foot care. Ordinary hygiene is quite enough. Foot baths can be relieving for tired, healthy feet and there are no restrictions for children or teenagers with diabetes in this case. It is only if you already have nerve damage that foot baths with massage should be avoided. If you are in any doubt about this ask your doctor.

Nerve damage: Diagnosis

① Test of vibratory sense (tuning-fork).

② Test of sensation with a thin plastic fiber (monofilament).

③ Tests with special instruments.

Treatment

① Improved glucose control.

② Foot care, good shoes that don't hurt.

③ Treatment of foot and leg ulcers.

④ Oxygen treatment in pressurized chambers is sometimes tried if ulcers are slow to heal.

⑤ Drug treatment — ongoing research.

when barefoot, compared to 19% of people without diabetes.

The part of our nervous system that is self-regulatory (uncontrollable by willpower) is called the autonomic nervous system. This can also be damaged by diabetes but the symptoms will be different. They include disturbances in sweating, diarrhea, constipation, impotence (see page 277) or delayed emptying of the stomach.

Difficulties in emptying the bladder properly may be caused by diabetes. Individuals who have had diabetes for many years should therefore empty their bladder thoroughly and often.

Delayed stomach emptying can lead to hypoglycemia one or two hours after a meal. At that time, the insulin level will be at its highest if you are using premeal injections. However, when the peaks of glucose from the meal are delayed, the timing with premeal insulin injections will not match, especially if you are using rapid acting insulins (NovoLog/NovoRapid or Humalog). One idea is to try taking insulin after rather than before the meal. Other symptoms of delayed stomach emptying are an early feeling of being full and a sense of the stomach being distended. The emptying rate of the stomach can be examined by a special type of X-ray (scintigraphy). A decreased A1C with the avoidance of high blood glucose levels can lead to a

reduction of these types of symptoms. If problems are pronounced, you should try to exclude everything that decreases the emptying rate of the stomach (fat, dietary fiber, very cold or very hot food, see page 203). Special drugs may also help.

The cells in the brain can pick up glucose directly from the blood without using insulin, but despite this they seem to be relatively immune to the long-term toxic effects of glucose. This may be due to the so called blood-brain barrier that prevents substances from the blood to be freely transported into the brain. The brain cells normally have much lower glucose levels than the blood.

Treatment

As for the other complications of diabetes, the most important treatment for nerve damage is improved diabetes control. Good foot care is also important. If the skin lesions are slow to heal, oxygen treatment in a pressurized chamber can be effective.[257]

Delayed emptying of the stomach: Diagnosis [44]

① Typical symptoms:
Hypoglycemia 1 hour after a meal.
Early feeling of satiety (no more hunger).
Feeling of being full.
Distended stomach.

② Special X-ray (scintigraphy).

Treatment

① Improved glucose control.

② Change in diet:
Less fiber.
Less fat.
Small but frequent meals.
Temperature of food should be not less than 4°C (39°) or more than 40°C (104° F).

③ Take insulin injection after eating.

④ Drug treatment.

Foot care if you have nerve damage

① Don't walk around barefoot.

② Always use clean and dry socks. Wear them inside out (less risk of blisters from the seams).

③ Inspect your feet daily or twice daily for redness or blisters. Use a mirror to view the soles.

④ Wear shoes that fit well and don't hurt. Empty them of gravel often.

⑤ Wash your feet carefully and rub them with moisturizing cream in order to avoid chapping.

⑥ See a doctor as an emergency if you see redness, callous growth, blisters, ingrown toenails or signs of infection.

⑦ Ensure you have regular foot care at the diabetes clinic. Learn how to manicure your toenails to avoid sore skin.

⑧ If you smoke, stop!

Other complications

Limited joint mobility (LJM) can be a complication of diabetes.[761] The elbow and finger extension, and wrist flexion, can be decreased. The mobility can also be decreased in the feet and other joints. The mobility in the finger joints can be tested by the "prayer sign", i.e. putting the hands together in a praying position with the fingers fanned. LJM is present if there is a missing joint contact between the fingers. This is most common in the little finger.

Lowering the risk of complications

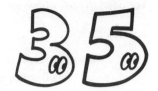

Constantly trying to achieve a good blood glucose level can be very tiresome. Many people, including teenagers, are pessimistic about the benefits of keeping the blood glucose low believing that: "Things will go to pot anyway," whatever they do.

However, there is convincing scientific evidence that good glucose control will pay off by postponing and preventing complications. While it may be impossible to avoid every type of long term complication of diabetes completely (despite today's improved treatment methods), it is quite clear that a person with a higher A1C risks earlier and more severe complications. Of course there are always exceptions. Some people do have complications in spite of meticulous control while others, who have never "managed well", are spared. This may seem very unfair, but it can also be of some comfort to those individuals who do develop complications since there is no guarantee that, had they achieved better blood glucose levels, the problems would have been completely avoided.

An unusual example comes from Kuwait, where a person with kidney disease (without diabetes) received a kidney donated from a person with diabetes who was killed in a traffic accident. The kidney had been severely damaged by diabetes but no other suitable kidney was available for him. The transplanted kidney now was exposed to perfect glucose control since the person who received it as a transplant did not have diabetes. Two years later, new tests were performed on the transplanted kidney, and the diabetes lesions were found to have gone!

The DCCT study

A large US study clearly shows that a lower A1C will decrease the development of compli-

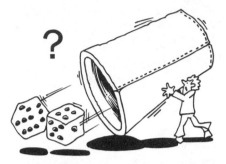

Many people believe that complications strike randomly among the population with diabetes. Others feel that it does not matter if you "manage well", complications will arise anyway. In fact, modern research has clearly shown that the degree of long-term complications depends directly upon the blood glucose levels over the course of the years that a person has diabetes.

cations.[191] In the course of a nine-year period, 1441 individuals with diabetes (aged between 13-39 years) were compared. They were divided into two groups, one with an average A1C of 7% (intensive treatment using insulin pumps (42% at the end of the study) or multiple daily injections, and one with a level of 9% (conventional treatment with 1 or 2 doses/day).

The insulin treatment was not the only factor that differed between the two groups. In the intensive treatment group, blood glucose was measured four times a day, and the doses of insulin adjusted if necessary. Clinic visits were scheduled once a month with telephone contacts in between on at least a weekly and often a daily basis. A1C was measured every month. The aim was specifically to attain low blood glucose readings (70-120 mg/dl, 3.9-6.7 mmol/l, before meals) and an A1C of 6%, at the highest. In the group using 1-2 doses per day, the goal of treatment was to feel well including the absence of symptoms from high or low blood glucose levels. Clinic visits were scheduled every three months, urine or blood glucose was monitored

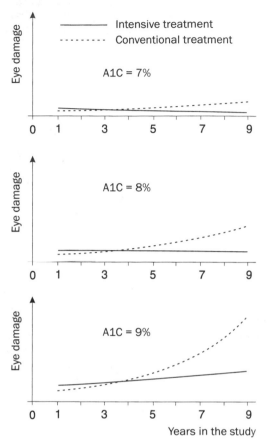

Intensive treatment

Conventional treatment

A1C = 7%

A1C = 8%

A1C = 9%

Years in the study

Patients in the DCCT study with the same average A1C throughout the 9 study years but different types of insulin treatment, were compared.[193] Somewhat surprisingly there was a clear difference, i.e. a considerably increased risk of visual impairment when on conventional treatment (1-2 doses/day) compared to intensive treatment. With 1-2 doses/day the average A1C must be reduced to 7% to avoid visual impairment while in the intensive treatment group (pump or multiple injections) A1C was above 8% before impaired vision was observed. The figures are redrawn from reference.[193]

Many parents ask us if it is healthy for the blood glucose level to swing up and down throughout the day as often happens when multiple injections or insulin pump treatments are used to maintain an optimal A1C value. The graphs above imply that there may be some further factor besides A1C that affects the development of complications. A possible explanation is that with swinging blood glucose levels, there are longer periods of normal glucose levels, compared to when the glucose levels are slightly above 180 mg/dl (10 mmol/l) for the greater part of the day, although A1C remains the same.

daily and regular education was given at the visits. A1C values were taken but the results were not revealed to this group.

In the group receiving intensive treatment, the risk of developing eye damage was lowered by 76%, early kidney damage (microalbuminuria) by 39%, severe kidney damage (albuminuria) by 54% and nerve damage by 60%. The risk of severe hypoglycemia (requiring help from another person) increased by 2-3 fold in the intensively treated group. Neuro psychological tests did not show any permanent damage from the hypoglycemic incidents.[195] The individuals in the group with intensive insulin treatment gained more weight (on average 4.6 kg, 10.1 lb). There was a 46% reduction in vaginal infections in the intensive treatment group, but no differences in the rates of other infections.[194]

Another way of presenting the data is that intensive treatment will give a person with diabetes 7.7 additional years of sight, 5.8 years of renal function, 6.0 years of limb preservation, and 5.3 additional years of life. In summary, each 10% fall in A1C (for example from 9.0 to 8.1%) decreased complications by 43-45%.[193] Neither of the two groups experienced a deterioration in the quality of their personal lives despite the increasing demands of their diabetes care and the frequency of hypoglycemia.[197] When analyzing quality of life issues and psychiatric symptoms, data showed no differences between the intensive and the conventional group despite the fact that the intensive group spent considerably more time on injections, blood glucose testing and visits to the clinic.[194] Only those individuals who had experienced repeated (three or more) episodes of severe hypoglycemia resulting in unconsciousness or seizures, scored lower on life quality. The overall conclusion was that the decreased risk of long-term complications more than compensates for the increased risk of severe hypoglycemia.

The individual's own insulin production was better sustained in the intensive treatment group (measured by level of maintained C-peptide, see page 320) which, in turn, allowed for better glucose control, less frequent hypoglycemia and fewer long-term complications.[199] These observations emphasize the importance of implementing intensive treatment, even during the early years of living with diabetes.

In the group of adolescents between the ages 13-17 years in the DCCT study, those with 1-2 doses had an average A1C of 9.8% and those with intensive treatment 8.1%.[192] After between 4 and 7 years of treatment, the group who had received intensive treatment had 53-70% fewer eye complications and 55% fewer kidney complications than the group on 1-2 doses of insulin per day. The intensively treated adolescents had a risk of severe hypoglycemia with unconsciousness or seizures of 27% in one year.[192] The corresponding figure for adults was 16%.[194]

An Australian study showed that the risk of severe hypoglycemia increased when the average A1C of the clinic went down from 10% to 8%.[189] However, European studies have not shown the same increase in risk for severe hypoglycemia when using intensive insulin treatment.[107,575,591,689] In a Swedish study of intensively treated individuals with diabetes aged 1-18 years, the risk was 15% despite a mean A1C of 7.9%[508] (DCCT numbers). See also page 47. The reason for this may lie in the fact that there is a longer tradition of using intensive treatment in Europe and that patients eventually learn, at least in part, how to avoid dangerously low blood glucose values. The frequency of hypoglycemia in the DCCT study decreased slightly towards the end of the study,[194] an observation that supports this hypothesis. More recent studies from the US show lower figures of severe hypoglycemia.[85,524]

In another American study, the average number of years until complications from different organs developed was calculated with different HbA$_1$ levels (older A1C method). For most microvascular complications to develop, it would take, on average, 83 years with an average A1C unit at 1% above normal (7%), 42

years at 8%, 28 years at 9%, 21 years at 10%, and 18 years at 11%.[584] From this follows that every percentage decline in A1C is important, even if you are in the high range.

The Oslo study

Knut Dahl-Jørgensen and collaborators in Oslo performed a long-term study comparing 2-dose treatment, multiple daily treatment and pump treatment.[342] This study showed clearly that the risk for complications decreased considerably as the A1C was lowered (see figures on previous page).

The Stockholm study

A Swedish study performed by Per Reichard showed that good glucose control pays off.[637] Two groups with diabetes were followed for 8 years, one with A1C 8.4% and the other with a level of 9.8% (DCCT numbers). The risk of kidney damage, nerve damage and progression of eye damage decreased with lower blood glu-

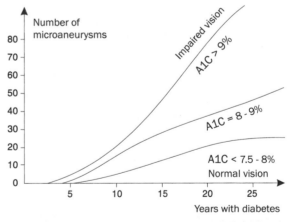

This graph is from a Norwegian study showing how the number of microaneurysms increase considerably with increased average A1C in the course of many years.[342] With a lower A1C the changes will probably not be severe enough to affect your vision. The A1C levels in this study are approximately the same as in the DCCT study (see page 105).

cose levels. In the group with higher A1C levels, 27 participants developed serious eye damage, and 9 participants developed kidney damage. In the group with lower A1C levels, however, only 12 participants developed eye damage and only one had kidney damage.

Heredity appears to play a part in the degree to which some people will develop complications at an A1C of 10-11% whereas others are unaffected until their A1C reaches 13-14%. This is very unfair and, unfortunately, we do not know why it should be the case. If your A1C is less than 10.2%, serious kidney damage can be avoided but you must have an even lower A1C if you are to avoid eye damage. Under a level of 8.1%, the risk of serious complications are minimized according to Per Reichard.[638]

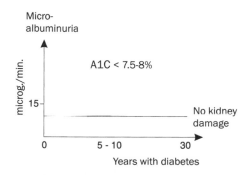

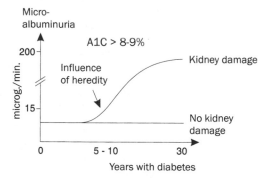

In the same Norwegian study, it was shown that kidney damage will only develop in individuals with a high A1C. But not all people with diabetes are susceptible to kidney damage as there seems to be a hereditary "sensitivity". With an average A1C below 7.5-8% you will probably not develop kidney damage even if you have such hereditary "sensitivity".

The Berlin eye study

In Berlin, 346 individuals with diabetes, aged between 8 and 35 years, were studied with a special type of X-ray displaying the vessels of the retina (fluorescence angiography). The conclusion was that if the average A1C was lower during the previous years, retinal vessel changes developed later.[181]

Average A1C	Years before eye changes
< 7%	25
7-8%	16
8-9%	13
> 9%	12

A1C levels are shown in DCCT numbers (approximately 1% lower than in the Berlin study).[181]

Every percentage lowering of A1C means a decreased risk of eye lesions. With an A1C above 9%, the risk of eye damage increased considerably.

The Linköping studies

The risk of being affected by long term complications has been studied in a series of investigations from Linköping in Sweden.[97,98,99] Children and adolescents whose diabetes developed during the 20 year period, 1961-1980, have been studied and a decreased risk in later years has been demonstrated. See their results in the figures on the next page.

The Hvidøre Study

The Hvidøre Study Group on Childhood diabetes collected data from 2,873 children and adolescents from 18 countries in Europe, Japan and North America.[558] The patients took part in the routine care program which at all centers had a multidisciplinary approach involving pediatric diabetologists. All tests for A1C were analyzed at a central laboratory.

The average A1C was 8.3% (DCCT numbers). However, the average A1C among the centres varied significantly, both between and within countries, from 7.3% to 9.9%. Of the children who had had diabetes for two years or longer, 34% had an A1C below 7.7% (DCCT numbers). A1C increased with age, reaching a maximum at 16-17 years.

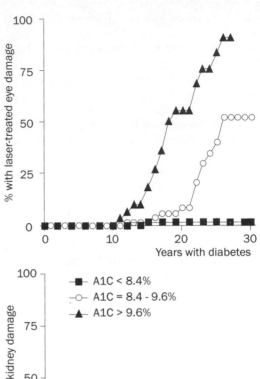

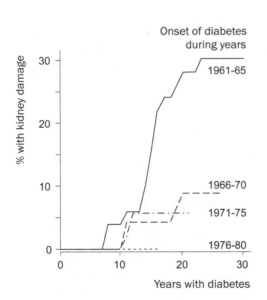

A study from Sweden shows that the risk of developing kidney damage (albuminuria) has decreased considerably in recent years.[97] Amongst those who developed diabetes before the age of 15 (between the years 1961-65), 30% developed kidney damage after 25 years of diabetes. Less than 10% of those who developed diabetes from 1966 and onwards have developed kidney damage.

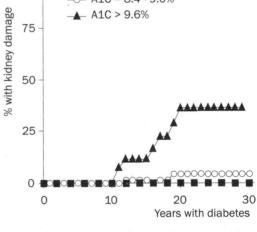

In a study of 213 individuals who had developed their diabetes before the age of 15 years (and who had been diabetic for 11-30 years), only one person with average A1C < 8.4% (DCCT numbers) needed laser treatment of their eyes.[99] Only two individuals with an average A1C < 9.6% had permanent kidney damage (so called macroalbuminuria). The conclusion is that it takes slightly lower average blood glucose to avoid eye damage than kidney damage. However, with an A1C of 8.2% or less, the risk of serious long-term complications is very low.

Research and new developments

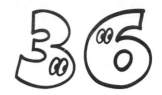

Huge efforts are put into diabetes research around the world and more than 10,000 scientific studies are published every year. A large part of this is basic research, trying to throw light upon the causes of diabetes and why different things take place in the body when a person has diabetes. Even if you hear of new treatment for diabetes from newspapers or the television, you must remember that it usually takes several years before such methods become available outside the research clinics and unfortunately many new "wonder drugs" never become established treatments.

New treatments for diabetes

Implantable insulin pumps

Insulin pumps that can be implanted into the belly (abdominal cavity) are being used as part of research programs in some centers. These pumps are refilled with insulin by the insertion of a syringe through the skin into a membrane on the pump. Premeal bolus doses are given by using a small transmitter. Insulin from the pump is injected into the abdominal cavity (called intraperitoneal delivery) and is quickly absorbed into the bloodstream. Contrary to what one may think, the risk of hypoglycemia is reduced by this type of insulin treatment.[569] This is because the insulin administered in this way passes through the liver *before* it reaches the other parts of the body, just like insulin secreted from a pancreas without diabetes.

Another research project involves an artificial pancreas which can be connected to a blood

Ongoing research projects

※ Artificial pancreas.

※ Blood glucose meters that measure without blood specimens.

※ Implantable or subcutaneous insulin pump with continuous monitoring of blood glucose levels (sensor) that regulates the insulin doses automatically ("closed loop").

※ Transplantation of pancreas or islets.

※ Alternative (noninvasive) methods of delivering insulin.

※ Immune modulation at the onset of diabetes.

※ Adding C-peptide to insulin.

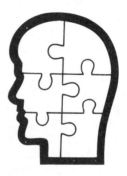

vessel. This device both measures blood glucose levels and injects insulin directly into the bloodstream. Such an approach is still very complicated and, at present, is found only in research laboratories.

Blood glucose meters

The possibility of measuring one's blood glucose at home has brought a revolution in diabetes treatment. We are now waiting for the next generation of blood glucose meters which can measure without obtaining a blood sample. Promising results have been shown using a ray of infrared light,[522] even during hypoglycemic episodes.[289] It is also possible to measure the glucose content of the fluid within the skin, using a needle that penetrates less than 1.5 mm (1/16 inch).[695]

Glucose sensor

A device that can measure the blood glucose levels continuously over a longer period of time is called a glucose sensor. So far such devices have only been shown to give reliable readings for a couple of days or a week at a time. One type of sensor is implanted into the subcutaneous fat. Glucose is measured either by an enzymatic method that generates an electrical current (MiniMed® CGMS,[89] see page 97) or by a special method called microdialysis [101] that measures the glucose content in a saline solution circulating slowly through the inserted catheter. Another method (GlucoWatch®) is to measure the glucose content of fluid extracted across the skin with an electro-osmotic method (called reverse iontophoresis).[233] After a 2 hour warm-up period and calibration with a blood glucose measurement, the device provides readings up to six times an hour for up to 13 hours, and has alarms for high, low, and rapidly falling glucose levels. An emerging technique is the use of electromagnetic waves to monitor changes in the impedance of the wrist that reflects blood glucose levels (Pendra®).[687]

With these types of devices we can measure night time blood glucose levels relatively easily, thereby gaining a better understanding of how to adjust bedtime doses. Many parents of small children (and other relatives) would sleep much better with an alarm for hypoglycemia. Implantable sensors with a lifetime of several months have successfully been used in animal studies.[773] The readings can be transmitted to a receiver, for example in the shape of a wrist watch.

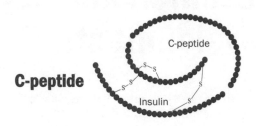

C-peptide

In a pancreas without diabetes, insulin is produced in the form of proinsulin. Before insulin is secreted to the blood stream, a part called C-peptide (connecting peptide) is cut off. By measuring C-peptide, one can estimate how much a person with diabetes has left of his or her own insulin production. Early data suggested that C-peptide was of no use in the body but recently positive effects on metabolism have been shown in the form of a decreased A1C. During a month's treatment with C-peptide, leakage of protein into the urine decreased and capillary function in the retina improved.[411] C-peptide stimulates the uptake of glucose into the muscle cells and thereby improves the effect of insulin (decreased insulin resistance). Nerve function in patients with diabetes-related nerve damage is improved as well.[412] Long-term studies have been started and it is possible that in the future C-peptide will be given along with insulin, though more research is still needed.

Vaccinations

Vaccinations have been proposed as one of the causes of diabetes. Some children have developed diabetes shortly after MMR vaccination (against measles, mumps and German measles/rubella) at the age of 18 months. However, scientific studies have not been able to show a correlation between vaccination and the onset of diabetes.[254] Indeed, it appears that vaccination against measles results in a slightly lower risk of developing diabetes.[80] BCG-vaccination (against tuberculosis) has been thought to have a protective effect but this has not been confirmed in studies.[170,593] The risk of acquiring diabetes is not affected by vaccination for pertussis (whooping cough),[351] varicella (chicken-

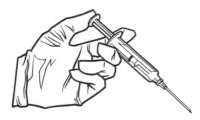

There is no scientific evidence that childhood vaccinations cause diabetes.

pox)[254] or other early childhood immunizations.[311] Vaccinations for hepatitis B and Hemophilus type b have not been shown to increase the risk for diabetes.[210]

Vaccination against diabetes would obviously be the ideal solution. If a virus could be identified that triggers diabetes it might be possible to vaccinate against it. If cows' milk protein plays a part in the cause of diabetes, a vaccine could perhaps prevent the onset of diabetes.[248]

Through vaccination, it may be possible to redirect the autoimmune reaction to another track so that the insulin-producing beta cells in the pancreas will not be destroyed. Animal studies vaccinating with the protein GAD (see page

327), which is found in beta cells, have been very promising and have succeeded in inducing a tolerance for GAD. Investigations in humans have just started. Trials have also been done where insulin is given to people with a very high risk of developing diabetes, in order to influence the immune system before all beta cells have been destroyed. In the US Diabetes Prevention Trial (DPT-1), insulin was given as twice daily subcutaneous injections to close relatives of a person with diabetes (both children and adults) with a high risk of developing diabetes. Unfortunately, this type of insulin therapy over the course of 2-4 years did not succeed in preventing the development of diabetes.[213] In the other part of the DPT-1 study, insulin was given as tablets but this did not prevent the development of diabetes either. In an ongoing Finnish study insulin is given as a nasal spray.

Salicylic acid

Salicylic acid (aspirin, a component of many over the counter painkillers), has been used in trials to lessen the risk of heart disease as a complication of long-term diabetes.[231] The current policy is to use it for individuals with type 1 diabetes and established heart disease, but it is also recommended as a preventative measure in people with diabetes who are above the age of 30, as long as there are no known medical reasons why they should not be taking it.[21]

What causes diabetes?

As of today we do not know what causes type 1 diabetes. However, we do know that it is not caused by eating too much candy. A common view is that about 60-70% of type 1 diabetes is caused by non-hereditary factors, i.e. risk factors due to life-style habits, infections or being exposed to environmental factors.[166] But it is still unclear what those factors, infections or exposures are. The risk of developing diabetes is very different in different countries (see

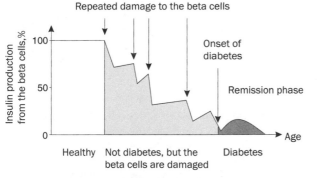

It is believed that the first attack on the beta cells in the pancreas (the cells that produce insulin) takes place many years before a person shows symptoms of diabetes. By the time diabetes is diagnosed, 80-90% of the beta cells are already damaged. The illustration is from reference [452].

"How common is diabetes?" on page 14). The reason for this is unclear but there are many proposed theories.

Many parents feel that: "If we had only done this or that our child would probably not have developed the disease." It is important to realize that diabetes was not caused by something that you or your family have done or failed to do.

An autoimmune disease

Part of the explanation for the abnormal reaction of the body's immune defense is heredity. Certain signals or "markers" that can be measured in the blood are present in almost all children and teenagers with diabetes (such as HLA-antigens on chromosome number 6). However, these markers are also present in 20-60% of people who do not have diabetes.[166,699] Certain gene components have a protective effect in that they appear to prevent a person who has them from developing diabetes.

A viral disease is believed to induce antibodies that, in addition to killing the virus, cross-react with and damage the insulin producing beta cells in the pancreas. As the damage is caused by a defect in one's own immune system, diabetes is considered to be an autoimmune disease. One theory is that other agents having a structure similar to the GAD protein (see page 327) in the beta cells will react with the immune system at some time, causing the production of antibodies that also can react with GAD. Much later, perhaps many years later, when the immune system is exposed to GAD, the autoimmune "memory" will be activated, attacking the beta cell. Example of agents that have a protein structure partly similar to GAD are viruses (enterovirus [366], rotavirus [385]) and cows' milk.[787] Both of these viruses are common among children, and cause viral symptoms and gastroenteritis.

The beta cells will usually partly recover after some time, but if the initial attack is repeated

---

Possible causes of diabetes

➠ To get type 1 diabetes, you need to be genetically predisposed.

➠ A viral disease can trigger the onset of diabetes.

➠ If a mother has certain viral infections during pregnancy, her child may have an increased risk of developing diabetes.[169]

➠ Impaired insulin production in the beta cells of the pancreas can be found several years before the onset of diabetes.

➠ Drinking cows' milk during the first 6 months of life or even later, may be a factor.

➠ Fathers eating smoked mutton (contains nitrose-amines) at the time of conception has been found to be a risk factor in Iceland.[352] High dietary intake of nitrite and nitrate [165] and nitrate in drinking water [594] have also been shown to be risk factors.

➠ Overweight is an important factor, but only for the development of type 2 diabetes.

➠ Psychological stress, such as severe life events, have been found to occur more often both during the first two years of life [751] and during the year before the onset of diabetes.[323,643] They are not believed to be the cause of the disease,[13] but may increase the risk by affecting the autoimmune process. [751]

➠ A very high standard of hygiene [456] and fewer infections [299,596] during infancy may lead to the immune defense not being "trained" correctly.

---

several times, insulin production will decrease enough to raise the blood glucose level. Antibodies directed against the insulin producing islets of Langerhans in the pancreas (ICA, islet cell antibodies and GAD antibodies), can be detected several years prior to the onset of diabetes, and are an early sign of cell damage. However, screening for these antibodies is usually not done since, in people who do not yet have diabetes, there is at present no way of pre-

When one identical twin has type 1 diabetes, the risk of the other twin developing diabetes before the age of 35 was 70% in a Danish study.[467] The risk for diabetes in nonidentical twins was 13% in this study. This indicates that more than half the explanation for the development of diabetes is inherited and the rest depends on environmental factors.

venting the onset of the disease even if you know the risks in advance. The antibodies can even disappear spontaneously without the child developing diabetes. Most children and adolescents who develop diabetes have measurable levels of antibodies. In adults, it is common to measure ICA and GAD antibodies to determine if an autoimmune type 1 diabetes or a type 2 diabetes.

Heredity

At most, only 13% of children and adolescents who develop diabetes have a parent or sibling with diabetes.[164] The risk of developing diabetes by age 30 for first-degree relatives (brother/sister or parent/child) is between 3% and 10%.[221] Of children with newly diagnosed diabetes, 2-3% have a mother with type 1 diabetes, 5-6% have a father with type 1 diabetes, and 4-5% have a brother or sister with type 1 diabetes.[164] In this study only 1.5% had a first-degree relative with type 2 diabetes.[164] (See also "Will the child have diabetes?" on page 276.) Studies in identical twins have found that the risk for the other twin to develop diabetes can be as high as 50-70%.[55,467]

Environmental factors

Environmental factors that trigger the disease process may start early in life, many years before the onset of diabetes.[486] It is believed that the increase in the number of new cases of diabetes is caused by environmental factors as the genetic markers have not changed over time.

A low groundwater content of zinc, which may reflect long-term exposure through drinking water, was associated with later development of diabetes in one study.[324] Another fact that points to an early influence is that an increased risk for diabetes has been correlated to the time and place of birth.[172] An explanation for the different ages at which diabetes occurs may be that the rate of decline in insulin production, once the disease process has started, is quite variable from one person with diabetes to another.

Sometimes children living close to each other develop diabetes at the same time which may indicate that viral infections trigger the onset (called clustering).[666] One theory is that diabetes and other autoimmune diseases are caused by so called slow viruses, i.e. viruses that can reside in the body for many years, while avoiding detection and destruction by the immune system.[109]

In countries with lower standards of hygiene, where there are more infections around, the immune system is activated to a greater degree at an earlier age. This has been shown to decrease the risk of diabetes in animal studies.[456] In Northern Ireland, the risk for diabetes was decreased in areas with higher population density which may be explained by a higher frequency of infections early in life.[596] In a British study the risk of developing diabetes also decreased by 20% if the child had had an infection during the first year of life.[299] Pre-school day-care attendance (a marker for an increased number of infections) decreased the risk of developing diabetes in a European study.[254] Infections in the newborn period seem to increase the risk of diabetes, probably due to an immature immune system.[254] Pinworm infec-

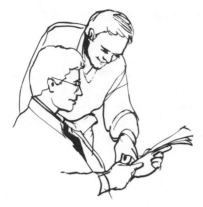

Bring newspaper clippings to your healthcare team when you have read something interesting, such as diabetes research, so you can discuss it together. You may both learn something!

tions are very common but with an increased standard of hygiene, the numbers of infected children decrease. Pinworms can protect mice from developing diabetes, and it has been proposed that the decreased number of infected children could contribute to the rise in incidence of diabetes risk that is common in many countries.[290]

If a mother has German measles (rubella) during pregnancy, the risk of the child developing diabetes is around 20%.[486] If the mother has a particular type of virus infection (enterovirus) during pregnancy, the child will have an increased risk of developing diabetes later in life.[169,395]

There may be a link between coffee drinking during pregnancy and the baby's risk of developing diabetes. Finland has the highest incidence of type 1 diabetes in the world and the highest coffee consumption as well.[766] Another risk factor is an increased height gain, seen in boys mainly, several years before the onset of diabetes.[81,622] Weight gain and obesity, on the other hand are not risk factors for developing type 1 diabetes.[81] However, children who developed diabetes later had a more rapid weight gain early in life (before 2-2.5 years of age) according to one study.[410] No difference was found in height or weight at birth in children who later developed diabetes.

Environmental factors affect the individual, causing the risk for developing diabetes to change in families that have emigrated.[571] Asian children living in Great Britain and children from the Samoan Islands living in New Zealand have a higher risk of acquiring diabetes than children in their home countries.[265,781] Most of the population of Iceland originate from Norway and have the same type of hereditary disposition.[47] Despite this, the risk for developing diabetes in Iceland is only between one third and half of what it is in Norway.[353] One might believe that this variation is caused by differences in environment and climate. However, Iceland and parts of Norway are located on the same latitude and have the same average temperature.

It is more common to develop diabetes during the winter months and during the years of puberty. While climate and puberty could certainly not be described as the causes of diabetes, they may very well be triggering factors as both growth spurts and cold weather increase the body's insulin requirements.[486]

Cows' milk

The number of new cases of diabetes per year (incidence) in different countries coincides well with the consumption of cows' milk.[177] Increased levels of antibodies against cows' milk have been found in children who have developed diabetes.[167,674] In the Samoan Islands where children do not drink milk at all, there is essentially no childhood diabetes. Sardinia has about the same risk of diabetes as the Nordic countries. The consumption of milk is not as high as in Finland but on the other hand it is much higher than in the rest of Italy.[262]

Studies on rats have shown that whey protein from cows' milk increases the risk of developing diabetes.[245] When rats were fed with soya formula instead of milk they did not get diabetes.

It seems that only certain types of cows (our ordinary milk cow) have the protein components which affect the risk of developing diabetes. Breast-feeding as such does not seem to affect the risk of diabetes,[665] but the time when the child is first introduced to cows' milk seems to be significant.[781,786] However, there are traces of cows' milk in breast milk and even children who have been fully breast-fed can have antibodies against cows' milk.[737] This might explain why even children who have been breast-fed for a long time still can develop diabetes. In an Australian study, children who developed diabetes after the age of 9 had ingested more milk the year immediately before the onset of diabetes when compared to other children of the same age.[781]

Since it is not yet proven that cows' milk causes diabetes, most authorities do not currently recommend any changes in infant diet.[506,677] However, The American Academy of Pediatrics recommends avoidance of cows' milk during the first year of life in families with a strong history of type 1 diabetes, particularly if a sibling has diabetes.[17] A Finnish study showed a five-fold risk of diabetes in siblings of children with type 1 diabetes with a high consumption

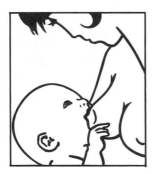

Some studies indicate an increased risk of acquiring diabetes if a child is not breast-fed at all or for only 3 months or less.[781] Other studies indicate that it may not be the short period of breast-feeding as such, but the child's early introduction to cows' milk that increases the risk for diabetes. At the present time, however, there is insufficient data available to advise people in the general population against drinking milk during pregnancy or early infancy.[677]

(three or more glasses per day) of cows' milk during childhood.[788]

Climate

There is a higher risk for diabetes in northern countries and onset is more common during the winter. A cold climate increases the need for insulin, which in turn increases the risk of triggering the onset of diabetes. Fewer hours of sunlight can lead to an increased risk of diabetes through higher turnover of calcium and reduced production of vitamin D.[168]

AGE

AGE stands for Advanced Glycation End products and represents an irreversible binding between glucose and different substances like protein, fat and nucleic acids (see illustration on page 305). Food chemists have known for a long time that a high concentration of glucose will cause protein-containing compounds to discolor and turn gluey. The proteins will become "sticky" with an increased tendency for cross-bindings. Ordinary caramel is an example of this reaction, between glucose and milk proteins or fat. The chemical structure of the compound will be altered. If this happens inside a cell, its function may change, contributing to the development of diabetes complications, for example in the eyes.[70] AGE products in food have not been shown to contribute to diabetes complications.[66]

In Italy [141] and Norway [65] increased levels of AGE have been measured in children and adolescents before clinical signs of diabetes complications have started. In the Italian study, the levels decreased after two years of intensified diabetes treatment and lowered A1C. An increased level of AGE has been found in the retina and in the blood vessels of eyes affected with retinopathy.[328] An increased deposition of AGE in skin, tendons, connective tissue and joint capsules can lead to a reduced tissue flexibility. This can give rise to symptoms in the hands, hips or feet, and make problems such as foot ulcers more likely.[225]

The damage done by AGE may be counteracted at several levels by:

① Blocking the production of AGE.

② Removing AGE from the blood.

③ Breaking AGE, i.e. breaking the bond to glucose.

④ Blocking the AGE receptor on the cell surface.

Research is now being carried out to develop drugs that have these effects. Promising experiments have been done with people who have kidney damage. Their blood was passed through a kind of dialysis apparatus containing a protein that binds AGE.[549] One study with pimagedine, an aminoguanide type of drug that breaks AGE bindings, showed a slowing down in the progression of both eye damage and kidney damage.[705]

Glucose may also bind to different proteins in the blood, forming AGE that can bind to receptors on the cell wall. This can cause damage to the function, for example of cells in the blood

vessel walls, in the retina and the smooth muscle cells in our inner organs.[83] Smokers have higher levels of AGE in the blood.[83] At present, it is difficult to measure AGE in blood and no routine method has yet been developed.

Blocking the immune process

At the onset of diabetes, 10-20% of the insulin-producing beta cells in the pancreas are still functioning (see illustration on page 321). If it were possible to stop the autoimmune attack on these cells it might also be possible to preserve a degree of insulin production for a long time, thereby prolonging the honeymoon phase (see page 193).

Immune treatment

Immune-modulation in the form of cell toxin drugs has been tried early in the course of diabetes. Cyclosporin A is a compound that has been used successfully and has even made it possible to stop using insulin for some time.

In a study of 188 people with newly diagnosed diabetes, 25% managed without insulin after one year of cyclosporin treatment compared to 10% of those who had not received cyclosporin.[126] However, when cyclosporin treatment is stopped, insulin production always decreases again. Cyclosporin can have serious side effects including kidney damage and is therefore not used as a routine treatment at the present time. The International Study Group of Pediatric and Adolescent Diabetes (ISPAD) has stated that cyclosporin has no place in the treatment of diabetes in children except for clinical trials addressing questions that cannot be answered in adults.[400]

Immunotherapy

In France and Canada, cell toxins (Cyclosporin A) have been used for experimental treatment at the onset of diabetes.

➡ Some people can do without insulin.

➡ BUT — the need for insulin always returns when the medication is stopped.

➡ These drugs carry a risk of serious side effects (such as damage to the kidneys).

Light treatment

In a Swedish study, the white blood cells were treated with ultraviolet light (called photopheresis) at the onset of diabetes after the children and teenagers had received a special medication (psoralen).[510] The aim was to make it easier for the immune defense to recognize the cells that are causing damage to the beta cells. Patients needed less insulin but there was no difference in A1C after three years.

Diazoxide

At the onset of diabetes, the immune defense attacks the body with antibodies directed against a special protein (called GAD) in the beta cell. When insulin treatment is started, the beta cells do not need to work as hard and therefore the production of the protein that triggers the antibodies decreases as well, leading to a less intense immune attack. This is believed to be part of the mechanism behind the remission or "honeymoon" phase.

Diazoxide is a compound that puts a powerful block on the activity of the beta cells, thereby decreasing insulin production. The production of the GAD protein that is attacked by the antibodies decreases as well, therefore decreasing the damage to the beta cells. When treatment with diazoxide is stopped after a couple of months, the hope is that the immune defense will no longer react as strongly. A Swedish study of adults has shown a higher residual production of insulin up to 1½ years after the onset of diabetes in a group with newly diagnosed diabetes that was treated with diazoxide for 3 months.[76] When the study was repeated in children, the same effect was seen after 1 year but after 2 years it was no longer so prominent.[586] However, diazoxide is not suitable for treating children with new-onset diabetes, as it is associated with a high rate of side effects.

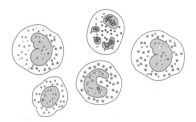

The white blood cells are the "soldiers" in your body's army of defenders against bacteria and virus infections. When a person develops diabetes, the body thinks it is under attack, so the immune defense launches a "counter-attack" on the insulin producing beta cells. Immune-modulating treatment is used in research studies to influence this process.

Nicotinamide

Nicotinamide is a type of vitamin B (niacin) that is thought to lessen the risk of developing diabetes by protecting the beta cells from attack by the immune system. In New Zealand, this substance has been given to brothers and sisters of children who have recently been diagnosed with diabetes, for a period of couple of years, in order to prevent them from developing diabetes too.[247] It has also been given to whole classes of schoolchildren, resulting in a 60-70% reduction in the risk of developing diabetes.[246]

In a large-scale study looking at parents and siblings of children with diabetes, nicotinamide was given to those with a high risk of developing diabetes indicated by a blood test (the ENDIT study). Unfortunately, the study failed to show any benefit from nicotinamide treatment.[291] The study was done with a so called double-blind technique, i.e. half of the participants were treated with nicotinamide and half with placebo (non-active tablets). Neither patients nor doctors knew who was given the nicotinamide and who the placebo. The same number of people developed diabetes in both groups.

It may seem strange that half of the people in a trial like this get medication that does not work, but this is the only scientific way to do the study to see if nicotinamide has a protective effect. It is common to conduct a double-blind study when the effect of a new drug is being tested.

Nicotinamide has been tried at the onset of diabetes to preserve the beta cell function. Only patients older than 15 years seem to be definitely affected, as their C-peptide levels did not decrease as much after 12 months as they did without the nicotinamide.[621] This indicates that residual insulin production was continued for a longer time. Nicotinamide has also been tried on a group of people who have been known to have diabetes for a period of 1-5 years, and who are still able to produce a certain amount of their own insulin.[776] The group receiving nicotinamide had a better A1C and a higher C-peptide level which indicates an improved production of insulin by the beta cells.

Transplantation

Pancreas

Pancreas transplants have been performed for many years. Today most pancreas transplants are done at the same time as kidney transplants but pancreas only transplants are also available. Kidney transplants are done on a routine basis. If a pancreas transplant works well, there is no need for further insulin injections. The patient can eat a normal diet and their A1C will normalize.

Problems can arise after transplantation due to rejection of the transplant (the immune defense does not like "foreign" things in the body and tries to reject them). After one year, about 80% of the pancreas transplants function well when a kidney is transplanted at the same time.[808] However, the results of transplanting a pancreas alone are not particularly satisfactory. The reason for this is that the rejection of a pancreas is less easy to discover than a rejection of the kidney where urine tests can be very informative.

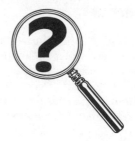

More than 5,000 articles on diabetes research are produced every year. Many small advances have resulted but so far no one has been able to solve the question of why a person develops diabetes or how to cure it. However, there is every reason to be optimistic about the future. There have been discussions about the way some of the body's own stem cells (developing stages of the beta cells) could be manipulated using gene technology to start producing insulin.

When a kidney transplant is threatened by rejection, medication can be started early, thereby protecting the pancreas transplant as well. Another problem is the possibility of tissue damage by digestive enzymes from the transplanted pancreas.

After a transplant, several drugs are needed, including cortisone which counteracts rejection. Cortisone increases the level of glucose in the blood, leading to a complicated situation. Drugs used to prevent rejection (called cytotoxic agents or immune-modulating drugs) can also result in numerous side effects, some of which are serious.

The beta cells in the new pancreas are susceptible to attack by the immune defense, causing diabetes to recur, especially if the transplant comes from an identical twin.[486] However, this is effectively prevented by the immune-modulating drugs that are given to prevent rejection reactions.[730]

Even if all problems with rejection were solved, pancreas transplantation can never be the method of choice for routine treatment of diabetes because there will simply never be enough human pancreases available for transplantation.

Islet transplantation

The islets of Langerhans (see illustration on page 23) that contain insulin producing beta cells can be extracted from a donor. These islets can be injected into the liver of the person with diabetes and will then produce a certain amount of insulin. This method is still at the research stage and only a couple of hundred individuals with diabetes around the world have tried it.

Previously, only 12% of patients receiving new islets have been able to manage without insulin for more than a week at a time.[808] A breakthrough was published in 2000 from Edmonton in Canada where a cortisone-free immunosuppression program was used (although cortisone increases blood glucose it has always been a necessary part of the immunosuppression program).[697] Seven people received islets from two or three donors, and these were injected into the portal vein in the liver. They were able to manage without insulin for an average of 9 months and the mean A1C dropped from 8.4% to 5.7%. This "Edmonton Protocol" has been mirrored in Canada, the US and Europe, and about 200 people have been treated worldwide. The success rate in 46 patients from Edmonton as of 2003 is 80% insulin-free.

One problem with islet transplants is that antibodies and rejection reactions can strike these islets as well as complete transplanted organs. Methods where the islets are put into small tubes or sealed within a plastic film have been tried to prevent the antibodies from attacking the islets.[718]

Engineered cells

Experiments have been conducted where so called stem cells are manipulated genetically to produce insulin.[572] The thought is very appealing because if some of your own cells were be able to produce insulin there would be no rejection problems.

Engineered rat muscle cells have been able to secrete insulin at a constant level, independent of the blood glucose level.[318] This would be an effective substitute for the night time and basal insulins used today and could produce a very stable level of insulin in the bloodstream. Cells from the pituitary gland have been engineered to recognize different levels of glucose and to produce insulin at sufficient levels to cure diabetes in mice.[261] In contrast to transplanted islet cells, these pituitary cells were resistant to autoimmune attack.

Other ways of administering insulin

Nasal spray

Insulin given as nasal spray is absorbed more quickly through the lining of the nose than when injected subcutaneously. Many studies have been performed on humans but it is still unclear whether this can become a clinical reality.[365] Problems may arise with the insulin absorption in people who have hay fever or other allergies, or who are suffering from a cold. Also, we do not yet know how insulin might affect the nose lining in the long run. Twenty times more insulin was needed for administration via the nose than for an injection, according to one study.[365] However, 7 of the 31 participants interrupted the study prematurely due to problems with high or low blood glucose levels. A1C increased slightly in this study, from 7.1 to 8.1%.

Tablets

The problem with insulin in tablet form is that it is degraded by the acid in the stomach. This can be solved by putting a capsule around the insulin tablets in order to release insulin only after the tablets reach the intestines.[387] Insulin can then be absorbed into the blood, but this is a slow process with a risk of an irregular insulin effect. One advantage is that insulin which is absorbed into the blood from the intestines, passes the liver before it enters the general blood circulation in the same way as insulin that is produced in a healthy pancreas. Insulin in tablets is extremely long-acting and one single dose can work for up to one week. This may cause difficulties in working out appropriate doses.

Insulin as suppositories

Insulin is absorbed from the rectum when administered as suppositories. Due to poor absorption, more than 10 times the ordinary dose is needed to obtain the appropriate blood glucose lowering effect.[364]

Inhalation of insulin

Experiments with administering insulin as an aerosol spray (in the same way as people with asthma take their drugs) has been tried successfully in adults.[709] Clinical trials in teenagers and children with inhaled insulin appear to be as promising as those in adults. Insulin is absorbed rapidly through the thin lung lining. There may be some practical limitations to this method: in people with asthma, the absorption from inhaled insulin is decreased [357] while in smokers it is enhanced.[367] However, the long term effects on the lungs of inhaling insulin will not be known for many years.

Chemical alteration of the insulin molecule

Changing the composition of the insulin molecule can result in both more short-acting and

Alternative ways of administering insulin	
⇒ Nasal spray	Quick effect, good for premeal injections. However, unlikely to become clinical reality.
⇒ Oral insulin (tablets)	Slow effect, good for basal insulin.
⇒ Suppositories	Quick effect but large doses are needed.
⇒ Aerosol for inhalation	Quick effect but difficult to administer.
⇒ Chemically bound insulin	Released only at high blood glucose levels. Technically difficult.
⇒ Altered insulin structure	Quicker or slower action.
⇒ C-peptide (see page 320)	Produced in the human pancreas but not included in today's insulin.

more long-acting insulin. Examples of this are the new rapid-acting insulin analogs, Novo-Log/NovoRapid, Humalog and Apidra, which have a much quicker effect than regular short-acting insulin (see page 70).

There is a great need for better night time and basal insulins with a more even action profile.[654] This has been achieved by replacing some of the amino acids in the insulin molecule as in insulin glargine (Lantus) that now is registered in several countries (see page 71). Insulin has also been made more long-acting by binding it to a protein in the bloodstream (albumin). Insulin is released slowly to maintain a steady level between meals and throughout the night. This insulin analog is called detemir (Levemir, see page 71).

Psychology

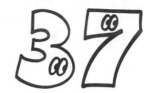

The onset of diabetes

When any child, teenager or adult develops a long term illness, the situation for the whole family is always a difficult one. Adjusting to a new life poses challenges and takes time. Most people go through the same stages when faced with crisis. Professor Johnny Ludvigsson describes the different phases of crisis:[504]

Shock phase

During the shock phase, it is difficult to think clearly. Thoughts will whirl around in your head. Everything seems unreal. This cannot really be happening, it can't be true. Maybe it will all turn out to have been a dream? It is common to experience a sense of walking around in a kind of haze. You cannot take in information. You see your doctor, you watch the doctor's body language and see just how serious the situation is. You listen out for hope, consolation, belief in the future, but shut out all details of the disease, its likely progression and treatment, all the accompanying practicalities. You want to ask questions but find it difficult to keep your thoughts focused, or see a way forward. The doctor should listen, you think, the nurse should listen, everybody should LISTEN to your inner thoughts of what is most important right now.

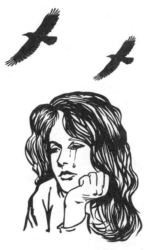

"You cannot stop the birds of sorrow from flying over your head – but you can stop them from building a nest there."

Chinese saying

Reaction phase

A reaction of sorrow with tears, sleeplessness, aggression and bitterness will also take time. Consolation is important but should be honest, not hearty and unrealistic. "You need not feel sad" seems false and "You should not be sad" feels like a punch in the face. Why shouldn't one feel sad? Everybody has the right to be sad in this situation. It is only natural to feel sorrow, bitterness and disappointment. You grieve for the healthy person you used to be, and life seems unfair. It is always unfair when someone is stricken by a severe disease, but the sorrow will eventually fade away. You will feel better. You have had no part in developing the disease, it is not your fault. We must have the strength to listen, to face up to reality, to allow and acknowledge grief and fear.

The different phases of crisis

① Shock phase.

② Reaction phase.

③ Repair phase.

④ Reorientation phase.

Repair phase

After some time, you will enter the repair phase. Somebody must be able to do something about this disease. Now you need knowledge. What do you do if your blood glucose level falls too low? How do you give yourself these dreaded injections? You won't be able to relax or breathe easily again until you have got to grips with this. Now the worst part is over. You can learn more about insulin, testing, diet, and hypoglycemia. Systematically, a little bit at a time, you can absorb facts and start to rebuild your life.

Reorientation phase

It takes a long time before a crisis moves on to the reorientation phase, and a different but acceptable life style is established — one where diabetes is an important part but by no means everything. At times, those around you will have difficulties in understanding that it takes time to go through the different phases of a cri-

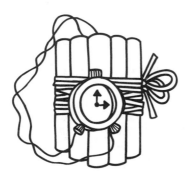

When the first baby is born into a family, some parents feel as if there is an unexploded bomb in their midst. They never know when the baby will start crying, need their diapers changed, or get hungry. As time goes by, the parents relax, learn what to do, and become more secure in their new role. There is a parallel situation when parents first discover their child has diabetes. They thought they knew what to expect, now they find they know nothing at all. What will happen when the child becomes hypoglycemic? What can they do as a family? But in the same way as adjusting to a new baby, parents will soon learn to accommodate their child again in this new situation.

sis, but this is inevitable when someone in a family develops diabetes. Of course it is unfair, the treatment can be difficult, life has changed, you might be afraid of dying or being different from others. But there will still be Saturday afternoons, song, laughter, dancing, good food, school or work, picnics, vacations and friends. Life will never be the same again but it can still be exciting and enjoyable even if some of the rules have changed.

There are people who come to a standstill in their grief and are unable to move on. Such people will need professional help. Continuing denial inhibits people from absorbing knowledge and adjusting life to accommodate diabetes.

Regardless of whether a crisis is caused by the death of someone near and dear, a divorce, developing diabetes or something else, there will always remain a memory of what happened, much like a scar. But when you have worked yourself through the crisis and accepted what has happened, it will be like looking at a wound that has completely healed: you can see the scar but most of the time you are unaware of its existence.

"You cannot teach a person anything — just help him or her to find it within themselves."

Galileo Galilei 1564-1642

Diabetes rules or family rules?

Diabetes can be a "thorn in the side" in different ways depending in part on the age of the person concerned. If, as a parent, you are discussing what the "rules" are at home, it is important to consider what is actually provoked by your son or daughter having diabetes, and what is a part of a normal upbringing. If you are always referring to diabetes when it comes to rules and prohibitions, the young person will hate the very thought of diabetes since it puts an end to so many nice things. However, if you think about it, most rules and methods of upbringing are influenced by other factors and

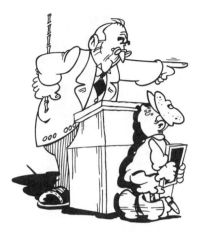

We must cooperate on equal terms when you come to see us at the diabetes clinic. If a visit feels like "a trip to the principal's office" something has gone badly wrong.

hold true just as much for a child with diabetes as for his or her brothers, sisters or friends without diabetes.

Many children are only allowed candy on special occasions, such as at weekends. Most children, on the other hand, would prefer to have candy every day if only it were allowed. This type of discussion goes on in families everywhere. However, if a child has diabetes it is very convenient just to refer to the effect on the blood glucose level when saying "No" to candy. I often argue that it is very important to return to normal rules between children and parents as soon as possible and to refer to diabetes as little as possible when it comes to child upbringing and setting limits. In the long run it is important to be on as friendly terms as possible with your diabetes. If many rules and prohibitions are put down to diabetes, it will have the opposite effect and cause the young person to start hating the disease.

It is important, therefore, to explain to younger children that most rules or limitations relating to food or treats are not caused by their diabetes, but would have applied anyway. The child will otherwise associate all prohibitions with diabetes.

Remember that there were both rules and limitations in the child's life even before diabetes entered the scene. Diabetes brings with it many restrictions, resulting in a lot of "not this and not that's". Try instead to encourage your child to do the things he or she still can — this will still include most aspects of everyday life. Give encouragement and praise. The praise is well-deserved, as a child with diabetes has to do many things on a daily basis that most adults would not be very keen to do. Praise the child for doing the necessary blood tests, and give due credit for giving injections. Encourage the child when he or she chooses to eat in a way appropriate for diabetes, show your appreciation when the child does not eat candy behind your back. (How many parents have not taken out their own candy from the cupboard when the children have gone to bed?) Praise and encouragement help everything to run so much more smoothly.

Even as a parent or an adult with diabetes, you will naturally need encouragement, praise and "positive reinforcement" when you visit the diabetes clinic. If it feels like "being called in to see the principal" something is wrong. You don't come to pass or fail a test. It is our job to cooperate and help you, in the best way possi-

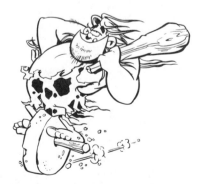

"We learn by our own mistakes", as the saying goes. But does one always have to invent the wheel again? You can learn a lot by discussing with other parents or friends who have diabetes. They can give you tips about day to day practicalities that the staff at the diabetes clinic is less familiar with, since most of us don't live with diabetes at home.

ble, to cope with diabetes as part of your family life.

How far would a soccer team advance without encouragement and praise? Any person, be they child or adult, who has diabetes needs a coach to motivate them, assess their abilities and potential, and adjust their diabetes training on a continuous basis. Let the young person know that you recognize just how difficult things are — often it is much more difficult for children or teenagers to manage life with diabetes well than it would be for their parents to give up smoking, for example. On the other hand, it is important not to embarrass the young person with an overload of praise and encouragement at times when everything is going smoothly. It is far too easy to be overprotective of children with diabetes. Sympathy is fine but pity is less helpful.

Making friends with your diabetes

Your diabetes will be with you 24 hours a day. So it is important that you find a way to make friends with it, or at least to avoid seeing it as an enemy. If you allow yourself to hate the illness, it will be difficult to get on with your life without being negatively affected by it. There are three common ways in which people view their diabetes:

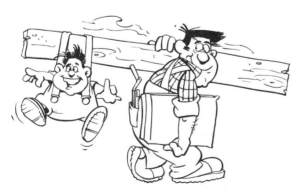

It may be a good idea to be apprenticed to someone who has had diabetes for many years and has had time to learn how to live with it in a positive way.

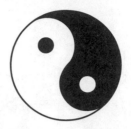

Yin and yang are conceptions in the Chinese philosophy for two principles that are in balance and harmony. Try to see your diabetes as a part of yourself which can melt into balance and harmony with the rest of your personality. Your attitude is a very important part of diabetes treatment. Those who hate their illness will soon begin fighting against it.

① Ignoring it, eating what they like and only taking enough insulin to avoid feeling bad at that moment.

Many teenagers will go through this phase for a shorter or longer period of time, and some will never be able to leave it because they hate their illness. If you have this attitude when you enter adulthood, there is a risk that you will never be able to change it. Try instead to see the end of the teenage years as an opportunity when you dare to take action, and can do something about your life style and your diabetes.

② Becoming absorbed and obsessed by diabetes, living only to take care of the illness as effectively as possible.

"Regulating illness" or "regulopathy" is the term used when you give up your ordinary life and your goals for the future.[271] Initially, both parents and caregivers at the clinic are under the impression that everything is going along very well. However, if the efforts to obtain a perfect glucose level prevent the young person from enjoying social activities, parties, being with friends or staying overnight with friends or at camps, things have gone too far. If this applies to you, it is high time to give yourself a break and allow yourself to start living life again.

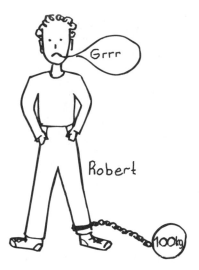

One may feel like this many times. It is difficult to live with diabetes, often very difficult. But if you hate your diabetes it will be difficult to make friends with it... It is important not to let diabetes take control. Decide instead what kind of life you want to live, and your diabetes team will help you to adjust your treatment according to your wishes.

If your diabetes is too strictly regulated, you are likely to end up having too many hypoglycemic episodes or hypoglycemia unawareness, (see page 48) which is far from healthy.

 ③ Making diabetes a natural part of everyday life.

This is easier said than done, as everyone knows who has tried. But it is possible to accept your illness without letting it take control of your life completely. If taking insulin becomes like brushing your teeth, something you do daily without really thinking about it but that you would absolutely not want to be without, then you have come a long way.

How do you go about making diabetes a part of your daily life? Learn from your friends, observe others with diabetes and you will probably find someone who has an attitude worth learning from. Just as young people used to have a period of apprenticeship when learning a profession, so you now may need to "be apprenticed" to someone who manages their diabetes in a good way.

Diabetes affects the whole family

Different people will feel differently about the relative difficulty of various aspects of diabetes. For a small child, the injections are often the hardest part. Older children and teenagers often find the need to be punctual, and explaining diabetes to others more bothersome. Adults often find food issues and weight control to be the most difficult thing.

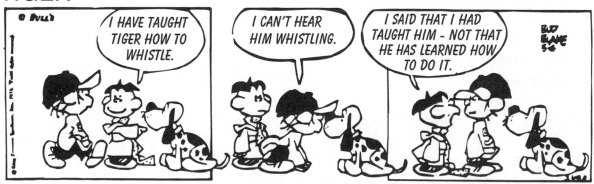

Teaching something to someone is not the same as the other person learning it...

"Treatment of insulin dependent diabetes — art or science?" was the title of a lecture by the British physician, Robert Tattersall, from Nottingham. He described what happens in a family when a child develops diabetes:

— A good recipe for putting the "thumb-screws" on someone is to let a family member, preferably a child, develop a chronic disease.

— The disease should have an unclear cause but with a hereditary component so that family members are forced to check the family tree to find a "scapegoat", Robert Tattersall continues. The treatment should be an important part of the disease, time consuming and preferably painful.

— To put further pressure on the family, the management of the disease should affect the life of all other family members. Self control and self management should be important components.

— The future outlook completes the picture. Terrible results of an unwise life style can be indicated perhaps by sitting the family members in a waiting room together with other sufferers from the same disease who are showing obvious and drastic consequences such as amputations. Better still, if health professionals are uncertain about treatment goals and regimes, they will give contradictory information which of course will make the situation even worse. Don't forget, says Professor Tattersall, that a family where someone has developed diabetes will be in exactly this situation.

Being a relative or friend of someone with diabetes

People close to you only want what is best for you but it may not always look like this. It is important to know what kind of help individuals with diabetes want, and what they can manage on their own. At the same time a child, a teenager or a spouse must understand how

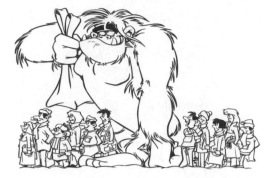

Diabetes is an invisible handicap, and can't be seen from the outside. You may sometimes feel better if nobody knows. However, both you and your friends will find it easier in the long run if you let everyone know. If, for instance, you become hypoglycemic, everyone will understand what is going on and what to do if you have informed them beforehand. Many people have described how embarrassing and troublesome they found it, having to explain their diabetes for the first time when they became hypoglycemic and needed help.

much those closest to them need to know about their everyday life, for them to feel secure and confident.

It can be easy for parents to become overprotective, and the young person can then react by wanting to manage too much by themselves, or rebel by, for example, eating too much candy. Try to be as open as possible about each others' needs in the family. A "family council", where you put aside time to sit down together, can be an ideal forum to discuss how to come to agreement on different subjects within the family.

Friends need to know how they can help, otherwise they may turn into "candy policemen" who, with the best of intentions, will go on about this or that being unhealthy to eat. It becomes a balance between saying: "I don't care about your diabetes, it is your problem" and "Are you really going to eat that bag of candies?" It is a good idea to talk things over and decide upon "how much or how little" help and support you want from those close to you.

Family and friends must also be sufficiently knowledgeable about diabetes if they are to offer any help or understanding. Treatment of hypoglycemia is an obvious example, and it would be useful if they could also give an injection of glucagon. The more your friends know, the more help you will be able to receive from them. Try to explain what you are doing and why. Explain how insulin works, how exercise works, why sometimes you can eat sugar and sometimes you can't.

Telling your friends

Many people do not want to talk about their diabetes since it is not visible from the outside. At the same time it is evident that you have not accepted your diabetes if you do not want to tell your friends. It is important your friends understand why you might be feeling unwell, and what they can do about it. It is best to tell everybody as soon as possible after you have been diagnosed. Then it is over with and things will not feel so strange any more. It is much worse to walk around wondering to yourself what or how much any individual knows.

My earliest memory of diabetes is when I was 8 years old. The girl living next door was my age and had diabetes. The only thing I knew about

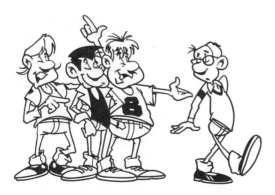

You may drift away from your friends if they do not understand why you must do certain things at particular times. Try to make diabetes a natural part of your life by telling friends at school or work about it. It is important that they know what to do if you need help, for example if you have a difficult hypoglycemic episode.

it was that she was not allowed to eat sugar. But I also observed sugar packs in her pocket that she would eat from time to time. It was very difficult for me to understand this and, as nobody explained to me why she did it, I thought she was cheating.

How do you change your life style?

Many people ask themselves this question. It is not easy to persuade someone that they must change their habits to feel better. Persuasion may not even be the best way of getting a person to do what is best for his or her health. And what is really "best", from the person's own perspective?

Elisabeth Arborelius, Ph.D. in Psychology, has studied how to change people's life habits.[128]

— It is all about concentrating the information on behavior instead of knowledge. It is not always true that knowledge will affect attitudes which in turn will affect behavior. We assume that human beings are rational but they are not, she claims. Something that is disadvantageous to a person's health, from an objective point of view, will not necessarily be experienced that way by the person concerned.

— I once heard a nurse say: "I am not a fanatic, but I see no reasons why people should smoke!" Of course she was right if she disregarded the patient's point of view. If the objective is to change behavior, the person with diabetes must have the opportunity to explain the advantages and disadvantages he or she will experience on account of a change of habits.

— We have come to believe that the balance between an individual's experienced advantages and disadvantages is very important in whether or not that person will change his or her behavior. If the disadvantages seem to outweigh the advantages, it will not help that there is a threat of worsening health. The person with diabetes will not change his or her life style habits anyway.

Diabetes at different developmental stages

The psychological effect of diabetes in the family will be different at different ages and depends very much on the child's development and basic needs for that age. Naturally, parents will often feel unsure about how to handle specific situations, and may on occasion need expert help to address particular issues. Sometimes the help of a child psychologist will be appropriate. It is a good idea to let all children and adolescents see the psychologist at least once during the early months after diagnosis. That way, if parents feel psychological help is necessary at a later date, the initial contact will already have been made.

Marianne Helgesson who is a psychologist at the Department of Pediatrics in Linköping, Sweden, lectures on psychology and diabetes in individuals at different ages. She teaches the following: [488]

— It is not always easy to accommodate three people in a marriage. The first crack between spouses often appears when the first child is born. Discussions and disputes begin to focus on how to organize time, something that may not have been an issue before.

— It will become a question of balance as to how much time and care one should devote to the child, to one's partner and to oneself. The parents must come to an agreement on how work at home should be divided, and whether one of them or both will be able to pursue a career.

— Child raising is for the most part a repetition of how you were brought up yourself, since this is the only model you are familiar with. But usually there are two parents, both with their own upbringing behind them. Conflicts are inevitable and the result will be a combination of both parents' previous experiences.

— However, if the child has a chronic illness, there is usually a lack of role models and this will make parents feel insecure. The balance between dependency and responsibility is difficult to establish and the question arises as to how much to help the child without being over-protective.

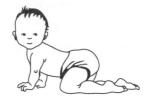

Infants (0-1½ years)

This period is characterized by a so called symbiosis, at first between mother and child and later on the father is also included. During this time it is very important that the parent subordinates his or her own needs in favor of the child's needs. The child, after all, is not in any position to give priority to the parent's needs. When the child is able to move around unaided, after about one year of age, he or she will begin to explore the world.

Risks from diabetes

Diabetes at this age will inevitably bring stress into the family. If parents find it difficult to handle this without feeling tense and uncertain towards the child, they will also find it difficult to communicate security and confidence to the child. Security and confidence will depend very much on the issues of food and diabetes. Young children do not understand why they should eat if they are not hungry and vice versa, so there is considerable risk of feeding problems at this age. Multiple injections or pump therapy can help to address such problems.

Children need to feel their parents display trust and confidence in various situations, but clearly this may be difficult when a child has diabetes. Over-protectiveness may lead to a child anxiously staying by the parent's side instead of looking outwards to the world beyond. Young children cannot understand injections and blood testing, or the pain, anger and anxiety that go with them. We cannot explain to them why they must be hurt in this way. Usually, the best approach is to get the injection out of the way as quickly as possible, and then comfort the child. Injection aids may be very helpful for this age group (see page 122).

Toddlers (1½-3 years)

Toddlers start to explore the world more actively. Around the age of 2, the child will often take a step "backwards", becoming more attached to the mother again. This is quite normal and is not due to inappropriate parental attitudes towards the child.

The "obstinate age" (the age of practicing one's own free will) begins between 2 and 3 years of age. Children will first test the parents' and then their own ability to set limits. All children will show quite a lot of anger and frustration during this time. They must experience their own limitations which can be unpleasant. It is important that parents engage in such "battles of will" as it is through these that children learn how to stand up for something, to compromise and to give in.

Risks from diabetes

It can be difficult to know whether or not a child's bad temper is caused by a low or high blood glucose level. Should the child be given something to eat every time he or she is angry? It may be difficult to take a blood test every time. A child with diabetes will have more limitations than other children due to injections, meal times and monitoring. There is always a tendency with a chronic illness that parents will want to compensate for the restrictions caused by the illness by letting the child decide about everything else. In doing this the parent shows pity for the child and becomes less effective in setting limits in other areas. The child then becomes insecure and disorderly, continuously testing the limits in order to provoke a parental reaction. However, if the parents do not have enough strength to deal with such aggressiveness the child may turn inwards, becoming passive and insecure, with a low feeling of self confidence. Parents, too, need understanding, as this period may be very challenging. But they also need encouragement because a child with diabetes needs a normal upbringing just as much as any other child.

A fear of strange environments (such as the hospital) can be even greater than the fear of injections. Some children of this age will become very anxious if they feel they are being restrained. Try to give injections and take blood tests in as secure an environment as possible.

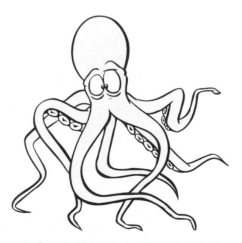

Any parent of small children knows that it is difficult enough to find time for everything. But when there is diabetes to cope with as well, parents can feel they need as many arms as an octopus in order to cope with blood glucose monitoring, injections, meal planning and all the other adjustments of daily life that have to be made.

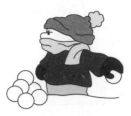

Pre-school children (3-6 years)

The child in this age group begins to understand more about the outside world and will be conscious of the fact that his or her body can experience both desire and pain. The child will role play and have a very rich imaginative life.

During this period the differentiation of sex roles takes place. The child wants to imitate the parent of the same sex and falls in love, often wanting to marry the parent of the opposite sex. A child of 4-5 years will be "the king of the universe", knowing and being able to do everything, especially knowing what he or she wants and does not want. Children feel powerful when they discover how to control others. A six year old is usually more willing to fit in with what the parent wants.

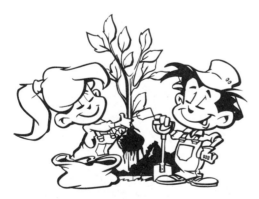

Plant the tree of knowledge early within children. Children who have grown up with diabetes often find it easier to manage during puberty compared to those developing diabetes in prepubertal or pubertal years. When children grow up, they will be trained by their parents to take responsibility for themselves. The goal should be that they will be able to take responsibility for important aspects of their diabetes before entering puberty.

Children begin to develop a conscience, thinking about crime and punishment in a "primitive way" in terms of "an eye for an eye and a tooth for a tooth". They become aware of the boundaries of the body. Bandages have a magic ability to restore and heal. See also "Children and blood glucose tests" on page 97.

Risks from diabetes

Children in this age group may believe they have developed diabetes as a punishment for doing something wrong, or that a blood glucose test is a punishment. This must be brought up and into the open with the child even if he or she does not ask about it. After all, even adults ask themselves "What have I done to deserve this?" when something unpleasant or unfortunate occurs. We all try to find a logical connection between things that have happened.

Children can be limited in the amount of freedom they have on account of the parents' fear of hypoglycemia. It may be difficult to give insulin and take tests when children refuse to cooperate. They will have definite views on what they do and don't want to eat. It may be very difficult to know in advance how much of the meal a child will eat. Try letting him or her decide about some other details of daily life instead. Multiple injections or an insulin pump give children more freedom over what they eat and how much.

Don't tell a child in this age group too far in advance about injections, testing or other unpleasant things. They can easily build this up to unrealistic proportions in their imagination.

In a family where the children are of different sexes, diabetes may be linked to gender in the child's mind. For example, a girl might believe it would be better to be a boy since her brother does not have diabetes (or vice versa).

"Consider what the restrictions may cost in terms of development before you say no ..."
                              Marianne Helgesson, child psychologist

Elementary children

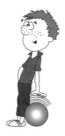

Starting school is stressful for all children, and many will find it difficult to adjust in the beginning. School-age children are occupied with understanding and exploring the world. They like to take things apart and understand how everything works. They will also be interested in understanding how their diabetes works. Friends become increasingly important and it is important to do the same sort of things as they do. Children in this age group like to keep track of how long an activity takes, such as running an errand. They are interested when they know something is going to happen but really cannot yet understand how long it will take. They expand their relationships from parents to other adults, including teachers and other caregivers at school. During the elementary school years, children learn how to master impulse control and to behave within acceptable limits and guidelines.[34]

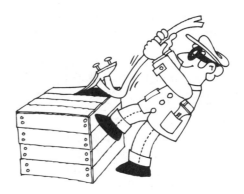

Stealing candy from the cupboard behind the parent's back is not uncommon behavior for pre-school children. It is important to avoid over dramatizing this — even children who do not have diabetes will do it. I think it is important that the result is not a total ban on candy. It is often more practical to give some extra candy once in a while, perhaps with the afternoon snack for 1-2 weeks, and give some extra insulin as well (see page 228). Explain that you are making an exception and that you expect the child to be able to choose more wisely about candy-eating as he or she grows older. The child will usually get over the craving for candy after a while.

Risks from diabetes

The fear of the unknown is still there even if the child seems interested in exploring. It is important to adapt the information to the age of the child. "Normalize", i.e. tell the child that it is quite normal and fully understandable ("Other

THE SINGLE MOTHER

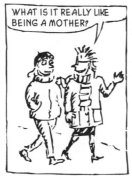 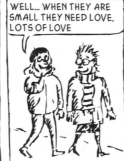 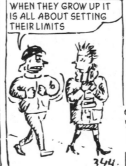 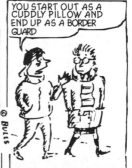

Being a good parent for a toddler is not the same as being a good parent for a teenager. The important, but difficult issue is to adjust the demands to the child's age in order to promote maturity. Children of all ages need lots of love, but it must be adapted to the age of the child. "Toddler love" to a teenager is experienced as overprotection and prevents liberation.

children would feel the same way") to feel the way he or she does in different situations, such as taking an injection or a blood test. Keeping track of time will often help, for instance when administering an injection. Food at school does not taste the same as it does at home, and sometimes the child will not eat at all. It is important to find someone at school who is able and willing to help the child take insulin at lunchtime. At first you may feel very insecure — what happens if my child becomes hypoglycemic at school? Try to ensure that one parent is always contactable by telephone and can come to school if necessary, especially early on. It is important that school teachers know how to deal with hypoglycemia. They will often take the child's illness more seriously after seeing a hypoglycemic episode.

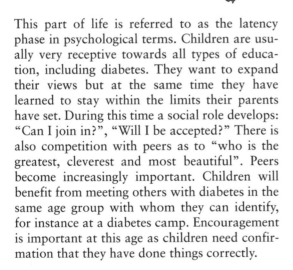

Middle-school children

This part of life is referred to as the latency phase in psychological terms. Children are usually very receptive towards all types of education, including diabetes. They want to expand their views but at the same time they have learned to stay within the limits their parents have set. During this time a social role develops: "Can I join in?", "Will I be accepted?" There is also competition with peers as to "who is the greatest, cleverest and most beautiful". Peers become increasingly important. Children will benefit from meeting others with diabetes in the same age group with whom they can identify, for instance at a diabetes camp. Encouragement is important at this age as children need confirmation that they have done things correctly.

Risks from diabetes

All children wonder about their role in life during this period. At the age of 10 or 11, a child

with a chronic disease will usually start to reflect upon and react to their illness in a new way. "Why did this happen to me?" is a common question. There will often be a time when the child experiences everything that has to do with diabetes as difficult and strenuous. For the first time the child understands that having diabetes means having it for the rest of his or her life. It will take some time to accept this.

During this time it is important to talk openly and often to the child about what diabetes entails, as this will help him or her to move towards acceptance. Show that you as a parent also feel concerned, and confirm that life with diabetes is both difficult and unfair. Children usually pass through this phase after a while but some may, on occasion, need help from a psychologist or counsellor.

As children in this age group are very receptive to learning without defying their parents' authority, it is important to make diabetes management a natural part of daily life during the years leading up to puberty. Children who are confident about managing their diabetes before the onset of puberty will be less likely to feel their diabetes prevents their growth and independence.

When should children take over responsibility for diabetes control?

During the early school years, all children expand their skills across a wide range of areas: athletic, artistic, academic, and self-control. As a natural part of this generalized increased ability in many fields, children will also gradually increase their participation in, and responsibility for, various diabetes-related tasks. However, current research indicates that parents should continue to take part in diabetes tasks throughout these years.[34] It is helpful if the expectation for continued parental involvement throughout the elementary school years and into adolescence is introduced to children and families by the diabetes team as early as possible.[34] Don't hand over responsibility too early!

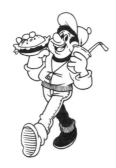

Puberty

During puberty, the teenager should begin the development of an adult identity, having independence and an equal standing with other adults. This increasing independence is fragile, which is why teenagers need to defend their integrity so strongly.

In a way, earlier stages of development are repeated. Teenagers often vacillate between behaving like children and being grown up. It is important to realize that they have the chance to "revisit" areas that have not been completed during earlier phases of development. Many parents look upon the teenage period with horror, but if you try instead to see puberty as a "final run through" of the childhood and adolescent years before embarking upon adulthood, your view may be more positive.

Friends are very important, and as it is only natural to want to be able to do the same things as everyone else. Teenagers like to go out in the evening to have a hamburger or pizza with their friends, instead of staying at home to eat the usual evening meal. It is important that young people are given both the freedom and responsibility to experiment with insulin doses on such occasions. Teenagers are very interested in their own body, especially during early adolescence, and are well aware just who that body belongs to. They want to be well informed about the way diabetes affects their body. At the same time they are often shy about exposing their body and, in this sense, are not at all as open-minded as might be expected.

We encourage older teenagers to come to some of the visits without their mother or father. An alternative is to let the parent enter the room at the end of the consultation and then only raise issues that the teenager has consented to. It is important for teenagers to understand that the professional confidentiality also applies to parents. If a young person wants to raise personal issues, he or she should be able to do so without fear of the information being passed on.

Teenagers often bring a buddy or a boyfriend/girlfriend to the visits. They appreciate someone's support but feel too old to bring their mother or father.

It may be a difficult for parents to know just how much involvement with the teenager's diabetes is appropriate. It can be difficult to remain sufficiently well informed as you are less and less involved with your child's diabetes and clinic visits.

Most teenagers prefer to manage without their parents' input but at the same time want them to be informed. One 18 year old girl said: "Of course I want them to know how my diabetes is managed — who else can jump in and help me if I fail?"

"Teenagers are impossible to raise, but it doesn't matter as long as parents do not stop trying."

Ackerman

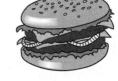

Risks from diabetes

The teenage years are a difficult period in which to develop diabetes. Teenagers are not mature enough to take sole responsibility for their diabetes but find it hard to let their parents do it. Children who are younger at the onset of diabetes find it easier for the parents to take full control, and then gradually let go as the child matures. Children who develop diabetes early in life are likely therefore to have better diabetes control and adherence to the treatment during the years of puberty than those developing it in the early teens.[403]

Learning to stand on their own two feet will be more difficult for a teenager with diabetes. They feel that they will never quite become an adult and will never have complete control over their own body. Just when it is time to cut the umbilical cord, it is securely tied again. In addition, their body will be inspected on regular visits to the clinic.

Of course, teenagers with diabetes will be concerned about the future. They will worry about what sort of job they can do, how to find a partner, whether they will be able to have children, as well as about complications of diabetes and so on. It is quite natural to become depressed about these things if you look towards the future in a negative way. It is not uncommon to have existential thoughts in general, but it is important to be on the look-out for suicidal thoughts as well.

At the same time, teenagers will often not think beyond the next few days. The risk of having eye damage or renal complications at the age of 40 if their blood glucose level continues to be high, matters less: "Then I will be so old that it will not matter anyway".

Most teenagers want to take injections in an adult way, that is to say without showing emotions. They hate it if this can't be managed and they are forced to be "a baby" again by crying or being unable to take the injection by themselves. It is just as important to "normalize" for teens as it is for younger children, that is to reassure them that many adults also find injec-

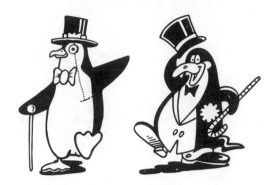

Friends are very important in the teenage years. When you start seeing your diabetes healthcare team without your parents it is a good idea to bring a buddy or girl/boyfriend instead.

tions difficult. Teenagers who can feel their behavior is accepted are likely to grow in self confidence.

Remember that being a good parent to a teenager is not the same as being a good parent to a younger child. Inappropriate adjustment by the teenager to diabetes has been found to be related to inappropriate adjustment on the part of the parents to the child's increasing need for independence during the years leading up to puberty.

Let your teenager practice as much as possible on his or her own. However, it is equally important to discuss afterwards how things went and why. Although the onset of puberty marks a dramatic change in a child's development and level of independence, children with diabetes and their parents must protect diabetes responsibilities (for example, the task of remembering blood glucose tests and injections) from excessive independence, handing over responsibility in a very gradual manner.[34]

In the interplay between children and parents, negotiation and agreement are essential. When young people say they want to assume the responsibility for something, let them give it a try. It is natural for parents always to want to know where their children are when they are away from home. If a young person has diabe-

---

How to handle a teenager

①   Don't be too understanding during early puberty. Setting limits is another way of showing that you care.

②   You may have to accept that certain things take precedence over diabetes for a year or two.

③   Try to argue about things other than diabetes when "fighting" in the family.

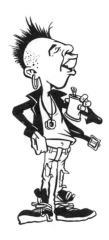

When teenagers have control over their diabetes, other subjects can be brought up as they grow in independence.

tes it is even more important. It is a good idea therefore to come to some agreement about having contact at certain times. A cellular phone may be a practical and popular way of keeping in touch with a child or teenager with diabetes.

Many teenagers demonstrate so called "risk behavior in that they like to do things that are slightly (or very) risky to test their ability. This is often more pronounced in boys than in girls. If this is the case, try connecting this behavior with the diabetes treatment and encourage experimenting with insulin dosages for example. There may very well be an element of risk included (such as how to dose insulin when staying up all night) but it is equally important that there be a "protective network" in the form of friends or adults whom the teenager can trust if something goes wrong.

A serious type of risk behavior is forgetting or skipping insulin injections. In an American interview study, 25% of the teenagers (11-19 years of age) stated that they had missed one or more insulin injections during the last 10 days, mainly due to forgetfulness.[805] Of these, 29% missed taking blood glucose tests which had been previously agreed upon and a further 29% had entered a lower blood glucose reading in their logbook than was actually registered. The adolescents who had missed insulin injections had a higher A1C value. If insulin doses are missed, blood glucose levels will start swinging around and the diabetes will become difficult to regulate.[557]

"Puberty is a necessary good. A person that does not pass through all the phases of puberty will risk becoming a bad copy of their parents."

Torsten Tuvemo, pediatric diabetologist

Healthy siblings

Being a healthy brother or sister to a child with a chronic disease can be difficult at times. Siblings often see many of the "advantages" that the ill child has, not to mention all the increased attention from the parents. At the same time it is difficult for a brother or sister totally to understand the situation of the child with diabetes. They will need help in answering some questions even if they don't bring them up by themselves:

— Is it my fault that my brother/sister has developed diabetes?

— Is it contagious? Will I get it as well?

— Who will take care of me when my parents are busy with my brother's/sister's diabetes?

It is important to listen to healthy siblings and accept that they can sometimes feel that "It is difficult to be the one not ill". Parents may find it easy to say: "You should be grateful that you are healthy" or "Would you want to be in that position?" Often it will be enough just to confirm the feelings of the child not having diabetes by saying: "I understand that it can be difficult at times".

Take it seriously when a sibling complains for instance about a headache or abdominal pain, even if you as a parent have the impression that it is not so serious. The brother or sister may benefit from seeing a doctor of his or her own. They may certainly benefit from being able to discuss stress and worry, and how these can cause headaches and other physical symptoms.

You can give a healthy sibling some extra attention. For example, the two of you could do something together on your own. It will not matter much what you do. Being alone with a parent is always something special. Take the opportunity to eat something tasty together and keep it "a secret" from the other family members. Do something else secretly together with the child with diabetes, like visiting a special playground, or, if the child is older, a theatre or exhibition. The purpose of keeping it "a secret" is to avoid envy between the siblings (regardless of whether they have diabetes or not).

It is difficult for siblings always having to hear that they cannot eat this or that because their brother or sister has diabetes and must not be tempted. One method, practiced in most families, is to allow something special to be eaten when the child with diabetes is not at home. As the child with diabetes gets older, he or she must become accustomed to not having the same arrangements as everyone else. Children with other diseases or problems (such as celiac disease, allergies or a tendency to put on weight) must learn that they cannot eat like their friends. Try to find something else that is desirable for the child with diabetes in order to avoid unfair treatment within the family. The goal is that, as children get older, they become increasingly able to withstand temptation on their own, for instance at school or during leisure times.

When a healthy brother or sister has a birthday party, parents should make an exception and let this child make all the decisions about what the treats should be. The child with diabetes can take some extra insulin that day in order to be able to join the party.

As brothers and sisters grow older, a strong feeling of friendship often develops. In many instances a good relationship develops between older teenagers with diabetes and their siblings, providing a springboard from which they can take the step towards adulthood, assuming

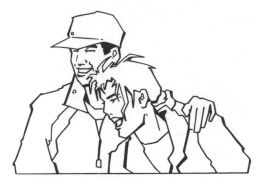

As a teenager you want to spend time with your friends. It is important that your diabetes doesn't stop you from doing this. Practice taking responsibility for adjusting your insulin doses and meal times so they will fit with the type of life you want to live.

responsibility for their diabetes. This can be particularly helpful, for example, in situations where parents are caught up in divorce, other conflict or are too overprotective, leading to difficulties in letting a maturing teenager take over responsibility and control.

Divorced families

More and more children these days do not live with both their parents. About one quarter of all children and teenagers in the UK and US live with only one biological parent. Divorced parents often have difficulties communicating and the children can end up delivering messages between them.

When a child develops a chronic illness, great demands are put on both parents to cooperate and trust each other. If the parents are divorced, the best approach is for both to obtain the same information from the very onset of diabetes. If they have new partners, these partners will also need information. The situation between the parents may be tense, but it will always be better for children if the parents can remain on speaking terms and cooperate with regard to the child's diabetes as much as possible.

Fathers' involvement

In a Swedish study, different factors, were investigated characterizing families where the children had different diabetic adjustment (high/l ow A1C and psychological adjustment to disease).[660] In families with poorer adjustment, the fathers were more impulsive and dependent. The children were also more impulsive. In families with better adjustment, the fathers were more independent and because of this, in a better position to support the mother and the child in coping with the diabetes. Children, especially boys, will find it easier to identify with their father and be inspired to take a greater responsibility for their diabetes.

It is difficult to generalize from a single study. However, from a clinical point of view it is clear that things work best in families where both mother and father are engaged with the child and his or her diabetes. Two people can usually find it easier to deal with a problem than one person alone, especially if they are able to discuss how different situations can be managed. If the father is not involved, but lets the mother take care of diabetes, it does appear that boys, in particular, are likely to have problems in their teens. It is important that fathers be with their child as much as possible at the time of diagnosis and that both parents be allowed to take an active part in the diabetes management from the very beginning.

The above applies also to divorced families where it is still important for both parents to cooperate and share the care of their child's diabetes (see above) as far as possible. Sometimes this is impossible for practical reasons and a single parent will have to take full responsibility for the child. This is of course an extra stress for that parent, and they may need additional support from extended family networks or friends. But in the overwhelming majority of cases it works very well.

"One cannot be cautious enough when choosing one's parents."

Henrik Pontoppidan

Brittle diabetes

Brittle diabetes can be caused by many different factors. It is defined as a diabetes that is so difficult to control "that life is constantly being disrupted by episodes of high or low blood glucose levels, whatever their cause".[743] In spite of great efforts from everyone, the swinging blood glucose levels continue. Swinging unstable blood glucose levels happen in all young people but "brittleness" may have contributing physical causes (such as insulin antibodies, decreased insulin sensitivity, puberty, delayed emptying of the stomach, missed insulin doses, incorrect injection technique) but also psychological where chronic stress (as in a divorce situation) may create a high or swinging blood glucose level.

When a person has brittle diabetes, the insulin doses will often be very large, even if the sensitivity for intravenously administered insulin is normal.[414] Ketones may be produced even when the levels of counter regulatory hormones are normal, and these patients will often have ketoacidosis.[414]

Sometimes a person with "brittle" diabetes deliberately manipulates the insulin doses for various reasons, creating widely varying blood glucose levels. This can create a vicious cycle which is difficult both to understand and to break. Afterwards, when looking back at this behavior, people often find it hard to believe that they really did this. If you think about it as a temporary coping response when the world is difficult to live in, it is not all that strange. Most adults have done things in their younger years that they are not all that proud of.

What is worrying is if the manipulative behavior continues, leading to dangerously unstable glucose control with many episodes of hypoglycemia and/or ketoacidosis. If you recognize yourself in this, you definitely need help to straighten things out. The most important starting point is "to put the cards on the table" by beginning to enter correct readings in your logbook, take your insulin doses regularly, and

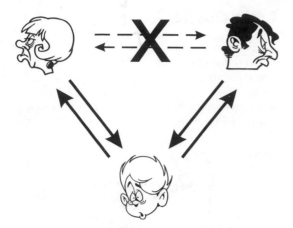

If the parents cannot agree, after a divorce for example, there is a risk that the child will act as a "messenger" between them. "Tell your Father that..." or "Ask your Mother about...". This is a role that will put the child in an awkward situation, causing distress and ultimately a high A1C value.

note in your logbook when you miss or forget an insulin dose. Otherwise your diabetes team has no way of knowing what is going on in your body and, because of this, may give you quite incorrect advice. For example, if you have a lot of high blood glucose readings, and give no indication that you have missed a lot of doses, your doctor is likely to advise you to increase your doses. But if you take these higher doses, you may end up with severe hypoglycemia.

It may not be necessary at this point to actually state that you have been "forgetting" doses — we all find it difficult "to lose face" and the most important thing right now is to get a new start. Just one little wish: if you sometimes (perhaps many years later) do tell your doctor or nurse what really happened, they will have a better chance of finding clues and helping someone else in your situation to get out of that vicious cycle.

Occasionally, sexual abuse from an adult in the child's or teenager's close surroundings, sometimes even by their father, can be the reason for a "brittle diabetes".[573] Remember that if something like this happens it is NEVER the young person's fault. Sexual abuse is always the fault of the adult and it is illegal. Something like this is very difficult to think about and even more difficult to reveal to anyone else. However, if you recognize yourself when reading this you must confide in someone whom you trust. This is the only way to make it stop, the only way to start over again and to have the opportunity once again to feel safe.

All doctors and nurses at your doctor's office or diabetes clinic are sworn to professional secrecy. This means that anything you tell your doctor or nurse stays between you, in confidence. Wherever you live, your diabetes team is under professional and legal obligation to guard every secret disclosed. Another alternative may be to speak to a priest, counsellor or teacher who you feel you can trust.

Quality of life

Diabetes is an illness that affects you 24 hours of every day, and will therefore have a substantial influence on your quality of life. In an international study from 17 countries, including 2101 adolescents aged 10-18 years, the main conclusion was that a lower A1C was associated with a better quality of life (as judged by the young people themselves).[375] Parents also found the family burden of diabetes to be lower. Teenagers from single-parent families and ethnic minority groups showed both higher A1C and poorer quality of life. Teenage girls had more difficulties with diabetes control than boys from the same age group. The message is that young people who try hard to improve their diabetic control also find that their overall quality of life is better, not worse.

Needle-phobia

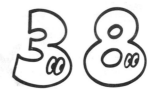

Phobia for injections and blood tests will show up in different ways at different ages (see page 338). Injection aids (such as Insuflon, see page 122) or a pump, can help many children take injections, though blood tests are still impossible to avoid. If you "get stuck" in these matters it is important to see a psychologist as quickly as possible to prevent needle-phobia from becoming a permanent problem for you, your child, or your family. See also page 97 and 111.

Topical anesthetic cream (EMLA®, ELA-Max®) gives effective pain relief and can be used to make some blood tests less unpleasant. It can be used for insulin injections on isolated occasions but, in practice, it is impossible to use for every insulin injection. Creams like this do not work on the fingertips as the skin there is too thick.

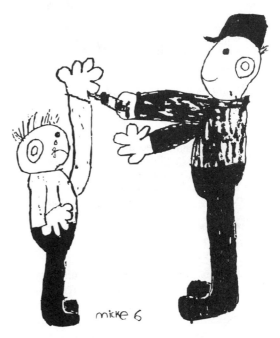

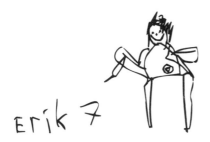

Children who are asked how they feel about injections often say they wonder why adults look so happy when they stick needles in children. "Do they enjoy hurting us?" It is easy to misinterpret an adult's smile, which is meant to comfort the child, as something else.

Needle-phobia: general advice

(adapted from Marianne Helgesson)

① Parents' attitudes to needle stabs are very important. You must be sure the finger prick or needle stab is necessary, otherwise you can never convey this to the child. If you, as a parent, have a needle-phobia of your own, it will be difficult to stick a needle into your child.

② The child must know exactly what is going to happen and why. Many children (even older ones) may believe that the injection or blood test is a punishment for something done wrong. You must state clearly that the needle is necessary, and not because anyone has behaved badly. Remember that the person sticking the needle in is not "being mean". He or she is only doing what has to be done.

③ Be honest about the pain. A needle prick can be painful, no matter how much we would like it not to be.

④ Indicate the acceptable limits of protest, such as: "You can cry if you feel like it, but you must not pull your hand away."

Needle-phobia, cont.

⑤ Offer realistic choices. They lessen the child's feeling of being a victim. But do not offer to give the injection another time as you cannot do that. The child will only remember being tricked and things will be even more difficult the next time around.

⑥ Suggest diverting activities, such as choosing a bandage.

⑦ The phase of persuasion should be short. When dealing with smaller children it is best to hold them firmly, do the needle prick, and then comfort. If inserting the needle takes time, the child will suffer for longer. Use a firm grip if you must hold the child, so that the injection is over quickly.

⑧ Don't smile to encourage. The child may believe that you are laughing.

⑨ **Afterwards:** Comfort, praise, and talk to the child. Dealing with what has been difficult through drawing or play may help. Stay with the child when playing in order to be able to correct misunderstandings and help the child come to terms with the experience.

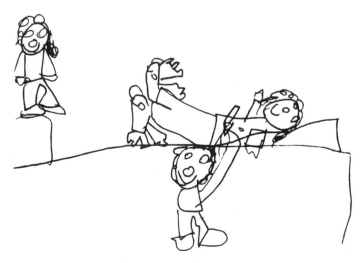

It need not always be difficult to start taking injections. Elin was 5 years old when she was diagnosed with diabetes. She did not mind the nurse giving her injections as she had an injection aid (Insuflon) inserted subcutaneously in her belly (see page 122). Her mother does not seem to be upset by this either.

Well-known people with diabetes

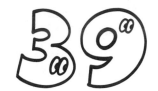

People with diabetes can be found in most professions. You probably know prominent people with diabetes in your home town or country. Below are some examples of how successful people cope with their diabetes.

Jay Leeuwenburg

Now in his eighth season of professional football, in September 1999 Jay was signed to a one-year contract with Cincinnati to help shore up the Bengals' offensive front line.[547] Jay had played at Indianapolis for three years as a starter. He was diagnosed with diabetes at the age of 12.

"I listen to what my body tells me. I use my blood glucose monitoring system a lot. On game days, I'll check my blood sugar 20 to 30 times. I'll check it every fifteen minutes for two hours before a game, so I can get a mental picture of what my blood sugar is doing. I've never been hospitalized or had an emergency on the field in my 14 years playing football, and I feel really fortunate. But I've worked really hard at it, too. I always keep a monitor on the sidelines, and Gatorade is always there for me to drink, too."

"I have the same advice for everyone with diabetes. It's my motto. "You need to control your diabetes, not let your diabetes control you." So many people feel "I can't do this, I won't do this, I shouldn't do this." You can do whatever you want, as long as you manage your blood sugar. It shouldn't keep you from doing anything."

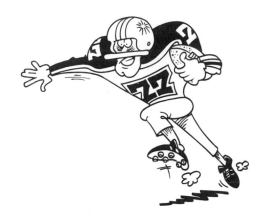

Bret Michaels

Bret Michaels from the US is a singer in the rock group Poison. He has had diabetes from the age of 6.[533] Today he says: "I accept having diabetes. Besides I try to live my life as normally as possible. It is like everything else you accept — you must know the rules. Of course you break them at times, but you must know them before you can break them". He can practise for hours to reach musical perfection but tries almost as hard to manage his diabetes. He takes blood glucose tests 6 - 10 times per day, "I must always know my actual blood glucose level as my working schedule is so irregular".

His appearance shocks many adults. This is what he wants to say to an adolescent who has just had the message of acquiring diabetes:

— It is difficult. You have already lived part of your life and suddenly you will be stricken by this disease. OK, sit down, cry, hit the sand bag, hit the door, crush a window or make a hole in the wall - whatever is needed to make that day pass. Then realize that you have diabetes and start taking care of yourself.

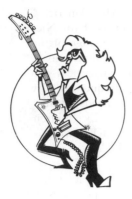

For young people he recommends a life without anxiety:

— Some young people with diabetes whom I meet are so scared. I want to tell them that there is nothing wrong with being scared, but you can't live a life of fear. One just can't say "Help - I have diabetes, I can't do anything". I want children to be taught to be prepared rather than scared.

— It is like this: go out and take hold of life and do your best. Just take care of yourself and always be prepared, wherever you go, whatever you do, partying or otherwise. Check that your friends know that you have diabetes, tell them what symptoms they need to learn to recognize and exactly what to do if you don't look well or act abnormal. Remember that you are worth something to yourself and your friends. If they are the type of people you can't tell that you have diabetes, or if they are such that will not help you, then they are not your friends!

— I always carry dextrose. No matter where I am I check that someone knows how to help me if I have a hypoglycemic reaction.

— Otherwise my opinion is that young persons with diabetes should continue to do what all adolescents do - ride skateboard or motorbike, play basketball or whatever they like.

.

Michelle McGann

Michelle McGann has been thrilling her fans on the women's pro-golf circuit for 11 years now, booking seven Ladies Professional Golf Association (LPGA) wins.[214] When Michelle was 13 she was afraid she'd never play golf again. Like any 13-year old she didn't understand what it meant to be diagnosed with something called type 1 diabetes. She fought her concerns about the disease, determined that it would not break up her love affair with golf. "In fact, I knew almost as soon as I got back to the course that my diabetes wasn't going to handicap me," she says.

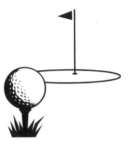

Diabetes sometimes throws her life into the rough, however. "I have ups and downs, of course. At times the adrenaline is really flowing, and it is hard to know how much insulin to take. Other times I know something is wrong because I feel tired and my swing gets weaker. But when you're a professional you have to keep going."

Nicole Johnson

Nicole Johnson came upon diabetes as most people with the disease do: unexpectedly and uninformed. In 1993, as a 19 year-old, she and her family were shocked when she was diagnosed with diabetes.[149] Rather than give in to the condition, she cast off the warnings that she would be prevented from realizing her dreams and goals. Ignoring her diabetes was not an option. Instead she challenged herself to learn all she could about the disease and how to manage it effectively.

Immediately, Nicole embarked upon a program of intensive diabetes management, requiring up to five shots a day. After several years of hard work, the control she knew she required had eluded her. Her life was a virtual roller coaster of glucose. It was then she decided to try insulin pump therapy. "I gained a sense of freedom that I thought I had lost forever!" was her observation. "The first day I got the pump I cried myself to sleep because I was so afraid, but I want kids not to worry about it because everything will be all right.[544] But it won't be perfect, and it doesn't solve all the problems — it's a lot of work and a big commitment."

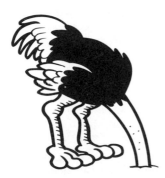

Ostrich strategy, i.e. not caring about diabetes and not taking any responsibility for its management, is among the most dangerous things a person with diabetes can do. Your diabetes team can contribute with knowledge, tips and advice — but living with your diabetes is something only YOU can do.

Winning the Miss America crown for 1999 was not a goal in itself for Nicole. She viewed the visibility and prestige of the honor as a means to further her greater goal of speaking out to raise greater awareness of diabetes, its symptoms and consequences. "I will use my voice to represent the needs of all persons living with diabetes, especially children with diabetes and their families who work tirelessly to ensure their care."

"With young people, I'm trying to give them hope and a new perspective, a new lease on life — because when you have diabetes you can have a bad attitude and almost be defeated by the disease, and we don't want that to happen. We want you to understand that regardless of the circumstances in your life, you can accomplish all you want to. It comes down to good control, and if you're in good control, you can achieve your dreams. You also don't have to be perfect. Nobody is perfect or has perfect blood sugars every single day, so don't get discouraged about that. Just try as hard as you can."

There are many other famous people in the world who take insulin for their diabetes. They include sportsmen and women, film stars, professors, captains of industry. All of them prove how you can live with diabetes successfully with a bit of courage and motivation.

"If you become a teacher, by your pupils you will be taught."

Hammerstein and Rogers 1951 [327]

Epilogue

When diabetes occurs in a family, life will naturally become difficult. If the person with diabetes is a child or teenager, issues of dependence and independence will be heightened. Parents will find themselves facing the dilemma of how to be sufficiently supportive without being overprotective.

When one family member has a chronic disease, extra demands fall on every other family member, and conflicts can result. When a child is sick, parents may find it extremely difficult to find enough time, as well as to balance the time needed for the child and his or her illness, time for other siblings, time for him or herself as well as time to have an adult relationship with a spouse or partner. Try to remember though, that all families have problems, especially if the children are in their teen years. Diabetes is not the only reason for stress. It can be helpful to try to think through how you might have handled the situation if the family member concerned had not had diabetes.

Artwork and other credits

In addition to the acknowledgments made at the beginning of this book, I wish to express my gratitude to the following authors and medical journals (© owners) who kindly gave me permission to print their illustrations (the full credit line is in the reference list on page 366):

Acta Paediatrica Scandinavia
(Scandinavian University Press):
Cedermark et al 1990 (p. 234)

American Journal of Medicine
(Elsevier Science)
Weinger et al 1995 (p. 94)

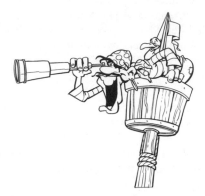

Land ahead! As an adult, one will often continue with the same attitude towards diabetes as one had when leaving the teens. But don't forget that "today is the first day of the rest of your life". It is never too late to decide to do something radical about your diabetes if you have high A1C values. Every percentage decrease in A1C will reduce your risk of complications in the future!

Archives of Diseases in Childhood
(BMJ Publishing Group):
Sackey et al. 1994 (p. 76)

Clinical Science (The Biochemical Society and Medical Research Society):
Welch et al. 1987 (p. 208)

Diabetologia (Springer-Verlag GmbH & Co. KG):
Malherbe et al. 1969 (p. 22)
Wahren et al 1978 (p. 245)
Maran et al. 1995 (p. 49)
Amiel et al 1998 (p. 44)
Tuominen et al 1995 (p. 249)

Diabetes (American Diabetes Association):
The DCCT Study Group 1995 (p. 315)

Diabetes Care (American Diabetes Association):
Bantle et al. 1993 (p. 113)

Frid et al. 1988 (p. 81)
Guerci et al 2003 (p. 175)
Hildebrandt et al 1986 (p. 165)
Linde 1986 (p. 81)
Schiffrin et al. 1982 (p. 109)

Diabetic Medicine (John Wiley & Sons Ltd):
Hanssen et al. 1992 (p. 317)
Bojestig et al 1998 (p. 318)

Endocrine Reviews
(The Endocrine Society):
Yki-Järvinen 1992 (p. 197)

European Journal of Paediatrics
(Springer-Verlag GmbH & Co. KG):
Cedermark et al. 1993 (p. 234)

JAMA (American Medical Association):
Brodows et al. 1984 (p. 65)
Nathan et al. 1984 (p. 230)

Journal of Pediatrics (Mosby, Inc)
Hanas et al 2002 (p. 125)

New England Journal of Medicine
(Massachusetts Medical Society):
Bojestig et al. 1994 (p. 318)

Nordic Medicine (Nordisk Medicin):
Knip 1992 (p. 321)

Scandinavian Journal of Nutrition
(The Swedish Nutrition Foundation):
Andersson et al. 1986 (p. 204)

I am also thankful to the following authors and medical publications (© owners) for letting me adapt their tables for use in the book:

APEG handbook on childhood and adolescent diabetes (Australian Paediatric Endocrine Group):
Silink M. 1996 (p. 261)

Diabetes Reviews International (Macmillan):
Kassianos G. 1992 (p. 297)

Diabetes Care (American Diabetes Association):
Kullberg CE et al. 1996 (p. 105)
McCrimmon RJ et al 1995 (p. 43)
Hirsch IB et al. 1990 (p. 135)

SPRI and Swedish Medical Society 1989:
Berg K. (p. 282)
Sundkvist G. (p. 311)

The Insulin Pump Therapy Book (MiniMed):
Tanenberg RJ, Bode BW, Davidson PC, Sonnenberg GE (pp. 162, 166, 175)

Diving and Subaquatic Medicine (Arnold)
Edge C. 2002 (p. 254)

Dietetic Management of Diabetes (John Wiley)
Waldron S. (p. 218)

Special thanks to Diabetes, the official journal of the Swedish Diabetes Association, for letting me print quotations from their journal.

Drawings are reproduced with the permission of the individual artist. Comic strips are reproduced with the permission of the respective vendor. The clip art is published with permission from the following vendors (© owners):
3 G Graphics Inc., BeeLine ArtProfile, Corel Corporation, Image Club Graphics Inc., One Mile Up Inc. and Totem Graphics Inc. LifeART Images Copyright © 1989-1997 by TechPool Studios Inc. US.

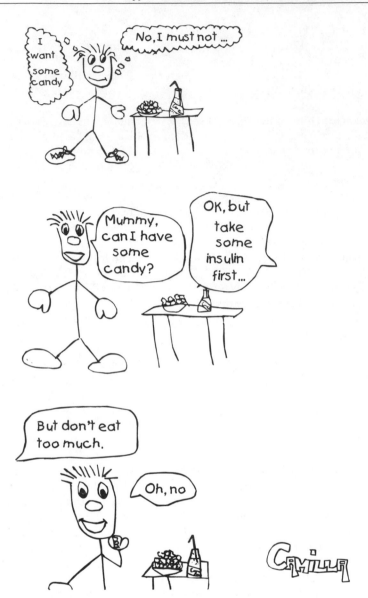

When using multiple injections or an insulin pump you will have increased freedom — but only if you take the responsibility that goes with it. One should not confuse this with an "anything goes" mentality where everything is allowed. It is a question of quantity as well — exceptions must be exceptions. If you make the exception every day it becomes a habit instead.

It is important to remember that it is not your blood glucose level today or tomorrow that counts in the long run, but your average blood glucose level over a long period of time to come, years and tens of years. As a parent (or teenager or adult with diabetes) you need to make some exceptions to learn and get used to the guidelines you should continue with in the future.

Today, Camilla is a young adult using an insulin pump and takes good care of her diabetes. As a teenager, she had strong support from her parents when she chose to make exceptions, but also clear limits on how much and how many exceptions she could allow herself. In my opinion this is a very good start of a long and well-managed life with diabetes. Thank you Camilla, for all the observations and good points about living with diabetes that you have given me throughout the years.

Glossary

<	Less than
>	More than
≥	Equal to or more than
≤	Equal to or less than
28	The references where the text is taken from are shown as small, superscript numbers. See page 366.

Units

Weight
1 kg (kilogram = 2.2 pounds (lb)
1 gram = 15.4 grains = 0.035 ounces
1 ounce = 28.35 grams = 1/16 pound

Length
1 cm (centimeter) = 0.4 inches
1 inch = 2.54 cm

Capacity
1 liter = 2.11 US pints = 0.26 US gallons
250 ml = ¼ liter ≈ 1 cup
1 US cup = 240 ml, 1 UK cup = 280 ml
1 US fluid oz. = 30 ml, 1 UK fluid oz. = 28 ml
1 tablespoon = 15 ml
1 teaspoon = 5 ml

Temperature
$° F = (9/5 \times °C) + 32$

Time
14 = 2 PM
02 = 2 AM

Terms

A1C
Blood test that measures how much glucose binds to red blood cells. Gives a measure of the average blood glucose level during the last 2-3 months. Also called HbA_{1c}.

ACE-inhibitors
Drugs that inhibit an *enzyme* (angiotensin converting enzyme) in the kidneys that increases the blood pressure.

Acesulfam K
Sweetener that provides negligible energy.

Acetone
Is produced when there is an excess of *ketones* in the blood. Acetone can be smelt on the breath when the level of ketones is raised.

Acidosis
Shifting of the pH in the blood towards being acidic.

Adrenaline
Stress hormone from the *adrenal glands* that increases the blood glucose level.

Adrenal glands
Small organs situated above the kidneys that produce a number of different hormones, including adrenaline and cortisol.

Adrenergic symptoms
Bodily symptoms of hypoglycemia caused mainly by adrenaline.

Albuminuria
A larger amount of albumin in the urine than the traces of albumin found with *microalbuminuria*. A sign of permanent kidney damage.

Aldose reductace inhibitors
Drugs that can affect nerve damage caused by diabetes.

Alpha cells
Cells in the *Islets of Langerhans* of the pancreas that produce the hormone *glucagon*.

Amino acid
Protein building blocks.

Amnesia
Loss of memory.

Amylase
An enzyme that is produced in the saliva and the pancreas. Amylase breaks down the starch in the food.

Anesthetic cream
Cream that numbs the skin (EMLA®, ELA-Max®). Can be used to reduce pain when inserting a pump catheter or Insuflon.

Antibiotics
Drugs that kill bacteria. Penicillin is one type of antibiotic.

Antibody
Produced by the *immune defense* to destroy viruses and bacteria.

Anorexia
Lack of appetite. Also commonly used to mean Anorexia Nervosa, an eating disorder in which a person starves him or herself.

Arteriosclerosis
Hardening, narrowing and eventually blocking of the blood vessels.

Aspartame
Sweetener that provides negligible energy.

Autoimmune
Sometimes things go wrong with the *immune defense* and the cells of your own body are attacked.

Autonomic nervous system
The "independent" part of the nervous system that is operated without one having to give it a thought, includes such aspects as breathing and the movements of the intestines.

Basal insulin
A low level of insulin that covers the body's need for insulin between meals and during the night. This insulin is given as *intermediate* or *long-acting insulin* or in a pump.

Basal rate
With an *insulin pump*, a low dose of basal insulin is infused every hour of the day and night.

Beta cells
Cells in the *Islets of Langerhans* of the pancreas that produce the hormone *insulin*.

Blood glucose level
The level of *glucose* in the blood. It is measured in mmol/l (SI-units) or mg/dl (mg%). For conversion table see page 90. Can be measured as *plasma glucose* or whole blood glucose. Earlier meters showed values in whole blood glucose but today, patient meters in most countries display *plasma glucose*. Unless otherwise mentioned, values in this book refer to plasma glucose (whole blood glucose values were used in the previous edition).

Brittle diabetes
Diabetes with very unstable blood glucose (rapid swings up and down) that prevents the person from living a normal life.

Bulimia
Eating disorder involving binge eating, i.e. sometimes eating huge amounts of food followed by purge (induced) vomiting or use of laxatives.

Capillary blood
The capillaries are the very fine blood vessels between arteries and veins where the blood delivers oxygen to the tissues. Blood tests from fingers contain capillary blood.

Carbohydrate
All compounds that are made up of different types of sugar, such as cane and beet sugar, grape sugar, syrup, starch, cellulose.

Cataract
Clouding of the lens in the eye.

Cellulose
Glucose molecules in long chains, present in all plants. Cannot be broken down in the intestines.

Chylomicrones
Small drops of fat that are being transported from the blood into the lymph drainage system.

Cyclosporin A
A *cytotoxic drug* that has been used to stop the immune process at the onset of diabetes.

Celiac disease
Illness where the person cannot tolerate *gluten*, a substance found in wheat, oats, barley and rye.

Coma
Unconsciousness. Can occur in people with diabetes when the blood glucose is very low (*insulin coma*) or very high (*diabetic coma*).

C-peptide
"Connecting peptide", a protein produced together with insulin in the *beta cells*. By measuring C-peptide, the residual insulin production of the pancreas can be estimated.

Cortisol
Stress hormone that is produced in the adrenal gland.

Counter-regulation
The body's defense against low levels of blood glucose. The excretion of the counter-regulating hormones (glucagon, adrenaline, growth hormone and cortisol) increases when the blood glucose level falls too low.

CSII
Continuous subcutaneous insulin infusion, treatment with an insulin pump.

Cyclamate
Sweetener that does not provide any energy.

Cytotoxic drugs
Drugs that affect the ability of cells to divide. Often used for cancer therapy.

Dawn phenomenon
The growth hormone level rises during the night, causing the blood glucose level to rise early in the morning.

Depot effect
Part of the insulin that is injected is stored in the fat tissue as a depot (a "spare tank" of insulin). The longer the action of the insulin, the larger the depot will be.

Dextrose
Pure glucose.

Diabetic coma
Severe *ketoacidosis* that has led to unconsciousness.

Diabetes ketones
Ketones that are produced when the cells in the body are starving due to a lack of insulin. The blood glucose level is high. See *ketones*.

Dialysis
The process of extracting harmful substances from the blood when the kidneys do not work properly.
See *uremia*.

Direct-acting insulin
Term for *rapid-acting insulin* used in some countries. Used in the previous edition of this book.

DNA
The genetic code inside the chromosomes is made of DNA.

Double-blind study
Technique to perform a study where neither the participant nor the investigator know who is treated with which type of medication or intervention.

EEG
Electroencephalography ("brain-wave"), a method for measuring the very weak electrical currents in the brain.

Enzyme
Protein compound that cleaves chemical bonds.

Fasting blood glucose
Blood glucose test taken before eating in the morning. In a person without diabetes, the plasma glucose result would not normally be higher than 100 mg/dl (5.6 mmol/l).

Fat pad
See *lipohypertrophy*.

Fatty acids
Substances produced when fat is broken down in the body.

Fluorescein angiography
Special type of X-ray technique to visualize the retinal blood vessels in the back of the eye.

Fructosamine
Blood test that measures how much glucose that is bound to proteins (mainly albumin) in the blood. Gives a measure of the average blood glucose level during the last 2-3 weeks.

Fructose
Fruit sugar.

Gastroparesis
Slower stomach emptying caused by diabetes complications (*neuropathy*).

Galactose
Sugar molecule. *Lactose* consists of galactose and *glucose*.

Gestational diabetes
Diabetes discovered during pregnancy. The symptoms usually disappear after childbirth but the woman has an increased risk of acquiring type 2 diabetes later on in life.

Glucagon
Hormone that raises the blood glucose level. It is produced in the *alpha cells* in the *Islets of Langerhans of the pancreas*.

Gluconeogenesis
Production of sugar (*glucose*) in the liver.

Glucose
Simple carbohydrate, *dextrose*, grape sugar, corn sugar.

Glucose tolerance test
Test to diagnosis early stages of diabetes. Tells how much the blood glucose level rises after orally ingested (OGTT) or intravenously given (IVGTT) glucose.

Gluten
Compound that makes dough sticky. Found in wheat, oats, rye and barley.

Glycemic index
A method to classify *carbohydrates* and foods according to how they affect the blood glucose level. Abbreviates to GI.

Glycogen
Glucose is stored as glycogen in the liver and muscles. The glucose molecules are connected in long chains. See illustration on page 204.

Glycogenolysis
The breakdown of the *glycogen* store in liver or muscles.

Glycosylated hemoglobin
See *A1C*.

Goiter
Enlarged thyroid gland.

Grape sugar
Glucose.

Growth hormone
Hormone that is produced in the pituitary gland. Increased growth is the most important effect. Increases the blood glucose level.

HbA₁
Older method of measuring A1C. Gives values approximately 2% higher than A1C.

HbA₁c
See A1C.

HLA-antigens
Genetic markers on chromosome 6 that are important when transplanting organs and for studying the heredity of different diseases.

Honeymoon phase
See *remission phase*.

Hormone
Protein compound that is produced in one of the glands in the body and that attains its target organ or tissue through the blood. Hormones work as "keys" to influence the cells in the body to perform different functions.

Hyperglycemia
High blood glucose level.

Hyperinsulinism
High level of insulin in the blood.

Hyperthyroidism
Excessively elevated levels of thyroid hormone in the blood. The thyroid gland is enlarged (toxic goiter).

Hypoglycemia
Too low a level of blood glucose. Usually defined as a blood glucose level below 3-3.5 mmol/l (55-65 mg/dl).

Hypophysis
See *pituitary gland*.

Hypothyroidism
Too low a level of thyroid hormone in the blood. The thyroid gland is often enlarged (goiter).

ICA
Islet cell antibodies. Antibodies directed against the *Islets of Langerhans*. Indicates an attack of the immune defense on the islets.

IDDM
Insulin dependent diabetes mellitus, former name for type 1 diabetes.

Immune defense
The defense in the body against foreign substances, such as bacteria and virus.

Implantable insulin pump
Insulin pump that is implanted under the skin in the subcutaneous tissue. Infuses insulin through a thin tubing into the abdominal (intraperitoneal) cavity.

Incidence
The number of diagnosed cases per year of a particular disease.

Incubation time
The time between when you have been infected with a contagious disease and when you show the first symptoms of the disease.

Insulin
Hormone produced in the pancreas' *beta cells*. Lowers the blood glucose level by "opening the door" of the cells.

Insulin antibodies
Antibodies in the blood that bind insulin. The insulin that is bound has no function, but can be released at a later time when the concentration of insulin in the blood is lower (e.g. during the night).

Indwelling catheter (Insuflon)
An aid to lessen the pain when injecting insulin. It consists of a soft teflon catheter which is inserted into the subcutaneous tissue.

Insulin analogs

Newer types of insulin where the structure of the insulin molecule has been changed to make the insulin action quicker (NovoLog/ NovoRapid, Humalog, Apidra) or slower (Lantus, Levemir).

Insulin coma

Unconsciousness caused by severe *hypoglycemia*.

Insulin depot

See *depot effect*.

Insulin pump

Insulin is infused into the *subcutaneous* tissue through a thin tubing continuously during day and night. Premeal doses are taken by pressing buttons on the pump.

Insulin receptor

Structure on the cell surface to which insulin binds. Initiates the signal that opens the cell membrane for glucose transport.

Insulin resistance

Decreased insulin sensitivity. A higher level of insulin than normal is needed to obtain the same blood glucose lowering effect.

Intermediate-acting insulin

Insulin that has an effective time action of 8-12 hours, corresponding to a normal night.

Intracutaneous injection

A very superficial injection into the skin that often leaves a small nodule (bubble) and is likely to hurt.

Intramuscular injection

Injection into a muscle.

Intraperitoneal delivery of insulin

Insulin is administered into the abdominal (intra-peritoneal) cavity where it is absorbed into the bloodstream leading to the liver.

Intravenous injection

Injection directly into a vein.

Islets of Langerhans

Small islets in the pancreas with cells that produce insulin (*beta cells*) and glucagon (*alpha cells*).

Jet injector

Injection without a needle. A thin jet of liquid is propelled using a very high pressure and penetrates the skin.

Jet-lag

Tiredness after long-distance flights when the day gets longer or shorter.

Juvenile diabetes

Diabetes in childhood and adolescence.

Ketoacidosis

The blood turns acidic from a high level of *ketones* when there is a deficiency of insulin. Can develop into *diabetic coma*.

Ketones

Fat is broken down to fatty acids when the cells are starving due to a lack of *glucose*. The fatty acids are transformed into ketones in the liver. This can occur when there is a lack of insulin ("high blood glucose, diabetes ketones") or when there is a lack of food (low blood glucose, "starvation ketones").

Ketosis

Increased amounts of ketones in the blood.

Kg

Kilogram, unit of weight. 1 kg = 2.2 lb.

Lactose

Milk sugar.

LADA

Latent Autoimmune Diabetes in the Adult. Onset of type 1 diabetes after the age of 35, usually with not so dramatic symptoms.

Langerhans
The scientist who discovered the *Islets of Langerhans* (in the pancreas) in 1869.

Latency phase
Psychological term for describing the years before puberty.

Lente insulin
Insulin made *intermediate* or *long-acting* with a mixture of zinc.

Lipoatrophy
Cavity in the *subcutaneous* tissue that can be caused by an immunologic reaction towards insulin.

Lipohypertrophy
Tissue build-up ("fat pad") that develops when you inject many times into the same area.

Long-acting insulin
Insulin with a very prolonged action, up to 24 hours.

Macroangiopathy
Diabetes complications in the large blood vessels (arteriosclerosis, cardiovascular disease).

Microalbuminuria
Small amounts of protein in the urine. The first sign of kidney damage (*nephropathy*) caused by many years of high blood glucose levels. Microalbuminuria is reversible if the blood glucose control is improved.

Microaneurysm
Small protuberances on the retinal blood vessels (see illustration on page 308). The first sign of eye damage caused by many years of high blood glucose levels. Microaneurysms are reversible if the blood glucose control is improved.

Microangiopathy
Diabetes complications in the small blood vessels (eyes, kidneys, nerves).

MODY
Maturity Onset Diabetes of the Young. A special kind of diabetes that is inherited.

Monocomponent insulin
Purified porcine (pig) insulin. Gives fewer problems with antibody formation than older types of insulin.

Multiple injection treatment
Treatment with injections of *short* or *rapid-acting insulin* before meals and *intermediate* or *long-acting insulin* to cover the night. When using rapid-acting insulin for meals you will need *basal insulin* during the day as well.

Nasal insulin
Insulin in aerosol form that is given via the nose.

Necrobiosis lipoidica diabeticorum
A special type of skin lesion that can be seen in individuals with diabetes.

Nephropathy
Kidney damage caused by many years of high blood glucose levels.

Neuroglycopenic symptoms
Symptoms of brain dysfunction caused by a low blood glucose level.

Neuropathy
Nerve damage caused by many years of high blood glucose levels.

NIDDM
Non-insulin dependent diabetes mellitus, former name for type 2 diabetes.

Nicotinamide
A vitamin B compound that has been shown to lower the risk of acquiring diabetes in some studies but a larger study showed no effect.

NPH insulin
Insulin made *intermediate-acting* by adding a protein (protamin).

Pancreas
An organ in the abdominal cavity that produces digestive *enzymes* (released into the intestines) and different *hormones* (released directly into the blood).

Pituitary gland
Small gland situated in the brain where many of the most important hormones in the body are produced.

Plasma glucose
A way of measuring the glucose content in the blood stream. Plasma glucose values are approximately 11-15% higher than whole blood glucose values. Check which type of readings your meter displays. In this book "blood glucose" refers to plasma glucose values.

Premeal injection
Injection with *short or rapid-acting insulin* prior to a meal.

Prevalence
The total number of existing cases of a disease at a given time.

Prospective study
A study that investigates what happens from now and onwards when giving a certain treatment. This is the best method of conducting a study of the effect of a new treatment.

Protamin
A protein from salmon that is added to protract the action time of insulin. *NPH insulin* is based on this method.

Proteinuria
Protein in the urine due to permanent kidney damage (*nephropathy*) from having high blood glucose levels for many years.

Pylorus
The lower sphincter (opening) of the stomach into the small intestine.

Rapid-acting insulin
Insulin analogs (NovoLog/NovoRapid, Humalog, Apidra) with a much quicker action than regular short-acting insulin. In some countries these are called ultra-rapid insulins, in others, direct-acting insulins.

Receptor
A special structure on the cell surface that fits with a hormone. The hormone ("the key") must fit into the receptor for it to mediate its effect to the cell.

Rebound phenomenon
After a hypoglycemic episode, the blood glucose may rise to high levels. This is caused both by the secretion of counteracting hormones (see *counterregulation*) and by eating too much when feeling hypoglycemic.

Regression
Psychological term to describe when a person temporarily regresses to an earlier stage of psychological development. An independent teenager who is hospitalized will often become more dependent and react as if he or she were several years younger.

Remission phase
Also called honeymoon phase. The need for insulin will often be lowered during the months after the onset of diabetes due to an increase of the residual insulin production in your pancreas.

Renal threshold
If the blood glucose level is above this level, glucose will show up in the urine when you test it.

Retinopathy
Eye damage caused by many years of high blood glucose levels.

Retrospective study
A study that investigates what happened when a certain treatment was given by looking backwards in time at treated individuals. Compare with *prospective* study.

Saccharin
Sweetener that does not provide any energy.

Sensor
Device to measure blood glucose continuously.

Short-acting insulin
Soluble insulin without additives.

Somogyi phenomenon
A special type of night time rebound phenomenon with high blood glucose level in the morning.

Sorbitol
Sugar alcohol, a sweetener that gives energy.

Starch
Complex *carbohydrates* found for example in potatoes, corn, rice and wheat.

Starvation ketones
Ketones that are produced when the cells starve due to a low blood glucose level. Caused by not eating enough food containing *carbohydrates*.

Subcutaneous
In the fatty tissue under the skin.

Sucrose
Cane or beet sugar, brown sugar, table sugar, powdered sugar, invert sugar, saccharose.

Transplantation
The implantation of a new organ in the body by surgery.

Type 1 diabetes
Previously called insulin-dependent diabetes (IDDM). Diabetes that needs to be treated with insulin from the onset. Is caused by a failure of the pancreas to produce insulin.

Type 2 diabetes
Previously called non insulin-dependent diabetes (NIDDM). Diabetes that initially can be treated with diet and oral drugs. Is caused by an increased resistance to the insulin produced by the pancreas.

U
Short for international units of insulin. Also short for Ultralente in Humulin U.

Unawareness of hypoglycemia
A hypoglycemic episode without having had warning symptoms associated with decreasing blood glucose.

Uremia
Urine poisoning when the body cannot get rid of its waste products. End stage of *nephropathy*.

Venous blood test
Test taken by puncturing a blood vessel (vein).

References

1) Aarø LE. Hauknes R, Berglund E-L. Smoking among Norwegian schoolchildren 1975-1980. II. The influence of the social environment. Scand J Psychology 1981;22:297-309.

2) Acerini CL, Patton CM, Savage MO, Kernell A, Westphal O, Dunger DB. Randomised placebo-controlled trial of human recombinant insulin-like growth factor I plus intensive insulin therapy in adolescents with insulin-dependent diabetes mellitus. Lancet 1997;350:1199-204.

3) Acerini CL, Cheetham TD, Edge JA, Dunger DB. Both insulin sensitivity and insulin clearance in children and young adults with type I (insulin-dependent) diabetes vary with growth hormone concentrations and with age. Diabetologia 2000;43:61-8.

4) Adamsson U, Lins PE. Hormonal counterregulation of hypoglycemia in insulin treated diabetics. Lakartidningen 1985;40:3369-70.

5) Adamsson U. Hypoglycemia. In the book: Diabetes. SPRI and Swedish Medical Society 1989: 238-47.

6) Adamsson U, Lins P-E. Clinical views on insulin resistance in type 1-diabetes. In the book: Agardh C-D, Berne C, Östman J. Diabetes. Almqvist & Wiksell, Stockholm 1992: 142-50.

7) Adlersberg MA, Fernando S, Spollett GR, Inzucchi SE. Glargine and lispro: two cases of mistaken identity. Diabetes Care 2002;25:404-5.

8) Ahlqvist J, Andersson K, Anzén B, von Bahr C, Endresen L, Hagenfeldt K et al. Contraception. Recommendations from a group of experts. Lakartidningen 40/1993;90:3456-64.

9) Ahmed AB, Home PD. The effect of the insulin analog lispro on nighttime blood glucose control in type 1 diabetic patients. Diabetes Care 1998;21:32-7.

10) Ahmed AB, Mallias J, Home PD. Optimization of evening insulin dose in patients using the short-acting insulin analog lispro. Diabetes Care 1998;21:1162-6.

11) Ahmed AM. Islamic pillars: possible adverse effects on diabetic patients. Pract Diab Internat 2000;17:96-97.

12) Airaghi L, Lorini M, Tedeschi A. The insulin analog aspart: a safe alternative in insulin allergy. Diabetes Care 2001;24:2000.

13) Åkerblom HK. Aetiological factors in type 1 diabetes. Nord Med 1992;107:204-6,230.

14) Åman J, Wranne L. Treatment of hypoglycemia in Diabetes: Failure of absorption of glucose through rectal mucosa. Acta Ped Scand 1984;73:560-61.

15) Åman J, Wranne L. Hypoglycemia in childhood diabetes: I. Clinical signs and hormonal counterregulation. Acta Ped Scand 1988;77:542-7.

16) Åman J, Wranne L. Hypoglycemia in childhood diabetes: II. Effect of subcutaneous or intramuscular injection of different doses of glucagon. Acta Ped Scand 1988;77:548-53.

17) American Academy of Pediatrics Work Group on Cows' Milk Protein and Diabetes Mellitus. Infant feeding practices and their possible relationship to the etiology of diabetes mellitus (RE9430). Pediatrics 1994/5;94:752-54.

18) American Diabetes Association. Diabetic retinopathy. Clinical Practice Recommendations 2003. Diabetes Care 2003;26(Suppl 1):S99-102.

19) American Diabetes Association. Clinical Practice Recommendations 2003. Diabetes Care 2003;26:Suppl 1.

20) American Diabetes Association. Report of the expert committe on the diagnosis and classification of diabetes mellitus. Diabetes Care 2003;26(Suppl 1):S5-20.

21) American Diabetes Association. Aspirin therapy in diabetes. Clinical Practice Recommendations 2003. Diabetes Care 2003;26(Suppl 1):S87-88.

22) American Diabetes Association. Diabetic Retinopathy. Diabetes Care 1998;21:157-59.

23) American Diabetes Association. Care of children with diabetes in the school and day care setting. Clinical Practice Recommendations 2003. Diabetes Care 2003;26 (suppl 1):S131-135.

24) American Diabetes Association: Hyperglycemic crisis in patients with diabetes. Diabetes Care 2001;24:154-161.

25) American Diabetes Association: Tests of glycemia in diabetes. Clinical Practice Recommendations 2003. Diabetes Care 2003;26(Suppl 1):S106-108.

26) American Diabetes Association: Physical Activity/Exercise and Diabetes Mellitus. Clinical Practice Recommendations 2003. Diabetes Care 2003;26(Suppl 1):S73-77.

27) American Diabetes Association: Diabetic Nephropathy. Clinical Practice recommendations 2003. Diabetes Care 2003;26(Suppl 1):S94-98.

28) American Diabetes Association: Standards of Medical Care for Patients With Diabetes Mellitus. Clinical Practice recommendations 2003. Diabetes Care 2003;26(Suppl 1):S33-50.

29) Amiel SA, Pottinger RC, Archibald HR, Chusney G. Effect of antecedent glucose control on cerebral function during hypoglycaemia. Diabetes Care 1991;14: 109-118.

30) Amiel S. Gale E. Physiological responses to hypoglycaemia. Counterregulation and cognitive function. Diabetes Care 1993;16, suppl 3:48-55.

31) Amiel SA, Maran A, Powrie JK et al. Gender differences in counterregulation to hypoglycaemia. Diabetologia 1993;36:460-64.

32) Amiel SA. Hypoglycaemia in diabetes mellitus - protecting the brain. Diabetologia 1997;40:S62-S68.

33) Amiel SA. Cognitive function testing in studies of acute hypoglycaemia: rights and wrongs? Diabetologia 1998;41:713-9.

34) Anderson B, Laffel L. Behavioral and psychosocial research with school-aged children with type 1 diabetes. Diabetes Spectrum 1997;10:277-81.

35) Anderson JH, Brunelle RL, Koivisto VA, Pfützner A, Trautmann ME, Vignati L, DiMarchi R et al. Reduction of postprandial hyperglycemia and frequency of hypoglycemia in IDDM patients on insulin-analog treatment. Diabetes 1997;46:265-70.

36) Andersson H, Asp N-G, Hallmans G. Diet and diabetes. Scand J Nutrition 1986;30:78-90.

37) Annersten M, Frid A. Insulin pens dribble from the tip of the needle after injection. Pract Diab Int 2000;17:109-111.

38) Anzén B, Zetterström J. Postcoital contraception, a forgotten and unused resource? Lakartidningen 1992;89:2948-2950.

39) Apelqvist J. Personal communication 1996.

40) Asp NG. Nutritional classification and analysis of food carbohydrates. Am J Clin Nutr 1994;59:679S-681S.

41) Attia N, Jones TW, Holcombe J, Tamborlane WV. Comparison of human regular and lispro insulins after interruption of continuous subcutaneous insulin infusion and in the treatment of acutely decompensated IDDM. Diabetes Care 1998;21:817-21.

42) Attvall S, Lager I, Smith U. Rectal glucose administration cannot be used to treat hypoglycemia. Diabetes Care 1985;8:412-13.

43) Attvall S, Fowelin J, Lager I, Schenck H, Smith U. Smoking induces insulin resistance - a potential link with the insulin resistance syndrome. J Intern Med 1993;233:327-32.

44) Attvall S, Abrahamsson H, Schvarcz E, Berne C. Gastric emptying is important for the patients with diabetes. Lakartidningen 1995;92(45):4166-72.

45) Avogaro A, Beltramello P, Gnudi L, Maran A, Valerio A, Miola M, Marin N, Crepaldi C, Confortin L, Costa F, Macdonald I, Tiengo A. Alcohol intake impairs glucose counterregulation during acute insulin-induced hypoglycemia in IDDM patients. Diabetes 1993;42:1626-34.

46) Axelsen M, Wesslau C, Lonnroth P, Arvidsson Lenner R, Smith U. Bedtime uncooked cornstarch supplement prevents nocturnal hypoglycaemia in intensively treated type 1 diabetes subjects. J Intern Med 1999;245:229-36.

47) Backman VM, Thorsson AV, Fasquel A, Andrason HS, Kristjansson K, Gulcher JR, Stefansson K. HLA class II alleles and haplotypes in Icelandic Type I diabetic patients: comparison of Icelandic and Norwegian populations. Diabetologia 2002;45:452-3.

48) Bagdade JD, Root RK, Bulger RJ. Impaired leukocyte function in patients with poorly controlled diabetes. Diabetes 1974;23:9-15.

49) Bancroft J. Sexual problems in diabetes. Diabetes Reviews International 1995;3:2-5.

50) Bantle JP, Weber MS, Rao SMS, Chattopadhyay MK, Robertson RP. Rotation of the anatomic regions used for insulin injections and day-to-day variability of plasma glucose in type 1 diabetic subjects. JAMA 1990;263:1802-6.

51) Bantle JP, Neal L, Frankamp LM. Effects of the anatomical region used for insulin injections on glycemia in type 1 diabetes subjects. Diabetes Care 12/1993;16:1592-97.

52) Bardhan PK, Salam MA, Molla AM. Gastric emptying of liquid in children suffering from acute rotavirus gastroenteritis. Gut 1992;33:26-29.

53) Barkai L, Peja M. Impaired work capacity in diabetic children with autonomic dysfunction. Lecture, ISPAD, Atami, Japan 1994.

54) Barkai L, Vámosi I, Lukács K. Prospective assessment of severe hypoglycemia in diabetic children and adolescents with impaired and normal awareness of hypoglycemia. Diabetologia 1998;41:898-903.

55) Barnett AH, Eff C, Leslie RDG, Pyke DA. Diabetes in identical twins. Diabetologia 1981;20:87-93.

56) Bastyr III EJ, Holcombe JH, Anderson JH, Clore JN. Mixing insulin lispro and ultralente insulin. Diabetes Care 1997;20:1047-8.

57) Beaser R. Fine-tuning insulin therapy. Postgraduate Medicine 1992;91:4.

58) Becker DJ. Management of insulin-dependent diabetes mellitus in children and adolescents. Curr Opinion Ped 1991;3:710-23.

59) Beer SF, Lawson C, Watkins PJ. Neurosis induced by home monitoring of blood glucose concentrations. BMJ;298:362.

60) Bendtson I, Gade J, Theilgaard A, Binder C. Cognitive function in Type 1 (insulin-dependent) diabetic patients after nocturnal hypoglycemia. Diabetologia 1992;35:898-903.

61) Bendtson I, Kverneland A, Pramming S, Binder C. Incidence of nocturnal hypoglycemia in insulin-dependent diabetic patients on intensive therapy. Acta Med Scand 1988;223:453-548.

62) Bennett PH, Haffner S, Kasiske BL, Keane WF, Mogensen CE, Parving HH, Steffes MW, Striker GE. Screening and management of microalbuminuria in patients with diabetes mellitus: Recommendations to the Scientific Advisory Board of the National Kidney Foundation from an Ad Hoc Committee of the Council on Diabetes Mellitus of the National Kidney Foundation. Am J Kidney Dis 1995;25:107-12.

63) Beregszàszi M, Tubiana-Rufi N, Benali K, Noel M, Bloch J, Czernichow P. Nocturnal hypoglycemia in children and adolescents with insulin- dependent diabetes mellitus: prevalence and risk factors. J Pediatr 1997;131:27-33.

64) Berg Kelly K. Living with diabetes. In the book: Diabetes. SPRI and Swedish Medical Society 1989: 285-90.

65) Berg TJ, Clausen JT, Torjesen PA, Dahl-Jørgensen K, Bangstad HJ Hanssen KF. The advanced glycation end product Nepsilon-(carboxymethyl)lysine is increased in serum from children and adolescents with type 1 diabetes. Diabetes Care 1998;21:1997-2002.

66) Berg TJ. Advanced glycation end products. Thesis, Aker University Hospital 1998.

67) Berger M, Cüppers J, Hegner H, Jörgens V, Berchthold P, Absorption kinetics and biologic effects of subcutaneously injected insulin preparations. Diabetes Care 1982;5:77-91.

68) Berne C, Hansson, Persson B. Pregnancy and diabetes. In the book: Diabetes. SPRI and Swedish Medical Society 1989: 119-134.

69) Berne C, Persson B. Pregnancy. In the book: Agardh C-D, Berne C, Östman J. Diabetes. Almqvist & Wiksell, Stockholm, 1992: 226-41.

70) Bierhaus A, Ziegler R Nawroth PP. Molecular mechanisms of diabetic angiopathy - clues for innovative therapeutic interventions. Horm Res 1998;50:1-5.

71) Biessels GJ, Kappele AC, Bravenboer B, Erkelens DW, Gispen WH. Cerebral function in diabetes mellitus. Diabetologia 1994;37:643-50.

72) Binder C, Lauritzen T, Faber O, Pramming S. Insulin pharmacokinetics. Diabetes Care 1984;7:188-199.

73) Birke G (Ed.) Drug Handbook. US English Pharmaceutical Company 1991-92, p 324.

74) Birkebaek NH, Johansen A, Solvig J. Cutis/subcutis thickness at insulin injection sites and localization of simulated insulin boluses in children with type 1 diabetes mellitus: need for individualization of injection technique? Diabet Med 1998;15:965-71.

75) Bjørgaas M, Sand T, Vik T, Jorde R. Quantitative EEG during controlled hypoglycaemia in diabetic and non-diabetic children. Diabet Med 1998;15:30-7.

76) Björk E, Berne C, Kämpe O, Wibell L, Oskarsson P, Karlsson FA. Diazoxide treatment at onset preserves residual insulin secretion in adults with autoimmune diabetes. Diabetes 1996;45:1427-30.

77) Blackett PR. Insulin pump treatment for recurrent ketoacidosis in adolescence. Diabetes Care 1995;18:881-2.

78) Bleich D, Polak M, Eisenbarth GS, Jackson RA. Decreased risk of type 1 diabetes in offspring of mothers who acquire diabetes during adrenarchy. Diabetes 1993;42:1433-39.

79) Blohmé G. Insulin treatment - possibilities and limitations. Swedish Diabetes Association, Booklet no. 6, 1987.

80) Blom L, Nyström L, Dahlquist G. The Swedish childhood diabetes study. Vaccinations and infections as risk determinants for diabetes in childhood. Diabetologia 1991;34/3: 176-81.

81) Blom L, Persson LÅ, Dahlquist G. A high linear growth is associated with an increased risk of childhood diabetes mellitus. Diabetologia 1992;35:528-33.

82) Bloomgarden ZT. American Diabetes Association Postgraduate Course, 1996: Monitoring glucose, defining diabetes, and treating obesity. Diabetes Care 1996;19:676-79.

83) Bloomgarden ZT. The 32nd annual meeting of the European Association for the Study of Diabetes. Neuropathy, health care, and glycation. Diabetes Care 1997;20:1037-9.

84) Bodansky HJ, Staines A, Stephenson C, Haigh D, Cartwright R. Evidence for an environmental effect in the aetiology of insulin dependent diabetes in a transmigratory population. Bmj 1992;304:1020-2.

85) Bode B, Steed D, Davidson P. Long-term pump use and SMBG in 205 patients. Diabetes 1994;43 (Suppl 1):220A.

86) Bode BW. Establishing & Veryfying Basal Rates. In the book: Fredrickson L (Ed.). The Insulin Pump Therapy Book. Insights from the experts. MiniMed, Los Angeles 1995.

87) Bode BW, Steed RD, Davidson PC. Reduction in severe hypoglycemia with long-term continuous subcutaneous insulin infusion in type 1 diabetes. Diabetes Care 1996;19:324-27.

88) Bode BW, Strange P. Efficacy, safety, and pump compatibility of insulin aspart used in continuous subcutaneous insulin infusion therapy in patients with type 1 diabetes. Diabetes Care 2001;24:69-72.

89) Bode BW, Gross TM, Thornton KR, Mastrototaro JJ. Continuous glucose monitoring used to adjust diabetes therapy improves glycosylated hemoglobin: a pilot study. Diabetes Res Clin Pract 1999;46:183-90.

90) Bode BW, Gross TM, Ghegan MB, Davidson PC. Factors Affecting the Reduction of Starting Insulin Dose in Continuous Subcutaneous Insulin Infusion (CSII): A Review of 389 Pump Initiations. Diabetes 2000;48(suppl. 1):abstract 264.

91) Bode BW, Strange P. Efficacy, safety, and pump compatibility of insulin aspart used in continuous subcutaneous insulin infusion therapy in patients with type 1 diabetes. Diabetes Care 2001;24:69-72.

92) Bode B, Weinstein R, Bell D, McGill J, Nadeau D, Raskin P, Davidson J, Henry R, Huang WC, Reinhardt RR. Comparison of insulin aspart with buffered regular insulin and insulin lispro in continuous subcutaneous insulin infusion: a randomized study in type 1 diabetes. Diabetes Care 2002;25:439-44.

93) Bode BW. Schleusener DS, Strange P. Switch from Continuous Subcutaneous Insulin Infusion (CSII) with Insulin Lispro (Humalog) to Multiple Daily Injections (MDI) with Insulin Glargine (Lantus) and Insulin Lispro. Diabetes 2003;52(suppl 1):439P (abstract).

94) Boëthius G, Gilljam H. Out of 1000 youngsters who smoke today 500 will die from smoking. Is further documentation necessary? Lakartidningen 119;92:375.

95) Bohannon N. Benefits of lispro insulin: control of postprandial glucose levels is within reach. Postgrad Med 1997 ;101/2:73-6, 79-80. (http://www.postgradmed.com/issues/1997/02_97/bohannon.htm).

96) Bohannon NJV. Treatment of vulvovaginal candidiasis in patients with diabetes. Diabetes Care 1998;21:451-56.

97) Bojestig M, Arnqvist H, Hermansson G, Karlberg B, Ludvigsson J. Declining incidence of nephropathy in insulin-dependent diabetes mellitus. New Engl J of Medicine 1994;330:15-18.

98) Bojestig M, Arnqvist H, Karlberg B, Ludvigsson J. Glycemic control and prognosis in type 1 diabetic patients with microalbuminuria. Diabetes Care 1996;19:313-17.

99) Bojestig M, Arnqvist HJ, Karlberg BE, Ludvigsson J. Unchanged incidence of severe retinopathy in a population of Type 1 diabetic patients with marked reduction of nephropathy. Diabet Med 1998;15:863-9.

100) Boland E, Ahern J, Ahern J, Vincent M. Pumps and kids: basal requirements for excellent metabolic control. Diabetes 2002:51(Suppl 2):A3 (abstract).

101) Bolinder J, Hagström-Toft E, Ungerstedt U, Arner P. Self-monitoring of blood glucose in type 1 diabetic patients: Comparison with continous microdialysis measurements of glucose in subcutaneous adipose tissue during ordinary life conditions. Diabetes Care 1997;20:64-70.

102) Bolli GB, De Feo P, De Cosmo S et al. Demonstration of a dawn phenomenon in normal human volunteers. Diabetes 12/1984;33:1150-3.

103) Bolli G, Fanelli C, Periello G, De Feo P. Nocturnal blood glucose control in type 1 diabetes. Diabetes Care 1993;16:suppl 3, 71-89.

104) Bolli GB, Di Marchi RD, Park GD, Pramming S, Koivisto VA. Insulin analogues and their potential in the management of diabetes mellitus. Diabetologia 1999;42:1151-67.

105) Bonfanti R, Bazzigaluppi E, Calori G, Riva MC, Viscardi M, Bognetti E, Meschi F, Bosi E, Chiumello G, Bonifacio E. Parameters associated with residual insulin secretion during the first year of disease in children and adolescents with Type 1 diabetes mellitus. Diabet Med 1998;15:844-50.

106) Borch-Johnsen K. Improving prognosis of type 1 diabetes. Mortality, accidents, and impact on insurance. Diabetes Care 1999;22 Suppl 2:B1-3.

107) Bott S, Bott U, Berger M, Mühlhauser I. Intensified insulin therapy and the risk of severe hypoglycaemia. Diabetologia 1997;40:926-32.

108) Bottalico JN. Diabetes in pregnancy. J Am Osteopath Assoc 2001;101:S10-3.

109) Bottazo, GF. On the honey disease. Diabetes 1993;42:778-800.

110) Boyle PJ, Schwartz NS, Shah SD, Clutter WE, Cryer PE. Plasma glucose concentrations at the onset of hypoglycemic symtoms in patients with poorly controlled diabetes and in nondiabetes. N Engl J Med 1988;318:1487-92.

111) Boyle PJ, Kempers SF, O'Connor AM, Nagy RJ. Brain glucose uptake and unawareness of hypoglycemia in patients with insulin-dependent diabetes mellitus. N Engl J Med 1995;333:1726-31.

112) Braatvedt GD, Mildenhall L, Patten C, Harris G. Insulin requirements and metabolic control in children with diabetes mellitus attending a summer camp. Diabet Med 1997;14:258-61.

113) Brackenridge BP, Reed JH. Counting carbohydrates - the key to proper bolusing. In the book: Fredrickson L (Ed.). The Insulin Pump Therapy Book. Insights from the experts. MiniMed, Los Angeles 1995;73-83.

114) Brand-Miller J, Hayne S, Petocz P, Colagiuri S. Low-glycemic index diets in the management of diabetes: a meta-analysis of randomized controlled trials. Diabetes Care 2003;26(8):2261-7.

115) Brink SJ, Miller M, Moltz KC. Education and multidisciplinary team care concepts for pediatric and adolescent diabetes mellitus. J Pediatr Endocrinol Metab 2002;15:1113-30.

116) Brodows G, Williams C, Amatruda J. Treatment of insulin reactions in diabetics. JAMA 24/1984;252:3378-3381.

117) Brown B. The effects of exercise on gastric emptying. Motility 1995/31:4-6.

118) Brunelle BL, Llewelyn J, Anderson JH, Jr., Gale EA, Koivisto VA. Meta-analysis of the effect of insulin lispro on severe hypoglycemia in patients with type 1 diabetes. Diabetes Care 1998;21:1726-31.

119) Brunner GA, Hirschberger S, Sendlhofer G, Wutte A, Ellmerer M, Balent B, Schaupp L, Krejs GJ, Pieber TR. Post-prandial administration of the insulin analogue insulin aspart in patients with Type 1 diabetes mellitus. Diabet Med 2000;17:371-5.

120) Bryden KS, Neil A, Mayou RA, Peveler RC, Fairburn CG, Dunger DB. Eating habits, body weight, and insulin misuse. A longitudinal study of teenagers and young adults with type 1 diabetes. Diabetes Care 1999;22:1956-60.

121) Burdick

122) Burge MK, Castillo KR, Schade DS. Meal composition is a determinant of Lispro-induced hypoglycemia in IDDM. Diabetes Care 1997;20/2:152-55.

123) Buyken AE, Toeller M, Heitkamp G, Vitelli F, Stehle P, Scherbaum WA, Fuller JH and the EURODIAB IDDM Complications Study Group. Relation of fibre intake to HbA1c and the prevalence of severe ketoacidosis and severe hypoglycaemia. Diabetologia 1998;41(8):882-90.

124) Byrne HA, Tieszen KL, Hollis S, Dornan TL, New JP. Evaluation of an electrochemical sensor for measuring blood ketones. Diabetes Care 2000;23:500-3.

125) Campbell LV, Ashwell SM, Borkman M, Chrisholm DJ. White coat hyperglycemia: disparity between diabetes clinic and home blood glucose concentrations. BMJ 1992;305:1194-6.

126) The Canadian-European Randomized Control Trial Group. Cyclosporin-induced remission of IDDM after early intervention: association of 1 year of cyclosporin treatment with enhanced insulin secretion. Diabetes 1988; 37:1574-82.

127) Canadian Diabetes Association. Clinical Practice Guidelines for the prevention and management of diabetes in Canada. Can J Diab 2003;27(suppl 2):S84.

128) Carpelan C. Why don't they change life-style? Diabetes (Swed. Diab. Ass.) 3/93:34

129) Cars O, Uhnoo I, Linglöf T, Svenungsson B, Burman L. Self administration of antibiotics in traveller's diarrhea. Advantages are not in balance with the risk. Lakartidningen 36/1990;87:2751-52.

130) Casella SJ, Mongilio MK, Plotnick LP, Hesterberg MP, Long CA. Accuracy and precision of low-dose insulin administration. Pediatrics 1993;91/6:1155-57.

131) Cedermark G. Selenius M. Tullus K. The postprandial blood glucose response to sucrose/glucose intake in a mixed snack in diabetic teenagers. Acta Pediatr Scand 1990;79: 473-474.

132) Cedermark G. Selenius M. Tullus K. Glycaemic effect and satiating capacity of potato chips and milk chocolate bar as snacks in teenagers with diabetes. Eur J Pediatr 1993;152:635-39.

133) Cersosimo E, Garlick P, Ferretti J. Renal glucose production during insulin-induced hypoglycemia in humans. Diabetes 1999;48:261-6.

134) Chase HP, Crews KR, Garg S, Crews MJ, Cruickshanks KJ, Klingensmith G, Gay E, Hamman, RF. Outpatient management vs in-hospital management of children with new-onset diabetes. Clinical Ped 1990:29:450-56.

135) Chantelau E, Heinemann L, Ross D. Air bubbles in insulin pens. Lancet 1989;336:387-88.

136) Chantelau E, Lee DM, Hemmann DM, Zipfel U, Echterhoff S. What makes insulin injections painful? BMJ 1991;303:26-7.

137) Charron-Prochownik D, Maihle T, Siminerio L, Songer T. Outpatient versus inpatient care of children newly diagnosed with IDDM. Diabetes Care 1997;20:657-60.

138) Chase HP, Saib SZ, MacKenzie T, Hansen MM, Garg SK. Post-prandial glucose excursions following four methods of bolus insulin administration in subjects with Type 1 diabetes. Diabet Med 2002;19:317-21.

139) Chaturvedi N, Stevens L, Fuller JH, WHO Multinational Study Group. Which features of smoking determine mortality risk in former cigarette smokers with diabetes? Diabetes Care 1997;20:1266-72.

140) Chew I, Brand JC, Thorburn AW, Truswell AS. Application of glycemic index to mixed meals. Am J Clin Nutr 1988;47:53-6.

141) Chiarelli F, de Martino M, Mezzetti A, Catino M, Morgese G, Cuccurullo F, Verrotti A. Advanced glycation end products in children and adolescents with diabetes: relation to glycemic control and early microvascular complications. J Pediatr 1999;134:486-91.

142) Chiasson, J L. Ducros, F. Poliquin-Hamet, M. Lopez, D. Lecavalier, L. Hamet, P. Continous subcutaneous insulin infusion (Mill-Hill Infuser) versus multiple injections (Medi-Jector) in the treatment of insulindependent diabetes mellitus and the effect of metabolic control on microangiopathy. Diabetes Care 1984 ;4: 331-37.

143) Chng HH, Leong KP, Loh. Primary systemic allergy to human insulin: recurrence of generalized urticaria after successful desensitization. Allergy 1995;50/12:984-87.

144) Christiansson J. The diabetic eye. Swedish Diabetes Association, Booklet no. 1, 1992.

145) Chlup R, Marsálek E, Bruns W. A prospective study of multiple use of disposable syringes and needles in intensified insulin therapy. Diabet Med 1990;7:624-7.

146) Ciofetta M, Lalli C, Del Sindaco P, Torlone E, Pampanelli S, Mauro L, Chiara DL, Brunetti P, Bolli GB. Contribution of postprandial versus interprandial blood glucose to HbA1c in type 1 diabetes on physiologic basal insulin replacement therapy with lispro insulin at mealtime. Diabetes Care 1999;22:795-800.

147) Cohen M. Changing from regular to lispro insulin: Lessons after 2 years. Diabetes 1999;48(Suppl 1):abstract 1562.

148) Combs CA, Gavin AL, Gunderson E, Main EK, Kitzmiller JL. Relationship of fetal macrosomia to maternal postprandial glucose control during pregnancy. Diabetes Care 1992;15:1251-57.

149) Congress Daily News 1. IDF New mexico 2000.

150) Conrad SC, McGrath MT, Gitelman SE. Transition from multiple daily injections to continuous subcutaneous insulin infusion in type 1 diabetes mellitus. J Pediatr 2002;140:235-40.

151) Consensus Guidelines for the Management of Insulin-dependent (Type 1) Diabetes. Implementing the St Vincent Declaration. European IDDM Policy Group, Medicom Europe BV, Bussum, The Netherlands 1993.

152) Cox DJ. Gonder-Frederick L, Clarke W. Driving decrements in type 1 diabetes during moderate hypoglycemia. Diabetes 1993;42:239-43.

153) Cox D, Taylor A, Nowdeek G, Holley-Wilcox P, Pohl SN. The relationship between psychological stress and insulin-dependent diabetic blood glucose control: preliminary investigations. Health Psychol 1994;3:63-75.

154) Cox D, Gonder-Frederick L, Polonsky W, Schlundt D, Julian D, Clarke W. A multicenter evaluation of blood glucose awareness training-II. Diabetes Care 1995;18:523-28.

155) Coustan DR. Gestational Diabetes. Diabetes Care 1993;16 (Suppl 3):8-15.

156) Cryer P, Gerich J. Hypoglycemia in insulin-dependent diabetes mellitus. In the book: Rifkin H, Porte D. Diabetes Mellitus, Theory and Practice. Elsevier 1990:526-46.

157) Cryer P. Iatrogenic hypoglycemia as a cause of hypoglycemia-associated autonomic failure in IDDM. A vicious cycle. Diabetes 1992;41:255-60.

158) Cryer P. Perspectives in Diabetes. Hypoglycemia begets hypoglycemia in IDDM. Diabetes 1993;42:1691-93.

159) Cryer PE. Hypoglycemia unawareness in IDDM. Diabetes Care 1993;16, suppl 3:40-47.

160) Cryer P, Fisher J, Shamoon H. Hypoglycemia. Diabetes Care 1994;17:734-55.

161) Cutfield WS, Peart JM, Thompson JMD, Holt J, Jefferies CA, Lawton SA, Hofman P. Prepubertal children are at high risk of intramuscular insulin administration based upon subcutaneous fat thickness. JPEM 2002;15(Suppl 4):1076(abstract).

162) The DAFNE study group. Training in flexible, intensive insulin management to enable dietary freedom in people with type 1 diabetes: dose adjustment for normal eating (DAFNE) randomised controlled trial. BMJ 2002;325:746.

163) Dagogo-Jack S, Craft S, Cryer P. Hypoglycemia-associated autonomic failure in insulin-dependent diabetes mellitus. J Clin Invest. 1993;91:819-28.

164) Dahlquist G, Blom L, Holmgren G, Hägglöf B, Wall S. Epidemiology of diabetes in Swedish children 0-14 years of age. A six year prospective study. Diabetologia 1985; 28:802-8.

165) Dahlquist G, Blom L, Persson LÅ, Sandström A, Wall S. Dietary factors and the risk of developing insulin dependent diabetes in childhood. BMJ 1990;300:1302-6.

166) Dahlquist G. Epidemiology of type 1-diabetes. In the book: Agardh C-D, Berne C, Östman J. Diabetes. Almqvist & Wiksell, Stockholm 1992:50-55.

167) Dahlquist G, Savilahti E, Landin-Olsson M. An increased level of antibodies to β-lactoglobulin is a risk determinant for early-onset type-I (insulin dependent) diabetes mellitus independently of islet cell antibodies and early introduction of cows' milk. Diabetologia 1992;35:980-84.

168) Dahlquist GG, Mustonen LR. Clinical onset characteristics of familial versus nonfamilial cases in a large population-based cohort of childhood-onset diabetes patients. Diabetes Care, 1995;18/6,:852-4.

169) Dahlquist G, Frisk G, Ivarsson SA, Svanberg L, Forsgren M, Diderholm H. Indications that maternal coxsachie B virus infection during pregnancy is a risk factor for childhood-onset IDDM. Diabetologia 1995;38:1371-73.

170) Dahlquist G, Gothefors L. The cumulative incidence of childhood diabetes mellitus in Sweden unaffected by BCG-vaccination. Diabetologia 1995;38:7, 873-4.

171) Dahlquist G, Frisk G, Ivarsson SA et al. Indications that maternal Coxsackie B virus infection during pregnancy is a risk factor for childhood-onset IDDM. Diabetologia 1995;38:1371-3.

172) Dahlquist GG, Kallen BAJ. Time-space clustering of date at birth in childhood-onset diabetes. Diabetes Care 1996;19:328-32.

173) Dahlquist G, Mustonen L. Analysis of 20 years of prospective registration of childhood onset diabetes time trends and birth cohort effects. Swedish Childhood Diabetes Study Group. Acta Paediatr 2000;89:1231-7.

174) Dahl-Jørgensen K, Brinchmann-Hansen O, Hanssen KF, Sandvik L, Aagenaes O. Rapid tightening of blood glucose control leads to transient deterioration of retinopathy in insulin dependent diabetes mellitus: the Oslo study. Br Med J (Clin Res Ed) 1985;290:811-5.

175) Dahl-Jørgensen K, Brinchmann-Hansen O, Hanssen K, Ganes T, Kierulf P, Smeland E. Effect of near normoglycaemia for two years on progression of early diabetic retinopathy, nephropathy and neuropathy: the Oslo study. BMJ 1986; 293: 1195-9.

176) Dahl-Jørgensen K, Torjesen P, Hanssen KF, Sandvik L, Aagenaes O. Increase in insulin antibodies during continuous subcutaneous insulin infusion and multiple-injection therapy in contrast to conventional treatment. Diabetes 1987;36:1-5.

177) Dahl-Jørgensen K, Joner G, Hanssen KF. Relationship between cows' milk consumption and incidence of IDDM in childhood. Diabetes Care 1991;14:1081-83.

178) Daly ME, Vale C, Littlefield A, Walker M, Alberti KGMM. Altering food preparation decreases glycemic response with a greater decrease in insulin response. Diab Med 2000;17(Suppl 1):Abstract P132.

179) Dammacco F, Torelli C, Frezza E, Piccinno E Tansella F. Problems of hypoglycemia arising in children and adolescents with insulin-dependent diabetes mellitus. The Diabetes Study Group of The Italian Society of Pediatric Endocrinology & Diabetes. J Pediatr Endocrinol Metab 1998;11 Suppl 1:167-76.

180) Daneman D, Olmsted M, Rydall A, Maharaj S, Rodin G. Eating disorders in young women with type 1 diabetes. Prevalence, problems and prevention. Horm Res 1998;50:79-86.

181) Danne T, Weber B, Hartmann R, Enders I, Burger W, Hovener G. Long-term glycemic control has a nonlinear association to the frequency of background retinopathy in adolescents with diabetes. Diabetes Care 1994;17:1390-96.

182) Danne T, Mortensen HB, Hougaard P, Lynggaard H, Aanstoot HJ, Chiarelli F, Daneman D, Dorchy H, Garandeau P, Greene SA, et al. Persistent differences among centers over 3 years in glycemic control and hypoglycemia in a study of 3,805 children and adolescents with type 1 diabetes from the Hvidore Study Group. Diabetes Care 2001;24:1342-7.

183) Danne T, Aman J, Schober E, Deiss D, Jacobsen JL, Friberg HH, Jensen LH. A comparison of postprandial and preprandial administration of insulin aspart in children and adolescents with type 1 diabetes. Diabetes Care 2003;26:2359-64.

184) Datta V, Swift PG, Woodruff GH, Harris RF. Metabolic cataracts in newly diagnosed diabetes. Arch Dis Child 1997;76:118-120.

185) Davidson PC. Bolus & Supplemental Insulin. In the book: Fredrickson L (Ed.). The Insulin Pump Therapy Book. Insights from the experts. Mini-Med, Los Angeles 1995.

186) Davis EA, Soong SA, Byrne GC, Jones TW. Acute hyperglycaemia impairs cognitive function in children with IDDM. J Pediatr Endocrinol Metab 1996;9:455-61.

187) Davis EA, Jones TW. Hypoglycemia in children with diabetes: incidence, counterregulation and cognitive dysfunction. J Pediatr Endocrinol Metab 1998;11 Suppl 1:177-82.

188) Davis EA, Keating B, Byrne GC, Russel M, Jones TW. Hypoglycemic incidence and clinical predictors in a large population-based sample of children and adolescents with IDDM. Diabetes Care 1997;20:22-25.

189) Davis EA, Keating B, Byrne GC, Russell M, Jones TW. Impact of improved glycaemic control on rates of hypoglycaemia in insulin dependent diabetes mellitus. Arch Dis Child 1998;78:111-5.

190) The DCCT Research group. Diabetes control and complications study (DCCT): Results of feasibility study. Diabetes Care 1987;10:1-19.

191) The DCCT Research Group. The effect of intensive treatment of diabetes on the development and progression of long-term complications in insulin-dependent diabetes mellitus. N Engl J Med 1993;329:977-986.

192) The DCCT Research Group. Effect of intensive diabetes treatment on the development and progression of long-term complications in adolescents with insulin-dependent diabetes mellitus: Diabetes Control and Complications Trial. J Ped 1994;125:177-88.

193) The DCCT Research Group. The relationship of glycemic exposure (HbA$_{1c}$) to the risk of development and progression of retinopathy in the Diabetes Control and Complications Trial. Diabetes 1995;44:968-83.

194) The DCCT Research Group. Adverse events and their association with treatment regimens in the Diabetes Control and Complications Trial. Diabetes Care 1995;18:1415-27.

195) The DCCT Research Group. Effects of intensive diabetes therapy on neuropsychological function in adults in the Diabetes Control and Complications Trial. Ann Intern Med 1996;124:379-88.

196) The DCCT Study Group. Pregnancy outcomes in the Diabetes Control And Complications Trial. Am J Obstet 1996;174/4;1343-53.

197) The DCCT Study Group. Influence of intensive diabetes treatment on quality-of-life outcomes in the Diabetes Control and Complications Study. Diabetes Care 1996;19:195-203.

198) The DCCT Research Group. Clustering of long-term complications in families with diabetes in the diabetes control and complications trial. The Diabetes Control and Complications Trial Research Group. Diabetes 1997;46:1829-39.

199) The DCCT Research Group. Effect of intensive therapy on residual beta-cell function in patients with type 1 diabetes in the diabetes control and complications trial. A randomized, controlled trial. Ann Intern Med 1998;128:517-23.

200) The DCCT Research Group. Early worsening of diabetic retinopathy in the Diabetes Control and Complications Trial. Arch Ophtalmol 1998;116:874-76.

201) The DCCT Research Group. Effect of pregnancy on microvascular complications in the diabetes control and complications trial. Diabetes Care 2000;23:1084-91.

202) Debrah K, Sherwin RS, Murphy J, Kerr D. Effect of caffeine on recognition of and physiological responses to hypoglycaemia in insulin-dependent diabetes. Lancet 1996;347:19-24.

203) Dedorsson I, Eye complications. In the book: Diabetes. SPRI and Swedish Medical Society 1989:135 - 42.

204) Deeb LC, Holcombe JH, Brunelle R, Zalani S, Brink S, Jenner M, Kitson H, Perlman K, Spencer M. Insulin lispro lowers postprandial glucose in prepubertal children with diabetes. Pediatrics 2001;108:1175-9.

205) DeFronzo RA, Hendler R, Christensen N. Stimulation of counterregulatory hormonal response in diabetic man by a fall in glucose concentration. Diabetes 1980;29:125-131.

206) DeFronzo RA, Matsuda M, Barret EJ. Diabetic ketoacidosis. A combined metabolic-nephrologic approach to therapy. Diabetes Reviews 1994;2:209-38.

207) Del Sindaco P, Ciofetta M, Lalli C, Perriello G, Pampanelli S, Torlone E, Brunetti P, Bolli GB. Use of the short-acting insulin analogue lispro in intensive treatment of type 1 diabetes mellitus: importance of appropriate replacement of basal insulin and time-interval injection-meal. Diabet Med 1998;15:592-600.

208) Delahanty LM, Halford BN. The role of diet behaviors in achieving improved glycemic control in intensively treated patients in the Diabetes Control and Complications Trial. Diabetes Care 1993;16:1453-8.

209) Denker P, Leonard D, DiMarco P, Maleski P. An easy sliding scale formula. Diabetes Care 1995;18:278.

210) DeStefano F, Mullooly JP, Okoro CA, Chen RT, Marcy SM, Ward JI, Vadheim CM, Black SB, Shinefield HR, Davis RL, et al. Childhood vaccinations, vaccination timing, and risk of type 1 diabetes mellitus. Pediatrics 2001;108:E112.

211) Detlofsson I, Kroon M, Aman J. Oral bedtime cornstarch supplementation reduces the risk for nocturnal hypoglycaemia in young children with type 1 diabetes. Acta Paediatr 1999;88:595-7.

212) Diabetes in Canada. National Statistics and Opportunities for Improved Surveillance, Prevention, and Control. Minister of Public Works and Government Services Can ada 1999.

213) Diabetes Prevention Trial. Effects of insulin in relatives of patients with type 1 diabetes mellitus. N Engl J Med 2002;346:1685-91.

214) Diabetes Voice 1999. Global initiatives: Famous sportspeople with diabetes.

215) DiaMond Project Group on Social Issues. Global regulations on diabetics treated witn insulin and their operation of commercial motor vehicles. BMJ 1993;307:250-53.

216) Dinneen S, Alzaid D, Rizza. Failure of glucagon suppression contributes to postprandial hyperglycemia in IDDM. Diabetologia 1995;38:337-43.

217) Domargard A, Sarnblad S, Kroon M, Karlsson I, Skeppner G, Aman J. Increased prevalence of overweight in adolescent girls with type 1 diabetes mellitus. Acta Paediatr 1999;88:1223-8.

218) Donaghue KC, King J, Fung ATW, Chan A, Hing S, Howard NJ, Fairchild J, Silink M. The effect of prepubertal diabetes duration on diabetes microvascular complications in early and late adolescence. Diabetes Care 1997;20:77-80.

219) Donaghue KC, Pena MM, Chan AK, Blades BL, King J, Storlien LH, et al. Beneficial effects of increasing monounsaturated fat intake in adolescents with type 1 diabetes. Diabetes Res Clin Pract 2000;48:193-9.

220) Dorchy H. What level of HbA$_{1c}$ can be achieved in young patients beyond the honeymoon period? Diabetes Care 1993;16:1311-13.

221) Dorman JS, O'Leary LA, Koehler AN. Epidemiology of childhood diabetes. In the book: Childhood and adolescent diabetes. Chapman & Hall Medical, London 1995.

222) Douvin C, Zinelabine H, Wirquin V, Perlemuter C, Dhumeaux D. An outbreak of hepatitis B in an endocrinology unit traced to an capillary-blood-sampling device. N Engl J Med 1991;322:57.

223) Draelos MT, Jacobson AM, Weinger K, Widom B, Ryan CM, Finkelstein DM, Simonson DC. Cognitive function in patients with insulin-dependent diabetes mellitus during hyperglycemia and hypoglycemia. Am J Med 1995;98:135-144.

224) Drexler AJ. Pump therapy in preconception and pregnancy. In the book: Fredrickson L (Ed.). The Insulin Pump Therapy Book. Insights from the experts. MiniMed, Los Angeles 1995.

225) Duffin AC, Donaghue KC, Potter M, McInnes A, Chan AK, King J, Howard NJ, Silink M. Limited joint mobility in the hands and feet of adolescents with Type 1 diabetes mellitus. Diabet Med 1999;16:125-30.

226) Dunger DB, Edge JA. Diabetes and endocrine changes of puberty. Pract Diab Internat 1995;12:63-66.

227) Dunger DB, Sperling MA, Acerini CL, Bohn DJ, Daneman D, Danne TP, Glaser NS, Hanas R, Hintz RL, Levitsky LL, et al. ESPE/LWPES consensus statement on diabetic ketoacidosis in children and adolescents. Arch Dis Child 2004;89:188-94.

228) Dunn SM. Psychological issues in diabetes management: (I) Blood glucose monitoring and learned helplessness. Practical Diabetes 1987;4:108-10.

229) Schober E, Schoenle E, Van Dyk J, Wernicke-Panten K. Comparative trial between insulin glargine and NPH insulin in children and adolescents with type 1 diabetes mellitus. J Pediatr Endocrinol Metab 2002;15:369-76.

230) Eapen SS, Connor EL, Gern JE. Insulin desensitization with insulin lispro and an insulin pump in a 5-year-old child. Ann Allergy Asthma Immunol 2000;85:395-7.

231) Early Treatment Diabetic Retinopathy Study Group: Aspirin effects on mortality and morbidity in patients with diabetes mellitus. JAMA 1992;268:1292-300.

232) EASD, The Diabetes and Nutrition Study Group(DNSG). Recommendations for the nutritional management for patients with diabetes mellitus. Euro J Clin Nutr 2000;54:353-56.

233) Eastman RC, Chase HP, Buckingham B, Hathout EH, Fuller-Byk L, Leptien A, Wyhe MMV, Davis TL, Fermi SJ, Pechler H, et al. Use of the GlucoWatch biographer in children and adolescents with diabetes. Pediatric Diabetes 2002;3:127-134.

234) Ebeling P, Tuominen JA, Bourey R, Koranyi L, Koivisto VA. Athletes with IDDM exhibit impaired metabolic control and increased lipid utilization with no increase in insulin sensitivity. Diabetes 1995;44:471-7.

235) Ebeling P, Jansson PA, Smith U, Lalli C, Bolli GB, Koivisto VA. Strategies toward improved control during insulin lispro therapy in IDDM. Importance of basal insulin. Diabetes Care 1997;20:1287-9.

236) Eckert B, Ryding E, Agardh CD. The cerebral vascular response to a rapid decrease in blood glucose to values above normal in poorly controlled type 1 (insulin-dependent) diabetes mellitus. Diabetes Res Clin Pract, 1995; 27/3:221-7.

237) Eckert B, Rosén I, Stenberg G, Agardh CD. The recovery of brain function after hypoglycemia in normal man. Diabetologia 1992;35 (Suppl 1):abstract 161.

238) Edge C. Diving and diabetes. UK Sports Diving Medical Committee. http://www.ukdiving.co.uk/ukdiving/info/medicine/diabetes.htm

239) Edge C, Bryson P. Insulin-dependent diabetes mellitus. In the book: Edmonds C, Lowry C, Pennefather J, Walker R (Eds). Diving and Subaquatic Medicine. Arnold, London, 2002.

240) Edge JA, Ford-Adams ME, Dunger DB. Causes of death in children with insulin dependent diabetes 1990-96. Arch Dis Child 1999;81:318-23.

241) Ehtisham S, Barrett TG, Shaw NJ. Type 2 diabetes mellitus in UK children--an emerging problem. Diabet Med 2000;17:867-71.

242) Eizirik D. Damage and repair in human islet cells. Diabetes in the XXI century; Part II. 1995:21-22.

243) Ekholm L, Björk E, Åman J. Insulin pens have the best precision when injecting small dosages of insulin. Lakartidningen 22/1991;88:2050.

244) Eliasson B, Attvall S, Taskinen MR, Smith U. The insulin resistance syndrome in smokers is related to smoking habits. Arterioscler Thromb, 1994 Dec, 14:12, 1946-50.

245) Elliott RB, Martin JB. Dietary protein: A trigger of insulin-dependent diabetes in the BB rat? Diabetologia 1984;26:297-9.

246) Elliott RB, Pilcher CC. Prevention of diabetes in normal school children. Diab Res Clin Pract 1991;14, suppl 1:85.

247) Elliott RB, Chase HP. Prevention or delay of Type I (insulin-dependent) diabetes mellitus in children using nicotinamide. Diabetologia 1991;34:362-5.

248) Elliott RB. Lecture, ISPAD Annual Meeting, Greece 1993.

249) Ellison JM, Stegmann JM, Colner SL, Michael RH, Sharma MK, Ervin KR, Horwitz DL. Rapid changes in postprandial blood glucose produce concentration differences at finger, forearm, and thigh sampling sites. Diabetes Care 2002;25:961-4.

250) Enzlin P, Mathieu C, Vanderschueren D, Demyttenaere K. Diabetes mellitus and female sexuality: a review of 25 years' research. Diabet Med 1998;15:809-15.

251) Ernström U. High price for a pinch of snuff. Diabetes (Swed. Diab. Ass.) 4/91:32-33.

252) Engström I, Kroon M, Arvidsson CG, Segnestam K, Snellman K, Aman J. Eating disorders in adolescent girls with insulin-dependent diabetes mellitus: a population-based case-control study. Acta Paediatr 1999;88:175-80.

253) Escalante D, Davidson J, Garber A. Maximizing glycemic control. How to achieve normal glycemia while minimizing hyperinsulinemia in insulin-requiring patients with diabetes mellitus. Clinical Diabetes Jan/Feb 1993:3-6.

254) EURODIAB Substudy 2 Study Group. Infections and vaccinations as risk factors for childhood type I (insulin-dependent) diabetes mellitus: a multicentre case-control investigation. Diabetologia 2000;43:47-53.

255) Evans ML, Pernet A, Lomas J, Jones J, Amiel SA. Delay in onset of awareness of acute hypoglycemia and of restoration of cognitive performance during recovery. Diabetes Care 2000;23:893-7.

256) Ewing FME, Deary IJ, McCrimmon RJ, Strachan MWJ, Frier BM. Auditory information processing during acute hypoglycaemia in IDDM. Diab Med 1998 (Suppl 1):S36 (abstract).

257) Faglia E, Favales F, Aldeghi A et al. Adjunctive systemic hyperbaric oxygen therapy in treatment of severe prevalently ischemic diabetic foot ulcer: a randomized study. Diabetes Care 1996;19/12:1338-43.

258) Fanelli CG, Epifano L, Rambotti AM, Pampanelli S, DiVincenzo A, Modarelli F, Lepore M, Annibale B, Ciofetta M, Bottini P, Porcellati F, Scionti L, Santeusanio F, Brunetti P, Bolli GB. Meticulous prevention of hypoglycemia (near-)normalizes the glycemic thresholds and magnitude of most neuroendocrine responses to, symptoms of and cognitive function during hypoglycemia in intensively treated patients with short-term IDDM. Diabetes 1993;42:1683-89.

259) Fanelli C, Pampanelli S, CalderoneS, Lepore M, Annibale B, Compagnucci P, Brunetti P, Bolli GB. Effects of recent, short-term hyperglycemia on responses to hypoglycemia in humans. Relevance to the pathogenesis of hypoglycemia unawareness and hyperglycemia-induced insulin resistance. Diabetes 1995;44:513-19.

260) Fanelli CG, Paramore DS, Hershey T, Terkamp C, Ovalle F, Craft S, Cryer PE. Impact of nocturnal hypoglycemia on hypoglycemic cognitive dysfunction in type 1 diabetes. Diabetes 1998;47:1920-7.

261) Faradji RN, Havari E, Chen Q, Gray J, Tornheim K, Corkey BE, Mulligan RC, Lipes MA. Glucose-induced toxicity in insulin-producing pituitary cells that coexpress GLUT2 and glucokinase. Implications for metabolic engineering. J Biol Chem 2001;276:695-702.

262) Fava D, Leslie D, Pozzilli P. Relationship between dairy product consumption and incidence of IDDM in childhood in Italy. Diabetes Care 1994;17:1488-90.

263) Feldt-Rasmussen B, Mathiesen ER, Jensen T, Lauritzen T, Deckert T. Effect of improved metabolic control on loss of kidney function in type 1 (insulin-dependent) diabetic patients: an update of the Steno studies. Diabetologia 1991;34:164-70.

264) Felig P, Bergman M. Integrated physiology of carbohydrate metabolism. In the book: Rifkin H, Porte D. Diabetes Mellitus, Theory and Practice. Elsevier 1990:51-60.

265) Feltbower RG, Bodansky HJ, McKinney PA, Houghton J, Stephenson CR, Haigh D. Trends in the incidence of childhood diabetes in south Asians and other children in Bradford, UK. Diabet Med 2002;19:162-6.

266) Feltbower RG, McKinney PA, Parslow RC, Stephenson CR, Bodansky HJ. Type 1 diabetes in Yorkshire, UK: time trends in 0-14 and 15-29-year-olds, age at onset and age-period-cohort modelling. Diabet Med 2003;20:437-41.

267) Flanagan DE, Watson J, Everett J, Cavan D, Kerr D. Driving and insulin--consensus, conflict or confusion? Diabet Med 2000;17:316-20.

268) Fleming DR, Jacober SJ, Vanderberg MA, Fitzgerald JT, Grunberger G. The safety of injecting through clothing. Diabetes Care 1997;20:244-47.

269) Fogh-Andersen N, D'Orazio P. Proposal for standardizing direct-reading biosensors for blood glucose. Clin Chem 1998;44:655-9.

270) Fort P, Waters S, Lifshitz F. Low-dose insulin infusion in the treatment of diabetic ketoacidosis: Bolus versus no bolus. Journal of Pediatrics 1980;96:36-40.

271) Fortunat W, Binter E. Do young diabetic patients benefit from functional insulin therapy in the long run? Wien Med Wochenschr 1991;141:53-5.

272) Foster-Powell K, Holt SH, Brand-Miller JC. International table of glycemic index and glycemic load values: 2002. Am J Clin Nutr 2002;76:5-56.

273) Fowelin J, Attvall S, v Schenck H, Bengtsson BÅ, Smith U, Lager I. Effect of prolonged hyperglycemia on growth hormone levels and insulin sensitivity in Insulin-dependent diabetes mellitus. Metabolism 1993;42:387-94.

274) Franz MJ, Bantle JP, Beebe CA, Brunzell JD, Chiasson JL, Garg A, Holzmeister LA, Hoogwerf B, Mayer-Davis E, Mooradian AD, et al. Evidence-based nutrition principles and recommendations for the treatment and prevention of diabetes and related complications. Diabetes Care 2002;25:148-98.

275) Franz MJ, Bantle JP. Response to Wolever. Diabetes Care 2002;25:1264-5.

276) Franzén I, Ludvigsson J. Specific instructions gave reduction of lipomas and improved metabolic control in diabetic children. Diabetologia 1997;40 (Suppl 1):A615, abstract 2421.

277) Frayn K. Metabolic Regulation. A human perspective. In the book: Snell K. (Ed.). Frontiers in Metabolism. Portland Press Ltd, London 1996, p 229-36.

278) Fredrickson DD, Guthrie DW, Nehrling JK, Guthrie R. Effects of DKA and severe hyperglycemia in cognitive functioning: a prospective study. Diabetes 1995;44(suppl. 1) abstract 97.

279) Freeman SL, O'Brien PC, Rizza RA. Use of human ultralente as the basal insulin component in the treatment of patients with IDDM. Diab Res Clin Pract 1991;12:187-92.r

280) Frid A, Gunnarsson R, Günther P, Linde B. Effects of accidental intramuscular injections on insulin absorption in IDDM. Diabetes Care 1988;11:41-45.

281) Frid A, Östman J, Linde B. Hypoglycemia risk during exercise after intramuscular injection of insulin in thigh in IDDM. Diabetes Care 1990;13:473-77.

282) Frid A. Injection and absorption of insulin. Thesis, Lund, Sweden 1992.

283) Frid A, Linde B. Intraregional differences in the absorption of unmodified insulin from the abdominal wall. Diabetic Med 1992;9:236-39.

284) Friedrich I, Levy Y. Diabetic ketoacidosis during the Ramadan fast. Harefuah 2000;138:19-21, 86.

285) Fritsche A, Schnauder G, Eggstein M, Schmülling RM. Blood glucose perception (BGP) in type 1 diabetic patients during exercise and after consumption of alcohol. Diabetologia 1993;36 (Suppl 1):abstract 582.

286) Frohnauer MK, Liu K, Devlin JT. Adjustment of Basal Lispro insulin in CSII to minimize glycemic fluctuations caused by exercise. Diab Res Clin Pract 2000;50(suppl 1): S80(abstract).

287) Frost G. Is carbohydrate a complex problem? Pract Diab Internat 1995;12:160-63.

288) Fruhstorfer H. Pain and diabetes monitoring. Diabetes NEWS 1998;19:7-8.

289) Gabriely I, Wozniak R, Mevorach M, Kaplan J, Aharon Y, Shamoon H. Transcutaneous glucose measurement using near-infrared spectroscopy during hypoglycemia. Diabetes Care 1999;22:2026-32.

290) Gale EA. A missing link in the hygiene hypothesis? Diabetologia 2002;45:588-94.

291) Gale EA. Intervening before the onset of Type 1 diabetes: baseline data from the European Nicotinamide Diabetes Intervention Trial (ENDIT). Diabetologia 2003;46:339-46.

292) Ganrot PO. Insulin resistance syndrome: posiible key role of blood flow in resting muscle. Diabetologia 1993;36:876-79.

293) Gardner SG, Pingley PJ, Sawtell PA et al. Rising incidence of insulin dependent diabetes in children aged under 5 years in the Oxford region: time trend analysis. The Bart's-Oxford Study Group. Br Med J (Clin Res Ed) 1997;315/7110:713-17.

294) Garg SK, Chase PH, Marshall G, Hoops SL, Holmes DL, Jackson WE. Oral contraceptives and renal and retinal complications in young women with insulindependent diabetes mellitus. J Am Med Assoc. 1994;271:1099-102.

295) Geerlings SE, Stolk RP, Camps MJ, Netten PM, Hoekstra JB, Bouter PK, Braveboer B, Collet TJ, Jansz AR, Hoepelman AM. Asymptomatic bacteriuria can be considered a diabetic complication in women with diabetes mellitus. Adv Exp Med Biol 2000;485:309-14.

296) George E, Marques JL, Harris ND, Macdonald IA, Hardisty CA, Heller SR. Preservation of physiological responses to hypoglycemia 2 days after antedecent hypoglycemia in patients with IDDM. Diabetes Care 1997;20:1293-98.

297) Georgakopoulos K, Katsilambros N, Fragaki M, Poulopoulou Z, Kimbouris J, Sfikakis P, Raptis S. Recovery from insulin-induced hypoglycemia after saccharose or glucose administration. Clin Physiol Biochem 1990;8:267-72.

298) Giacco R, Parillo M, Rivellese AA, Lasorella G, Giacco A, D'Episcopo L, Riccardi G. Long-term dietary treatment with increased amounts of fiber-rich low-glycemic index natural foods improves blood glucose control and reduces the number of hypoglycemic events in type 1 diabetic patients. Diabetes Care 2000;23:1461-6.

299) Gibbon C, Smith T, Egger P, Betts P Phillips D. Early infection and subsequent insulin dependent diabetes. Arch Dis Child 1997;77:384-5.

300) Gilbertson HR, Brand-Miller JC, Thorburn AW, Evans S, Chondros P, Werther GA. The effect of flexible low glycemic index dietary advice versus measured carbohydrate exchange diets on glycemic control in children with type 1 diabetes. Diabetes Care 2001;24:1137-43.

301) Gill GV, Redmond S, Garratt F, Paisey R. Diabetes and alternative medicine: cause for concern. Diabetic Med. 1994;11:210-13.

302) Gill G, Durston J, Johnston R, MacLeod K, Watkins P. Insulin-treated diabetes and driving in the UK. Diabet Med 2002;19:435-9.

303) Gillespie SJ, Kulkarni KD, Daly AE. Using carbohydrate counting in diabetes clinical practice. J Am Diet Assoc 1998;98:897-905.

304) Ginsburg BH, Parkes JL, Sparacino C. The kinetics of insulin administration by insulin pens. Horm Metab Research 1994;26:584-87.

305) Glasier A, Thong KJ, Dewar M, Mackie M, Baird DT. Mifepristone (RU 486) compared with high-dose estrogen and progesterone for emergency postcoital contraception. N Engl J Med 1992;327:1041-4.

306) Gold AE, Reilly C, Walker JD. Transient improvement in glycemic control. The impact of pregnancy in women with IDDM. Diabetes Care 1998;21:374-8.

307) Golden SH, Peart-Vigilance C, Kao WH, Brancati FL. Perioperative glycemic control and the risk of infectious complications in a cohort of adults with diabetes. Diabetes Care 1999;22:1408-14.

308) Goldstein DE, Little RR, Lorenz RA, Malone JI, Nathan D, Peterson CM. Tests of glycemia in diabetes. Diabetes Care 1995;18:896-909.

309) Graff M, Rubin RR, Walker EA. How diabetes specialists treat their own diabetes: findings from a study of the AADE and ADA membership. Diabetes Educ 2000;26:460-7.

310) Grajower MM, Fraser CG, Holcombe JH, Daugherty ML, Harris WC, De Felippis MR, Santiago OM, Clark NG. How long should insulin be used once a vial is started? Diabetes Care 2003;26:2665-6; discussion 266-9.

311) Graves PM, Barriga KJ, Norris JM, Hoffman MR, Yu L, Eisenbarth GS, Rewers M. Lack of association between early childhood immunizations and beta-cell autoimmunity. Diabetes Care 1999;22:1694-7.

312) Gray RO, Butler PC, Beers TR, Kryshak EJ, Rizza RA. Comparison of the ability of bread versus bread plus meat to treat and prevent subsequent hypoglycemia in patients with insulin-dependent diabetes mellitus. J Clin Endocrinol Metab 1996;81:1508-11.

313) Green A, Gale EAM, Patterson CC, the EURODIAB ACE Study Group. Incidence of childhood-onset insulin-dependent diabetes mellitus: the EURODIAB ACE Study. Lancet 1992;339:905-909.

314) Green A, Patterson CC. Trends in the incidence of childhood-onset diabetes in Europe 1989-1998. Diabetologia 2001;44 Suppl 3:B3-8.

315) Gregory R, Edwards S, Yateman NA. Demonstration of insulin transformation products in insulin vials by High-performance liquid chromatography. Diabetes Care 1991;14:42-48.

316) Grey M, Boland EA, Tamborlane WV. Use of lispro insulin and quality of life in adolescents on intensive therapy. Diabetes Educ 1999;25:934-41.

317) Griffin ME, Fedor A, Tamborlane WV. Lipoatrophy associated with lispro insulin in insulin pump therapy: an old complication, a new cause? Diabetes Care 2001;24:174.

318) Gros L, Riu E, Montoliu L, Ontiveros M, Lebrigand L, Bosch F. Insulin production by engineered muscle cells. Hum Gene Ther 1999;10:1207-17.

319) Gscwend S, Ryan C, Atchinson J, Arslanian S, Becker D. Effects of acute hyperglycemia on mental efficiency and counterregulatory hormones in adolescents with insulin-dependent diabetes mellitus. J Pediatrics 1995;126:178-184.

320) Guerci B, Benichou M, Floriot M, Bohme P, Fougnot S, Franck P, Drouin P. Accuracy of an electrochemical sensor for measuring capillary blood ketones by fingerstick samples during metabolic deterioration after continuous subcutaneous insulin infusion interruption in type 1 diabetic patients. Diabetes Care 2003;26:1137-41.

321) Gunning R, Garber A. Bioactivity of Instant Glucose - Failure of absorption through oral mucosa. JAMA 1978;240:1611-12.

322) Gunton JE, Davies L, Wilmshurst E, Fulcher G, McElduff A. Cigarette smoking affects glycemic control in diabetes. Diabetes Care 2002;25:796-7.

323) Hägglöf B, Blom L, Dahlquist G, Lönnberg G, Sahlin B. The Swedish Childhood Diabetes Study: Indications of severe psychological stress as a risk factor for type 1 (insulin-dependent) diabetes mellitus in childhood. Diabetologia 1991;34:579-83.

324) Haglund B, Ryckenberg K, Selenius O, Dahlquist G. Evidence of a relationship between childhood-onset type 1 diabetes and low groundwater concentration of zinc. Diabetes Care 1996;19:873-75.

325) Halberg IB, Jacobsen LV, Dahl UL. A study on self-mixing insulin aspart with NPH insulin in the syringe before injection. Diabetes 1999;48(Suppl 1):abstract 448.

326) Hamann A, Matthaei S, Rosak C, Silvestre L. A randomized clinical trial comparing breakfast, dinner, or bedtime administration of insulin glargine in patients with type 1 diabetes. Diabetes Care 2003;26:1738-44.

327) Hammerstein O, Rogers R. The King and I. Williams music, Hel Leonard Publications, Milwaukee 1951.

328) Hammes HP, Alt A, Niwa T, Clausen JT, Bretzel RG, Brownlee M, Schleicher ED. Differential accumulation of advanced glycation end products in the course of diabetic retinopathy. Diabetologia 1999;42:728-36.

329) Hanas R, Ludvigsson J. Side effects and indwelling times of subcutaneous catheters for insulin injections: A new device for injecting insulin with a minimum of pain in the treatment of insulin-dependent diabetes mellitus. Diabetes Res Clin Pract 1990; 10:73-83.

330) Hanas R, Ludvigsson J. Metabolic control is not altered when using indwelling catheters for insulin injections. Diabetes Care 1994;17:716-18.

331) Hanas R, Ludvigsson J. Experience of pain from insulin injections and needle-phobia in young patients with IDDM. Practical Diabetes 1997;14:95-99.

332) Hanas, R. Carlsson S, Frid A, Ludvigsson J. Unchanged insulin absorption after 4 days' use of subcutaneous indwelling catheters for insulin injections. Diabetes Care 1997;20:487-90.

333) Hanas R. Dead-in-bed syndrome in diabetes mellitus and hypoglycemic unawareness. Lancet 1997;350:492-3 (letter). Lancet 1997;350:1032-33 (reply).

334) Hanas R, Stanke CG, Ostberg H. Diagnosis of the cause of malfunction of indwelling catheters for insulin injections by the use of digital fluoroscopy. Pediatr Radiol 2000;30:674-6.

335) Hanas R, Lytzen L, Ludvigsson J. Thinner needles do not influence injection pain, insulin leakage or bleeding in children and adolescents with type 1 diabetes. Pediatric Diabetes 2000;1:142-49.

336) Hanas R. Low Risk of Hypoglycemia Despite Metabolic Control at DCCT Level in a Population of Children and Adolescents Using Intensified Insulin Treatment. Diabetes 2000;49 (Suppl 1):Abstract 540.

337) Hanas R, Adolfsson P, Andreasson C, Johansson E. Decreased HbA$_{1c}$ and low risk of hypoglycemia when using insulin pumps in a pediatric population. Diab Res Clin Pract 2000;20(suppl. 1); Abstract 1622.

338) Hanas R. Reducing injection pain in children and adolescents with diabetes. Studies on indwelling catheters and injection needles. Linköpings Universty Medical Dissertations # 700, Linköping 2001.

339) Hanas R, Adolfsson P, Elfvin-Akesson K, Hammaren L, Ilvered R, Jansson I, Johansson C, Kroon M, Lindgren J, Lindh A, Ludvigsson J, Sigstrom L, Wiik A, Aman J. Indwelling catheters used from the onset of diabetes decrease injection pain and pre-injection anxiety. J Pediatr 2002;140:315-20.

340) Hanson U, Persson B, Thunell S. Relationship between haemoglobin A$_{1c}$ in early type 1 (insulin-dependent) diabetic pregnancy and the occurrence of spontaneous abortion and fetal malformation in Sweden. Diabetologia l990;33:100-4.

341) Hanssen KF. Pregnancy in insulin-dependent diabetis. Nord Med 8-9/ 1992;107:211-12.

342) Hanssen KF, Bangstad HJ, Brinchmann-Hansen O, Dahl-Jørgensen K. Blood glucose control and diabetic microvascular complications. Long term effects of near-normoglycaemia. Diabetic Medicine 1992;9:697-705.

343) Hansson SL, Pichert JW. Perceived stress and diabetes control in adolescents. Health Psychol 1986;5:439-52.

344) Haycock P. Insulin Absorption: Understanding the Variables. Clinical Diabetes Sept/Oct 1986:98-118.

345) Haymond MW, Schreiner B. Mini-dose glucagon rescue for hypoglycemia in children with type 1 diabetes. Diabetes Care 2001;24:643-5.

346) Hayward LM, Burden ML, Burden AC, Blackledge H, Raymond NT, Botha JL, Karwatowski WS, Duke T, Chang YF. What is the prevalence of visual impairment in the general and diabetic populations: are there ethnic and gender differences? Diabet Med 2002;19:27-34.

347) Hawthorne G, Irgens LM, Lie RT. Outcome of pregnancy in diabetic women in northeast England and in Norway, 1994-7. BMJ 2000;321:730-1.

348) Heine RJ, Bilo HJG, Fonk T, Van der Veen EA, Van der Meer J. Absorption kinetics and action profiles of mixtures of short- and intermediate acting insulins. Diabetologia 1984; 27:558-62.

349) Heise T, Berger M Sawicki PT. Non-evidence-based concepts are still established in the treatment of IDDM. Horm Res 1998;50:74-8.

350) Heise T, Nosek L, Ronn BB, Endahl L, Heinemann L, Kapitza C, et al. Lower within-subject variability of insulin detemir in comparison to NPH insulin and insulin glargine in people with type 1 diabetes. Diabetes 2004;53:1614-20.

351) Heijbel H, Chen RT, Dahlquist G. Cumulative incidence of childhood-onset IDDM is unaffected by pertussis immunization. Diabetes Care 1997;20:173-5.

352) Helgasson T, Jobnasson MR, Evidence for a food additive as cause of ketosis-prone diabetes. Lancet 1981;11:716-20.

353) Helgasson T, Danielsen R, Thorsson AV. Incidence and prevalence of Type 1 (insulin-dependent) diabetes mellitus in Icelandic children 1970-89. Diabetologia 1992;35:880-3.

354) Heller SR, Amiel SA, Mansell P. Effect of the fast-acting insulin analog lispro on the risk of nocturnal hypoglycemia during intensified insulin therapy. U.K. Lispro Study Group. Diabetes Care 1999;22:1607-11.

355) Henriksen JE, Djurhuus MS, Vaag A, Thye-Rønn P, Knudsen D, Hother-Nielsen O, Beck-Nielsen H. Impact of injection sites for soluble insulin on glycaemic control in Type 1 (insulin-dependent) diabetes mellitus treated with a multiple insulin injection regimen. Diabetologia 1993;36:752-58.

356) Henriksen JE, Vaag A, Ramsgaard Hansen I, Lauritzen M, Djurhuus MS, Beck-Nielsen H. Absorption of NPH (Isophane) insulin in resting diabetic patients: evidence for subcutaneous injection on the thigh as the preferred site. Diabetic Medicine 1991;8:453-57.

357) Henry RR, Mudaliar SR, Howland IW, Chu N, Kim D, An B, Reinhardt RR. Inhaled Insulin Using the AERx Insulin Diabetes Management System in Healthy and Asthmatic Subjects. Diabetes Care 2003;26:764-9.

358) Herold KC, Polonsky KS, Cohen RM, Levy J, Douglas F. Variable deterioration in cortical function during insulin-induced hypoglycemia. Diabetes 1985;34:677-85.

359) Hershey T, Bhargava N, Sadler M, White NH, Craft S. Conventional versus intensive diabetes therapy in children with type 1 diabetes: effects on memory and motor speed. Diabetes Care 1999;22:1318-24.

360) Hildebrandt P, Sestoft L, Nielson RL. The absorption of subcutaneously injected short-acting soluble insulin:influence of injection-technique and concentration. Diabetes Care 1983;6:459-62.

361) Hildebrandt P, Birch K. Subcutaneous insulin infusion: Change in basal rate infusion has no immediate effect on insulin absorption rate. Diabetes Care 1986;9:561-64.

362) Hildebrandt P. Skinfold thickness, local subcutaneous blood flow and insulin absorption in diabetic patients. Acta Physiol Scand. 1991;143 (Suppl. 603):41-45.

363) Hildebrandt P, Vaag A. Local skin-fold thickness as a clinical predictor of depot size during basal rate infusion. Diabetes Care 1993;16:1-3.

364) Hildebrandt P, Ilius U, Schliack V. Effect of insulin suppositories in type 1 diabetic patients (preliminary communication). Exp Clin Endocrinol 1984;83(2):168-72.

365) Hilsted J, Madsbad S, Hvidberg AM, Rasmussen MH, Krarup T, Ipsen H, Hansen B, Pedersen M, Djurup R, Oxenbøll. Intranasal insulin therapy: The clinical realities. Diabetologia 1995;38:680-84.

366) Hiltunen M, Hyoty H, Knip M, Ilonen J, Reijonen H, Vahasalo P, Roivainen M, Lonnrot M, Leinikki P, Hovi T, et al. Islet cell antibody seroconversion in children is temporally associated with enterovirus infections. Childhood Diabetes in Finland (DiMe) Study Group. J Infect Dis 1997;175:554-60.

367) Himmelmann A, Jendle J, Mellen A, Petersen AH, Dahl UL, Wollmer P. The impact of smoking on inhaled insulin. Diabetes Care 2003;26:677-82.

368) Hirsch IB, Farkas-Hirsch R, Skyler JS. Intensive insulin therapy for treatment of type 1 diabetes. Diabetes Care 12/1990;13:1265-1283.

369) Hirsch IB, Boyle PJ, Craft S, Cryer PE. Higher glycemic thresholds for symptoms during ß-adrenergic blockade in IDDM. Diabetes 1991;40:1177-88.

370) Hirsch IB, Farkas-Hirsch R, Cryer PE. Continuous subcutaneous insulin infusion for the treatment of diabetic patients with hypoglycemia unawareness. Diab Nutr Metab 1991;4:41-43.

371) Hirsch IB, Heller SR, Cryer PE. Increased symptoms of hypoglycaemia in the standing position in insulin-dependent diabetes mellitus. Clinical Science 1991;80:583-86.

372) Hirsch IB, Paauw DS, Brunzell J. Inpatient management of adults with diabetes. Diabetes Care 1995;18:870-78.

373) Hirsch IB, Polonsky WH. Hypoglycemia and its prevention. In the book: Fredrickson L (Ed.). The Insulin Pump Therapy Book. Insights from the experts. MiniMed, Los Angeles 1995.

374) Hoelzel W, Miedema K. Development of a reference system for the international standardization of HbA1c/Glycohemoglobin determinations. J Internat Fed Clin Chem 1996;9:62-67.

375) Hoey H, Aanstoot HJ, Chiarelli F, Daneman D, Danne T, Dorchy H, Fitzgerald M, Garandeau P, Greene S, Holl R, et al. Good metabolic control is associated with better quality of life in 2,101 adolescents with type 1 diabetes. Diabetes Care 2001;24:1923-8.

376) Hofman PL, Peart JM, Holt J, Jefferies CA, Thompson JMD, Cutfield WS, Lawton SA. Angled 6 mm needles and a pinch technique dramatically reduce intramuscular injections in children. JPEM2002;15(Suppl 4):1079(abstract).

377) Hollander P, Pi-Sunyer X, Conif R. Acarbose in the treatment of type 2 diabetes. Diabetes Care 1995;20:248-253.

378) Holleman F, van den Brand JJ, Hoven RA, van der Linden JM, van der Tweel I, Hoekstra JB, Erkelens DW. Comparison of LysB28, ProB29-human insulin analog and regular human insulin in the correction of incidental hyperglycaemia. Diabetes Care1996;19/12,:1426-9.

379) Holm J, Koellreutter B, Wursch P. Influence of sterilization, drying and oat bran enrichment of pasta on glucose and insulin responses in healthy subjects and on the rate and extent of in vitro starch digestion. Eur J Clin Nutr 1992;46:629-40.

380) Holmes GK. Coeliac disease and Type 1 diabetes mellitus - the case for screening. Diabet Med 2001;18:169-77.

381) Holzmeister, LA. The Diabetes Carbohydrate and Fat Gram Guide. The American Diabetes Association, Alexandria, Virginia 2000.

382) Home PD. Potency of insulin. Diabetes Care 1988;11:604.

383) Home PD, Lindholm A, Hylleberg B, Round P. Improved glycemic control with insulin aspart: a multicenter randomized double-blind crossover trial in type 1 diabetic patients. UK Insulin Aspart Study Group. Diabetes Care 1998;21:1904-9.

384) Home PD, Lindholm A, Riis A. Insulin aspart vs. human insulin in the management of long-term blood glucose control in Type 1 diabetes mellitus: a randomized controlled trial. European Insulin Aspart Study Group. Diabet Med 2000;17:762-70.

385) Honeyman MC, Coulson BS, Stone NL, Gellert SA, Goldwater PN, Steele CE, Couper JJ, Tait BD, Colman PG, Harrison LC. Association between rotavirus infection and pancreatic islet autoimmunity in children at risk of developing type 1 diabetes. Diabetes 2000;49:1319-24.

386) Hopkins DFC, Cotton, SJ, Williams G. Effective treatment of insulin-induced edema using ephedrine. Diabetes Care 1993;16:1026-28.

387) Hosny EA, Ghilzai NM, al-Najar TA, Elmazar MM. Hypoglycemic effect of oral insulin in diabetic rabbits using pH- dependent coated capsules containing sodium salicylate without and with sodium cholate. Drug Dev Ind Pharm 1998;24:307-11.

388) Houghton LA, Magnall YF, Read NW. Effect on incorporating fat into a liquid test meal on the relation between intragastric distribution and gastric emptying in human volunteers. Gut 1990;31:1126-29.

389) Houtzagers CMGJ, Visser AP, Berntzen PA, Heine RJ, van der Veen EA. The Medi-Jector II: Efficacy and acceptability in insulin dependent diabetic patient with and without needle-phobia. Diabet Med 1988;5:135-8.

390) Houtzagers CMGJ, Berntzen PA, van der Stap H, et al. Efficacy and acceptance of two intensified conventional insulin therapy regimens: a long-term crossover comparison. Diabetic Med 1989; 6:416-21.

391) Houtzagers CMGJ, Visser AP, Berntzen PA, et al. Multiple daily insulin injections improve self-confidence. Diabetic Med 1989; 6:512-519.

392) Houtzagers CMGJ. Subcutaneous insulin delivery: Present status. Diabetic Med 1989;6:754-61.

393) Howey DC, Bowsher RR, Brunelle RL,Woodworth JR. [Lys(B28,Pro(B29)]-human insulin: a rapidly absorbed analogue of human insulin. Diabetes 1994;43:396-402.

394) Hutchinson A, McIntosh A, Peters J, O'Keeffe C, Khunti K, Baker R, Booth A. Effectiveness of screening and monitoring tests for diabetic retinopathy - a systematic review. Diabet Med 2000;17:495-506.

395) Hyoety H, Hiltunen M, Knip M, Laakkonen M, Uaehaesalo P, Karjalainen J, Koskela P, Roivainen M, Lenikki P; Hovi T et al. A prospective study of the role of coxsackie B and other enterovirus infections in the pathogenesis of IDDM. Diabetes 1995;16:652-7.

396) Hyllienmark L, Ludvigsson J. Insulin pump - a realistic alternative for treatment of diabetes in children and adolescents. Lakartidningen 13/1992;89:1057-62.

397) Iafusco D, Angius E, Prisco F. Early preprandial hypoglycemia after administration of insulin lispro. Diabetes Care 1998;21:1777-8.

398) Iafusco D, Rea F, Prisco F. Hypoglycemia and reduction of the insulin requirement as a sign of celiac disease in children with IDDM. Diabetes Care 1998;21:1379-81.

399) International Diabetes Federation. Diabetes Atlas 2003.

400) International Study Group for Diabetes in Children (now ISPAD). Position statement, Diabetes in the Young 1989.

401) Inui A, Kitaoka H, Majima M, Takamiya S, Uemoto M, Yonenaga C, Honda M, Shirakawa K, Ueno N, Amano K, et al. Effect of the Kobe earthquake on stress and glycemic control in patients with diabetes mellitus. Arch Intern Med 1998;158:274-8.

402) Jackson A, Ternand C, Brunzell C, Kleinschmidt T, Dew D, Milla C, Moran A. Insulin glargine improves hemoglobin A1c in children and adolescents with poorly controlled type 1 diabetes. Pediatr Diabetes 2003;4:64-69.

403) Jacobson AM, Hauser ST, Lavori P, Wolfsdorf JI, Herskowitz RD, Milley JE, Bliss R, Gelfand E, Wertlieb D, Stein J. Adherence among children and adolescents with insulin-dependent diabetes mellitus over a four-year longitudinal follow-up: I. The influence of patient coping and adjustment. J Pediatr Psychol 1990;15:511-26.

404) Janssen MM, Casteleijn S, Devillé W, Popp Snijders C, Roach P, Heine RJ. Nighttime insulin kinetics and glycemic control in type 1 diabetes patients following administration of an intermediate-acting lispro preparation. Diabetes Care 1997;20(12):1870-73.

405) Jefferson IG, Swift PG, Skinner TC, Hood GK. Diabetes services in the UK: third national survey confirms continuing deficiencies. Arch Dis Child 2003;88:53-6.

406) Jehle PM, Micheler C, Jehle DR, Breitig D, Boehm BO. Inadequate suspension of neutral protamine Hagendorn (NPH) insulin in pens. Lancet 1999;354:1604-7.

407) Jelinek J. Skin disorders associated with diabetes mellitus. In the book: Rifkin H, Porte D. Diabetes Mellitus, Theory and Practice. Elsevier 1990:838-49.

408) Jensen-Urstadt KJ, Reichard PG, Rosfors JS et al. Early atherosclerosis is retarded by improved long-term blood glucose control in patients with IDDM. Diabetes 1996;45/9:1253-8.

409) Johannes CB, Araujo AB, Feldman HA, Derby CA, Kleinman KP, McKinlay JB. Incidence of erectile dysfunction in men 40 to 69 years old: longitudinal results from the Massachusetts male aging study. J Urol 2000;163:460-3.

410) Johansson C, Samuelsson U, Ludvigsson J. A high weight gain early in life is associated with an increased risk of Type 1 (insulin-dependent) diabetes mellitus. Diabetologia 1994;37:91-94.

411) Johansson BL, Kernell A, Sjoeberg S, Wahren J. Influence of combined C-peptide and insulin administration on renal function and metabolic control in diabetes type 1. J Clin. Endocrinol. Metab. 1993;77:976-81.

412) Johansson BL, Borg K, Fernqvist-Forbes E, Kernell A, Odergren T, Wahren J. Beneficial effects of C-peptide on incipient nephropathy and neuropathy in patients with Type 1 diabetes mellitus. Diabet Med 2000;17:181-9.

413) Johnston A. Diabetes and Food. Yorkhill Diabetes Service 1998.

414) Johnston DG, Alberti KGMM. Hormonal control of ketone body metabolism in the normal and diabetic state. Clin Endocrin Met 1982;11:329-361.

415) Jones KL, Horowitz M, Berry M, Wishart JM, Guha S. Blood glucose concentration influences postprandial fullness in IDDM. Diabetes Care 1997;20:1141-6.

416) Jones KL, Arslanian S, Peterokova VA, Park JS, Tomlinson MJ. Effect of metformin in pediatric patients with type 2 diabetes: a randomized controlled trial. Diabetes Care 2002;25:89-94.

417) Jones TW, Boulware SD, Kraemer DT, Caprio S, Sherwin RS, Tamborlane WV. Independent effects of youth and poor diabetes control on responses to hypoglycemia in children. Diabetes 1991;40:358-63.

418) Jones TW, Porter P, Sherwin RS, Davis EA, O'Leary P, Frazer F, Byrne G, Stick S, Tamborlane WV. Decreased epinephrine responses to hypoglycemia during sleep. N Engl J Med 1998;338:1657-62.

419) Jornsay DL. Continous subcutaneous insulin infusion (CSII) during pregnancy. Diabetes Spectrum 1998;11:26-32.

420) Joseph SE, Korzon-Burakowska A, Woodworth JR, Evans M, Hopkins D, Janes JM, Amiel SA. The action profile of lispro is not blunted by mixing in the syringe with NPH insulin. Diabetes Care 1998;21:2098-102.

421) Joslin Diabetes Center 2003. Correcting Internet Myths About Aspartame.
http://www.joslin.harvard.edu/education/library/aspartame.shtml

422) Jungheim K, Koschinsky T. Glucose Monitoring at the Arm: Risky delays of hypoglycemia and hyperglycemia detection. Diabetes Care 2002;25:956-60.

423) Määr ML, Mäenpää J, Knip M. Insulin administration via a subcutaneous catheter. Diabetes Care 1993;16:1412-13.

424) Kadiri A, Al-Nakhi A, El-Ghazali S, Jabbar A, Al Arouj M, Akram J, Wyatt J, Assem A, Ristic S. Treatment of type 1 diabetes with insulin lispro during Ramadan. Diabetes Metab 2001;27:482-6.

425) Kanc K, Janssen MM, Keulen ET, Jacobs MA, Popp-Snijders C, Snoek FJ, Heine RJ. Substitution of night-time continuous subcutaneous insulin infusion therapy for bedtime NPH insulin in a multiple injection regimen improves counterregulatory hormonal responses and warning symptoms of hypoglycaemia in IDDM. Diabetologia 1998;41:322-9.

426) Kaneto H, Ikeda M, Kishimoto M, Iida M, Hoshi A, Watari T, Kubota M, Kajimoto Y, Yamasaki Y, Hori M. Dramatic recovery of counter-regulatory hormone response to hypoglycemia after intensive therapy in poorly controlled type 1 diabetes mellitus. Diabetologia 1998;41:982-83.

427) Kaplan W, Rodriguez LM, Smith OE, Haymond MW, Heptulla RA. Effects of mixing glargine and short-acting insulin analogs on glucose control. Diabetes Care 2004;27:2739-40.

428) Karlander S, Efendic S. Rapid and slow carbohydrates in the diabetic diet - time for a reevaluation? Lakartidningen 39/1984;81:3463-64.

429) Karvonen M, Viik-Kajander M, Moltchanova E, Libman I, LaPorte R, Tuomilehto J. Incidence of childhood type 1 diabetes worldwide. Diabetes Mondiale (DiaMond) Project Group. Diabetes Care 2000;23:1516-26.

430) Kassianos G. Some aspects of diabetes and travel. Diabetes Reviews International 2/1992;3:11-13.

431) Kaufman FR, Devgan S, Roe TF, Costin G. Perioperative management with prolonged intravenous insulin infusion versus subcutaneous insulin in children with type 1 diabetes mellitus. J Diabetes Complications 1996;10/1: 6-11.

432) Kaufman FR, Devgan S. Use of uncooked cornstarch to avert nocturnal hypoglycemia in children and adolescents with type 1 diabetes. J Diabetes Complications 1996;10/2:84-7.

433) Kaufman FR, Epport K, Engilman R, Halvorson M. Neurocognitive functioning in children diagnosed with diabetes before age 10 years. J Diabetes Complications 1999;13:31-8.

434) Kaufman FR, Halvorson M, Miller D, Mackenzie M, Fisher LK, Pitukcheewanont P. Insulin pump therapy in type 1 pediatric patients: now and into the year 2000. Diabetes Metab Res Rev 1999;15:338-52.

435) Kaufmann FR, Halvorson M, Kim C, Pitukcheewanont P. Use of insulin pump therapy at nighttime only for children 7-10 years of age with type 1 diabetes. Diabetes Care 2000;23:579-82.

436) Kaufman FR, Gibson LC, Halvorson M, Carpenter S, Fisher LK, Pitukcheewanont P. A pilot study of the continuous glucose monitoring system: clinical decisions and glycemic control after its use in pediatric type 1 diabetic subjects. Diabetes Care 2001;24:2030-4.

437) Kaufman FR. Diabetes at school: What a child's health care team needs to know about federal disability law. Clin Diab 2002;20:91-92.

438) Kemp P, Staberg B. Smoking reduces insulin absorption from subcutaneous tissue. BMJ 1982;284:237.

439) Kernell A, Dedorsson I, Johansson B, Wickström CP, Ludvigsson J, Tuvemo T, Neiderud J, Sjöström K, Malmgren K, Kanulf P, Mellvig L, Gjötterberg M, Sule J, Persson LÅ, Larsson LI, Åman J, Dahlquist G. Prevalence of diabetic retinopathy in children and adolescents with IDDM. A population-based study. Diabetologia 1997;40:307-10.

440) Kerr D, Macdonald IA, Heller SR, Tattersall RB. Alcohol causes hypoglycaemic unawareness in healthy volunteers and patients with type 1 (insulin-dependent) diabetes. Diabetologia 1990;33:216-21.

441) Kida K, Mimura G, Ito T, Murakami K, Ashkenazi I, Laron Z. Incidence of Type 1 diabetes mellitus in children aged 0-14 in Japan, 1986-1990, including an analysis for seasonality of onset and month of birth: JDS study. The Data Committee for Childhood Diabetes of the Japan Diabetes Society (JDS). Diabet Med 2000;17:59-63.

442) Kimmerle R, Weiss R, Berger M, Kurz K. Effectiveness, safety, and acceptance of a copper intrauterine device (CU Safe 300) in type 1 diabetic women. Diabetes Care 1993;16:1227-30.

443) Kimmerle R, Zass RP, Cupisti S, Somville T, Bender R, Pawlowski B, Berger M. Pregnancies in women with diabetic nephropathy: long-term outcome for mother and child. Diabetologia 1995;38:227-35.

444) Kimmerle R, Heinemann L, Berger M. Intrauterine devices are safe and effective contraceptives for type 1 diabetic women [letter]. Diabetes Care 1995;18:1506-7.

445) King P, Kong MF, Parkin H, Macdonald IA, Tattersall RB. Well-being, cerebral function and physical fatigue after nocturnal hypoglycemia in IDDM. Diabetes Care 1998;21:341-45.

446) Kipps S, Bahu T, Ong K, Ackland FM, Brown RS, Fox CT, Griffin NK, Knight AH, Mann NP, Neil HA, et al. Current methods of transfer of young people with Type 1 diabetes to adult services. Diabet Med 2002;19:649-54.

447) Kirk JM, Kinirons MJ. Dental health of young insulin dependent diabetic subjects in Northern Ireland. Community Dent Health 1991;8:335-41.

448) Kitabchi AE, Umpierrez GE, Murphy MB, Barrett EJ, Kreisberg RA, Malone JI, Wall BM. Management of hyperglycemic crises in patients with diabetes. Diabetes Care 2001;24:131-53.

449) Kitzmiller JL, Gavin LA, Gin GD, Jovanovic-Peterson L, Main EK, Zigrang WD. Preconception care of diabetes. Glycemic contol prevents congenital anomalies. JAMA 1991;265:731-36.

450) Klein R, Klein BE, Lee KE, Moss SE, Cruickshanks KJ. Prevalence of self-reported erectile dysfunction in people with long-term IDDM. Diabetes Care 1996;19:135-41.

451) Klemp P, Staberg B. Smoking reduces insulin absorption from subcutaneous tissue. BMJ 1982;284:237.

452) Knip M. Prevention of Childhood type 1 diabetes. Nord Med 8-9/1992;107:207-210.

453) Kobold U, Jeppsson JO, Dülffer T, Finke A, Hoelzel W, Miedema K. Candidate reference methods for hemoglobin A_{1c} based on peptide mapping. Clin Chem, 1997;43:1944-51.

454) Koivisto VA. Various influences on insulin absorption. Neth J Med 1985;28 suppl 1:25-28.

455) Koivisto VA, Haapa E, Tulokas S, Pelkonen R, Toivonen M. Alcohol with a meal has no adverse effect on postprandial glucose homeostasis in diabetic patients. Diabetes Care 12/1993;16:1612-14.

456) Kolb H, Elliot RB. Increasing incidence of IDDM a consequence of improving hygiene? Diabetologia 1994;37:729.

457) Kollind M. Lins P-E. Adamsson U. The man behind the phenomenon. Michael Somogyi and blood glucose regulation in unstable diabetes. A controversial hypothesis still discussed. Lakartidningen 10/1991;88:878-879.

458) Kong MF, King P, Macdonald IA, Blackshaw PE, Horowitz M, Perkins AC, Armstrong E, Buchanan KD, Tattersall RB. Euglycaemic hyperinsulinaemia does not affect gastric emptying in type I and type II diabetes mellitus. Diabetologia 1999;42:365-72.

459) Kong N, Ryder RE. What is the role of between meal snacks with intensive basal bolus regimens using preprandial lispro? Diabet Med 1999;16:325-31.

460) Kordonouri O, Deiss D, Hopfenmüller W, Lüpke K, von Schutz W, Danne T. Treatment with Insulin Glargine (Lantus®) Reduces Asymptomatic Nightly Hypoglycemia Detected by Continuous Subcutaneous Glucose Monitoring (CGMS) in Children and Adolescents with Type 1 Diabetes (dm). Diabetes 2002:51 (suppl 2):A427 (abstract 1754).

461) Kousseff BG. Gestational diabetes mellitus (class A): a human teratogen? Am J Med Genet 1999;83:402-8.

462) Kramer L, Fasching P, Madl C, Schneider B, Damjancic P, Waldhausl W, Irsigler K, Grimm G. Previous episodes of hypoglycemic coma are not associated with permanent cognitive brain dysfunction in IDDM patients on intensive insulin treatment. Diabetes 1998;47:1909-14.

463) Krane E. Diabetic Ketoacidosis. Biochemistry, physiology, treatment and prevention. Ped Clin North Am 4/1987;34:935-60.

464) Kruger D, Owen S, Whitehouse F. Scuba Diving and diabetes. Practical guidelines. Diabetes Care 1995;18:1074.

465) Kullberg CE, Bergström A, Dinesen B, Larsson L, Little RR, Goldstein DE, Arnqvist HJ. Comparisons of studies on diabetic complications hampered by differences in GHb measurements. Diabetes Care 1996;7:726-29.

466) Kumar D. Lispro analog for treatment of generalized allergy to human insulin. Diabetes Care 1997;20:1357-59.

467) Kyvik KO, Gren A, Beck-Nilsen H. Concordance rates of insulin dependent diabetes mellitus: A population based study of young Danish twins. BMJ 1995;311:913-17.

468) Kølendorf K, Bojsen J, Deckert T. Clinical factors influencing the absorption of 125 I-NPH insulin in diabetic patients. Horm Metabol Res 1983;15:274-8.

469) Laffel L. Ketone bodies: a review of physiology, pathophysiology and application of monitoring to diabetes. Diabetes Metab Res Rev 1999;15:412-26.

470) Laffel LMB, Loughlin CA, Tovar A, Zuehlke JB, Brink S. Sick Day Management (SDM) Using Blood β-Hydroxybuyrate (βOHB) vs Urine Ketones Significantly Reduces Hospital Visits in Youth with T1DM: A Randomized Clinical Trial. Diabetes 2002;51(suppl 1):A105.

471) Lager I. Metabolic disturbances in diabetes. In the book: Agardh C-D, Berne C, Östman J. Diabetes. Almqvist & Wiksell, Stockholm 1992:205-25.

472) Lahtela JT, Knip M, Paul R, Antonen J, Salmi J. Severe antibody-mediated insulin resistance: Successful treatment with the insulin analog Lispro. Diabetes Care 1997;20:71-73.

473) Landin-Olsson M, Öhlin AC, Agardh CD. Blood glucose: influence of different methods for analysis and procedures for sampling. Pract Diab 1997;14:47-50.

474) Larkin J. Typical infections in diabetes and their treatment. In the book: Pharmacology of Diabetes. Walter de Greyter, Berlin 1991:325-42.

475) Larsen ML, Hørder M, Mogensen EF. Effect of long-term monitoring of glycosylated Hemoglobin levels in insulin-dependent IDDM. N Engl J Med 1990;323:1021-25.

476) Lauritzen T, Pramming S, Deckert T, Binder C. Pharmacokinetics of continous subcutaneous insulin infusion. Diabetologia 1983;24:326-29.

477) Lauritzen T. Pharmacokinetic and clinical aspects of intensified subcutaneous insulin therapy. Dan Med Bull 1985;32:104-18.

478) Lavery LA, Harkless LB, Walker SC, Felder-Johnson K. Infected puncture wounds in diabetic and nondiabetic adults. Diabetes Care 1995;18:1588-1591.

479) Lawler-Heavner J, Cruickshanks KJ, Hay WW, Gay EC, Hamman RF. Birth size and risk of IDDM. Diabetes Res Clin Pract 1994;24:153-9.

480) Lawson ML, Gerstein HC, Tsui E, Zinman B. Effect of intensive therapy on early macrovascular disease in young individuals with type 1 diabetes. A systematic review and meta-analysis. Diabetes Care 1999;22 Suppl 2:B35-9.

481) Leahy JL, Cooper HE, Deal DA, Weir GC. Chronic hyperglycemia is associated with impaired glucose influence on insulin secretion. A study in normal rats using chronic in vivo glucose infusions. J Clin Invest 1986;77:908-15.

482) Lebovitz HE. Diabetic ketoacidosis. Lancet 1995;345:767-71.

483) Lehmann R, Kaplan V, Bingisser R, Bloch KE, Spinas GA. Impact of physical activity on cardiovascular risk factors in IDDM. Diabetes Care 1997;20:1603-11.

484) Lepore M, Pampanelli S, Fanelli C, Porcellati F, Bartocci L, Di Vincenzo A, Cordoni C, Costa E, Brunetti P, Bolli GB. Pharmacokinetics and pharmacodynamics of subcutaneous injection of long-acting human insulin analog glargine, NPH insulin, and ultralente human insulin and continuous subcutaneous infusion of insulin lispro. Diabetes 2000;49:2142-8.

485) Lernmark Å, Sundkvist G. Etiology of type 1-diabetes. In the book: Agardh C-D, Berne C, Östman J. Diabetes. Almqvist & Wiksell, Stockholm 1992:56-64.

486) Leslie RD, Elliot RB. Early environmental events as a cause of IDDM. Diabetes 1994;43:843-50.

487) Lindberg A-S. Diving into the depth of prejudice - or ignorance? Diabetes (Swed. Diab. Ass.) 2/1990:22-25.

488) Lindberg A-S. Even children with diabetes need an upbringing. Diabetes (Swed. Diab. Ass.)2/1993:14-15.

489) Lindberg A-S. Adolescents breaking up. One must chop the umbilical cord. Diabetes (Swed. Diab. Ass.) 6/1993:18-20.

490) Linde B. Dissociation of insulin absorption and blood flow during massage of a subcutaneous injection site. Diabetes Care 1986;9:570-74.

491) Lindblad B. Data from the National Swedish Childhood Diabetes Registry 2001.

492) Lindholm A, McEwen J, Riis AP. Improved postprandial glycemic control with insulin aspart. A randomized double-blind cross-over trial in type 1 diabetes. Diabetes Care 1999;22:801-5.

493) Lingenfelser T, Renn W, Buettner U, Kaschel R, Martin J, Jakober B, Tobis M. Improvement of impaired counterregulatory hormone response and symtom perception by short-term avoidance of hypoglycemia in IDDM. Diabetes Care 1995;18:321-5.

494) Little RR, Goldstein DE. Measurements of glycated haemoglobin and other circulating glycated proteins. In the book: Research Methodologies in Human Diabetes. Walter de Greyter, Berlin 1994.

495) Litton J, Rice A, Friedman N, Oden J, Lee MM, Freemark M. Insulin pump therapy in toddlers and preschool children with type 1 diabetes mellitus. J Pediatr 2002;141(4):490-5.

496) Liu D, Moberg E, Wredling R, Lins PE, Adamson U. Insulin absorption is faster when keeping the infusion site in use for three days during continuous subcutaneous insulin infusion. Insulin Res Clin Pract 1991;12:19-24.

497) Lloyd CE, Dyer PH, Lancashire RJ, Harris T, Daniels JE, Barnett AH. Association between stress and glycemic control in adults with type 1 (insulin-dependent) diabetes. Diabetes Care 1999;22:1278-83.

498) Loeb J, Herold K, Barton K, Robinson L, Jaspan J. Systematic approach to diagnosis and managment of biphasic insulin allergy with local anti-inflammatory agents. Diabetes Care 6/1989;12:421-23.

499) Loghmani E, Rickard K, Washburne L, Vandagriff J, Fineberg N, Golden M. Glycemic response to sucrose-containing mixed meals in diets of children with insulin dependent diabetes mellitus. J Pediatrics 1991;119:531-537.

500) Lönnroth P. Insulin's effects. In the book: Agardh C-D, Berne C, Östman J. Diabetes. Almqvist & Wiksell, Stockholm 1992:29-37.

501) Look D, Strauss K. Reuse of sharps in diabetic patients: is it completely safe? Diabetes Journal 1998;10:31-34.

502) Lteif AN, Schwenk WF. Accuracy of pen injectors versus insulin syringes in children with type 1 diabetes. Diabetes Care 1999;22:137-40.

503) Ludvigsson J, Hermansson G, Häger A, Kernell A, Nordenskjöld K. Adequate substitution of insulin deficiency as a base in the treatment of diabetes in young people. Lakartidningen 22/1988;85:2004-08.

504) Ludvigsson J. Insulin, love & care. Horm Res 1989;31:204-09.

505) Ludvigsson J, Tuvemo T. Diabetes in children. In the book Agardh C-D, Berne C, Östman J. Diabetes. Almqvist & Wiksell, Stockholm 1992:205-25.

506) Ludvigsson J. Is diabetes in children caused by cows' milk? Lakartidningen 16/1993;90:1529-1531.

507) Ludvigsson J. Measurement of HbA₁c with a rapid method. Improved handling of patients with diabetes. Lakartidningen 21/1994;91:2135-36.

508) Ludvigsson J, Nordfeldt S. Hypoglycemia during intensified insulin therapy of children and adolescents. J Ped Endo & Met 1998;11(suppl 1):159-166.

509) Ludvigsson J. Pain and diabetes monitoring in children and teenagers. Diabetes NEWS 1998;19:3-5.

510) Ludvigsson J, Samuelsson U, Ernerudh J, Johansson C, Stenhammar L, Berlin G. Photopheresis at onset of type 1 diabetes: a randomised, double blind, placebo controlled trial. Arch Dis Child 2001;85:149-54.

511) Ludvigsson J, Hanas R. Continuous Subcutaneous Glucose Monitoring improved metabolic control in pediatric patients with type 1 diabetes: A controlled cross-over study. Pediatrics 2003:111:933-38.

512) Lüpke K, Glinda E, von Walter E, von Schütz W, Danne T. Alternate site blood glucose testing at the forearm or hand: Is it feasible and reliable in children with type 1 diabetes? JPEM 2002;15(suppl 4):1082(abstract).

513) Lunt H, Brown JLJ. Self-reported changes in capillary glucose and insulin requirements during the menstrual cycle. Diabetic Med 1996;13/6:525-30.

514) Lustman PJ, Anderson RJ, Freedland KE, de Groot M, Carney RM, Clouse RE. Depression and poor glycemic control: a meta-analytic review of the literature. Diabetes Care 2000;23:934-42.

515) Luzi L, Barrett EJ, Groop LC, Ferrannini E, DeFronzo RA. Metabolic effects of low-dose insulin therapy on glucose metabolism in diabetic ketoacidosis. Diabetes 1988;37:1470-7.

516) Lytzen L, Hansen B, Sørensen JP. Pain perception and frequency of bleeding. A single-blind, randomized investigation comparing NovoPen Needle gauge 27/12mm, 28/12mm and 30/12mm. Abstract, AIDSPIT, Igls, January 1993.

517) MacCuish AC. Treatment of hypoglycemia. In the book: Frier B, Fisher M. Hypoglycemia and diabetes: Clinical and physiological aspects. Edward Arnold, London 1993:212-21.

518) Macfarlane PE, Walters M, Stutchfield P. A prospective study of symtomatic hypoglycemia in childhood diabetes. Diabetic Med 1989;6:627-30.

519) MacKenzie RG. A practical approach to the drug-using adolescent and young adult. Ped Clin N Am 1973;20:1035-45.

520) MacLeod KM, Hepburn DA, Frier BM. Frequency and morbidity of severe hypoglycaemia in insulin-treated diabetic patients. Diabet Med 1993;10:238-45.

521) MacLeod KM. Diabetes and driving: towards equitable, evidence-based decision-making. Diabet Med 1999;16:282-90.

522) Malchoff CD, Shoukri K, Landau JI, and Buchert JM. A Novel Noninvasive Blood Glucose Monitor. Diabetes Care 2002;25: 2268-2275.

523) Malherbe C, de Gasparo M, de Hertogh R, Hoet J: Circadian variations of blood sugar and plasma insulin. Diabetologia 1969;5:397-404.

524) Maniatis AK, Klingensmith GJ, Slover RH, Mowry CJ, Chase HP. Continuous subcutaneous insulin infusion therapy for children and adolescents: an option for routine diabetes care. Pediatrics 2001;107:351-6.

525) Maran A, Lomas J, Macdonald IA, Amiel SA. Lack of preservation of higher brain function during hypoglycemia in patients with intensively-treated IDDM. Diabetologia 1995;38:1412-18.

526) Marcus AO, Fernandez MP. Insulin pump therapy. Postgraduate Medicine 1996;99/3:125-32.

527) Marklund U. Drugs and Influence. Pupil analysis as starting-point for drug education. Thesis, Göteborg Studies in Educational Science 42, 1983. Göteborgs University, Dept. of Pedagogics, Sweden.

528) Marshall SM, Barth JH. Standardization of HbA1c measurements - a consensus statement. Diabet Med 2000;17:5-6.

529) Mathiesen B, Borch-Johnsen K. Diabetes and accident insurance. A 3-year follow-up of 7,599 insured diabetic individuals. Diabetes Care 1997;20:1781-84.

530) Matyka KA, Wigg L, Pramming S, Stores G, Dunger DB. Cognitive function and mood after profound nocturnal hypoglycaemia in prepubertal children with conventional insulin treatment for diabetes. Arch Dis Child 1999;81:138-42.

531) Mawby M (editorial). Time for law to catch up with life. Diabetes Care 1997;20:1640-41.

532) Mazze RS, Lucido D, Shamoon H. Psychological and social correlates of glycemic control. Diabetes Care 1984;7:360-66.

533) Mazur M. Rock star Bret Michaels is in love with ... life, music and his health. Diabetes (Swed. Diab. Ass.) 1990/1:10-13.

534) McCarthy JA, Covarrubias B, Sink P. Is the traditional alcohol wipe necessary before an insulin injection? Diabetes care 1993;16/1:402.

535) McCrimmon RJ, Gold AE, Deary IJ, Kelnar CJH, Frier BM. Symptoms of hypoglycemia in children with IDDM. Diabetes Care 1995;18:858-61.

536) McCullough D, Kurtz A, Tattersall R. A new approach to the treatment of nocturnal hypoglycemia using alpha-glucosidase inhibition. Diabetes Care 5/1993;6:483-87.

537) McHugh PR, Moran TH. Calories and gastric emptying: a regulatory capacity with implications for feeding. Am J Physiology 1979;236:R254-60.

538) McNally PG, Raymond NT, Swift PGF, Hearnshaw JR, Burden AC. Does the prepubertal duration of diabetes influence the onset of microvascular complications? Diab Med 1993;10:906-8.

539) Mecklenburg RS, Benson EA, Benson W, Fredlund PN, Cuinn T, Metz RJ, Nielsen RL, Sannar CA. Acute complications associated with insulin infusion pump therapy. Report of experience with 161 patients. JAMA 1984;252:3265-69.

540) Melki V, Renard E, Lassmann-Vague, Boivin S, Guerci B, Hanaire-Broutin H, Bringer J, Belicar P, Jeandidier N, Meyer L, Blin P, Augendre-Ferrante B, Tauber JP. Improvement of HbA₁c and blood glucose stability in IDDM patients treated with lispro insulin analog in external pumps. Diabetes Care 1998;21:977-86.

541) Meltzer S, Leiter L, Daneman D, Gerstein HC, Lau D, Ludwig S, Yale JF, Zinman B, Lillie D. 1998 clinical practice guidelines for the management of diabetes in Canada. Canadian Diabetes Association 1998;159 Suppl 8:S1-29.

542) Mendosa R. On-line Resources for Diabetics. Glycemic Index Lists. 1997 (http://www.mendosa.com/gilists.htm)

543) Mendosa R. The GI factor. 1997 (http://www.mendosa.com/gifactor.htm)

544) Mettenburg J. Role Models: Nicole Johnson, Miss America 1999. Countdown for Kids Spring 1999.

545) The Microalbuminuria Captopril Study Group. Captopril reduces the risk of nephropathy in IDDM patients with microalbuminuria. Diabetologia 1996;39:587-93.

546) Mitchell TH, Abraham G, Schiffrin A, Leiter LA, Marliss EB. Hyperglycemia after intense exercise in IDDM subjects during continuous subcutaneous insulin infusion. Diabetes Care 1988;11:311-7.

547) Mettenburg J. Role Models: Jay Leeuwenberg, Muscle Man. Countdown For Kids Winter 1997.

548) Mitrakou A, Platanisiotis D, Partheniou C, Kytelis E, Livadas S, Raptis SA. Glucose fall from hyper- to normoglycemia triggers norepinephrine secretion in type 1 diabetes. Diabetologia 1993;36 (Suppl 1):abstract 575.

549) Mitsuhashi T, Li YM, Fishbane S, Vlassara H. Depletion of reactive advanced glycation endproducts from diabetic uremic sera using a lysozyme-linked matrix. J Clin Invest 1997;100:847-54.

550) Moberg E, Kollind M, Lins P-E, Adamsson U. Acute mental stress impairs insulin sensitivity in IDDM patients. Diabetologia 1994;37:247-251.

551) Mohn A, Strang S, Wernicke-Panten K, Lang AM, Edge JA, Dunger DB. Nocturnal glucose control and free insulin levels in children with type 1 diabetes by use of the long-acting insulin HOE 901 as part of a three-injection regimen. Diabetes Care 2000;23:557-9.

552) Mohn A, Cerruto M, Iafusco D, Prisco F, Tumini S, Stoppoloni O, Chiarelli F. Celiac Disease in Children and Adolescents with Type I Diabetes: Importance of Hypoglycemia. J Pediatr Gastroenterol Nutr 2001;32:37-40.

553) Mohn A, Di Michele S, Di Luzio R, Tumini S, Chiarelli F. The effect of subclinical hypothyroidism on metabolic control in children and adolescents with Type 1 diabetes mellitus. Diabet Med 2002;19:70-3.

554) Montoro MN, Myers VP, Mestman JH, Xu Y, Anderson BG, Golde SH. Outcome of pregnancy in diabetic ketoacidosis. Am J Perinatology 1993;10:17-20.

555) Moore K, Vizzard N, Coleman C, McMahon J, Hayes R, Thompson CJ. Type 1 diabetes and extreme altitude mountaineering: lessons from the Diabetes Federation of Ireland Kilimanjaro Expedition. Diab Med 2000:17(Suppl 1):P145.

556) Morain WD, Colen BC. Wound healing in diabetes. Clin Plast Surg 1990;17:493-501.

557) Morris AD, Boyle DI, McMahon AD, Greene SA, MacDonald TM, Newton RW. Adherence to insulin treatment, glycaemic control, and ketoacidosis in insulin-dependent diabetes mellitus. Lancet 1997;350:1505-10.

558) Mortensen HB, Hougaard P and the Hvidøre Study Group on Childhood Diabetes. Comparison of metabolic control in a cross-sectional study of 2,873 children and adolescents with IDDM from 18 countries. Diabetes Care 1997;20:714-720.

559) Mortensen HB, Lindholm A, Olsen BS, Hylleberg B. Rapid appearance and onset of action of insulin aspart in paediatric subjects with type 1 diabetes. Eur J Pediatr 2000;159:483-8.

560) Moss SE, Klein R, Kessler SD, Richie KA. Comparison between ophthalmoscopy and fundus photography in determining severity of diabetic retinopathy. Ophthalmology 1985;92:62-7.

561) Moss SE, Klein R, Klein BE. Ten-year incidence of visual loss in a diabetic population. Ophthalmology 1994;106:1061-70.

562) Mudaliar SR, Lindberg FA, Joyce M, Beerdsen P, Strange P, Lin A, Henry RR. Insulin aspart (B28 asp-insulin): a fast-acting analog of human insulin: absorption kinetics and action profile compared with regular human insulin in healthy nondiabetic subjects. Diabetes Care 1999;22:1501-6.

563) Mühlhauser I, Koch J, Berger M. Pharmacokinetics and bioavailability of injected glucagon: differences between intramuscular, subcutaneous, and intravenous administration. Diabetes Care 1985;8:39-42.

564) Mühlhauser I. Cigarette smoking and diabetes: An update. Diabetes 1994;11:336-43.

565) Mulec H, Blohmé G, Grände B, Björck S. The effect on metabolic control on rate of decline in renal function in insulin dependent diabetes mellitus with overt diabetic nephropathy. Nephrol Dial Transplant 1998;13:651-5.

566) Murphy NP, Keane KK, Ford-Adams ME, Edge JA, Dunger DB. A Randomized Cross-Over Trial Comparing Insulin Glargine Plus Lispro with NPH Insulin Plus Soluble Insulin in Adolescents with Type 1 Diabetes. Diabetes 2002;51(suppl2):A54(abstract 218).

567) Murtaugh MA, Ferris AM, Capacchione CM, Reece EA. Energy intake and glycemia in lactating women with type 1 diabetes. J Am Diet Assoc 1998;98:642-8.

568) Nathan DM, Godine JE, Guthier-Kelley C, Kawahara D, Grinvalsky M. Ice cream in the diet of insulin-dependent diabetes. JAMA 1984;251:2825-27.

569) Nathan DM, Dunn FL, Bruch J et al. Postprandial insulin profiles with implantable pump therapy may explain decreased frequency of severe hypoglycemia, compared with intensive subcutaneous regimens, in insulin-dependent diabetes mellitus patients. Am J Med 1996;100/4:412-17.

570) Nathan DM, Lachin J, Cleary P, Orchard T, Brillon DJ, Backlund JY, O'Leary DH, Genuth S. Intensive diabetes therapy and carotid intima-media thickness in type 1 diabetes mellitus. N Engl J Med 2003;348:2294-303.

571) Neu A, Willasch A, Ehehalt S, Kehrer M, Hub R, Ranke MB. Diabetes incidence in children of different nationalities: an epidemiological approach to the pathogenesis of diabetes. Diabetologia 2001;44 Suppl 3:B21-6.

572) Newgard C. Cellular engineering and gene therapy for insulin replacement in diabetes. Diabetes 1994;43:341-350.

573) Newton RW, Greene SA. Diabetes in the adolescent. In the book: Kelnar CJH (Ed.). Childhood and adolescent diabetes. Chapman & Hall 1995:367-74.

574) Nielsen S, Emborg C, Molbak AG. Mortality in concurrent type 1 diabetes and anorexia nervosa. Diabetes Care 2002;25:309-12.

575) Nordfeldt S, Ludvigsson J. Severe hypoglycemia in children with IDDM. A prospective population study, 1992-94. Diabetes Care 1997;20:497-503.

576) Nordfeldt S, Ludvigsson J. Seasonal variation of HbA1c in intensive treatment of children with type 1 diabetes. J Pediatr Endocrinol Metab 2000;13:529-35.

577) North RV, Farell U, Banford D, Jones C, Gregory JW, Butler, Ownes DR. Visual function in young IDDM patients over 8 years of age. Diabetes Care 1997;20:1724-30.

578) Northam EA, Anderson PJ, Werther GA, Warne GL, Andrewes D. Predictors of change in the neuropsychological profiles of children with type 1 diabetes 2 years after disease onset. Diabetes Care 1999;22:1438-44.

579) Nutall F. Dietary fibers in the management of Diabetes. Diabetes 1993;42:503-508.

580) Nyström L, Dahlquist G, Rewers M, Wall S. The Swedish childhood diabetes study. An analysis of the temporal variation in diabetes incidence 1978-87. Int J Epidemiol 1990;19:141-46.

581) Nyström, Ostman J, Wall S, Wibell L. Mortality of all incident cases of diabetes mellitus in Sweden diagnosed 1983-87 at age 15-34 years. Diabetes incidence Study in Sweden (DISS) Group. Diabetic Med. 1992;9:422-7.

582) Olsson PO. Insulin treatment. In the book: Diabetes. SPRI and Swedish Medical Society 1989:226-32.

583) Olsson PO, Arnqvist H, Asplund J. No pharmacokinetic effect of retaining the infusion site up to four days during continuous subcutaneous insulin infusion therapy. Diabet Med 6/1993;10:477-80.

584) Orchard TJ, Forrest KY, Ellis D, Becker DJ. Cumulative glycemic exposure and microvascular complications in insulin- dependent diabetes mellitus. The glycemic threshold revisited. Arch Intern Med 1997;157:1851-6.

585) Östman J, Andersson D. Diabetes mellitus. In the book: Drugs. Swedish Pharmaceutical Company 1993-94:474.

586) Örtqvist E, Björk E, Wallensteen M, Ludvigsson J, Åman J, Forsander G, Lindgren F, Berne C, Persson B, Karlsson FA. Diazoxide treatment at onset in childhood type 1 diabetes. JPEM 2001;14(Suppl 3):1044(abstract).

587) O'Sullivan JB. Subsequent morbidity among gestational diabetic women. In the book: Sutherland HW, Stowers JM (Eds) Carbohydrate metabolism in pregnancy and the newborn. New York: Churchill Livingstone 1984;174-80.

588) Owens DR, Coates PA, Luzio SD, Tinbergen JP, Kurzhals R. Pharmacokinetics of ^{125}I-labeled insulin glargine (HOE 901) in healthy men: comparison with NPH insulin and the influence of different subcutaneous injection sites. Diabetes Care 2000;23:813-9.

589) Packer SC, Dornhorst A, Frost GS. The glycaemic index of a range of gluten-free foods. Diabet Med 2000;17:657-60.

590) Pampanelli S, Torlone E, Lalli C, Sindaco PD, Ciofetta M, Lepore M, Bartocci L, Brunetti P, Bolli GB. Improved postprandial metabolic control after subcutaneous injection of a short-acting insulin analog in IDDM of short duration with residual pancreatic β-cell function. Diabetes Care 1995;18(11):1452-59.

591) Pampanelli S, Fanelli C, Lalli C, Ciofetta M, Sindaco PD, Lepore M, Modarelli F, Rambotti AM, Epifano L, Di Vincenzo A, et al. Long-term intensive insulin therapy in IDDM: effects on HbA$_{1c}$, risk for severe and mild hypoglycaemia, status of counterregulation and awareness of hypoglycaemia. Diabetologia 1996;39:677-86.

592) Pampanelli S, Lepore M, Fanelli C, Del Sindaco P, Lalli C, Ciofetta M, Calabrese G, Brunetti P, Bolli GB. Intensive treatment maintains normal glucagon response to hypoglycemia in short-term IDDM. Diabetologia 1998;41(Suppl 1):A68.

593) Parent ME, Siemiatycki J, Menzies R, Fritschi L, Colle E. Bacille Calmette-Guérin vaccination and incidence of IDDM in Montreal, Canada. Diabetes Care 1997;20:767.

594) Parslow RC, McKinney PA, Law GR, Staines A, Williams R, Bodansky HJ. Incidence of childhood diabetes mellitus in Yorkshire, northern England, is associated with nitrate in drinking water: an ecological analysis. Dabetologia 1997;40:550-56.

595) Partanen TM, Rissanen A. Insulin injection practices. Pract Diab Int 2000;17:252-54.

596) Patterson CC, Carson DJ and the Northern Ireland Diabetes Study Group. Epidemiology of childhood IDDM in Northern Ireland 1989-1994: Low incidence in areas with highest population density and most household crowding. Diabetologia 1996;39:1063-69.

597) Pearson J, Chase HP, Wightman C, Klingensmith G, Walravens P, Rewers M, Garg S. Reduction of severe hypoglycemic episodes in children and adolescents with type 1 diabetes using insulin-glargine therapy. Diabetes 2002;51(suppl 2):A425 (abstract 1744).

598) Pedersen M. Lecture EASD 1993. In: Madsbad S, Dejgaard A. Highlights of the 29th EASD meeting, Istanbul 6-9 September 1993. NovoCare.

599) Pedrini MT, Levey AS, Lau J et al. The effect of dietary protein restriction on the progression of diabetic and nondiabetic renal diseases: a meta-analysis. Ann Intern Med 1996;124/7:627-32.

600) Perez M, Kohn S. Cutaneous manifestations of diabetes mellitus. J Amer Acad Derm 1994;30:519-531.

601) Periello G, Torlone E, Di Santo S, Fanwelli C, De Feo P, Santeusanio F, brunett P, Bolli GB. Effect of storage temperature on insulin on pharmacokinetics and pharmacodynamics of insulin mixtures injected subcutaneously in subjects with type 1 (insulin-dependent) diabetes mellitus. Diabetologia 1988;31/11:811-15.

602) Persson B, Hansson U. Diabetes and pregnancy. Swedish Diabetes Association, Booklet no. 5, 1987.

603) Persson B. Long term morbidity in infants of diabetic mothers. Acta Endocrinol 1986;suppl 1:156.

604) Persson B, Hanson U. Neonatal morbidities in gestational diabetes mellitus. Diabetes Care 1998;21 Suppl 2:B79-84.

605) Peters AL, Davidson MB, Eisenberg K. Effect of isocaloric substitution of chocolate cake for potato in type 1 diabetic patients. Diabetic Care 1990:888-92.

606) Peters AL, Davidson MB. Protein and fat effects on glucose responses and insulin requirements in subjects with insulin-dependent diabetes mellitus. Am J Clin Nutr 1993;58:555-60.

607) Petersen KR, Skouby SO, Vedel PV, Haaber AB. Hormonal contraception in women with IDDM. Diabetes Care 1995;18(6):800-806.

608) Peto R, Lopez AD, Boreham J, Thun M, Heath C Jr. Mortality from smoking in developed countries 1950-2000: indirect estimates from national vital statistics. Oxford: Oxford University Press, 1994.

609) Peveler R, Boller I, Fairburn C, Dunger D. Eating disorders in adolescents with IDDM. Diabetes Care 10/1992;15:1356-60.

610) Peyrot MF, Pichert JW. Stress buffering and glycemic control. Diabetes Care 1992;7:842-846.

611) Pezzarossa A, Taddei F, Cimicchi MC, Rossini E, Contini S, Bonora, Gnudi A, Uggeri E. Perioperative management of diabetic subjects. Subcutaneous versus intravenous insulin administration during glucose-potassium infusion. Diabetes Care 1988;11/1:52-58.

612) Pfützner A, Kustner E, Forst T, Schulze-Schleppinghoff B, Trautmann ME, Haslbeck M, Schatz H, Beyer J. Intensive insulin therapy with insulin lispro in patients with type 1 diabetes reduces the frequency of hypoglycemic episodes. Exp Clin Endocrinol Diabetes 1996;104:25-30.

613) Pieber TR, Eugene-Jolchine I, Derobert E. Efficacy and safety of HOE 901 versus NPH insulin in patients with type 1 diabetes. The European Study Group of HOE 901 in type 1 diabetes. Diabetes Care 2000;23:157-62.

614) Pinelli L, Mormile R, Alfonsi L, Gonfiantini E, Piccoli R, Chiarelli F. The role of nutrition in prevention of complications in insulin-dependent diabetes mellitus. Acta Paediatr 1999;88(Suppl):39-42.

615) Pinson M, Hoffman WH, Garnick JJ, Litaker MS. Periodontal disease and type I diabetes mellitus in children and adolescents. J Clin Periodontol 1995;22:118-23.

616) Plank J, Wutte A, Brunner G, Siebenhofer A, Semlitsch B, Sommer R, Hirschberger S, Pieber TR. A direct comparison of insulin aspart and insulin lispro in patients with type 1 diabetes. Diabetes Care 2002;25:2053-7.

617) Pocecco M, Ronfani L. Transient focal neurologic deficits associated with hypoglycaemia in children with insulin-dependent diabetes mellitus. Italian Collaborative Paediatric Diabetologic Group. Acta Paediatr 1998;87:542-44.

618) Polak M, Beregszaszi M, Belarbi N, Benali K, Czernichow P, Tubiana-Rufi N. Subcutaneous or intramuscular injections of insulin in children; Are we injecting where we think we are? Diabetes Care 1996;19:1434-36.

619) Polonsky WH. Diabetes Burnout. McGraw-Hill Professional Publishing 1999.

620) Porter PA, Byrne G, Stick S Jones TW. Nocturnal hypoglycaemia and sleep disturbances in young teenagers with insulin dependent diabetes mellitus. Arch Dis Child 1996;75:120-3.

621) Pozzilli P, Visalli N. Signore A et al. Double blind trial of nicotinamid in recent-onset IDDM (the IMDIAB III study). Diabetologia 1995;38:848-52.

622) Price DE, Burden AC. Growth of children before onset of diabetes. Diabetes Care 1992; 15:1393-95.

623) Puczynski M, Puczynski S, Reich J, Kaspas JC, Emanuele MA. Mental efficiency and hypoglycemia. J Dev Behav Pediatr 1990;11:170-74.

624) Pundziute-Lycka A, Dahlquist G, Nystrom L, Arnqvist H, Bjork E, Blohme G, Bolinder J, Eriksson JW, Sundkvist G, Ostman J. The incidence of Type I diabetes has not increased but shifted to a younger age at diagnosis in the 0-34 years group in Sweden 1983-1998. Diabetologia 2002;45:783-91.

625) Putz D, Kabadi UM. Insulin glargine in continuous enteric tube feeding. Diabetes Care 2002;25:1889-90.

626) Quillian WC, Cox DJ, Gonder-Frederick LA, Driesen NR, Clarke WL. Reliability of driving performance during moderate hypoglycemia in adults with IDDM. Diabetes Care 1994;17:1367-68.

627) Rabasa-Lhoret R, Garon J, Langelier H, Poisson D, Chiasson JL. Effects of meal carbohydrate content on insulin requirements in type 1 diabetic patients treated intensively with the basal-bolus (ultralente-regular) insulin regimen. Diabetes Care 1999;22:667-73.

628) Rabasa-Lhoret R, Burelle Y, Ducros F, Bourque J, Lavoie C, Massicotte D, Peronnet F, Chiasson JL. Use of an alpha-glucosidase inhibitor to maintain glucose homoeostasis during postprandial exercise in intensively treated Type 1 diabetic subjects. Diabet Med 2001;18:739-44.

629) Rami B, Zidek T, Schober E. Influence of a beta-Glucan-Enriched Bedtime Snack on Nocturnal Blood Glucose Levels in Diabetic Children. J Pediatr Gastroenterol Nutr 2001;32:34-36.

630) Rangawala S, Shah P, Hussain SZ, Goenka S, Pillai KK. Insulin Stored in Matka (Earthen Pitcher) with Water for 60 Days Does Not Reduce in Bioactivity. J Ped Endocrinol and Metab 1997;10 (suppl 2); 347 (abstract).

631) Rassam AG, Zeise TM, Burge MR, Schade DS. Optimal administration of lispro insulin in hyperglycemic type 1 diabetes. Diabetes Care 1999;22:133-6.

632) Rathod M, Saravolatz L, Pohlod D, Whitehouse F, Goldman J. Evaluation of the sterility and stability of insulin from multidose vials used for prolonged periods. Infect Control 1985;6:491-4.

633) Ratner RE, Hirsch IB, Neifing JL, Garg SK, Mecca TE, Wilson CA. Less hypoglycemia with insulin glargine in intensive insulin therapy for type 1 diabetes. U.S. Study Group of Insulin Glargine in Type 1 Diabetes. Diabetes Care 2000;23:639-43.

634) Rave K, Heise T, Herrnberger J, Bender R, Hirschberger S, Heinemann L. Intramuscular versus subcutaneous injection of soluble and lispro insulin: Comparison of effects in healthy subjects. Diab Med 1998;15:747-51.

635) Read NW, Welch IM, Austen CJ. Barnish C et al. Swallowing food without chewing; a simple way to reduce postprandial glycemia. Br J Nutrition 1986;55:43-7.

636) Reichard P, Britz A, Rosenqvist U. Intensified conventional insulin treatment and neuropsychological impairment. Br Med J 1991;303:1439-42.

637) Reichard P, Nilsson B-Y, Rosenqvist U. The effect of long-term intensified insulin treatment on the development of microvascular complications of diabetes mellitus. N Engl J Med 1993;329:304-309.

638) Reichard P. Are there any glycemic thresholds for the serious microvascular diabetic complications? J Diab Compl 1995;9:25-30.

639) Reichard P, Pihl M, Rosenqvist U, Sule J. Complications in IDDM are caused by elevated blood glucose level: the Stockholm Diabetes Intervention Study (SDIS) at 10-year follow up. Diabetologia 1996;39:1483-8.

640) Reichel A, Rietzsch H, Kohler HJ, Pfutzner A, Gudat U, Schulze J. Cessation of insulin infusion at night-time during CSII-therapy: comparison of regular human insulin and insulin lispro. Exp Clin Endocrinol Diabetes 1998;106:168-72.

641) Rendell MS, Rajfer J, Wicker PA, Smith MD. Sildenafil for treatment of erectile dysfunction in men with diabetes: a randomized controlled trial. Sildenafil Diabetes Study Group. JAMA 1999;281:421-6.

642) Rizzo TA, Dooley SL, Metzger BE, Cho NH, Ogata ES, Silverman BL. Prenatal and perinatal influences on long-term psychomotor development in offspring of diabetic mothers. Am J Obstet Gynecol 1995;173:1753-8.

643) Robinson N, Lloyd CE, Fuller J, Yateman NA. Psychosocial factors and the onset of type 1 diabetes. Diabetic Med 1989;6:53-8.

644) Rodin G, Craven J, Littlefield C, Murray M, Daneman D. Eating disorders and intentional undertreatment in adolescent females with diabetes. Psychosomatics 1991;32:171-6.

645) Rodin GM, Danman D. Eating disorders and IDDM. Diabetes Care 1992;15:1402-12.

646) Rohlfing CL, Wiedmeyer HM, Little RR, England JD, Tennill A, Goldstein DE. Defining the relationship between plasma glucose and HbA1c: analysis of glucose profiles and HbA1c in the Diabetes Control and Complications Trial. Diabetes Care 2002;25:275-8.

647) Rönnemaa T, Viikari J. Reducing snacks when switching from conventional soluble to lispro insulin treatment: effects on glycaemic control and hypoglycaemia. Diabet Med 1998;15:601-7.

648) Roper NA, Bilous RW. Resolution of lipohypertrophy following change of short-acting insulin to insulin lispro (Humalog). Diabet Med 1998;15:1063-4.

649) Rosenbloom A, Beverly P, Giordano RN: Chronic overtreatment with insulin in children and: Am J Dis Child 1977;131:881-885.

650) Rosenbloom A, Hanas R. Diabetic Ketoacidosis (DKA): Treatment Guidelines. Clin Ped 1996;35:261-266.

651) Rosenbloom AL. The cause of the epidemic of type 2 in children. Current Opinion in Endocrinology & Diabetes 2000;7:191-96.

652) Rosenn BM, Miodovnik M, Khoury JC, Siddiqi TA. Counterregulatory hormonal responses to hypoglycemia during pregnancy. Obstet Gynecol 1996;87/4:568-74.

653) Rosenstock J, Park G, Zimmerman J. Basal insulin glargine (HOE 901) versus NPH insulin in patients with type 1 diabetes on multiple daily insulin regimens. Diabetes Care 2000;23:1137-42.

654) Rosskamp RH, Park G. Long-acting insulin analogs. Diabetes Care 1999;22 Suppl 2:B109-13.

655) Rovet J, Alvarez M. Attentional functioning in children and adolescents with IDDM. Diabetes Care 1997;20:803-810.

656) Rutledge KS, Chase HP, Klingensmith GJ, Walravens PA, Slover RH, Garg SK. Effectiveness of postprandial Humalog in toddlers with diabetes. Pediatrics 1997;100:968-72.

657) Ryan C, Yega A, Drash A. Cognitive deficits in adolescents who developed diabetes early in life. Pediatrics 1985;75:921-927.

658) Ryan CM, Atchison J, Puczynski SS et al. Mild hypoglycemia associated with deterioration of mental efficiency in children with insulin-dependent diabetes mellitus. J Pediatr 1990;117:32-38.

659) Ryan C. Lecture, IDF 2000, Mexico City.

660) Rydén O, Nevander L, Johnsson P, Westbom L, Sjöblad S. Diabetic Children and Their Parents: Personality Correlates of Metabolic Control. Acta Paediatr Scand 1990;79:1204-1.

661) Sackey AH, Jefferson IG. Interval between insulin injection and breakfast in diabetes. Arch Dis Child 1994;71:248-50.

662) Sacks DB, Bruns DE, Goldstein DE, Maclaren NK, McDonald JM, Parrott M. Guidelines and recommendations for laboratory analysis in the diag-

nosis and management of diabetes mellitus. Diabetes Care 2002;25:750-86.

663) Saleh TY, Cryer PE. Alanine and terbutaline in the prevention of nocturnal hypoglycemia in IDDM. Diabetes Care 1997;20:1231-36.

664) Salerno M, Argenziano A, Di Maio S, Gasparini N, Formicola S, De Filippo G, Tenore A. Pubertal growth, sexual maturation, and final height in children with IDDM. Diabetes Care 1997;20:721-24.

665) Samuelsson U, Johansson C, Ludvigsson J. Breast-feeding seems to play a marginal role in the prevention of IDDM. Diabetes Res. Clin. Pract 3/1993;3:203-10.

666) Samuelsson U, Johansson C, Carstensen J, Ludvigsson J. Space-time clustering in insulin dependent diabetes mellitus (IDDM) in south-east Sweden. Int. J Epidemiol. 1994;23:138-142.

667) Samuelsson U, Ludvigsson J. When should determination of ketonemia be recommended? Diabetes Technol Ther 2002;4:645-50.

668) Sandelin O, Rogberg N. Diving into the depth of prejudice. The Diving Journal 4/1989:28-29.

669) Sane T, Koivisto VA, Nikkanen P, Pelkonen R. Adjustment of insulin doses of diabetic patients during long distance flights. BMJ 1990;301:421-22.

670) Sank A, Wei D, Reid J, Ertl D, Nimni M, Weaver F, Yellin A, Tuan TL. Human endothelial cells are defective in diabetic vascular disease. J Surg Res 1994;57:647-53.

671) Santiago J. Lessons from the Diabetes Control and Complications Trial. Diabetes 1993;42:1549-1554.

672) Sartor G, Dahlquist G. Short-term mortality in childhood onset insulin-dependent diabetes mellitus: a high frequency of unexpected deaths in bed. Diabet Med 1995;12:607-11.

673) Saukkonen T, Vaisanen S, Akerblom HK, Savilahti E. Coeliac disease in children and adolescents with type 1 diabetes: a study of growth, glycaemic control, and experiences of families. Acta Paediatr 2002;91:297-302.

674) Savilahti E, Åkerblom HK, Tainio V-M, Koskimies S. Children with newly diagnosed insulin dependent diabetes mellitus have increased levels of cows' milk antibodies. Diabetes Res 1988;7:137-40.

675) Sawicki P, Didjurgeit U, Mühlhauser I, Bender R, Heinemann L, Berger M. Smoking is associated with progression of diabetic nephropathy. Diabetes Care 1994;17:126-131.

676) Sawka AM, Burgart V, Zimmerman D. Loss of awareness of hypoglycemia temporally associated with selective serotonin reuptake inhibitors. Diabetes Care 2001;24:1845-6.

677) Schatz DA, Maclaren NK. Cows' milk and insulin-dependent diabetes. Innocent until proven guilty. JAMA 1996;276(8):647-8.

678) Schernthaner G, Wein W, Sandholzer K, Equiluz-Bruck S, Bates PC, Birkett MA. Postprandial insulin lispro. A new therapeutic option for type 1 diabetic patients. Diabetes Care 1998;21/4:570-3.

679) Scherstén B, Alm A, Berne C, Blohmé G, Eckerlund I, Edman L et al. A consensus document: vision-threatening retinal changes in diabetes. Lakartidningen 51-51/1991;88:4475-4478.

680) Schiavi RC, Stimmel BB, Mandeli J, Rayfield EJ. Diabetes mellitus and male sexual function: a controlled study. Diabetologia 1993;36:745-751.

681) Schiffrin A, Belmonte M: Multiple daily self-glucose monitoring: its essential role in long-term glucose control in insulin-dependent patients treated with pump and multiple subcutaneous injections. Diabetes Care 1982;5:479-84.

682) Schiffrin A, Suissa S. Predicting nocturnal hypoglycemia in patients with type 1 diabetes treated with continous insulin infusion. Am J Med 1987;82:1127-32.

683) Schmauss S, König A, Landgraf R. Human insulin analogue [Lys(B28), Pro(B29)]: the ideal pump insulin? Diabetic Med 1998;15:247-9.

684) Schober E, Borkenstein M, Frisch H. Basic-bolus therapy of diabetic children and adolescents using Novo Pens. Wien Klin Wochenschr 1987;99:312-3.

685) Schober E, Schoenle E, Van Dyk J, Wernicke-Panten K. Comparative trial between insulin glargine and NPH insulin in children and adolescents with type 1 diabetes mellitus. J Pediatr Endocrinol Metab 2002;15:369-76.

686) Schoenle EJ, Schoenle D, Molinari L, Largo RH. Impaired intellectual development in children with Type I diabetes: association with HbA(1c), age at diagnosis and sex. Diabetologia 2002;45:108-14.

687) Schrepfer T, Caduff A, Buschor S, Dewarrat R, Moricz A, Kapitza C, Heinemann L. Evaluation of a non-invasive, continuous glucose monitoring system in patients with diabetes: results of a home use study. Diab Metab 2003;29:4S195.

688) Schroeder B, Hertweck SP, Sanfilippo JS, Foster MB. Correlation between glycemic control and menstruation in diabetic adolescents. J Reprod Med 2000;45:1-5.

689) von Schütz W, Fuchs S, Stephan S, Lange K, Heiming R, Hürter P. Incidence of severe hypoglycemia under conventional and intensive insulin therapy in diabetic children and adolescents. Diabetologia 1994;37 (Suppl 1):abstract 66.

690) Schuler G, Peltz K, Kerp L. Is the reuse of needles for insulin injection systems associated with a higher risk cutaneous complications? Diabetes Res Clin Pract 1992;16/3:209-12.

691) Schvarcz E, Palmér M, Åman J, Lindqvist B, Beckman K-W. Hypoglycemia increases the gastric emptying rate in patients with type-1 diabetes mellitus. Diabetic Med 1993;10:660-63.

692) Schvarcz E, Palmer M, Aman J, Horowitz M, Stridsberg M, Berne C. Physiological hyperglycemia slows gastric emptying in normal subjects and patients with insulin-dependent diabetes mellitus. Gastroenterology 1997;113:60-6.

693) Seidl R, Birnbacher R, Hauser E, Bernert G, Freilinger M, Schober E. Brainstem auditory evoked potentials and visually evoked potentials in young patients with IDDM. Diabetes Care 1996;19:1220-4.

694) Sells CJ, Robinson NM, Brown Z, Knopp RH. Long-term developmental follow-up of infants of diabetic mothers. J Pediatr. 1994;125:1,S9-17.

695) Service FJ, O'Brien PC, Wise SD, Ness S, LeBlanc SM. Dermal interstitial glucose as an indicator of ambient glycemia. Diabetes Care 1997;20:1426-9.

696) Shah S, Malone J, Simpson N. A randomized trial of intensive insulin therapy in newly diagnosed insulin-dependent diabetes mellitus. N Engl J Med 1989; 320:550-54.

697) Shapiro AM, Lakey JR, Ryan EA, Korbutt GS, Toth E, Warnock GL, Kneteman NM, Rajotte RV. Islet transplantation in seven patients with type 1 diabetes mellitus using a glucocorticoid-free immunosuppressive regimen. N Engl J Med 2000;343:230-8.

698) Shehadeh N, Kassem J, Tchaban I, Ravid S, Shahar E, Naveh T, Etzioni A. High incidence of hypoglycemic episodes with neurologic manifestations in children with insulin dependent diabetes mellitus. J Pediatr Endocrinol Metab 1998;11 Suppl 1:183-7.

699) Shield JPH, Baum JD. Advances in childhood onset diabetes. Arch Dis Child 1998;78:391-94.

700) Silink M. Sick day rules. In the book: Baba S, Kaneko T (Ed.). Diabetes 1994. Elsevier Science BV 1995.

701) Silink M (Ed.). APEG handbook on childhood and adolescent diabetes. Australian Pediatric Endocrine Group 1996.

702) Silva SR, Clark L, Goodman SN, Plotnick LP. Can caretakers of children with IDDM accurately measure small insulin doses and dose changes? Diabetes Care 1996;19:56-59.

703) Silverstein J, Klingensmith G, Copeland K, Plotnick L, Kaufman F, Laffel L, Deeb L, Grey M, Anderson B, Holzmeister LA, et al. Care of children and adolescents with type 1 diabetes: a statement of the American Diabetes Association. Diabetes Care 2005;28:186-212.

704) Sindelka G, Heinemann L, Berger M, Frenck W, Chantelau E. Effect of insulin concentration, subcutaneous fat thickness and skin temperature on subcutaneous insulin absorption in healthy subjects. Diabetologia 1994;37:377-80.

705) Singh R, Barden A, Mori T, Beilin L. Advanced glycation end-products: a review. Diabetologia 2001;44:129-46.

706) Sjöblad S. Hypoglycemia in children. Paediatricus 1988;18:90-101.

707) Sjöblad S (Ed.). Consensus guidelines for the treatment of childhood and adolescent diabetes. Swedish Pediatric Association 1996.

708) Sjolie AK, Stephenson J, Aldington S, Kohner E, Janka H, Stevens L, Fuller J. Retinopathy and vision loss in insulin-dependent diabetes in Europe. The EURODIAB IDDM Complications Study. Ophthalmology 1997;104:252-60.

709) Skyler JS, Cefalu WT, Kourides IA, Landschulz WH, Balagtas CC, Cheng SL, Gelfand RA. Efficacy of inhaled human insulin in type 1 diabetes mellitus: a randomised proof-of-concept study. Lancet 2001;357:331-5.

710) Slama G. Unpublished results 1990, personal communication.

711) Smith CP, Sargent MA, Wilson BPM, Price DA. Subcutaneous or intramuscular insulin injections. Arch Dis Childhood 1991;66:879-82.

712) Solomon CG, Willett WC, Carey VJ, Rich-Edwards J, Hunter DJ, Colditz GA, Stampfer MJ, Speizer FE, Spiegelman D, Manson JE. A prospective study of pregravid determinants of gestational diabetes mellitus. JAMA 1997;278:1078-83.

713) Soltész G, Ascádi G. Association between diabetes, severe hypoglycemia and electroencephalographic abnormalities. Arch Dis Child. 1989;64:992-96.

714) Somogyi M. Insulin as a cause of extreme hyperglycemia and instability. Weekly Bulletin of the St Louis Medical Society 1938;32:498-510.

715) Sonnenberg GE, Fredrickson L. DKA Prevention. In the book: Fredrickson L (Ed.). The Insulin Pump Therapy Book. Insights from the experts. MiniMed, Los Angeles 1995.

716) Sönksen PH, Tompkins CV, Srivastava MC, Nabarro JDN. A comparative study on the metabolism of human insulin and porcine proinsulin in man. Clin Sci Mol Med 1973;45:633-54.

717) Søvik O, Thordarson H. Dead-in-bed syndrome in young diabetic patients. Diabetes Care 1999;22 Suppl 2:B40-2.

718) Soon-Shiong P, Heintz RE, Meredith N, Yao QX, Zheng T, Murphy M, Moloney MK, Schmehl M, Harris M et al. Insulin independence in a type-1 diabetic patient after encapsulated islet transplantation. Lancet 1994;343:950-51.

719) Steindel BS, Roe TR, Costin G, Carlson M, Kaufman FR. Continous subcutaneous insulin infusion (CSII) in children and adolescents with chronic poorly controlled type 1 diabetes mellitus. Diabetes Research and Clinical Practise 1995;27:199-204.

720) Stenninger E, Åman J. Intranasal glucagon treatment relieves hypoglycemia with Type 1 (insulin-dependent) diabetes mellitus. Diabetologia 1993;36:931-35.

721) Stewart NL, Darlow BA. Insulin loss at the injection site in children with type 1 diabetes mellitus. Diabetic Medicine 1994;11:802-05.

722) Stickelmeyer MP, Graf CJ, Frank BH, Ballard RL, Storms SM. Stability of U-10 and U-50 dilutions of insulin lispro. Diabetes Technol Ther 2000;2:61-6.

723) Stiller R, Kothny T, Gudat UHK, Anderson JH, Seger M, Johnson RD, Richardson MS, Haslbeck M. Intravenous administration of insulin lispro ver-

sus regular insulin in patients with type 1 diabetes. Diabetes 1999; 48(suppl 1):abstract 0497.

724) Strauss K. Guidelines for using short insulin needles. Becton-Dickinson 1996.

725) Strauss K. Insulin delivery devices and correct injection techniques. Becton-Dickinson 1997.

726) Strauss K. Insulin injection techniques. Report from the 1st international Insulin Injection Technique Workshop, Strasbourg, France - June 1997. Pract Diab Int 1998;15:181-184.

727) Suhonen L, Hiilesmaa V, Teramo K. Glycaemic control during early pregnancy and fetal malformations in women with type I diabetes mellitus. Diabetologia 2000;43:79-82.

728) Sun WM, Houghton LA, Read NW, Grundy DG, Johnson AG. Effect of meal temperature on gastric emptying of liquids in man. Gut 1988; 29: 302-305.

729) Sundkvist G. Autonomic neuropathy. In the book: Agardh CD, Berne C, Östman J (Ed.). Diabetes. Liber, Stockholm 2002;265-271.

730) Sutherland D, Moudry-Munns K, Elick B. Pancreas Transplantation. In the book: Rifkin H, Porte D. Diabetes Mellitus, Theory and Practice. Elsevier 1990:869-79.

731) Svenungsson B, Jertborn M, Wiström J. Prophylaxis and therapy of travelers' diarrhea. Nord Med 11/1992;107:272-73.

732) Swedish National Board of Health and Welfare. Recommendations from an expert meeting: Treatment of insulin-dependent diabetes mellitus. Lakartidningen 42/1989;86:3585-3589.

733) Swift PG, Hearnshaw JR, Botha JL, Wright G, Raymond NT, Jamieson KF. A decade of diabetes: keeping children out of hospital. Bmj 1993;307:96-8.

734) Swift PGF, Waldron S, Glass S. A child with diabetes: distress, discrepancies and dietetic debate. Pract Diab Internat 1995;12:59-62.

735) Swift PGF (Ed.). ISPAD (International Society for Pediatric and Adolescent Diabetes) consensus guidelines for the management of type 1 diabetes mellitus in children and adolescents. Medforum, Zeist, Netherlands 2000.

736) Swift PGF. Personal communication 2003.

737) Tainio VM, Savilahti E, Arjomaa P, Salmenperä L, Perheentupa J, Siimes MA. Plasma antibodies to cows' milk are increased by early weaning and consumption of unmodified milk, but production of plasma IgA and IgM cows milk antibodies is stimulated even during exclusive breast feeding. Acta Paediatr Scand 1988;77:807-11.

738) Tahara Y, Shima K. Response to Chantelau and Rech. Diabetes Care 1994;17:345.

739) Tahara Y, Shima K. Kinetics of HbA1c, glycated albumin, and fructosamine and analysis of their weight functions aganst preceding plasma glucose levels. Diabetes Care 1995;18:440-47.

740) Tallroth G, Karlson B, Nilsson A, Agardh CD. The influence of different insulin regimens on quality of life and metabolic control in insulin-dependent diabetics. Diabetes Res Clin Pract 1989;6:37-43.

741) Tamás G, Tabák AG, Vargha P, Kerényi Z. Effect of menstrual cycle on insulin demand in IDDM women. Diabetologia 1996;39 (Suppl 1):A52 (abstract 188).

742) Tanenberg RJ. Candidate Selection. In the book: Fredrickson L (Ed.). The Insulin Pump Therapy Book. Insights from the experts. MiniMed, Los Angeles 1995.

743) Tattersall R. Brittle diabetes. Clin Endocr Metabol 1977;6:403-19.

744) Tattersall RB, Gill GV. Unexplained death of type-1 diabetic patients. Diabetic Med. 1991;8:49-58.

745) Temple MYM, Riddell MC, Bar-Or O. The reliability and repeatability of the blood glucose response to prolonged exercise in adolescent boys with IDDM. Diabetes Care 1995;18:326-332.

746) Tenovuo J, Alanen P, Larjava H, Viikari J, Lehtonen OP. Oral health of patients with insulin-dependent diabetes mellitus. Scand J Dent Res 1986;94:338-46.

747) ter Braak EW, Woodworth JR, Bianchi R, Cerimele B, Erkelens DE, Thijssen JHH, Kurtz D. Injection site effects on the pharmacokinetics and glucodynamics of insulin lispro and regular insulin. Diabetes Care 1996;19:1437-40.

748) ter Braak EW, Appelman AM, van de Laak M, Stolk RP, van Haeften TW, Erkelens DW. Clinical characteristics of type 1 diabetic patients with and without severe hypoglycemia. Diabetes Care 2000;23:1467-71.

749) Tesfaye S, Cullen DR, Wilson RM, Wooley PD. Diabetic ketoacidosis precipitated by genital herpes infection. Diab Res Clin Pract 1991;13:83-84.

750) Tesfaye S, Malik R, Ward JD. Vascular factors in diabetic neuropathy. Diabetologia 1994;37:847-54.

751) Thernlund GM, Dahlquist G, Hansson K, Ivarsson SA, Ludvigsson J, Sjöblad S, Hägglöf B. Psychological stress and the onset of IDDM in children. Diabetes Care 1995;18:/10:1323-29.

752) Thernlund G, Dahlquist G, Hägglöf B, Ivarsson SA, Lernmark B, Ludvigsson J, Sjöblad S. Psychological reactions at the onset of insulin-dependent diabetes in children and later adjustment and metabolic control. Act Pediatr 1996;85:947-53.

753) Thorburn A, Brand J, Truswell S: The glycaemic index of foods: The Medical Journal of Australia, 1986;144:580-82.

754) Thorburn AW, Brand JC, Truswell AS. Salt and the glycaemic response. Br Med J (Clin Res Ed) 1986;292:1697-9.

755) Thow JC, Johnson AB, Antsiferov M, Home PD. Effect of raising injection-site insulin temperature on isophane (NPH) insulin crystal dissociation. Diabetes Care 1989;12:432-4.

756) Thow J, Home P. Insulin injection technique. BMJ 1990;301:3-4.

757) Thow JC, Johnson AB, Marsden S, Taylor R, Home PD. Morphology of palpably abnormal injection sites and effects on absorption of isophane (NPH) insulin. Diabetic medicine 1990;7:795-99.

758) Thrailkill KM, Quattrin T, Baker L, Kuntze JE, Compton PG, Martha PM, Jr. Cotherapy with recombinant human insulin-like growth factor I and insulin improves glycemic control in type 1 diabetes. RhIGF-I in IDDM Study Group. Diabetes Care 1999;22:585-92.

759) Torlone E, Pampanelli S, Lalli C, Del Sindaco P, Di Vincenzo A, Rambotti AM, Modarelli F, Epifano L, Kassi G, Perriello G, Brunetti P, Bolli G. Effects of the short-acting insulin analog [Lys(B28),Pro(B29)] on postprandial blood glucose control in IDDM. Diabetes Care 1996;19/9:945-52.

760) Torsdottir I, Andersson H. Effect on the postprandial glycaemic level of the addition of water to a meal ingested by healthy subjects and type 2 (non-insulin-dependent) diabetic patients. Diabetologia 1989;32:231-5.

761) Tubiana-Rufi N, Levy-Marchal C, Mugnier E, Czernichow P. Long term feasibility of multiple daily injections with insulin pens in children and adolescents with diabetes. Eur J Pediatr 1989;149:80-3.

762) Tubiana-Rufi N, Prieur AM, Bourden R, Priollet P, Czernichow P. Early detection of limited joint mobility in diabetic children and adolescents. Diabete Metab 1991;17:504-11.

763) Tubiana-Rufi N, de Lonlay P, Bloch J, Czernichow P. Remission of severe hypoglycemic incidents in young diabetic children treated with subcutaneous infusion. Arch Fr Pediatr 1996;3:969-76.

764) Tubiana-Rufi N, Belarbi N, Du Pasquier-Fediaevsky L, Polak M, Kakou B, Leridon L, Hassan M, Czernichow P. Short needles (8 mm) reduce the risk of intramuscular injections in children with type 1 diabetes. Diabetes Care 1999;22:1621-25.

765) Tubiana-Rufi N, Coutand R, Bloch J, Munz-Licha G, Delcroix C, Limal JM, Czernichow P. Efficacy and tolerance of insulin lispro in young diabetic children treated with CSII. Diabetologia 2000;43(suppl. 1):762 (abstract 762).

766) Tuomilehto J, Tuomilehto-Wolf E, Virtala E, LaPorte RE: Coffee consumption as trigger for insulin-dependent diabetes mellitus in childhood. BMJ 1990;300:642-43.

767) Tuominen JA, Karonen SL, Melamies L, Bolli G. Koivisto VA. Exercise-induced hypoglycaemia in IDDM patients treated with a short- acting insulin analogue. Diabetologia 1995;38:106-11.

768) Tupola S, Rajantie J, Mäenpää J. Severe hypoglycemia in children and adolescents during multiple-dose insulin therapy. Diab Med 1998;15:695-99.

769) Tupola S, Rajantie J. Documented symptomatic hypoglycaemia in children and adolescents using multiple daily insulin injection therapy. Diabet Med 1998;15:492-6.

770) Turner BC, Jenkins E, Kerr D, Sherwin RS, Cavan DA. The effect of evening alcohol consumption on next-morning glucose control in type 1 diabetes. Diabetes Care 2001;24:1888-93.

771) Twyman S, Rowe D, Mansell P, Schapira D, Betts P, Leatherdale B. Longitudinal study of urinary albumin excretion in young diabetic patients–Wessex Diabetic Nephropathy Project. Diabet Med 2001;18:402-8.

772) Tylleskär K, Tuvemo T, Gustafsson J. Diabetes control deteriorates in girls at cessation of growth: relationship with body mass index. Diabet Med 2001;18:811-5.

773) Updike SJ, Shults MC, Gilligan BJ, Rhodes RK. A subcutaneous glucose sensor with improved longevity, dynamic range, and stability of calibration. Diabetes Care 2000;23:208-14.

774) U.S. Pharmacopeia, 21st Rev. In the book: US Pharmacopeial Convention, Rockville, MD, 1985; p 1180.

775) Vaag A, Handberg A, Lauritzen M, Henriksen JE, Damgaard Pedersen K, Beck-Nielsen H. Variation in absorption of NPH insulin due to intramuscular injection. Diabetes Care 1990;13:74-76.

776) Vague P, Picq R, Bernal M et al. Effect of nicotinamide treatment on the residual insulin secretion in type-I (insulin-dependent) diabetic patients. Diabetologia 1989;32:316-21.

777) Vague P, Selam JL, Skeie S, De Leeuw I, Elte JW, Haahr H, Kristensen A, Draeger E. Insulin detemir is associated with more predictable glycemic control and reduced risk of hypoglycemia than NPH insulin in patients with type 1 diabetes on a basal-bolus regimen with premeal insulin aspart. Diabetes Care 2003;26:590-6.

778) Valenzuela GA, McCallum R. Etiology and diagnosis of gastroparesis:An introduction. Motility 1988;1:10-14.

779) Velho G, Froguel P. Genetic, metabolic and clinical characteristics of maturity onset diabetes of the young. Eur J Endocrinol 1998;138:233-9.

780) Veneman T. Mitrakou A. Mokan M. Cryer P, Gerich J. Induction of hypoglycemia unawareness by asymptomatic nocturnal hypoglycemia. Diabetes 1993;42:1233-37.

781) Verge CF, Simpson JM, Howard NJ, Mackerras D, Irwig L, Silink M. Environmental factors in IDDM. Diabetes Care 1994;17:1381-89.

782) Verotti A, Chiarelli F, Blasetti A, Bruni E, Morgese G. Severe hypoglycemia in insulin-dependent diabetic children treated by multiple injection regimen. Acta Diabetol 1996;33/1:53-57.

783) Vervoort G, Goldschmidt HMG, van Doorn LG. Nocturnal blood glucose profiles in patients with type 1 diabetes mellitus on multiple (>1) daily insulin injection regimes. Diab Med 1996;13:794-99.

784) Vessby B, Gustafsson IB. Diet treatment. In the book: Diabetes. SPRI and Swedish Medical Society 1989:206-214.

785) Viberti G. Mogensen CE. Groop LC. Pauls JF. Effect of captopril on progression to clinical proteinuria in patients with insulin-dependent diabetes mellitus and microalbuminuria. European Microalbuminuria Captopril Study Group. JAMA 1994;271:275-79.

786) Virtanen SM, Räsänen L, Aro A, Ylönen K, Sippola H, Lounamaa R. Toumilehto J, Åkerblom HK. Feeding in infancy and the risk of type 1 diabetes mellitus in Finnish children. Diabetic Medicine 1992;9:815-19.

787) Virtanen SM, Saukkonen T, Savilahti E, Ylönen K, Räsänen L, Aro A, Knip M, Toumilehto J, Åkerblom HK and the Childhood Diabetes in Finland Study Group. Diet, cows' milk protein antibodies and the risk of IDDM in Finnish children. Diabetologia 1994;37:381-87.

788) Virtanen SM, Laara E, Hypponen E, Reijonen H, Rasanen L, Aro A, Knip M, Ilonen J, Akerblom HK. Cows' milk consumption, HLA-DQB1 genotype, and type 1 diabetes: a nested case-control study of siblings of children with diabetes. Childhood diabetes in Finland study group. Diabetes 2000;49:912-7.

789) Virtanen SM, Virta-Autio P, Rasanen L, Akerblom HK. Changes in food habits in families with a newly diagnosed child with type 1 diabetes mellitus. J Pediatr Endocrinol Metab 2001;14 Suppl 1:627-36.

790) Wahren J, Felig P, Hagenfeldt L. Physical exercise and fuel homeostasis in diabetes mellitus. Diabetologia 1978;14:213-22.

791) Waldron S. Childhood diabetes - current dietary management. Current Pediatrics 1993;3:138-41.

792) Waldron S, Swift P, Oliver L, Foote D. The nutritional management of children's diabetes. In the book: Frost GF (Ed.). Dietetic Management of Diabetes. John Wiley, London 2003.

793) Walker M, Marshall SM, Alberti KGMM. Clinical aspects of diabetic ketoacidosis. Diabetes/Metabolism Reviews 1989;5:651-63.

794) Wallace TM, Meston NM, Gardner SG, Matthews DR. The hospital and home use of a 30-second hand-held blood ketone meter: guidelines for clinical practice. Diabet Med 2001;18:640-5.

795) Wallberg-Henriksson H, Wahren J. Exercise. In the book: Agardh C-D, Berne C, Östman J. Diabetes. Almqvist & Wiksell, Stockholm 1992:97-107.

796) Walsh JM, Wheat ME, Freund K. Detection, evaluation, and treatment of eating disorders, the role of the primary care physician. J Gen Intern Med 2000;15:577-90.

797) Walsh PA, Roberts R. Pumping insulin. Everything you need for success with an insulin pump. Torrey Pines Press, San Diego, 2000.

798) Walton C, Allan BJ, Hepburn DA. Tight glycemic control should be avoided post-partum because of increased risk of severe hypoglycemia. Diab Med 2000;17(suppl 1):A84 (abstract).

799) Warram J, Martin BC, Krolewski AS. Risk of IDDM in children of diabetic mothers decreases with increasing maternal age at pregnancy. Diabetes 1991;40:1679-1684.

800) Warshaw HS, Kulkarni K. Complete Guide to Carb Counting. ADA 2001, Virginia, USA.

801) Wasserman D, Zinman B. Exercise in individuals with IDDM. Diabetes Care 1994;17:924-37.

802) Watson J, Kerr D. The best defense against hypoglycemia is to recognize it: is caffeine useful? Diabetes Technol Ther 1999;1:193-200.

803) Weinger K, Jacobson AM, Draelos MT, Finkelstein DM, Simonson DC. Blood glucose estimation and symptoms during hyperglycemia and hypoglycemia in patients with insulin-dependent diabetes mellitus. Am J Med, 1995 Jan, 98:1, 22-31.

804) Weinger K, Kinsley BT, Levy CJ, Bajaj M, Simonson DC, Cox DJ, Ryan CM, Jacobson AM. The perception of safe driving ability during hypoglycemia in patients with type 1 diabetes mellitus. Am J Med 1999;107:246-53.

805) Weissberg-Benchell J, Glasgow A, Tynan D, Wirtz P, Turek J, Ward J. Adolescent diabetes management and mismanagement. Diabetes Care 1995;18:77-82.

806) Welch IM, Bruce C, Hill SE, Read NW. Duodenial and ileal lipid suppresses postprandial blood glucose and insulin responses in man: possible implications for the dietary management of diabetes mellitus. Clinical Science 1987;72:209-16.

807) Wheeler ML, Fineberg SE, Gibson R, Fineberg N. Controlled portions of presweetened cereals present no glycemic penalty in persons with insulin-dependent diabetes mellitus. J Am Diet Assoc 1996;96:458-63.

808) White SA, Nicholson ML. Islet cell transplantation and type 1 diabetes mellitus. Diabet Med 2001;18 Suppl 1:6-9.

809) Widom B, Simonson DC. Intermittent hypoglycemia impairs glucose counter-regulation. Diabetes 1992;41:1597-602.

810) Willi SM. Type 2 diabetes mellitus in adolescents. Current Opinion in Endocrinolgy & Diabetes 2000;7:71-76.

811) Wise JE, Kolb EL, Sauder SE. Effect of glycemic control on growth velocity in children with IDDM. Diabetes Care 1992;15:826-30.

812) Wittesjö B, Stenström TA, Eitrem R, Rombo L. Every other traveller abroad risks diarrhea. Water and food are the most common sources of infection. Lakartidningen 1995;92:865-67.

813) Wolever TMS. The Glycemic index. In the book: Bourne GH (Ed.). Aspects of some vitamins, minerals and enzymes in health and disease. World Rev Nutr Diet. Basel, Karger 1990;62:120-85.

814) Wolever TM. American diabetes association evidence-based nutrition principles and recommendations are not based on evidence. Diabetes Care 2002;25:1263-4.

815) Woodworth J. Howey D, Bowsher R, Lutz S, Sanat P, Brady P. [Lys(B28), Pro(B29) Human Insulin (K): Dose ranging vs. Humulin R (H). Diabetologia 1993;42(Suppl)1:54A.

816) Wynne HA, Brown PM Sönksen PM. Acceptability and effectiveness of self-administered intramuscular insulin in juvenile-onset diabetes. Practical Diabetes 1985;2:32-33.

817) Wysocki T, Meinhold PM, Taylor A, Hough BS, Barnard MU, Clarke WL, Bellando BJ, Bourgeois MJ. Psychometric properties and normative data for the parent version of the diabetes independence survey. Diabetes Educ 1996;22:587-91.

818) Wysocki T, Harris MA, Mauras N, Fox L, Taylor A, Jackson SC, White NH. Absence of adverse effects of severe hypoglycemia on cognitive function in school-aged children with diabetes over 18 months. Diabetes Care 2003;26:1100-5.

819) Würsch P, Pi-Sunyer FX. The role of viscous soluble fiber in the metabolic control of diabetes. A review with special emphasis on cereals rich in ß-glucan. Diabetes Care 1997;20:1774-80.

820) Yki-Järvinen H, Helve E, Koivisto VA. Hyperglycemia decreases glucose uptake in type 1 diabetes. Diabetes 1987;36:892-96.

821) Yki-Järvinen H. Glucose toxicity. Endocrine Reviews 1992;13:414-431.

822) Yki-Järvinen H. Glucose toxicity - its pros and cons. Nord Med 1996;111:80-3.

823) Yosipovitch G, Hodak E, Vardi P, Shraga I, Karp M, Sprecher E, David M. The prevalence of cutaneous manifestations in IDDM patients and their association with diabetes risk factors and microvascular complications. Diabetes Care 1998;21:506-9.

824) Young RJ, Hannan WJ, Frier BM, Steel JM, Duncan LJP. Diabetic lipohypertrophy delays insulin absorption. Diabetes Care 1984; 7:479-80.

825) Zachrisson I, Brismar K, Hall K, Wallensteen M, Dahlquist G. Determinants of growth in diabetic pubertal subjects. Diabetes Care 1997;20:1261-65.

826) Zimmet P, Turner R, McCarty D, Rowley M, Mackay I. Crucial points at diagnosis. Type 2 diabetes or slow type 1 diabetes. Diabetes Care 1999;22 Suppl 2:B59-64.

827) Zinman B, Tildesley H, Chiasson JL, Tsui E, Strack TR. Insulin Lispro in CSII: Results of a double-blind, crossover study. Diabetes 1997;46:440-43.

828) Zinman B, Ross S, Campos RV, Strack T. Effectiveness of human ultralente versus NPH insulin in providing basal insulin replacement for an insulin lispro multiple daily injection regimen. A double-blind randomized prospective trial. The Canadian Lispro Study Group. Diabetes Care 1999;22:603-8.

Index